The Physics of
Radiology and Imaging

The Physics of
Radiology and Imaging

(Targeted to postgraduate students of MD/DNB/FRCR, MSc, Medical Physics/PG Diploma in Radiation Physics, BSc/MSc, Radiography and Imaging Technology, Nuclear Medicine Technology and Biomedical Engineering)

Second Edition

Kuppusamy Thayalan MSc DipRP (BARC) MPhil PhD
Honorary Professor, Department of Medical Physics, Anna University
Adjunct Faculty, Department of Engineering Design
Indian Institute of Technology Madras
Founder and President, Radiologic Physics Foundation
Former Professor, Madras Medical College
Former Consultant Medical Physicist
Dr Kamakshi Memorial Hospital
Chennai, Tamil Nadu, India

Foreword
S Arumugam

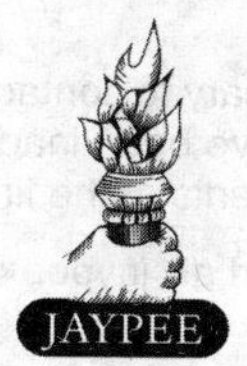

JAYPEE BROTHERS MEDICAL PUBLISHERS
The Health Sciences Publisher
New Delhi | London

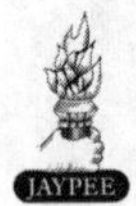 **Jaypee Brothers Medical Publishers (P) Ltd**

Headquarters
EMCA House
23/23-B, Ansari Road, Daryaganj
New Delhi 110 002, India
Landline: +91-11-23272143, +91-11-23272703
+91-11-23282021, +91-11-23245672
E-mail: jaypee@jaypeebrothers.com

Corporate Office
Jaypee Brothers Medical Publishers (P) Ltd.
4838/24, Ansari Road, Daryaganj
New Delhi 110 002, India
Phone: +91-11-43574357
Fax: +91-11-43574314
E-mail: jaypee@jaypeebrothers.com

Overseas Office
JP Medical Ltd.
83, Victoria Street, London
SW1H 0HW (UK)
Phone: +44-20 3170 8910
E-mail: info@jpmedpub.com

EU GPSR Authorised Representative
Logos Europe, 9 rue Nicolas Poussin
17000, La Rochelle, France
Phone: +33 (0) 6 67 93 73 78
E-mail: Contact@logoseurope.eu

Website: www.jaypeebrothers.com
Website: www.jaypeedigital.com

The Physics of Radiology and Imaging

First Edition: 2014

Second Edition: **2025**   Reprint : 2026
ISBN: 978-93-5696-589-8

Printed in India at K.K. Printers, Kundli, Haryana-131 028.

Dedicated to

My late mother K Arukkani
My late father K Kuppusamy
and

My late brother Pulavar K Krishnasamy

Foreword

I am happy to write foreword for the book titled *The Physics of Radiology and Imaging*, authored by Dr K Thayalan. Dr Thayalan has vast experience in radiological physics for over four decades as Medical Physicist, Radiological Safety Officer, and Professor. I do remember that he has been publishing a series of books in radiological sciences, and this is the second edition of the above title. There is a need for this kind of book for the benefit of postgraduates, since physics forms the foundation of radiological sciences.

The book has 15 chapters, including figures and tables. Chapter 1 discusses fundamental concepts such as atomic structure, electromagnetic radiation, and electricity and magnetism. Chapter 2 discusses radioactivity, production of gamma rays, and radioisotopes. Chapter 3 elaborates on production of X-rays, type of X-ray tubes, and quality of X-rays. Chapter 4 deals with interaction of radiation with matter and various radiation units.

Chapter 5 discusses radiation detectors used in medical radiology for measurements. In Chapter 6, screen-film radiography including cassette, intensifying screen, X-ray film, and film processing are discussed. Chapter 7 talks about computer and digital radiography and digital image quality. Chapter 8 discusses mammography including contrast-enhanced mammography and image quality. Chapter 9 talks about fluoroscopy including digital subtraction angiography.

Chapter 10 discusses computed tomography (CT) including image reconstruction, helical tomography, and radiation dose. Chapter 11 elaborates on nuclear imaging including Gamma camera, PET/CT, and PET/MRI. Chapter 12 discusses ultrasound imaging covering transducer design, image display, and Doppler ultrasound. Chapter 13 talks about magnetic resonance imaging, elaborating on equipment, relaxation times, and bio-effect and safety. Chapter 14 discusses various imaging sequences used in MRI and its clinical application. Chapter 15 talks about health and safety, natural exposure, biological effects, and regulatory requirements.

All the chapters are well designed, concise, and complete to cover all the topics needed for a hospital setup. The author has explained the physics and principles behind every medical equipment with relevant citations. I hope the students may be benefited by this book so that the quality of radiological education will improve across the country. It is also useful for healthcare providers of this region to plan a radiological facility in a medical college setup.

I appreciate Dr K Thayalan and wish him all success for his future endeavors.

S Arumugam PhD DSc
Vice-Chancellor and Professor
Tamil Nadu Open University
Chennai, Tamil Nadu, India

Preface to the Second Edition

Radiation has been used in medicine soon after the discovery of X-rays in 1896. Started with simple radiography, X-ray has widened its application in the form of real-time imaging, breast imaging, tomography, and digital radiography. On the other hand, ultrasonogram and magnetic resonance imaging play an additional role in imaging without using X-rays. Open radionuclides have also been used in diagnosis and therapy in the form of Gamma camera, Single photon emission computed tomography (SPECT), Positron emission tomography (PET), Hybrid Imaging, and High-Dose Therapy.

Understanding the physics of the above system is much important to produce good-quality images with minimal radiation. Establishment of medical X-ray facility requires license for an operation along with personnel training and standard operating procedure for each equipment. This will ensure an optimal image quality for interpretation, minimize retake, and reduce cost and time including personnel, patient, and public safety. Layout design, equipment selection, installation, quality assurance, and radiation survey form the basis, to establish a good radiology department within the regulatory requirement.

An attempt has been made to fulfil the essentials of the above in the form of "The Physics of Radiology and Imaging, as second edition". This book is targeted to postgraduate students of radiology (MD/DNB/FRCR), medical physics (MSc), radiography and imaging technology (BSc/MSc), and Biomedical Engineering (BE) of Indian Universities and abroad.

The book consists of 15 chapters with number of figures and tables. It addresses fundamental concepts, radioactivity and gamma rays, X-ray production, interaction of radiation with matter and radiation units, radiation detection and measurements, screen-film radiography, computed and digital radiography, mammography, fluoroscopy, computed tomography, nuclear imaging, ultrasound, magnetic resonance imaging, and radiation safety. Special attention is given to elaborate magnetic resonance imaging and image sequences. An attempt has been made to incorporate emerging technology. Clinical application with worked examples have been incorporated for easy understanding.

I hope that this book will be much useful to improve the standards of radiological education in this region and in turn the quality of patient service and safety.

I am looking forward to healthy comments and suggestions from the readers.

Kuppusamy Thayalan

Preface to the First Edition

Radiation has been used in medicine since from the discovery of X-rays in 1895 by the German physicist WC Roentgen. Over the period, its application has grown enormously and it is used today in the form of
radiography, fluoroscopy, mammography and computed tomography. Nonradiation tools are also competing in medicine in the form of ultrasound and magnetic resonance imaging. These tools not only provide early differential diagnosis of the disease but also improve the accuracy of clinical diagnosis. The uniqueness of the above tools is that they all work on the basis of physics principle.

Understanding the physics of the above instruments is very much essential, for those connected with radiological sciences. It helps not only the education, but also the equipment selection, its optimal use, maintenance, and safety. Hence, an attempt is made to explain the physical principle, instrumentation, function, its application and limitations in the form of a single book. Attempt is also made to incorporate nuclear imaging and radiological safety in the same book. Large number of figures and tables are incorporated wherever it is necessary, for better understanding of the concept. This book is intended for postgraduate students of medical physics, diagnostic radiology, Diplomate National Board (DNB), and FRCR. This is the first book of its kind from an Indian author, giving single solution for the entire range of radiology and imaging equipment.

I am very proud and happy to come out with this book, incorporating my three decades of experience in radiological/medical physics teaching. I am very happy and thankful to Dr R Ravichandran for writing the foreword to this book. I am also thankful to M/s Jaypee Brothers Medical Publishers (P) Ltd, New Delhi, for publishing this book as usual in a neat and elegant manner. Constructive comments are invited from the readers for the future betterment of the book.

I am very much thankful to my wife Tamilselvi, son Parthiban and daughter Kayal Vizhi for their support and cooperation during the book writing process.

I thank and acknowledge Dr Kamakshi Memorial Hospital, Chennai, especially the medical physics division for the support and assistance.

Kuppusamy Thayalan

Acknowledgments

I am thankful to my wife Tamilselvi, son Parthiban, and daughter Kayal Vizhi for their love, support, and cooperation. I am also thankful to my brothers K Ramaiyan and K Annadurai and sisters N Sulochana and T Vimala for their moral support. I acknowledge and thank the Department of Medical Physics, Anna University and Department of Engineering Design, Indian Institute of Technology Madras, Chennai, Tamil Nadu, for the recognition and support provided during the process of writing the book.

I am very thankful to Dr S Arumugam, the honorable Vice-Chancellor, Tamil Nadu Open University, and Former Senior Professor, Department of Physics and Director, Centre for High Pressure Research, Bharathidasan University, Tiruchirappalli, for having written Foreword to this book.

I am also thankful to Shri Jitendar P Vij (Group Chairman), Mr Ankit Vij (Managing Director), Mr MS Mani (Group President), Dr Madhu Choudhary (Director–Educational Publishing), Ms Pooja Bhandari [Director–Production (Books and Journals)], Mr Ajay Kumar Sharma [Deputy General Manager (Books and Journals)], Ms Sunita Katla (Executive Assistant to Group Chairman and Publishing Manager), Ms Samina Khan (Executive Assistant to Director–Educational Publishing), Mr Rajesh Sharma (Production Coordinator), Ms Seema Dogra (Cover Visualizer), Ms Neha Verma (Graphic Designer–Cover), Mr Rabindra Kumar Behera (Proofreader), Mr Mahesh Chand Joshi (Typesetter), Mr Manoj Pahuja (Graphic Designer), and all other staff of M/s Jaypee Brothers Medical Publishers (P) Ltd, New Delhi, India, for publishing this book in an elegant manner, as I wanted.

Kuppusamy Thayalan

Contents

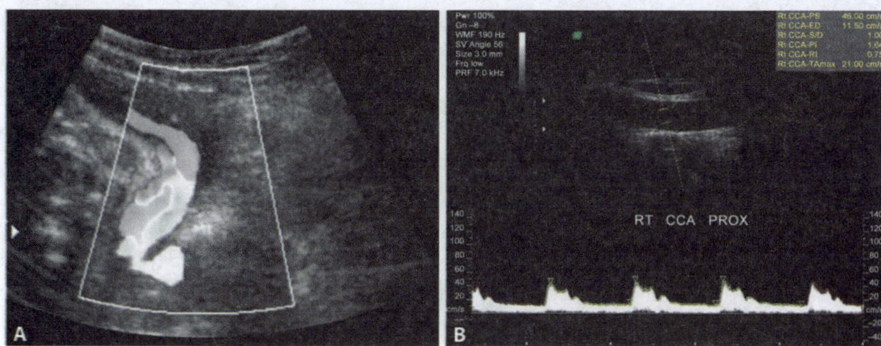

Figs. 12.18A and B: (A) Color Doppler of umbilical cord; (B) Doppler spectral display.

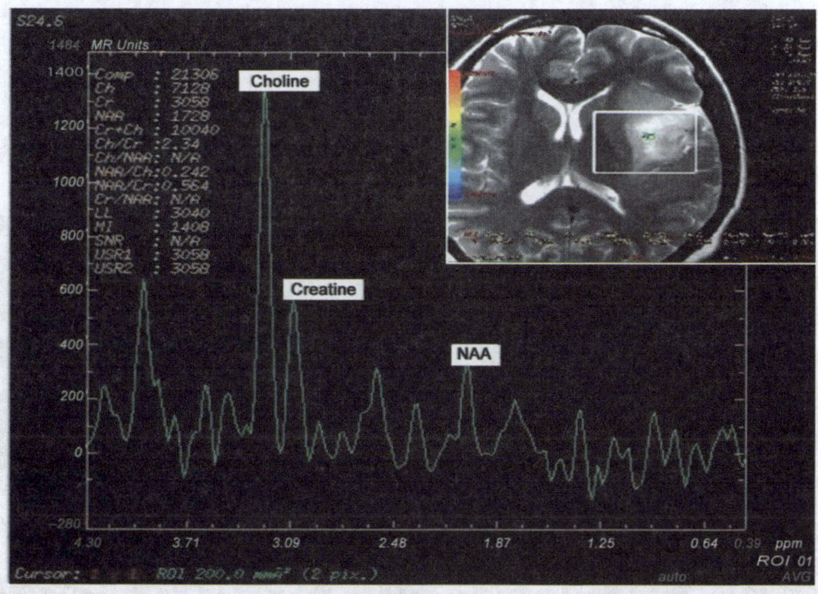

Fig. 14.13: MR spectroscopy of glioma with high T2 signal lesion of insular cortex shows raised choline peak, choline/creatine ratio with decreased N-acetylaspartate (NAA) peak.

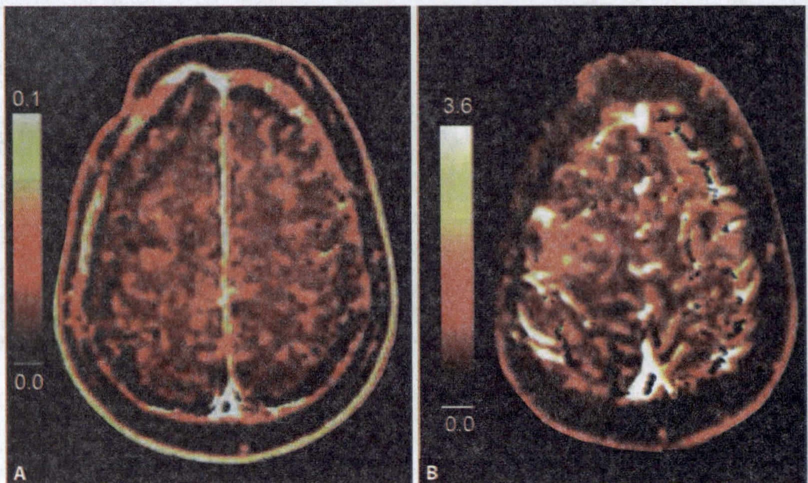

Figs. 14.17A and B: MR perfusion weighted imaging-Dynamic contrast-enhanced perfusion: (A) Axial volume transfer coefficient; (B) Plasma volume map shows mild increase in perfusion in recurrent metastasis in right frontal lobe. (*Courtesy:* David Fussell, 2013).

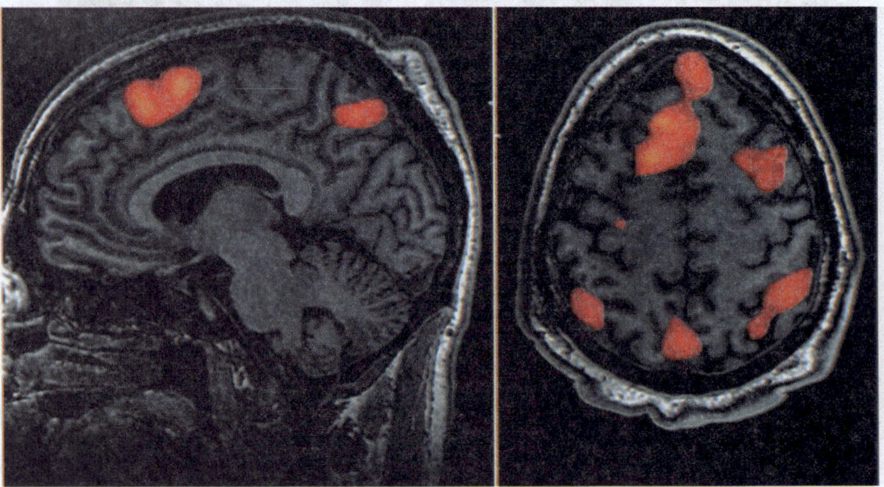

Fig. 14.18: fMRI shows activity of brain.

Fundamental Concepts

UNITS AND MEASUREMENTS

Physics is a science dealing with nature. It is concerned with the study of two concepts, matter, and energy, and how they interact with each other. Matter is one which occupies space, and it is made up of molecules or atoms, e.g., gold, wood, water, and air. Matter exists in four states, namely solid, liquid, gas, and plasma. Energy is the ability to do work, and it can be converted from one form to another, e.g., human body converts chemical energy (food) into kinetic energy (work). In general, physicists study the behavior of matter and energy under different physical conditions.

To study matter and energy and their various properties, measurement of physical quantities, such as length, mass, and time are required. Physical quantity is measured accurately in terms of its own standard, e.g., distance is measured in metre, mass in kilogram, and time in second.

Therefore, unit is a quantity adopted as a standard of measurement in terms of which similar quantities can be measured. The units which are independent of one another and have their own standard (base) is called *fundamental units*, e.g., kilogram, metre and second. The units, which do not have their own standard (base) and obtained from the fundamental units are called *derived units*, e.g., area; metre^2, velocity; metre per second, and density; kilogram per metre^3.

SI Units

In 1960, a new system of units called *International System of Units (SI Units)* was introduced. The SI system is superior to all other systems and more convenient in practice and is used throughout the world. There are 7 fundamental units and 2 supplementary units in the SI system **(Table 1.1)**.

Table 1.1: SI system of units.

Physical quantity	Unit	Symbol
Fundamental units		
Length	metre	m
Mass	kilogram	kg
Time	second	s
Electric current	ampere	A
Temperature	kelvin	K
Luminous intensity	candela	cd
Amount of substance	mole	mol
Supplementary units		
Plane angle	radian	rad
Solid angle	steradian	sr

(*Courtesy:* Kuppusamy Thayalan, 2017)

Prefixes

Though the SI units are a coherent system, they are found to be either too large or low in practice, e.g., the activity of an isotope for bone scan is expressed in billions of becquerel. Hence, prefixes are used to overcome the above difficulty **(Table 1.2)**. These prefixes are conveniently used to describe either very large or small physical quantities. In radiation physics, Mega becquerel (MBq), kilovolt (kV), centi-gray (cGy), milliampere (mA), nano-coulomb (nC) and nanometer (nm) are commonly used.

Radiological Units

In radiological science, units like kilovoltage (kV_p), milliampere (mA), milliampere-second (mAs), kilo electron volt (keV), heat units (HU), Hounsfield unit (HU) are used. Though they are not strictly SI units but are used in practice for convenience. One kV is equal to 1,000 volts that refers to potential difference applied between an anode and cathode of a X-ray tube.

Table 1.2: Prefixes used with SI units.

Prefix	Symbol	Factor	Prefix	Symbol	Factor
Exa	E	10^{18}	Deci	d	10^{-1}
Peta	P	10^{15}	Centi	c	10^{-2}
Tera	T	10^{12}	Milli	m	10^{-3}
Giga	G	10^{9}	Micro	μ	10^{-6}
Mega	M	10^{6}	Nano	n	10^{-9}
Kilo	k	10^{3}	Pico	p	10^{-12}
Hecto	h	10^{2}	Femto	f	10^{-15}
deka	da	10^{1}	Atto	a	10^{-18}

(*Courtesy:* John Ball et al, 2008)

The suffix P refers to peak value of the potential difference across the X-ray tube since the potential difference is varying in nature. In the case of high frequency generator or constant potential, P loses its meaning, it is simply kV.

One milliampere is equal to $\dfrac{1}{1,000}$ of amperes and refers to number of electrons flowing per second from cathode to anode. It is directly related to quantity of X-rays that are produced, in turn the blackening on the film. It depends on the duration of electron flow or exposure time in seconds. Hence, mAs means milliampere-second, refers not only the electron flow per second but also the duration of flow.

One keV is equal to 1,000 electron volt (eV) and refers to energy of X-ray photons. It is also the unit of energy, since joule is a larger unit. Heat unit is used to describe the heat produced in a X-ray tube. Hounsfield unit is used in CT to quantify attenuation of tissues relative to water.

Other SI units used in radiological sciences are, radioactivity; becquerel (Bq), exposure; roentgen (R), absorbed dose; grey (Gy), and effective dose; sievert (Sv).

MECHANICS

Velocity and Acceleration

Displacement (d) of a moving body is defined as the shortest distance between an initial and final positions of a body. The velocity (v) of a moving body is the rate of change of displacement of the body in a particular direction. Velocity is often referred as *speed* which describes how fast the body is moving. It is given by the relation: $v = \dfrac{d}{t}$, where d is the displacement in t seconds. The unit of velocity is m/s.

Acceleration (a) is defined as the rate of change of velocity and its unit is m/s². It is a measure of how quickly or slowly the velocity is changing. If the velocity is constant, the acceleration is zero:

$$a = \frac{(v_f - v_o)}{t}$$

where, v_o is the initial velocity and V_f is the final velocity, during the time interval t.

Force, Momentum and Pressure

Force

Force is an influence that changes the state of rest or uniform motion of a body along a straight line. As per **Newton's** second law of motion, if a force, F acts on a body of mass, m, and produces an acceleration, a, then F = m × a. The SI unit of force is *newton* (N). Weight (W) is a force acting on a body which pulls the body towards the earth. It is the product of mass (m) and acceleration due to gravity (g), W = mg, where, g = 9.8 m/sec².

Momentum

Momentum (P) of a moving body is the product of mass (m) and velocity (v):

$$P = m \times v$$

The momentum is a vector quantity, and its direction is the same as velocity, the unit is kg-m/s. *The total momentum before collision is equal to the total momentum after collision.*

Pressure

Total force acting on a liquid surface is called thrust. Pressure (p) is defined as the force (F) per unit area (A) and its unit is Nm^{-2} or pascal (Pa). The pressure is caused by the weight of material pressing on its surface. It may also be due to collisions of atoms or molecules of a gas within a container. In practice, *Psi, bar, Torr* and *atm* are used as units. Psi refers to pound-force per square inch, and 1 Psi = 6,895 Pa. 1 bar = 100,000 Pa, and 1 Pa = 0.00750062 Torr. Millibar (mbar) is often used as unit of pressure = 100 Pa. The atmospheric pressure (atm) is about 10^5 Pa or 760 Torr.

Work, Power and Energy

Work

If a force acts on a body and the point of application of force moves, then work is said to be done by the force. If force, *F* moves a body through a distance, *d*, in a direction, then the work done by the force is given by: W = F × d. If the direction of displacement, *d* is inclined to *F* at an angle of θ then the work done is:

$$W = F\cos\theta \times d$$

where, Fcos θ is the component of force. The SI unit of work is *joule* (J).

Power

The rate of doing work is called power. It is measured by the amount of work done in unit time. If *W* is the work done in time, *t*, then power, *P*:

$$P = \frac{W}{t}$$

The SI unit of power is *joule per second* (J/sec) equal to 1 *watt* (W). A larger unit of power is called *kilowatt*, which is equal to 1,000 watt. The unit of electrical energy consumption is *kilowatt-hour* (kWh). One kilowatt-hour is the power consumed at the rate of 1,000 watts for one hour. 1 kWh = 1,000 × 60 × 60 = 3,600,000 watts-second = 3,600,000 joules. British unit of power is *horsepower* (hp) and 1 hp = 746 W.

Energy

The energy of a body is its ability to do work. It is measured by the amount of work that it can perform. The SI unit of energy is *joule* (J). The electron volt (eV) is also used as unit of energy. *The law of conservation of energy states that energy can neither be created nor be destroyed, and the total energy in the universe is constant.* There are many forms of energy, such as mechanical energy, heat energy, light energy, electrical energy, chemical energy, atomic energy, etc. There are two forms of mechanical energy, namely (1) kinetic energy and (2) potential energy.

Kinetic Energy

Kinetic energy of a body is the energy associated with the motion of an object. It depends on the mass of the body and square of its velocity. Let us consider a body of mass, m moves with a velocity, v, then,

$$\text{Kinetic energy} = \frac{1}{2}\,mv^2\ \text{joule}$$

Potential Energy

Potential energy of a body is the stored energy of position or configuration, e.g., water stored in a tank, a wound spring, compressed air, etc. For a body of mass, m remaining at rest at a height, h above the ground, the potential energy is equal to the work done in raising the body from the ground to that height.

The work done or potential energy = force × displacement = mg × h, joule where, g is the acceleration due to gravity.

HEAT AND TEMPERATURE

Heat

Heat is a form of internal energy, which can be transferred from one part to an another part of a body. It is due to kinetic energy of random motion of molecules. There are three methods of heat transfer, namely (1) conduction, (2) convection, and (3) radiation. If a hot body and a cold body are placed in close contact, the hot body will transfer some of its heat energy to the cold body until the temperature of the two becomes equal. The difference in temperature creates temperature gradient. The SI unit of heat is *joule* and the special unit is *calorie*. One calorie is the amount of heat which will raise the temperature of one gram of water to one 1°C:

$$1\ \text{calorie} = 4.2\ \text{joules.}$$

Conduction

Conduction is the heat transfer through a material or by touching. It is the process in which heat energy is transferred by molecules, without visible motion of particles. Conduction takes place in solids, liquids, and gases. Heat transfer from the X-ray tube's anode to an oil through the rotor is by conduction.

Convection

Convection is the heat transfer in which heat energy is transferred by actual motion of particles of the body. Convection takes place in liquid and gases, e.g., trade winds, land, and sea breezes. Convection current in air removes heat from X-ray tube's housing to the atmosphere. Oil and water circulation remove heat from CT scan.

Radiation

Radiation is the heat transfer by the emission of infrared radiation. It is the process by which heat energy is transmitted from one place to another without the aid of any material medium, e.g., sun heat reaches the earth. X-ray tube's anode cooling is by radiation process.

Temperature

Molecules have regular movement in solids and random movement in liquids and gases. They possess potential energy as well as kinetic energy. The total energy of the molecules in the system is called *internal energy*. Kinetic energy is responsible for the hotness and coldness of the body.

Temperature is the measure of hotness and coldness of the body, and it is measured by a *thermometer*. Change of temperature may alter the electrical resistance, conductivity, viscosity, and rate of chemical reaction of the substance, e.g., change of human body temperature alters metabolism. There are three scales of temperature, namely, (1) *Celsius scale* (c), (2) *Kelvin scale* (K), and (3) *Fahrenheit scale* (F), and they are related as follows:

$$T_c = \frac{5}{9}(T_F - 32)$$

$$T_F = \frac{9}{2}T_c + 32$$

$$T_K = T_c + 273$$

ATOM

All matter is composed of elements and compounds. Elements are the simplest chemical entity, which cannot be broken further, e.g., Hydrogen, Carbon. Two or three elements form a compound, e.g., water. The smallest particle of an element is an atom, which forms the fundamental unit of matter (10^{-10m}). Every atom possesses a dense positively charged central core called *nucleus* (10^{-15m}). It is surrounded by revolving electrons in well-defined orbits **(Fig. 1.1)**.

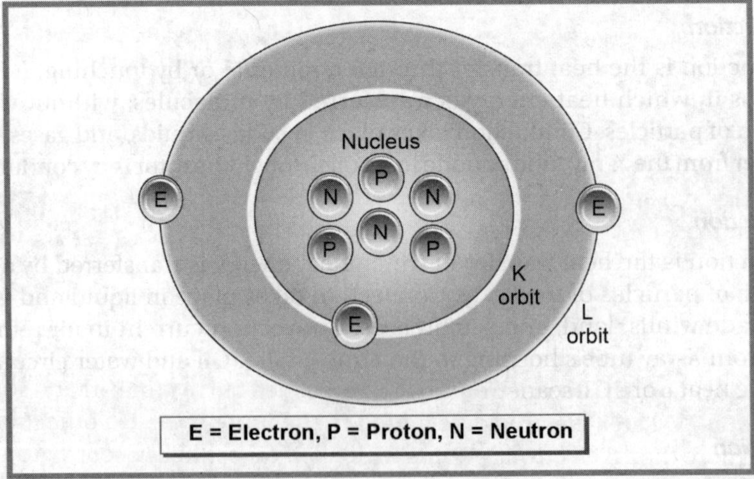

Fig. 1.1: Atomic structure.

The nucleus consists of protons and neutrons and collectively known as *nucleons*. The protons are positively charged, and neutrons have no charge, said to be neutral. The electrons are negatively charged particles and they circulate around the nucleus at varying distances, like planets rotate around the sun. *Centripetal force* keeps the electrons in an orbit. The number of electrons in an atom is equal to the number of protons, hence an atom is said to be neutral.

Fundamental Particles

There are more than 100 subatomic particles in an atom. However, electron, proton and neutron are the fundamental particles of the atom. The mass of one electron is 9.1×10^{-31} kg. Since atom is small, its mass is expressed in atomic mass unit (amu). One amu is equal to $\frac{1}{12}$ of mass of a Carbon-12 atom.

1 amu = 931 MeV and one electron mass is 0.000549 amu.

The proton and neutron in the nucleus are made up of *quarks* which are held together by *gluons*. They are 2,000 times higher mass than that of an electron. The mass of proton and neutron are 1.673×10^{-27} kg and 1.675×10^{-27} kg, respectively. Their mass in terms of amu is 1.

There are two types of forces that exist in the nucleus. The *electrostatic repulsive force* exists between particles of similar charge. The *strong attractive force* resulting from the exchange of pions among all nucleons, holds the nucleus together. These two forces act in opposite directions. The nucleus has an energy level, and the lowest energy state is called the *ground state*. Nuclei with energy excess of the ground state is said to be in an *excited state*. Excited states that exist $>10^{-12}$ s are referred to as *meta stable or an isomeric state*.

Atomic Structure

Atom is an empty space and all its mass is concentrated in the nucleus which is very small. Electron orbits are referred to as shells which reveal the chemical behavior and molecule formation. Shells are K, L, M, and N of different binding energies with *principal quantum number* (n = 1, 2, 3, etc.). The maximum number of electrons in a shell is: $2n^2$, where *n* denotes the shell number. The closer the electron to the nucleus, greater the binding energy.

Electron position in an atom is described by quantum numbers, namely (1) principal quantum number, (2) azimuthal quantum number, (3) magnetic quantum number, and (4) spin quantum number.

Elements are grouped in the *pediatric table* with increasing atomic numbers. The first element is Hydrogen, has one proton and one electron. The second element Helium has two protons, two electrons and two neutrons. Atoms that have one electron in the outer shell are in group-I of the pediatric table. Atoms with two electrons in the outer shell fall in group-II and so on, up to group-IV. Later, electrons are added to the inner shell. No outer shell can have more than 8 electrons. Atoms with filled outer shells occupy group-VIII, which are chemically stable and said to be noble gases.

Table 1.3: Symbol, Atomic number, and K-shell binding energy of few elements.

Element	Symbol	Atomic Number (Z)	K-Shell Binding Energy, keV
Beryllium	Be	4	0.11
Carbon	C	6	0.28
Oxygen	O	8	0.53
Aluminum	Al	13	1.56
Calcium	Ca	20	4.04
Copper	Cu	29	8.98
Molybdenum	Mo	42	20
Rhodium	Rh	45	23.2
Tin	Sn	50	29.2
Iodine	I	53	33.2
Cesium	Cs	55	36
Barium	Ba	56	37.4
Gadolinium	Gd	64	50
Tungsten	W	74	69.5
Rhenium	Re	75	71.7
Lead	Pb	82	88

(*Courtesy:* Stewart Carlyle Bushong, 2017)

Table 1.4: Density and Effective atomic number of few compounds.

Compound	Effective Atomic Number	Density (ρ), gcm^{-3}
Air	7.64	0.001293
Muscle	7.42	1.00
Water	7.42	1.0
Bone	13.8	1.85
Fat	5.92	0.916

(*Courtesy:* Johns and Gunningham JR, 1969)

Atomic number of an atom is the number of protons or electrons in the nucleus, denoted by Z. *Mass number* of an atom is the total number of protons and neutrons in the nucleus, denoted by A. An element (X) is symbolically described as $^{A}_{Z}X$ **(Table 1.3)**.

Effective atomic number (Z_{eff}) refers to a compound or mixture, which has more than one element. The Z_{eff} is the atomic number of an element with which photons interact the same way as with the given composite material **(Table 1.4)**.

One or more atoms combine and form molecules, e.g., sodium bicarbonate ($NaHCO_3$). A molecule is a smallest unit of a compound. Atoms combine and form compound in two ways: (1) covalent bond, e.g., H_2O and (2) ionic bond, e.g., NaCl.

Isotopes

Atoms composed of nuclei with same number of protons, but different number of neutrons is called an *isotope*. In other words, isotopes have same atomic numbers but different mass numbers, e.g., Hydrogen have three isotopes:

^1_1H have 1 proton (Hydrogen)

^2_1H have 1 proton and 1 neutron (Deuterium)

^3_1H have 1 proton and 2 neutrons (Tritium)

Isotopes of an element have same chemical properties but have different physical properties. If they perform radioactivity, they are called *radioisotopes* and their nucleus is said to be unstable.

Atoms having same mass numbers (nucleons), but different atomic numbers are called *isobars*, e.g., $^{17}_7N$ and $^{17}_8O$. It has different number protons and different number of neutrons, but the total number of nucleons are the same. Radioactive transition of such atom results in beta or positron particle.

Atoms having same number of neutrons, but different number of protons are called *isotones*, e.g., $^{37}_{17}Cl$ and $^{39}_{19}K$. They have different atomic numbers and different mass numbers, but a constant value of A–Z.

An *isomer* is an excited state of a nucleus, and it will have the same atomic number and same mass number. They are identical atoms but exists at different energy states, e.g., $^{99m}_{43}Tc$ decays to $^{99}_{43}Tc$ with emission of 140 keV gamma energy.

Ionization and Excitation

Removal of one or more electrons from a neutral atom is called an *ionization*. The atom is said to be ionized and it is not electrically neutral. After an ionization, the remainder of the atom is left with a positive charge, known as *positive ion*. The positive atom and the removed electrons are called *ion pairs*. About 34 eV energy is required to remove an electron and ionize an atom.

In an atom, if energy is supplied, the electrons can be moved from an inner orbit to an outer orbit. Now, the atom will have more energy than its normal state. It is said to be in an excited state and the process is known as an *excitation*. For example, to move an electron from K to L shell of a hydrogen atom, the energy required is: (–3.4 eV) – (–13.5 eV) = 10.1 eV.

Binding Energy

Binding energy of an electron in an atom is the energy required to remove an electron completely from the atom against the attractive force of positive nucleus. Magnitude of the binding energy depends on the atomic number and the shell from which the electron is being removed. It is greater for elements of higher atomic number, and greatest for K-shell, an inner most shell.

Binding energies are negative because they represent the amount of energy that must be supplied to remove an electron from an atom. Electron shells are often described in terms of binding energy of electrons occupying the shells. Binding energy of an electron in an atom is a form of potential energy and it is expressed in keV. The K-shell binding energies of various elements are given in **Table 1.3**.

Electron Volt

The electron volt (eV) is the unit of energy in atomic or radiation physics, where it deals with microscopic objects. One electron volt is the kinetic energy imparted to an electron, accelerated across a potential difference of one volt. In practice, we use *kiloelectron volt* (keV) and *million electron volt* (MeV):
$$1 \text{ eV} = 1.6 \times 10^{-19} \text{ J} = 1.6 \times 10^{-12} \text{ erg} = 4.4 \times 10^{-26} \text{ kWh}$$

The electron volt describes potential as well as kinetic energy. In practice, MeV and keV are used as units. $1 \text{ MeV} = 10^6 \text{ eV}$ and $1 \text{ keV} = 10^3 \text{ eV}$.

ELECTROMAGNETIC RADIATION

An electric charge is surrounded by an electric field and if the charge moves, a magnetic field is produced. When the charge undergoes an acceleration or deceleration, the magnetic and the electric fields of the charge will vary. The combined variation of an electric and magnetic fields result in loss of energy. The charge radiates this energy in the form known as an *electromagnetic energy* or *photons*. A photon is a smallest quantity of any form of an electromagnetic energy. It is also called *quanta,* which refers to a small bundle of energy.

Electromagnetic radiation moves in the form of sinusoidal waves **(Fig. 1.2)**. Its nature depends on the way in which the electric charges are disturbed. They are basically transverse waves that transfer energy away from an electric charge. They may be absorbed or scattered in a medium, resulting in loss of energy.

Wave Characteristics

Electromagnetic wave has wavelength (λ), frequency (ν), and velocity (c) and obey the relation:
$$c = \nu\lambda$$

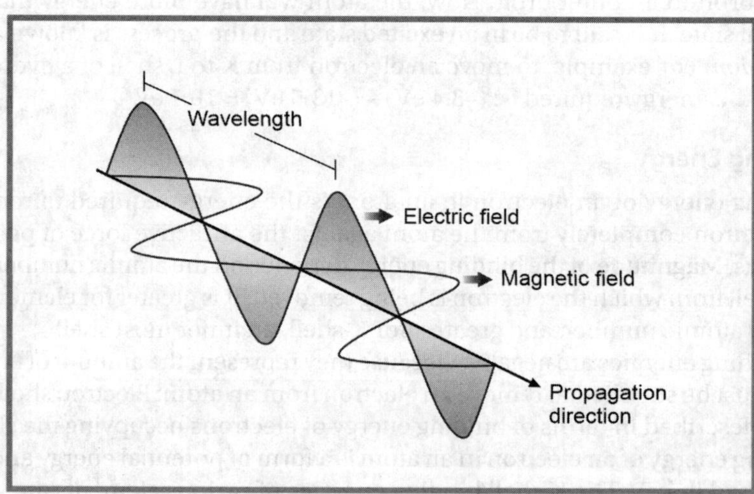

Fig. 1.2: Electromagnetic wave.

The distance between two consecutive positive peaks is known as *wavelength*. The number of cycles of the wave which pass a fixed point per second is known as *frequency* of the wave. *Velocity* of the wave is the distance traveled per second by the wave. All electromagnetic waves, travel with velocity of light = 3×10^8 m/sec. The wavelength of X-rays and gamma rays are in nanometers (nm).

Particle Characteristics

Though electromagnetic radiation has properties of waves, they also behave like particle during an interaction with matter. The actual amount of energy (E) carried by a photon is given by the equation E = hv, where *h* is **Planck's** constant = 6.63×10^{-34} J. Substituting the value of $v = \dfrac{c}{\lambda}$ in the above equation:

$$E(keV) = \frac{hc}{\lambda} = \frac{1.24}{\lambda}$$

where, λ is in nanometer (nm). It is seen that the energy of the photon is inversely proportional to its wavelength and as the wavelength decreases, the energy increases. Visible light tends to behave more like waves than particles, whereas, X-ray photons behave more like particles than waves.

Electromagnetic Spectrum

Electromagnetic spectrum includes radio waves, microwaves, infrared, visible light, ultraviolet (UV), X-rays, gamma rays and cosmic rays **(Fig. 1.3)**. Important spectrum for diagnostic radiology is visible light, X-rays, gamma rays and radio waves. Visible light wavelength ranges from 400 to 700 nm. Radio waves are described in terms of frequency, and they cover long rage of the spectrum. Radio and television broadcast frequencies are 960 kHz and 63.7 MHz, respectively. X-rays and gamma rays are identified by their energy, but their origin is different.

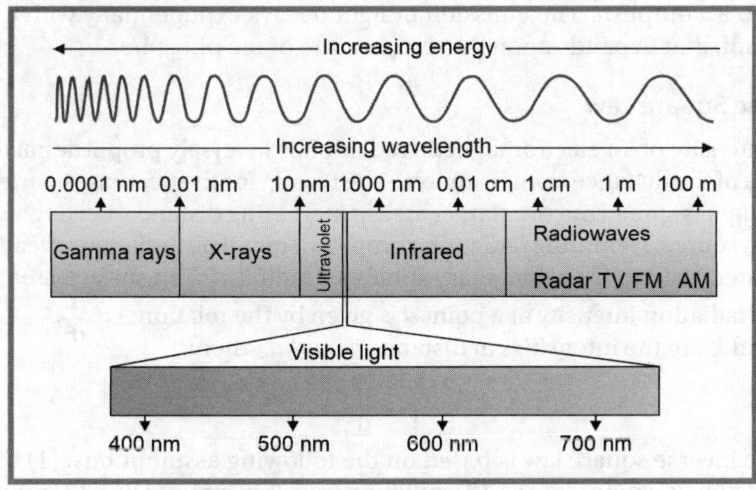

Fig. 1.3: Electromagnetic spectrum.

Ionizing and Non-ionizing Radiation

Ionization is the process of removal of an electron from a neutral atom. The radiation which does ionization in a medium, by removal of an electron is called *ionizing radiation*, e.g., UV, X-rays, and gamma rays have sufficient energy to do ionization. As a result, ionized atoms and molecules or ion-pairs are produced. This forms the basis for biological effects of radiation. Radiation that does not have sufficient energy to produce an ionization are called non-ionizing radiation, e.g., visible light, infrared, microwaves, and radio waves.

Fluorescence

When electromagnetic radiation incident on a phosphor, visible or ultraviolet light is emitted from the phosphor, and it is called *luminescence*. Electromagnetic radiation raises the valence electrons to the conduction band, which returns to the valence band to fill up the holes. As electrons fall through the luminescence centers, they emit the surplus energy in the form of flashes of light, called luminescence. If the luminescence is instantaneous, within 10^{-8} s, it is called *fluorescence*.

The energy of light emitted depends on the difference in energy across the luminescence centers. It is always less than the energy which originally stimulated the fluorescence, e.g., a phosphor exposed to ultraviolet may emit visible light. Fluorescent phosphors, such as *thallium activated sodium iodide* (Gamma camera), *terbium activated gadolinium oxysulfide* (intensifying screen) and *sodium activated cesium iodide* (image intensifier) are used in diagnostic radiology.

If the emission of light is delayed beyond 10^{-8} s, it is called *phosphorescence*. When the valence electrons are stimulated, they get trapped in the conduction band. They acquire energy from the atom (internal energy) and return to the valence band by emitting luminescence. It is a random process, which takes time to accomplish. The emission of light decays exponentially with a time constant, that depends upon the temperature of the phosphor.

Inverse Square Law

The intensity of an electromagnetic radiation is inversely proportional to the square of the distance from its source. The reason for the decrease in intensity is the light is spread out over larger area at increasing distance. Let us consider a point source, s, emitting radiation at constant rate. The radiation spread over the inner surface of an imaginary sphere of radius, d with surface area $4\pi d^2$.

Then, radiation intensity at a point d is given by the relation: $I \propto \dfrac{1}{d^2}$.

If I_1 and I_2 are the intensities at distance d_1 and d_2, then:

$$\frac{I_1}{I_2} = \frac{d_2^2}{d_1^2}$$

The inverse square law is based on the following assumptions: (1) source of radiation is a point source, (2) radiation travels in straight line, (3) radiation

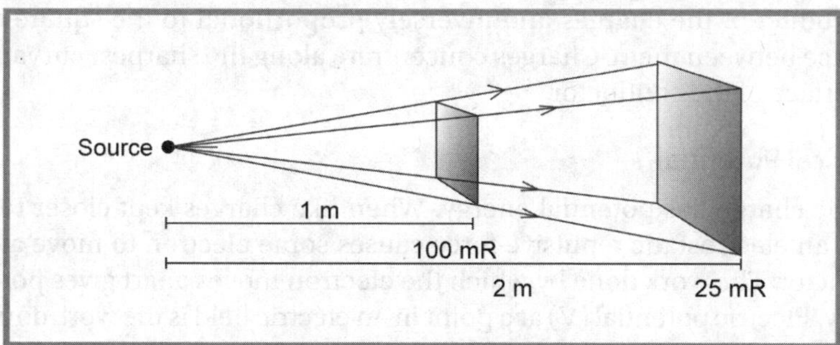

Fig. 1.4: Inverse square law.

is emitted equally in all directions, (4) energy is radiated at a constant rate, and (5) no radiation energy is lost on its way from the source to the point of measurement.

Let 100 mR be the radiation exposure at 1 m for a point source. The radiation exposure at 2 m is found to be 25 mR, by inverse square law **(Fig. 1.4).** Hence, if distance is doubled, the radiation is reduced by a factor of 4. Keeping a higher distance from the source, always reduce radiation exposure. Inverse square law can be applied to distances greater than seven times the longest dimension of the source. It is not applicable other than point source and distance nearer to the source.

ELECTROSTATICS

Electric Charge

Electrostatics is the study of stationary electric charges. The term electric is derived from the Greek word electron. Electric bodies are said to possess an electric charge (Q) and it is a basic property of any matter. There are two types of charges, namely, (1) positive charge, and (2) negative charge. The unit of charge is *coulomb (C)*. Electron and proton possess one unit of negative and positive charge, respectively. The amount of charge in an electron is equal to 1.6021×10^{-19}C.

To describe electric charges, electrostatic laws are given. Two like charges repel each other and two unlike charges attract each other. *Charges can neither be created nor be destroyed, and the total amount of charge in the system does not change.* While calculating the total charge in a system, the signs of the charge must be considered.

Electric charge is associated with an electric field. The electric field tends to point outward from a positive charge and inward from a negative charge. The force of attraction between unlike charges and repulsion from like charges is called *electrostatic force*, given by the **Coulomb's law**:

$$F = K \frac{Q_1 Q_2}{d^2}$$

where, Q_1 and Q_2 are the electrostatic charges separated by a distance, d, and K is a constant. Thus, an electrostatic force is directly proportional to the product of the charges and inversely proportional to the square of the distance between them. Charges concentrate along the sharpest curvature of the surface of the conductor.

Electrical Potential

Electric charge has potential energy. When like charges kept closer to each other, an electrostatic repulsive force causes some electron to move along a conductor. The work done by which the electron moves apart gives potential energy. Electric potential (V) at a point in an electric field is the work done (W) in taking a unit positive charge (Q) from infinity to that point:

$$V = \frac{W}{Q}$$

Positive charges flow from a point of higher potential to point of lower potential and negative charges flow in the reverse direction. The unit of potential is *volt* (V). The potential is a scalar quantity, and the potential of earth is taken as zero. Electric potential at our home service in India is 230 V. In practice, *kilovolt* (kV) and *megavolt* (MV) are used as units:

$1 \text{ kV} = 1{,}000$ volts and $1 \text{ MV} = 10^6$ volts.

ELECTRODYNAMICS

Electric Current

Electrodynamics is the study of electric charges under motion. The flow of an electric charge in a conductor is called an *electric current* or *electricity*. It is equal to the quantity of charge passing a given point in one second. The direction of current is opposite to the flow of electron. Unit of current is *ampere* (A), one ampere current consists of 6.281×10^{18} electrons/sec. In practice, milliampere (mA) and microampere (μA) are used as units, $1 \text{ mA} = 10^{-3}$ A, and $1 \text{ μA} = 10^{-6}$ A.

Charge flows through solid, liquid and gas or in vacuum. Substance in which electrons flow easily are called *conductors*. An *insulator* is a material which does not allow the flow of electrons. Copper and water are conductors, whereas glass and clay are insulators. *Semiconductor* is a material, partly behaves as conductor and insulator under some conditions, e.g., *Germanium and Silicon*.

Resistance

Resistance (R) is the property of a conductor by which it opposes the flow of an electric current (I). It is defined as the ratio of the potential difference (V) applied across a conductor to the current flowing through it:

$$R = \frac{V}{I}$$

Resistance decreases as temperature of the material decreases. The device which resists the flow of current is called *resister*. In a conductor, the atoms are vibrating, and the electrons move randomly. When a voltage is applied, the electrons move towards the positive terminal. During the process, they collide with vibrating atoms, resulting in resistance. Unit of resistance is *ohm* (Ω). In practice, *kilo ohm* (kΩ) and *mega ohm* (MΩ) are used as units, and 1 kΩ = 1,000 Ω, and 1 MΩ = 10^6 Ω.

Specific Resistance

The resistance of a resistor at a given temperature depends upon the material and its dimension. The resistance (R) is directly proportional to the length (L) and inversely proportional to the area (A) of cross section of resistor:

$$R \propto \frac{L}{A} = \frac{\rho L}{A} \quad \text{or} \ \rho = \frac{RA}{L}$$

where, ρ is a constant, called the *specific resistance or resistivity* and the unit is ohm-meter. The above relation reveals that the resistance of a thick wire would be lesser than that of a thin wire. The resistance is greater if the length is greater. The reciprocal of resistivity ($1/\rho$) is called conductivity (σ) and its unit is (*ohm-meter*)$^{-1}$.

Superconductivity

Superconductors are materials which offer no resistance to the flow of current below certain temperature. At very low temperatures, some metals, compounds, or alloys offer superconductivity, e.g., *Niobium and Titanium.* Conductors become superconducting at *super conducting transition temperature* (T_c). At transition temperature, electrical resistivity falls to zero, conductivity becomes infinity, material excludes its magnetic flux lines, and ohms law is not valid.

A material in a super conducting state requires no power to carry large currents. Since the resistance of the material in the super conducting state is zero, no thermal losses are associated with passage of large currents. Superconductors are used for generating strong magnetic fields, since they can withstand large magnetic fields and carry large currents.

Metal alloys like *Niobium-Titanium* become a superconductor below 10 K. It is used in magnetic resonance imaging equipment but requires *liquid Helium* as a coolant system. Ceramic *metal oxide compounds* become super conductors at higher temperatures, e.g., *Yttrium barium copper oxide* at 93 K and *Thallium-calcium-bismuth copper oxide* at 125 K. Since they operate at higher temperatures, liquid Nitrogen can be used as an effective coolant, which is cheaper than Helium.

Ohm's Law

Ohm's law describes the behavior of an electric current in an electrical circuit. Law states that voltage (V) across an electrical circuit is equal to the product of current (I) and resistance (R).

$$V = IR \text{ or } R = \frac{V}{I}$$

Electrical circuits with resistance can be made either series or parallel circuits.

Electrical Power

The electrical power (P) is the rate at which energy is expended and it is equal to the product of potential difference (V) and current (I) in a circuit, P = VI. It can be modified by using Ohm's law as P = (IR)I = I^2R, where *R* is the resistance. The unit of electrical power is *watt*, which is equal to one *joule per second* (Js^{-1}). If one ampere current flows through an electric potential of 1 volt, the consumed power is said to be 1 watt. In practice, *kilowatt*, and *kilowatt hour (kWh)* are used as units. The unit of electrical supply is kilowatt hour (kWh) = 3.6×10^6 J. X-ray machines require about 20–150 W of electric power.

Joule's Law of Heating

The heat (H) developed in a current carrying conductor is directly proportional to square of the current (I) passing through the conductor, resistance (R) of the conductor, and time (t) of flow of current:

$$H = I^2 \, Rt \text{ joule}$$

If the current is doubled, the heat generated is four times higher. This concept is applied in fuse wires, as the current goes to higher value, the heat generated in the circuit is sufficient to melt the fuse wire. The melting point of the fuse material is very critical for material selection.

MAGNETISM

Magnetism is a fundamental property of a matter, and it is produced by motion of electrical charges. Electrons are in random motion in materials and rotate about an axis either clockwise or anti-clockwise. This rotation creates electron spin which constitutes a *magnetic field*. This field is perpendicular to the motion of the particle. Atoms and molecules that have paired electrons cancel their magnetic fields and the net magnetic field is zero, but unpaired electron spins offer magnetic field. Thus, atoms having odd number of electrons in any shell gives small magnetic field.

A magnet possesses, two poles namely, *north pole* and *south pole* (**Fig. 1.5**). The term pole refers to end of a magnet in which the entire magnetism appears to be concentrated. The pole that points north under the influence of earth's magnetic field is called *north pole* and the other is called *south pole*. As in the case of an electric charge, like poles repel and unlike poles attract each other.

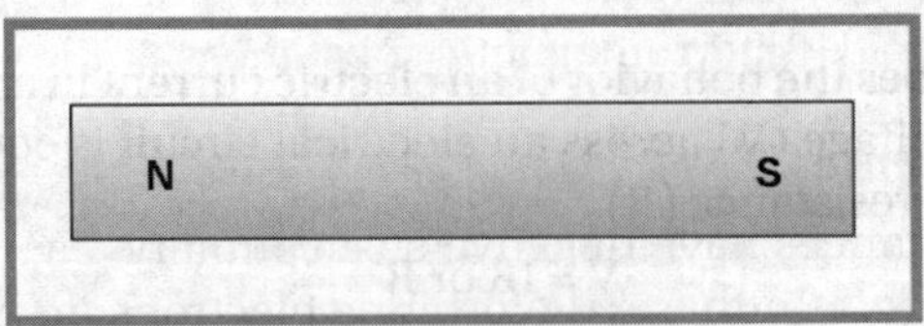

Fig. 1.5: Magnetic dipole.

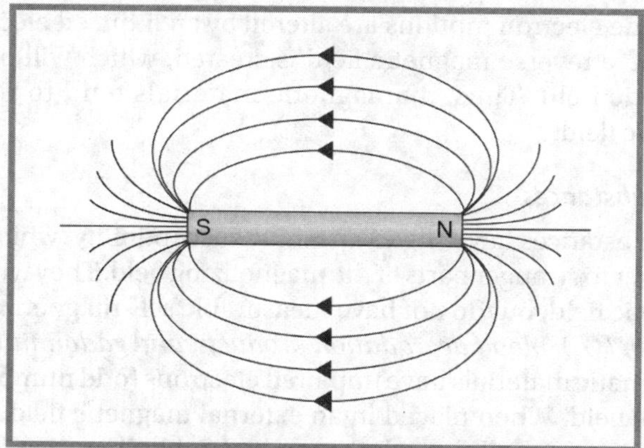

Fig. 1.6: Magnet and magnetic lines of force.

Magnetic field is visualized by an imaginary-lines, called *magnetic lines of force* (**Fig. 1.6**). The imaginary magnetic lines of force will leave the north pole and return to the south pole. The total number of lines of force at the pole expresses *magnetic field strength* and its unit is *weber* (Wb).

Magnetism obeys the laws of electrostatic and gravity forces. The force between the poles is proportional to the product of magnetic pole strengths and inversely proportional to the square of the distance between them. Magnets can be made by induction like an *electrostatic induction*.

SI unit of magnetic field strength is *tesla (T)* and one tesla = 1 Wbm^{-2}. The older unit of pole strength is *gauss* (G) and one tesla is equal 10,000 gauss. The earth's magnetic field strength is about 50–100 µT. Magnets used in MRI ranges from 0.3 to 3 T. There are three types of magnets, namely (1) natural magnet, (2) permanent magnet, and (3) electromagnet. Natural magnets get their magnetism from earth, whereas permanent magnets are artificially induced. An iron core wrapped by current carrying wire is used to produce an electromagnet.

Magnetic Properties

Magnetic properties of materials are determined by atomic and molecular structures in relation to electron behavior. *Magnetic permeability* is the ability by which the material attracts the lines of magnetic field intensity.

Magnetic susceptibility is another property which describes the extent to which the material becomes magnetized, when placed in a magnetic field. Based on susceptibility, the material can be classified as: (1) diamagnetic, (2) paramagnetic, and (3) ferromagnetic substances.

Diamagnetic Substances

Diamagnetic substances have negative susceptibility, e.g., *Calcium, water, and organic materials*. In these, the orbiting electrons do not lie in a plane and the net magnetic field is so small. When they are placed in an external magnetic field, the electron motions are altered by an induced electromotive force. As a result, a reverse magnetic field is created, which will oppose the applied magnetic field. Thus, diamagnetic materials tend to reduce the applied magnetic field.

Paramagnetic Substances

Paramagnetic substances have slightly positive susceptibility, which tends to move from weaker to stronger parts of the magnetizing field. They will enhance the local magnetic field, but do not have measurable self-magnetization, e.g., *molecular oxygen (O_2), blood degradation products, and gadolinium contrast agents.* Paramagnetic materials have unpaired electrons (odd number), which have a magnetic field. When placed in an external magnetic field, electron's magnetic field align themselves with the applied field. Thus, it enhances the applied field, but has slight attraction to the magnetic field. Contrast agents used in MRI are paramagnetic substances.

Ferromagnetic Substances

Ferromagnetic materials are those which are attracted by magnets and permanently get magnetized, e.g., *Iron, Cobalt, and Nickel.* The susceptibility of these materials is very high. Alloy of *Aluminum, Nickel, and Cobalt (alnico)* are ferromagnetic materials, used to produce magnets. Rare earth elements are also used to produce stronger magnets.

They are basically transition elements, in which electrons fill the outer orbital shells before inner shells are filled. When the spins are in random motion, usual cancellation of field does not take place, resulting in higher magnetic moment. When they are placed in an external magnetic field, the magnetic dipoles non-randomly align with an applied field. Thus, ferromagnetic materials enhance the applied magnetic field. Ferromagnetic materials can be made as magnets by induction.

ELECTROMAGNETISM

In 1831, **Michael Faraday** showed the production of an electric current from a magnetic field. According to Faraday, current can be induced in a closed conductor, if some part of that circuit is in a changing magnetic field. The current exists only so long as the change takes place. The *electromotive force* (emf), that produces the current is called an *induced emf.* The whole phenomenon is known as *electromagnetic induction.*

Laws of Electromagnetic Induction

- ❑ A change of magnetic flux linked with a conductor induces an electromagnetic force (emf) in the conductor.
- ❑ The magnitude of the induced emf is proportional to the rate of change of magnetic flux and to the area of the circuit.
- ❑ Induced emf is in such a direction that it always opposes the change of magnetic flux, which induced the emf.

The first two laws are called *Faraday's law,* while the third is called *Lenz's law.* The magnitude of the induced current depends on four factors, namely (1) strength of the magnetic field, (2) velocity of the magnetic field relative to the conductor, (3) angle of the conductor to the magnetic field, and (4) number of turns in the conductor.

Based on the laws of electromagnetic induction, *electric motors* and *generators* are employed. Electric current produces mechanical motion in an electric motor. Mechanical motion of a magnet near a coil induces electricity in the coil, is the principle used in an *electric generator.* Induction motor is used to induce current in the rotor of the rotating anode X-ray tube.

Transformer

A transformer is an electrical device, which can convert an electrical energy from one coil to another coil. It uses interacting magnetic fields and does not convert energy from form to another. Transformers convert potential and current into higher or lower intensity.

It consists of two coils, namely primary and secondary, and working on the principle *mutual induction* (**Figs. 1.7A and B**). These coils are wound on an iron core. An alternating voltage, which is to be transferred, is applied in the primary coil as input. This produces a changing magnetic flux in an iron core, which produces an alternating emf in the secondary coil. The induced emf in the coils are directly proportional to the respective number of turns of the coil.

Let N_P and N_S are the number of turns in the primary and secondary coils. Let V_P and V_S are the voltage in the primary and secondary coils. Let I_P and I_S are the current in the primary and secondary coils, then:

$$V_P \propto N_P, \; V_S \propto N_S$$

$$\text{or} \quad \frac{V_P}{V_S} = \frac{N_P}{N_S}$$

In a transformer, the turns ratio is equal to an *voltage ratio.* The power in put in the primary, $(P_P) = V_P I_P$ and the power output in the secondary,

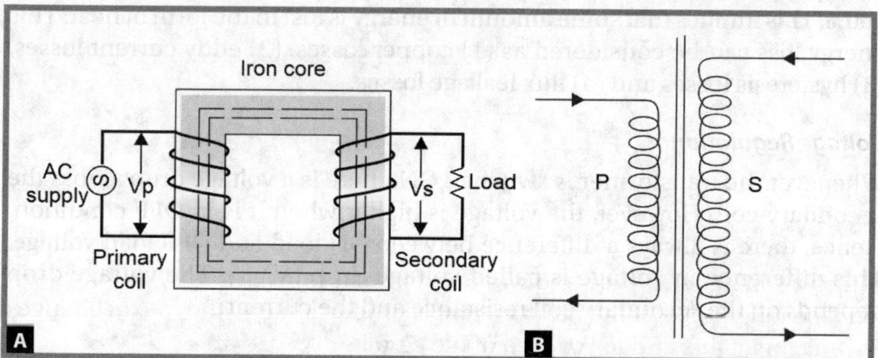

Figs. 1.7A and B: (A) Transformer principle; (B) Symbol.

$(P_S) = V_S I_S$. Based on the law of conservation of energy, power input is equal to the power output:

$$V_P I_P = V_S I_S$$

$$\text{or } \frac{V_P}{V_S} = \frac{I_S}{I_P} = \frac{N_P}{N_S}$$

This shows that the current in the coils is inversely proportional to the number of turns in the respective coils.

Basically, there are three types of transformers, namely *step-up, step-down* and *isolation* transforms. If a transformer transfers power of low voltage and high current into power of high voltage and low current, it is called *step-up transformer*. In this type, the secondary coil will have a greater number of turns than the primary, $N_S > N_P$ and the turns ratio is >1. If a transformer, transfer power of high voltage and low current into power of low voltage and high current, it is called *step-down* transformer. In this type, primary will have large number of turns than the secondary, $N_S < N_P$ and the turns ratio is <1. If, $N_S = N_P$, then the transformer is called an isolation transformer.

Efficiency

The efficiency of the transformer is the ratio between the output power and input power:

$$\text{Efficiency} = \frac{\text{Output power}}{\text{Input power}} = \frac{P_S}{P_P} \times 100$$

In actual transformer, the output power is always lesser than the input power due to some energy losses. Hence an efficiency is always less than <100% or 1.

Transformer Design and Losses

Transformers are designed as closed-core transformers, auto transformers and shell type transformers. In practice, the output power is always less than the input power and hence the efficiency of the transformer is always less than 100%. This implies that some amount of energy is lost in the form of heat. This energy loss can be considered as (1) copper losses, (2) eddy current losses, (3) hysteresis losses and (4) flux leakage losses.

Voltage Regulation

Whenever the transformer is switched ON, there is a voltage drop across the secondary coil. However, the voltage is higher when it is in OFF condition. Hence, there is always a difference between ON load and OFF load voltage. This difference in voltage is called voltage drop (V_{Drop}). The voltage drop depends on the secondary coil resistance and the current:

$$V_{Drop} = (V_{OFF\text{-}load} - V_{ON\text{-}load})$$

The voltage drop is usually expressed in percentage, and it is termed as voltage regulation as given below:

$$\text{Voltage regulation} = \frac{V_{Drop}}{V_{OFF\text{-}load}} \times 100$$

In practice, it is about 5% for 800 mA transformer.

Transformer Rating

The transformer rating refers to the maximum safe output that can be taken from the secondary winding. It specifies the maximum safe operating conditions, so that it is protected from damage. There are two ways of specifying ratings namely, (1) power rating and (2) voltage rating. Transformers can give high output power over a short period, without overheating. However, extended period of operation may overheat the system. Power rating prevents the transformer from overheating. It depends on the heat capacity of the transformer. This means that at what rate the transformer can dissipate heat and it mainly lies on the efficiency of the cooling system.

Usually, it is expressed as the maximum safe output of its secondary winding in kilowatts. For three-phase generators, ratings are calculated by:

$$kW = \frac{(kV) \times mA}{1,000}$$

For example, a three-phase generator operating at 100 kV and 500 mA, the rating is:

$$\text{Rating} = \frac{(100 \times 500)}{1,000} = 50 \, kW$$

For single-phase generators, the formula is:

$$kW = \frac{(kV \times mA \times 0.7)}{1,000}$$

The factor 0.7 comes from the root mean square (rms) value of the voltage. Kilowatt ratings of X-ray generators are determined when the generator is under load. Information about ratings is useful to compare X-ray generators.

Generally, transformers are designed with a specific electrical insulation, to withstand a particular voltage. Manufacturers usually specify this voltage up to which the transformer can be loaded. This is called *voltage rating*. If it exceeds, electrical insulation may breakdown and arcing may occur. This will subject the transformer to greater damage, which may be beyond repair.

The ratings are also specified in terms of (1) maximum current, which the transform can give on continuous running and (2) maximum current which the transformer can give for a period not exceeding one second.

RECTIFICATION

Rectification is the process of changing an alternating current into direct current. The device that produces the change is called a *rectifier*. A rectifier allows an electrical current to flow in one direction but does not allow

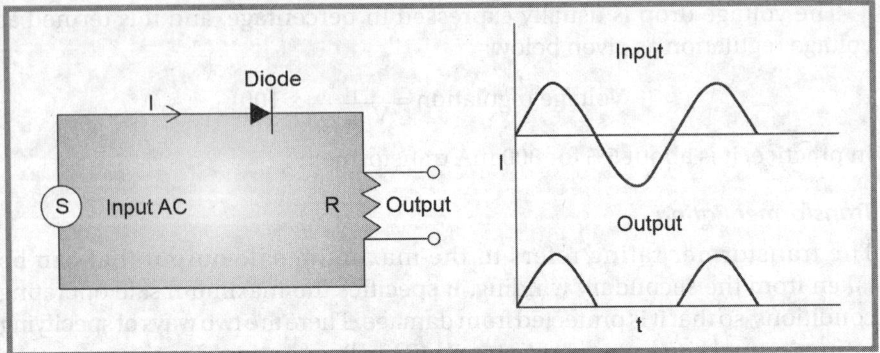

Fig. 1.8: Half-wave rectifier.

current to flow in the other direction. Rectifiers are connected into the X-ray circuit in series. They are mainly divided into (1) half-wave rectifier and (2) full-wave rectifiers.

Half-wave Rectifier

Vacuum tube diodes or solid state (semiconductor) diodes can be used for rectification. In a half-wave rectifier, a single diode is used (**Fig. 1.8**). An alternating voltage is applied to the diode as input. The output is obtained across the resistance R. When the plate is positive, the diode will allow the current to flow. When the plate is negative, the diode will not allow the current. The diode will allow the current only during those half cycles when the plate is positive. Hence, the output current is always in one direction. This circuit is known as *half-wave rectifier*, and it is mainly used in mobile and dental X-ray units. A single solid-state diode cannot prevent reverse current at higher voltages. Hence, many diodes are placed in series on a stick to do rectification.

Full-wave Rectifier

In the half-wave rectifier, the input voltage is used only in one half of the cycle. The other half of the cycle is not used. Hence, there is a need of a rectifier which will use the full cycle of the input AC voltage. This is possible by having two or more number of diodes (**Fig. 1.9**). The alternating voltage is applied between A and B. The output is obtained across the resistance R.

When end A is positive, $D1$ and $D3$ will conduct and a current flow through R. Since, the diode $D2$ and $D4$ are reverse biased, they do not pass current. During the next half of the cycle A is negative and end B is positive. Now, the diodes $D2$ and $D4$ will conduct, and a current flow through R. Since, the diode $D1$ and $D3$ are reverse biased, they do not pass current. Thus, the current flows through the resistance during the full cycle of the input voltage. The current is always flowing in the same direction—from C to D. Hence, this circuit is called full-wave rectifier, and it is mainly used in rotating anode X-ray tubes.

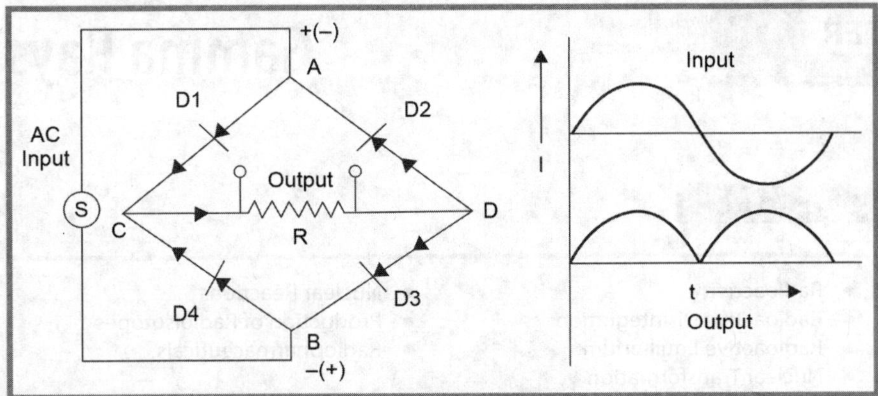

Fig. 1.9: Full-wave rectifier.

BIBLIOGRAPHY

1. Ball J, Moore AD, Turner S. Essential Physics for Radiographers, Balckwell Publishing, UK; 2008.
2. Bushberg JT, Seibert JA, Leidholdt EM, Jr, Boone JM. The Essential Physics of Medical Imaging, 3rd edn. Lippincott Williams and Wilkins; 2012.
3. Bushong SC. Radiological Science for Technologists, 11th ed. Elsevier; 2017.
4. Johns and Gunningham JR. The Physics of Radiology, 3rd edn. Springfield, IL: Charles C Thomas; 1969.
5. Thayalan K. Basic Radiological Physics, 2nd edn. Jaypee Brothers Medical Publishers (P) Ltd, New Delhi; 2017.

2

Radioactivity and Gamma Rays

RADIOACTIVITY

Henri Becquerel discovered the nuclear phenomenon Radioactivity (1896). He left some Uranium salt wrapped in a black paper, on a photographic plate which was lying in a dark room. When he developed the photographic plate, he found that the plate was affected. After repeating the experiment with other salts of Uranium, he concluded that Uranium and its salts emit invisible radiations which can pass through paper, wood, glass, etc., and affect photographic plate. Above radiations were found to have alpha (α), beta (β) particles and gamma (γ) radiations.

Radioactivity is the process by which a nucleus undergo disintegration and emits either alpha or beta and gamma radiations. During the radioactive process, atom changes its atomic number and chemical identity. An atom with an unstable nuclei and perform radioactivity is called *radioisotope*. Initial atom that undergoes disintegration is called *parent* and end product is called *daughter*. Radioactivity is classified as (1) *natural radioactivity* and (2) *artificial radioactivity*. The phenomenon of spontaneous emission of rays such as α, β and γ by heavy elements having atomic number >82 is called *natural radioactivity*, e.g., Radium-226.

Artificial or an induced radioactivity was discovered by **Curie and Joliet** (1934), when they were studying disintegration of light elements by α particles. They found that when light elements such as *Boron and Aluminum* were bombarded with α particles, an unstable nucleus was formed, which disintegrated spontaneously. Artificial radioactive substance emits electrons, neutrons, positrons and γ rays. They follow the same decay laws of natural radioactivity, e.g., Cobalt-60.

Nuclear Forces and Stability

If a nucleus wants to be stable, it should overcome the repulsive forces between protons. Stability of a nucleus requires certain combination of

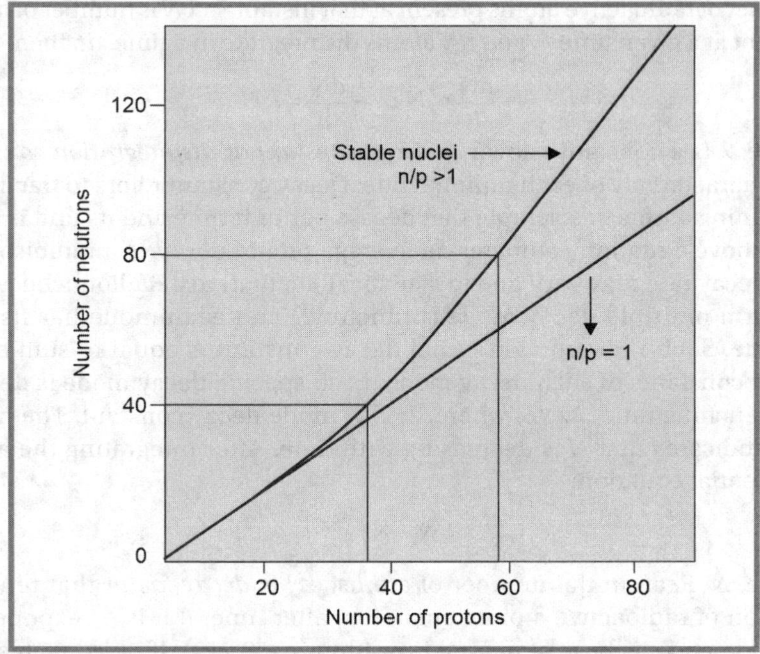

Fig. 2.1: Relation between proton and neutron in stable nuclei.

protons and neutrons. This means that neutrons (n) should be higher than protons (p) or n/p ratio must be higher. The n/p ratio is not linear for all elements of increasing order **(Fig. 2.1)**. The low atomic number elements (Z < 20) are called lighter elements, which are stable, and have n/p = 1. In this, number of protons is equal to number of neutrons. Elements with Z = 20 to 82 is called heavy elements. As atomic number increases, neutrons are more in number, and n/p ration is >1, leading to nuclear stability.

The elements having Z > 82 are said to be unstable nuclei, and majority of them are naturally radioactive. The neutron increases as Z increases. Above such atom requires n/p ratio of about 1.5 for stability. Hence, unstable nuclei perform radioactivity and attain stability. It is also found that greater proportion of nuclei are stable when proton and neutron are with even numbers, which is said to be *even-even nuclei*. Lower proportion of nuclei are stable when they have even Z and odd n or odd Z and even n. However, only four nuclei are stable in odd-odd nuclei.

RADIOACTIVE DISINTEGRATION

Rutherford and Soddy found that rate at which a radioactive material disintegrate was independent of physical and chemical conditions. Their law states that number of atoms that disintegrate in unit time is proportional to number of radioactive atoms present at that instant. Let N is number of atoms present at a given time, t, and dN atoms disintegrate in a time, dt, then:

$$-\frac{dN}{dt} \propto N \text{ or } -\frac{dN}{dt} = \lambda N$$

where, λ is a constant known as *decay constant* or *disintegration constant*. It is characteristic of each radionuclide. Decay constant refers to fraction of remaining atoms in a sample that decays per unit time and its unit is sec^{-1}. The above equation estimates an average rate of decay of a radioisotope. The decay rate may vary due to statistical fluctuations. Radionuclides may perform multiple decay mode (branching) and each mode has its own λ value. Such radionuclide's total decay constant is equal to sum of the decay constants of each decay mode. Each specific decay mode is defined by branching ratio = λ_i/λ, where, λ_i is i^{th} mode decay constant. The minus sign indicates that N is decreasing with time. After integrating the above differential equation:

$$N = N_0\, e^{-\lambda t}$$

where, N_0 is an initial number of atoms, $e^{-\lambda t}$ is *decay factor* that refers to fraction of radioactive atoms remaining, after time, t. It is an exponential function and e is base of natural logarithm (e = 2.719). If λt is much small, then approximated decay factor is $1 - \lambda t$. The equation shows that number of atoms of a given radioactive element decreases exponentially with time and approaches zero in a linear graph **(Figs. 2.2A and B)**. If it is drawn on a semi log paper, and it is a straight-line graph. From the graph it is found that disintegration takes place at much rapid rate initially, with gradual increase of time it decreases and reaches zero. Theoretically, an infinite time is required to disintegrate all the atoms.

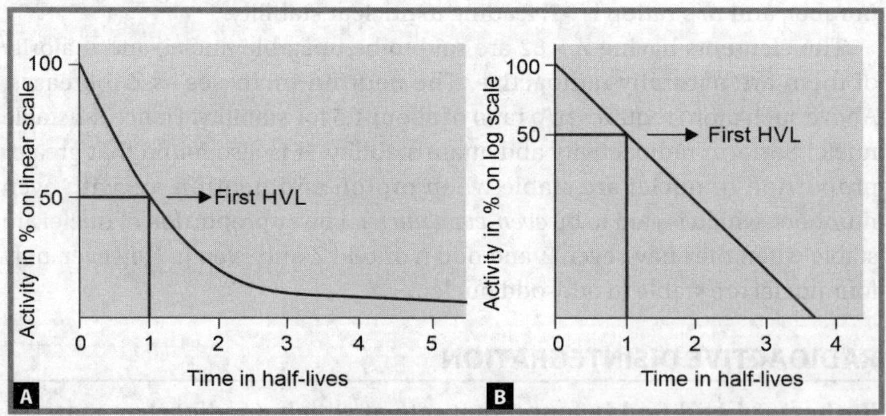

Figs. 2.2A and B: Decay curve of a radioisotope in terms of time in half-life vs activity in percentage: (A) Linear scale plot; (B) Semi-log scale plot.

Half-life and Mean Life Period

Half-life of a radioactive element is defined as the time taken for half of an initial number of atoms to disintegrate. From the law of radioactive disintegration, fundamental decay equation is:

$$N = N_0\, e^{-\lambda t}$$

If $T_{1/2}$ is half-life, then $t = T_{1/2}$, $N = N_0/2$, substituting this in the above equation,

$$N_0/2 = N_0\, e^{-\lambda T_{1/2}}$$

$$1/2 = e^{-\lambda T_{1/2}}$$

$$2 = e^{\lambda T_{1/2}}$$

$$\log_e 2 = \lambda T_{1/2},\ \text{or}\ T_{1/2} = \frac{\log_e 2}{\lambda} = 0.693/\lambda$$

The half-life of a radioactive element is inversely proportional to decay constant of that element. It is seen that after one half-life period, activity is reduced to ½ value, after two half-life period, it is $\frac{1}{2^2}$ value, and after n half-life period, activity is equal to $1/2^n$ value. Half-life values of some important radioisotopes used in medicine is given in **Table 2.1**.

In general, decay of all radioactive atoms will take infinite time, however as an imaginary concept one can define *mean life or average life* (τ) for a radioactive isotope. Mean life refers to an average lifetime for decay of all radioactive atoms. It is defined as the lifetime of an imaginary source which decays at a constant rate equal to an initial activity and produces same total number of disintegrations, as in its exponential decay. The mean life is related to half-life as, $\tau = 1.44 T_{1/2}$, so that mean life is directly proportional to half-life. It is always longer than half-life period and finds application in radiation dosimetry.

In 3D image reconstruction, multiple image frames are needed. During acquisition of counts for an image frame, radioisotope undergoes decay. If an image acquisition time is not small, compared to half-life of radioisotope, then an *image-frame decay correction* is required, e.g., FDG imaging in PET-CT. If an image frame acquisition starts at t sec and ends at $t + \Delta t$ sec, then effective decay factor (DF_{eff}) is given by:

$$DF_{eff} = DF(t) \times [(1 - e^{-x})/x]$$

where, *DF(t)* is decay factor at time, *t*, and $x = \ln 2 \times \Delta t/T_{1/2}$.

Table 2.1: Half-life periods of few radioisotopes used in medicine.

Radioisotope	Half-life period	Radioisotope	Half-life period
Radium-226	1,622 years	Phosphorus-32	14.26 days
Cesium-137	30 years	Iodine-131	8.04 days
Cobalt-60	5.26 years	Lutetium-177	6.64 days
Iridium-192	73.8 days	Samarium-153	1.93 days
Iodine-125	60 days	Technetium 99m	6 hours
Strontium-90	28.9 years	Gallium-68	68 minutes

(*Courtesy:* Kuppusamy Thayalan, 2023)

Effective Half-life

Physical half-life is the time required for a radionuclide to decay to half its original activity. It is expressed by the relation, $T_{1/2} = \dfrac{0.693}{\lambda}$, where, λ is decay constant. Biological half-life (T_b) is determined by clearance of radio nuclides from the organ, tissue, or body. Effective half-life (T_e) of a radio nuclide in any organ consists of both radioactive decay and biological decay **(Fig. 2.3)**. The relation between effective, biological, and physical half-life is given by:

$$\frac{1}{T_e} = \frac{1}{T_b} + \frac{1}{T_{1/2}}$$

For example, a radio nuclide has a physical half-life of 6 hours and a biological half-life of 3 hours, then, $\dfrac{1}{T_e} = \dfrac{1}{6} + \dfrac{1}{3}$, and $T_e = 2$ hours. The effective half-life is always lesser than the biological half-life, which is lesser than the physical half-life.

Activity

Rate of activity of a radioisotope is called *activity* of that isotope. The decay equation is multiplied by λ $(A = \lambda N)$ to express activity of a radioisotope:

$$A = A_0\, e^{-\lambda t}$$

where, A_0 is initial activity and A is activity at time, t. Activity refers to number of unstable nuclei that regains stability through radio-disintegration per unit time. This information is significant as the quantity of radiation released from radioactive material is directly proportional to its activity. Activity gives an idea about the quantity of radiation released per time (disintegration rate) from the radiation source.

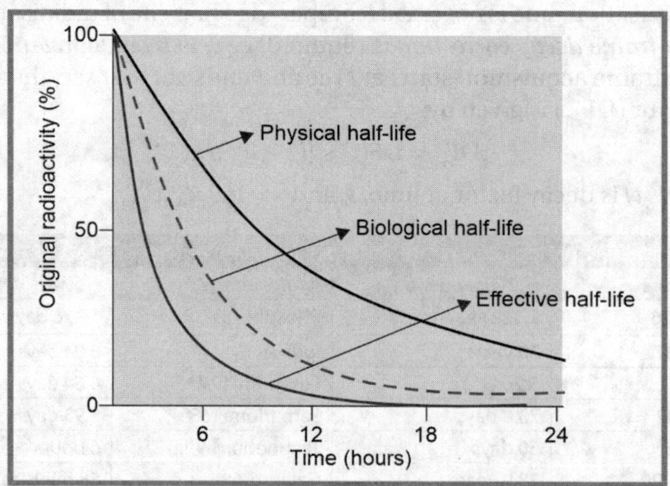

Fig. 2.3: The effective half-life is a function of biological and physical half-life.

Unit of Activity

The disintegration rate of a radioisotope is measured by the unit becquerel (Bq). Becquerel is the SI unit of activity, and it is equal to 1 disintegration per second (dps). In practice, mega becquerel (MBq) and giga becquerel (GBq) are used as units:

$$1 \text{ MBq} = 10^6 \text{ Bq, and } 1 \text{ GBq} = 10^9 \text{ Bq.}$$

The special and old unit of activity is curie. One curie (Ci) is the number of dps from 1 g of Radium (Ra-226) and it is found to be 3.7×10^{10} dps. Smaller units such as milli-curie (mCi), micro-curie (μCi), nano-curie (nCi) and pico-curie (pCi) are also used as unit:

$$1 \text{ mCi} = 3.7 \times 10^7 = 37 \text{ MBq,}$$
$$1 \text{ μCi} = 3.7 \times 10^4 = 37 \text{ kBq,}$$
$$1 \text{ nCi} = 3.7 \times 10^1 = 37 \text{ Bq,}$$
$$\text{and } 1 \text{ pCi} = 3.7 \times 10^{-2} = 0.037 \text{ Bq.}$$

The unit becquerel and curie is related as:

$$1 \text{ Bq} = 2.70 \times 10^{-11} \text{ Ci, and } 1 \text{ Ci} = 3.7 \times 10^{10} \text{ Bq} = 37 \text{ GBq}$$

Since activity deals with nuclear emissions, it does not have any practical application in diagnostic radiology, except in nuclear medicine. These units do not tell us the dose delivered to the biological system or patient. Hence, new quantities like exposure and absorbed dose are defined.

Specific Activity

Specific activity is defined as the activity per unit mass and its unit is Bqkg^{-1}. It is a useful quantity in designing radiation sources in nuclear medicine and radiotherapy. Small miniature size sources can be made if specific activity is higher. Radioisotopes may contain stable isotopes, which are called *carrier*. Radioisotopes without stable isotopes are called *carrier free isotopes* which may have highest specific activity. If the radioactive substance is liquid, specific activity is expressed in activity per unit volume (MBqml^{-1}). This is very useful to calculate the activity to be injected to the patient for nuclear imaging study. It also gives an information about presence of carrier (non-radioactive) material in the sample.

Worked Example-2.1

Iodine-131 radioisotope having a half-life of 8 days is used as iodine therapy in thyroid ablation and has initial activity of 100 mCi. What is the remaining activity after 10 days?

$$A_0 = 100 \text{ mCi, } T_{1/2} = 8 \text{ days}$$

$$T_{1/2} = 0.693/\lambda \text{ or } \lambda = \frac{0.693}{T_{\frac{1}{2}}} = \frac{0.693}{8 \text{ days}} = 0.0866 \text{ days}^{-1}$$

$$A = A_0 \, e^{-\lambda t} = 100 \text{ mCi} \times e^{-0.0866 \times 10} = 42 \text{ mCi}$$

This includes both physical and biological decay.

Radioactive Series

There are 103 elements in the periodic table, elements with Z = 1 to 92 are occurring naturally, whereas Z > 92 are produced artificially. Elements of Z > 82 are unstable and said to be radioactive elements. There are three group of naturally occurring radioactive elements:

- ❑ Uranium series
- ❑ Actinium series
- ❑ Thorium series

The uranium series starts from U-238, has a half-life of 4.51×10^9 years, and undergoes series of transformations with emission of α, β and γ rays, and end in Lead-206. Radium comes from the above series after fifth transformation with emission of Radon daughter. After undergoing 11 transformations, Radium is converted into a stable isotope, *Lead-206*. The Actinium series starts from U-235, has a half-life of 7.13×10^8 years, undergoes transformations, and end up with lead-207. Thorium series start from Thorium-232 with a half-life of 1.39×10^{10} years, undergoes transformation, and end in Lead-208.

RADIOACTIVE EQUILIBRIUM

Radioactive equilibrium exists when radioactive nuclide is decaying at same rate at which it is being produced. The disintegrating nucleus is called *parent* and the nucleus remaining after the event is called *daughter*. Daughter nucleus can be stable or radioactive, and decays into another daughter and so on. Thus, a series of decay arises with its own characteristic decay constant.

If half-life of parent is longer than daughter, an equilibrium may arise known as *radioactive equilibrium.* Radioactive equilibrium is not happing immediately, only after a transition period. This period may be in the order of few half-life periods. Concentration of daughter nuclei in the radioactive equilibrium depends on proportions of half-life of parent and daughter nuclei. The ratio of daughter activity to parent activity is constant over time. In addition, apparent decay rate of the daughter is controlled by the half-life of parent. There are two kinds of radioactive equilibrium **(Figs. 2.4A and B)**:

- ❑ Secular equilibrium
- ❑ Transient equilibrium

If the daughter half-life is longer than parent, there will be no equilibrium between them, e.g., ^{131m}Te.

Secular Equilibrium

Secular equilibrium is one, in which half-life of parent is much longer (>100 times) than that of daughter, e.g., ^{226}Ra ($T_{1/2}$ = 1,622 y) decays to ^{222}Rn ($T_{1/2}$ = 3.8 d). It occurs usually after 5–6 half-life of daughter and activity of parent (A_1) is equal to activity of daughter (A_2). Now daughter's apparent half-life is equal to that of parent.

$$A_1 = A_2 \text{ or } \lambda_1 N_1 = \lambda_2 N_2$$

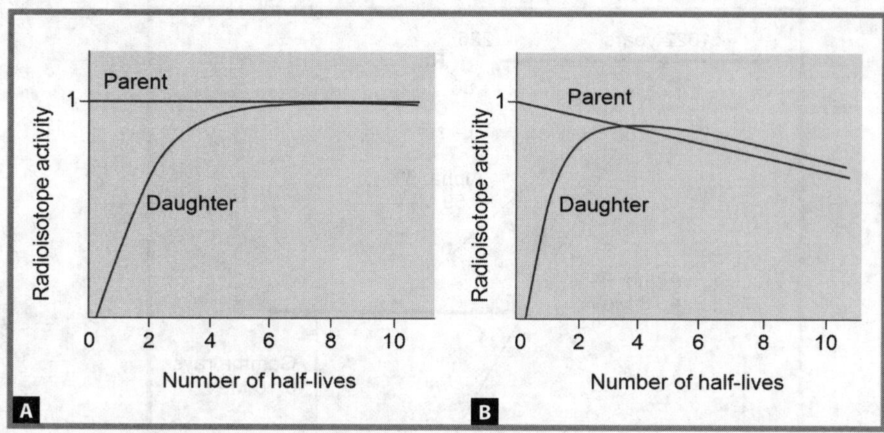

Figs. 2.4A and B: Radioactive equilibrium: (A) Secular equilibrium; (B) Transient equilibrium.

where, λ_1 and λ_2 are decay constants of the parent and daughter, respectively. This type of equilibrium is important in nature. Over a billion years, parent nuclei of Uranium-238, Uranium-235 and Thorium-232 have attained radioactive equilibrium with their daughters. For example, Radium is kept in sealed container, after a month time all the daughters are in secular equilibrium with parent.

Transient Equilibrium

In transient equilibrium, half-life of parent is not much longer than half-life of daughter, e.g., ^{99}Mo ($T_{1/2} = 67$ hours) decays to ^{99m}Tc ($T_{1/2} = 6$ hours). After 23 h of ^{99m}Tc activity, the production and decay rates of parent and daughter is equal. Now, ^{99m}Tc is said to be in transient equilibrium with parent. At equilibrium, daughter activity exceeds parent by about 10%. Later, the ^{99m}Tc activity decreases so that its apparent half-life is equal to its parent. Here, the ratio of the activity of the daughter to parent is constant, and is given by a relation:

$$\frac{A_1}{A_2} = \frac{T_1}{T_1 - T_2}$$

where, T_1 and T_2 are half-lives of parent and daughter, respectively. About 88% of Mo decays into ^{99}Tc through ^{99m}Tc, whereas its decay into ^{99}Tc without metastable state is about 12%. In equilibrium, ^{99m}Tc activity is only about 97%. The elusion efficiency of ^{99m}Tc is about 90%, combining both decay and elusion efficiency, the overall yield is only about 85%.

NUCLEAR TRANSFORMATION

Alpha Decay

Radioactive nuclides with high atomic numbers (Z >150) decay mostly with spontaneous emission of alpha (α) particle, followed by gamma rays and

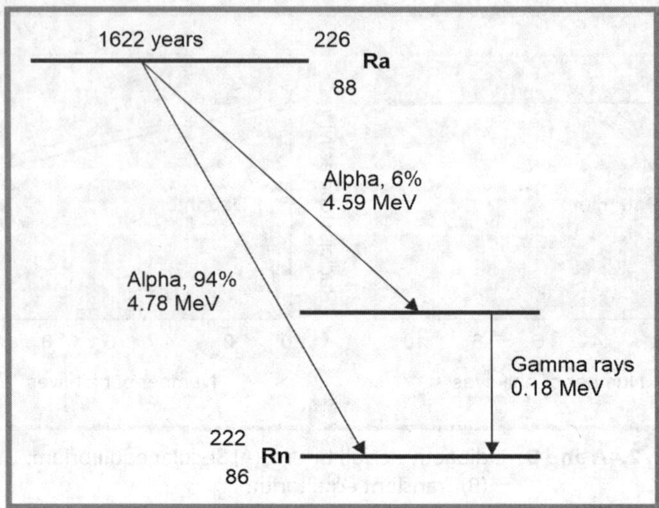

Fig. 2.5: Decay scheme of Radium-226.

characteristic X-rays. After α decay, atomic number is reduced by 2 and mass number is reduced by 4. A typical example of α decay is transformation of Radium (Ra) to Radon (Rn); Radium-226 has two decay modes, the first one accounts 6% and decays to an excited state of Radon with alpha energy 4.59 MeV. The second decay mode accounts 94%, directly reaches ground state of Radon with alpha energy 4.78 MeV. Excited Radon goes to the ground state with emission of gamma photons of energy 0.18 MeV **(Fig. 2.5)**:

$$^{226}_{88}\text{Ra} \rightarrow {}^{222}_{86}\text{Rn} + {}^{4}_{2}\text{He} + 6.4 \text{ MeV}$$

where, 6.4 MeV is transition energy released in the process. The α particle is a doubly ionized Helium atom with positive charge and about four times heavier than protons. They are emitted from nucleus with discrete energies of 2–10 MeV. The daughter Radon is also radioactive and performs further alpha emission. After nine transformations, it becomes stable nuclei of Lead-206.

Properties

Alpha particles are positively charged and cause intense ionization in matter. The electric and magnetic field influence alpha particles. They have much short range and get attenuated within few μm in tissue and 1 cm per MeV in air. A sheet of paper can cut off entire alpha particles. Hence, it is not used in medicine, however, research is ongoing to explore its therapeutic applications. Alpha is a high LET radiation and gives localized intense radiation in living organisms.

Beta Decay

Process of radioactive decay, in which an electron (negatron) or positron is ejected, is called beta (β) decay. Electron emission is denoted by β^- and

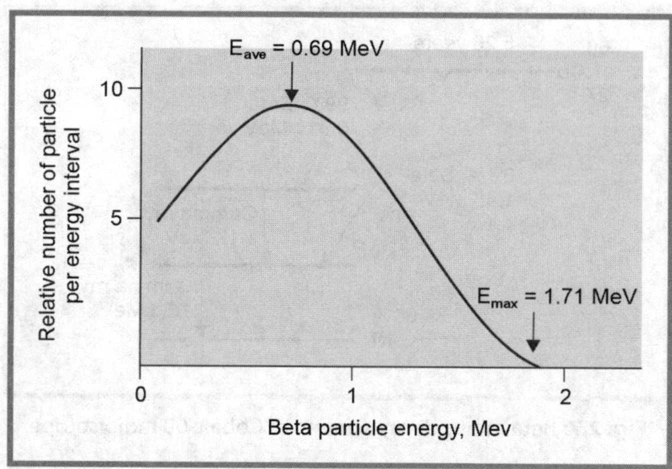

Fig. 2.6: Beta spectrum of ^{32}P, suggesting its polychromatic nature.

positron emission is denoted by β^+. Neither electron nor positron exists inside the nucleus, but it is created during radioactive decay.

Beta Minus Decay

Nuclei having excess neutron performs beta minus decay to attain nuclear stability. In this transformation, one neutron is converted into proton, beta, and antineutrino ($\bar{\nu}$). Neutrino is a subatomic particle, having neutral charge and mass lesser than an electron and antiparticle of neutrino is called antineutrino. Hence, number of neutrons is reduced by 1 and number of protons is increased by 1:

$$_0^1n \rightarrow {}_1^1p + {}_{-1}^0\beta^- \ (\bar{\beta} \ \text{decay}) + \bar{\nu} + \text{energy}$$

Beta minus decay decreases n/p ratio and bring the daughter nearer to stability. Beta energy is a poly energetic spectrum consisting of discrete maximum energy and lot of low energy **(Fig. 2.6)**. The mean energy is equal to $\frac{E_{max}}{3}$, and remaining energy is shared by antineutrino. Beta particle is identical to an electron having same mass and charge. When a β^- particle is emitted, resulting new atom has same mass number, but an atomic number increases by 1. Beta particle may carry the entire energy or part of released energy. A typical example for β^- decay is transformation of *Cobalt (Co) to Nickel (Ni)*, as shown in **Figure 2.7**. The Cobalt-60 decays to excited states of Nickel-60 with beta kinetic energies of 0.313 and 1.48 MeV, respectively. Excited Nickel-60 goes to ground state with emission of gamma rays of energy 1.17 and 1.33 MeV, respectively:

$$_{27}^{60}\text{Co} \rightarrow {}_{28}^{60}\text{Ni} + {}_{-1}^0\beta + \bar{\nu}$$

Properties

Beta particles are negatively charged, and cause an ionization in medium. They are deflected by an electric and magnetic fields. The range of beta

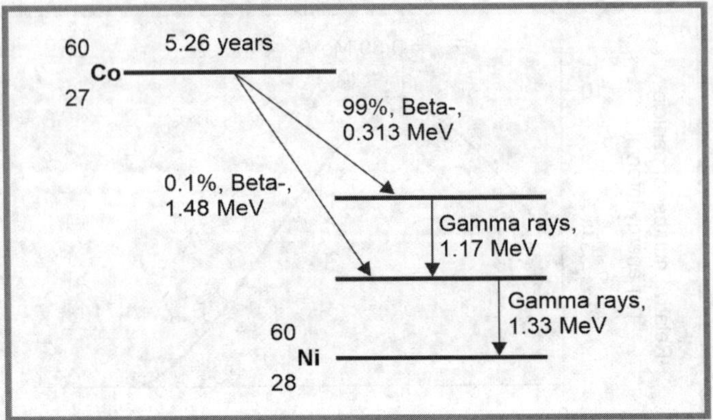

Fig. 2.7: Beta minus decay scheme of Cobalt-60 radioisotope.

particle is higher than an alpha and get absorbed by few mm thickness of an Aluminum. They perform localized biological effect on living tissues.

Beta Plus Decay

Nuclei having lesser neutron number performs beta plus decay to attain nuclear stability. In this transformation, one proton is converted into neutron, *beta plus and neutrino* (ν). Hence, number of neutrons is increased by 1 and number of protons is decreased by 1:

$$^1_1p \rightarrow {}^1_0n + {}^0_{+1}\beta \ (\beta^+ \ \text{decay}) + \nu + \text{energy}$$

The daughter will have more electrons initially, referred as negative ion. Later, it will emit excess electrons in an orbit and become neutral. When a β^+ particle is emitted, resulting new atom has same mass number, but atomic number decreases by 1. Beta plus particle is positively charged and is named as *positron*. It is an antiparticle of an electron having same mass, but opposite charge. Positrons are poly energetic like beta particle, and its mean energy is equal to $\dfrac{E_{max}}{3}$. Positron decay has threshold, the parent should have excess mass than the daughter which is equal to mass of two electrons. Radioisotopes that are produced by an accelerator is neutron deficient and they decay with positron by increasing the n/p ratio, e.g., *Nitrogen-13* (**Fig. 2.8**). Nitrogen-13 decays directly to ground state of Carbon –13 with positron energy of 1.19 MeV and no gamma is emitted:

$$^{13}_7N \rightarrow {}^{13}_6C + \beta^+ + \nu$$

The mass difference between parent and daughter nuclides should be at least equal to 1.022 MeV, for positron decay to happen. The positron does ionization and excitation in their path and comes to rest. They react violently with an electron and their entire mass (1.022 MeV) is converted into two gamma photons of energy of 0.511 MeV. This process is called *positron annihilation* in which two photons are emitted at 180° apart, to conserve momentum. This is a typical

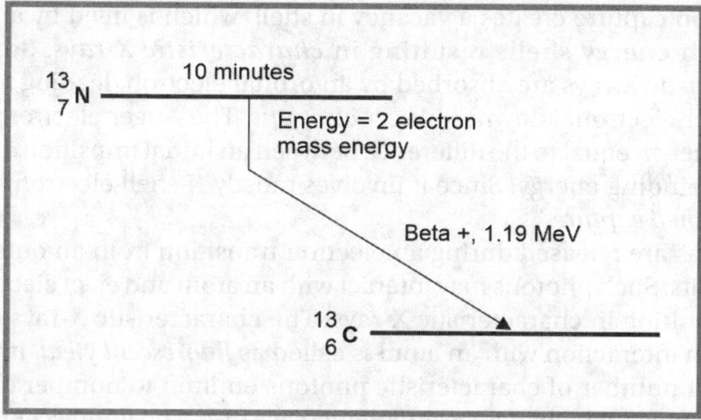

Fig. 2.8: Beta plus decay of Nitrogen-13 radioisotope.

example of **Einstein's** mass energy equivalence, $E = mc^2$ where m is the mass of the partricle and c is the velocity of light. This is the principle used in *positron emission tomography* (PET). Positron decay is likely in light, proton richer nucleus in which the parent-daughter transition energy is equal or > 1.02 MeV.

Electron Capture

Nuclei deficient of neutrons may undergo decay by absorbing its own K or L shell electron. When an electron is absorbed, it combines with a proton and is converted into a neutron with emission of neutrino:

$$_1^1p + e^{-1} \rightarrow {}_0^1n + v$$

The electron capture is like to that of positron decay. The atomic number decreases by 1 and mass number remains constant, thereby increasing the n/p ratio, e.g., *Chromium-51*. It decays to *Vanadium-51* through an electron capture process with emission of gamma rays of an energy of 0.32 MeV **(Fig. 2.9)**:

$$_{24}^{51}Cr + e \rightarrow {}_{23}^{51}V + v + energy$$

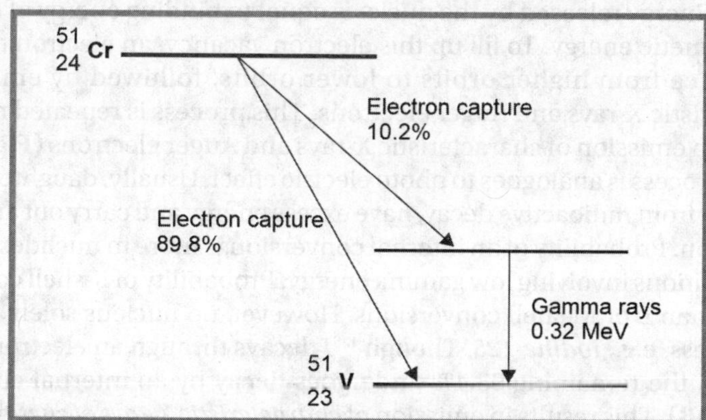

Fig. 2.9: Radioactive decay by electron capture process.

Electron capture creates a vacancy in shell, which is filled by an electron from high energy shells resulting in *characteristic X-rays*. Some time, characteristic X-rays are absorbed by an orbital electron, leading to ejection of another electron, known as *Auger electrons*. The Auger electron will have kinetic energy, equal to the difference between an initial transition energy and electron binding energy. Since it involves mostly K-shell electron, it is often called *K-shell capture*.

Photons are released during an electron transition from an outer orbit to inner orbits. Such photons may interact with an atom and eject electrons from orbits resulting in characteristic X-rays. The characteristic X-rays produced by photon interaction with an atom is called as *fluorescent yield*. It is defined as ratio of number of characteristic photons emitted to number of electron orbit vacancies, which increases with increase of Z. The fluorescent yield and Auger electron process are competing to each other. Atoms having Z > 30, favors probability of fluorescent yield, whereas atoms with Z < 30, tend to give Auger electrons. The fluorescent yield in soft tissue (Z = 7.42) is zero, whereas it is 0.93 for tungsten (Z = 74). Auger electron is more dominant in soft tissue.

If the nucleus is left in an excited state after an electron capture, an excess energy will be emitted as gamma rays. Characteristic X-rays and gamma rays are used in medical applications. Electron capture is common in nuclides with mass energy difference between parent and daughter atoms is <1.02 MeV. If energy difference between parent and daughter is >1.02 MeV, it may decay either by an electron capture or positron emission or both. Heavier proton rich nuclides likely to undergo an electron capture decay process, whereas lighter proton rich nuclides prefer positron emission.

Internal Conversion

Internal conversion is due to an emission of gamma rays by an excited nucleus, after beta decay or an electron capture. An excited daughter nucleus has excess energy and releases this nuclear energy to one of its bound orbital electrons. As a result, an electron is ejected from an atom, and a vacancy is created. Energy released by the nuclei is equal to binding energy of electrons plus its kinetic energy. To fill up this electron vacancy, an electron transition takes place from higher orbits to lower orbits, followed by emission of characteristic X-rays and Auger electrons. This process is repeated more and more with emission of characteristic X-rays and Auger electrons **(Fig. 2.10A)**.

This process is analogues to photo electric effect. Usually, daughter nucleus emerging from radioactive decay, have excess energy and carry out an internal conversion. Probability of an internal conversion is more in nuclides of high Z and transitions involving low gamma energy. Probability of K-shell conversion is more than L or M shell conversions. However, no nucleus solely performs this process, e.g., *Iodine-125*. Though ^{125}I decays through an electron capture by 6.66%, the remaining 93.4% undergoes decay by an internal conversion **(Fig. 2.10B)**. This results in emission of *characteristic X-rays of energy 31.8 keV and Auger electrons*. Auger electron emission is higher in magnitude, and it

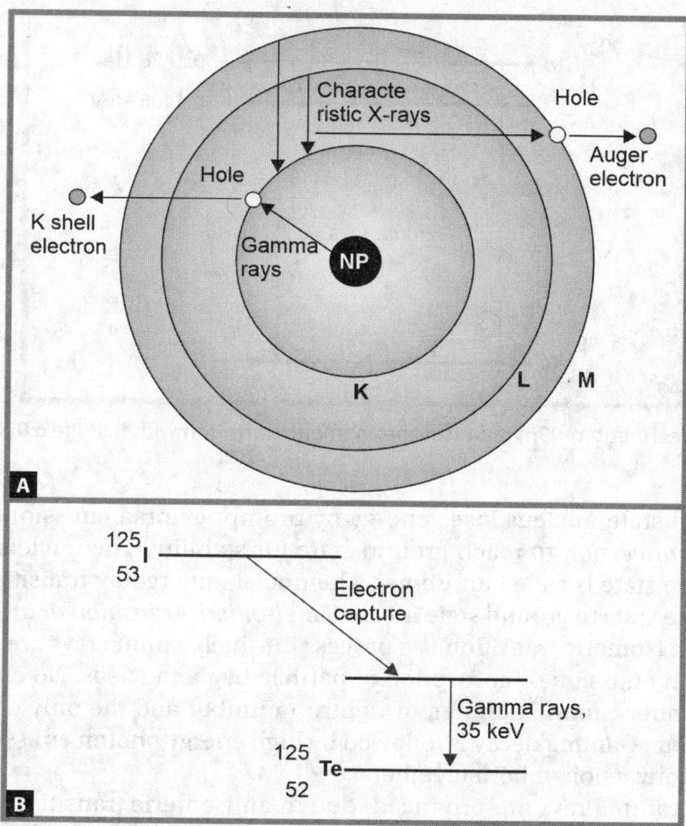

Figs. 2.10A and B: Internal conversion process: (A) Daughter Tellurium-125 nuclei is in excited state, ejects electron from the K-shell, resulting characteristic X-rays and Auger electrons; (B) Iodine-125 decay by electron capture.

is about 5.4 per decay. The energy spectrum is monoenergetic, compared to beta energy spectrum.

Gamma Emission

In most of the radioactive process, either alpha or beta, daughter nucleus exists in an excited state for an appreciable time. Duration of stay at an excited state depends upon shape of the nucleus, angular momentum difference, and quantum number parity between an initial and final energy states of nucleus. Some nucleus undergoes change in angular momentum of the order of one unit without change in parity. In such nuclei, the transition is instantaneous, of the order of 10^{-15} to 10^{-10} sec. Some nuclei undergo large change in angular momentum and stay for longer time in the excited state. Such excited states whose half-lives $>10^{-6}$ sec is known as *meta stable state or an isomeric state*, e.g., Technetium-99m, the letter *m* refers to metastable state **(Fig. 2.11)**.

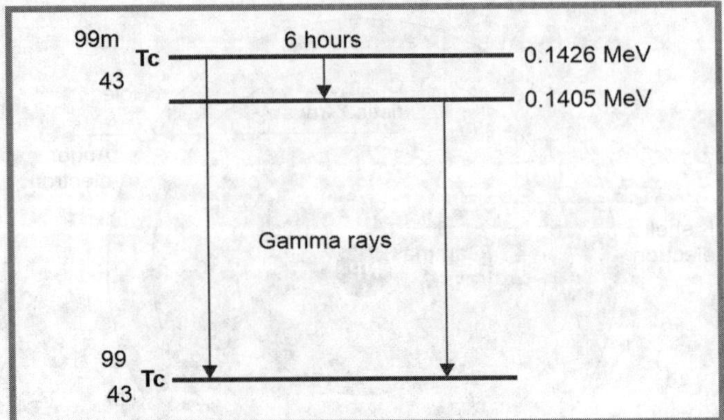

Fig. 2.11: Technetium-99m radioisotope: Isomeric transition with half-life 6.02 hours.

Excited state nucleus loses energy by prompt gamma emission and an *internal conversion* to reach ground state for stability. The nucleus in the metastable state is called an *isomer*. The nuclei undergoing transition from metastable state to ground state is called an *isomeric transition or an isotopic transition*. Isomeric transition is a process in which gamma rays are emitted without an emission or absorption of particle by the nucleus. No change in mass number, atomic number, or neutron number and the only change is energy state. Gamma decay is followed by high energy photon emission, and internal conversion or both together.

Thus, gamma rays are produced, due to an isomeric transition of radio nuclei from an excited state to ground state. For example, $^{137}_{55}$Cs nucleus decays to an exited state of $^{137}_{56}$Ba nucleus by 95%, with emission of β-particle of energy 0.514 MeV. Then it reaches stable ground state by emitting photon of energy 0.662 MeV by transition. About 5% of Cs-137 nucleus decays directly to ground state of Ba-137 with beta energy of 1.18 MeV **(Fig. 2.12)**.

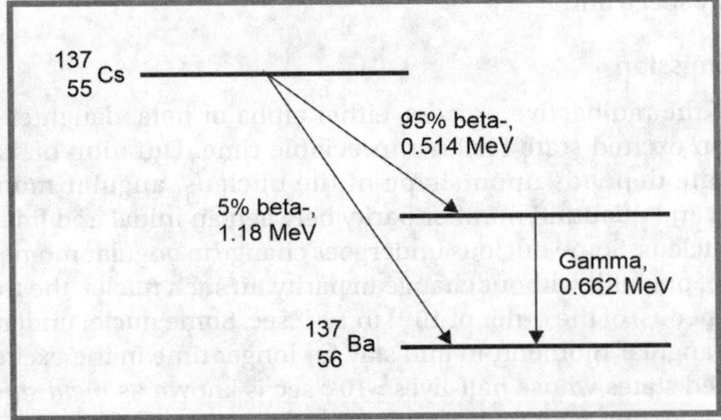

Fig. 2.12: Decay scheme of Cesium-137 by beta minus emission.

Properties of Gamma Rays

- ❏ Electromagnetic radiations of shorter wavelength (nm).
- ❏ No mass and charge.
- ❏ Not deflected by an electric or magnetic fields.
- ❏ Highly penetrating, and their penetrating power is about 100 times greater than that of beta particle. They can pass through several cm of Lead.
- ❏ Affects photographic plate/film and cause fluorescence in materials.
- ❏ Produce ionization in matter.
- ❏ Travels with velocity of light, $3 \times 10^8 \, ms^{-1}$.
- ❏ Capable of damaging biological cells and molecules.
- ❏ Gamma rays produce photoelectric effect when they incident on solid surfaces.

NUCLEAR REACTIONS

Alpha Bombardment

Rutherford (1919) had bombarded nitrogen gas with alpha particle from a radioactive source:

$$^{14}_{7}N + {}^{4}_{2}He \rightarrow {}^{17}_{8}O + {}^{1}_{1}H + Q$$

where, Q is energy either absorbed (*endoergic*) or released (*exoergic*) during the reaction. In this, alpha particle bombards a nucleus, later it is divided into an Oxygen nucleus and proton, this is known as *(α, p) reaction*. Instead of proton if neutron is released, it is called *(α, n) reaction*, e.g., ^{9}Be (α, n)^{12}C.

Proton and Deuteron Bombardment

Bombardment of *proton with Lithium* may yield *Beryllium* with emission of gamma rays: ^{7}Li (p, γ) ^{8}Be. Deuteron ($^2_1$H) is a combination of neutron and proton. When deuteron hits a compound nucleus, deuteron is not captured by nucleus. Instead, nucleus removes proton and the neutron and goes with higher speed. This is known as *stripping* since proton is stripped from the deuteron:

$$^{2}_{1}H + {}^{9}_{4}Be \rightarrow {}^{10}_{5}B + {}^{1}_{0}n$$

Neutron Bombardment

Neutrons have neutral charge in nature, much effective in penetrating the nuclei, without much kinetic energy. That is why *slow neutrons* (thermal neutrons) are mostly used in nuclear transformation. Type of neutron bombardment (fast or slow) depends on the mass difference between bombarded nucleus and product nucleus. During neutron bombardment, neutron is captured by the nucleus and the capture process is called n, α *reaction*:

$$^{10}_{5}B + {}^{1}_{0}n \rightarrow {}^{7}_{3}Li + {}^{4}_{2}He$$

Apart from this, neutron bombardment can produce (n, p) *reaction* and (n, γ) *reactions*. The latter is most common, and its end products are mostly radioactive with emission of β *particle*:

$$^{59}_{27}Co + \,^{1}_{0}n \rightarrow \,^{60}_{27}Co + \gamma, \text{ followed by,}$$

$$^{60}_{27}Co \rightarrow \,^{60}_{28}Ni + \,^{0}_{-1}\beta + \gamma_1 + \gamma_2$$

Fission

If neutron bombards a high atomic number nucleus and the nucleus split into nuclei of lower atomic number with additional neutrons which is known as *fission process*:

$$^{235}_{92}U + \,^{1}_{0}n \rightarrow \,^{236}_{92}U \rightarrow \,^{141}_{56}Ba + \,^{92}_{36}Kr + 3\,^{1}_{0}n + Q$$

where, Q is energy released during fission process, which appear as kinetic energy of product particles.

Chain Reaction

During fission, two or three neutrons are emitted in addition to fission fragments. These neutrons, in turn induce fission in other ^{235}U nuclei, with release of additional neutrons. Thus, number of fissions that takes place at each successive stage goes on increasing at a rapid rate, giving rise to a *chain reaction*. It can be set up only if mass of fissionable material is greater than a critical mass. This principle is employed in *nuclear reactors.*

Fusion

Fusion is the process in which two or more lighter nuclei combine to form a heavier nucleus:

$$^{2}_{1}H + \,^{3}_{1}H \rightarrow \,^{4}_{2}He + \,^{1}_{0}n + Q$$

where, Q is energy released, called *thermo-nuclear energy*. Since total mass of the product is less than mass of reactants, high energy (17.6 MeV) is released in this process. Similar reactions take place at much high temperatures of the order of few million degree Celsius. As a result, large quantity of heat is released during the reaction. This type of reaction is taking place in the sun and stars. The energy released during the reaction is responsible for higher temperature of the sun and emission of heat and light energy. *Hydrogen bomb* is made by using the *fusion principle*.

PRODUCTION OF RADIOISOTOPES

Naturally occurring radionuclides are long lived and do not have desirable characteristics required for medical applications. Hence, the majority of radioactive isotopes used in medicine are produced artificially by bombarding a stable target nucleus with suitable high energy particles. Radioisotope production methods are: (1) nuclear reactor, (2) accelerator, and (3) radionuclide generator.

Nuclear Reactor Production

Nuclear Reactor Principle

A typical nuclear reactor is shown in **Figure 2.13**. Core of the reactor consists of *fissionable material* (^{235}U and ^{238}U) which is enriched in ^{235}U. The ^{235}U undergoes spontaneous fission, resulting into two lighter elements and 2–3 neutron emission. These neutrons bombard ^{235}U and produce ^{238}U, which is unstable and undergo further nuclear fission with emission of stimulated neutrons. The neutron, either emitted by the spontaneous or stimulated event should have one additional fission event, is basic criteria for reactor. Thus, a controlled chain reaction is maintained.

Fissionable material is surrounded by *heavy water or graphite* as moderator, which slows down fission neutrons. *Control rods* made up of *Cadmium or Boron* are positioned so that they can either expose or shield *fuel cells*. This is achieved by inserting or removing the control rods. Control rods absorb excess neutrons and regulate number of neutrons for fission reaction. Thus, control rods and *fuel cells* are positioned so that critical conditions for chain reaction is established. In every nuclear fission, about 200–300 MeV energy per fission fragment is produced, which is used for thermal power production.

Neutrons being uncharged particle, have an advantage of penetrating through nucleus without being accelerated to high energies. Nuclear reactor uses two methods to produce radio nuclides, namely (1) nuclear fission fragments, and (2) neutron activation.

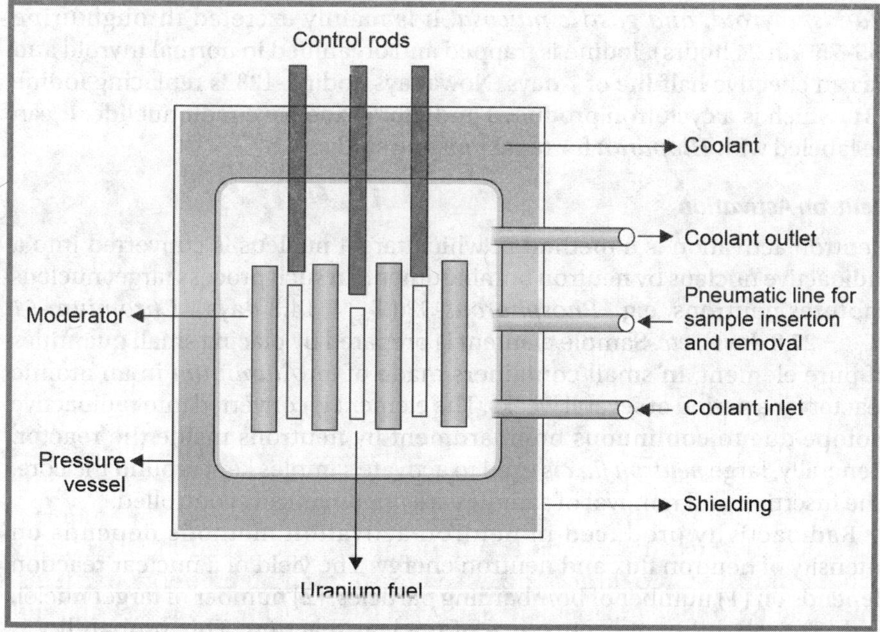

Fig. 2.13: Nuclear reactor model design.

Nuclear Fission Fragments

In this method, radionuclides are produced directly during fission process. Later, they are extracted by chemical separation from fission fragments. About 100 radionuclides corresponding to 20 different elements are obtained from nuclear fragments, e.g., *Molybdenum-99, Iodine-131, and Xenon-133.* Fragments of ^{238}U contains mass numbers of 85 to105 and 130 to 150, respectively, and they are rarely equal. Fission products have excess neutrons and undergo further radioactive decay with β emission. They are carrier free, and radionuclides of high specific activity can be produced by chemical separation. However, their specificity is low, in turn radionuclide yield is also low.

Iodine-131

Iodine-131 is a reactor produced radionuclide, highly reactive and can be labeled easily. It is easily trapped and metabolized by the thyroid organ. It is the first radionuclide used for imaging and it is inexpensive, and has long half-life of 8.06 d. It decays by beta emission to stable *Xenon-131*, average beta energy (90%) is 192 keV, and the dominant photon energy is 364 keV (82% abundance). It gives a whole-body dose of 0.5–3.5 rad per mCi and thyroid dose of 100–2,000 rad per mCi.

It is clinically administered as Iodide, much less satisfactory isotope for imaging today, because of high radiation dose to the patient. When Iodine is administered as Iodide ion, it is readily absorbed by the gastrointestinal (GI) tract and distributed in an extracellular fluid. It is concentrated in the *salivary glands, thyroid, and gastric mucosa.* It is mainly excreted through urine (35–75% in 24 hours). Iodine is trapped and organified in normal thyroid and has an effective half-life of 7 days. Nowadays, Iodine-123 is replacing Iodine 131, which is a cyclotron produced and more expensive radionuclide. It can be labeled with *Hippuran* for renal imaging study.

Neutron Activation

Neutron activation is a method in which target nucleus is converted into a radioactive nucleus by neutron bombardment. In such process target nucleus captures neutrons, e.g., *Phosphorous-32* ($T_{1/2}$ = 14.3 days), *Chromium-51* ($T_{1/2}$ = 27.8 days), *etc.* Sample element is prepared by placing small quantities of pure element, in small containers made of an *Aluminum* in an atomic reactor for a period of several weeks. The element is converted into radioactive isotope due to continuous bombardment by neutrons inside the reactor. Generally, large *neutron flux* is used to activate samples kept around the core. The insertion and removal of samples are pneumatically controlled.

Radioactivity produced in neutron activation methods depends on intensity of neutron flux and neutron energy. The yield of a nuclear reaction depends on (1) number of bombarding particles, (2) number of target nuclei, and (3) probability of occurrence of nuclear reaction. This probability is known as *cross-section,* and its unit is barn, one *barn = 10^{-24} cm^2*. Another parameter of importance is the *growth of activity*. Generally, activated nucleus grows exponentially and undergoes decay. If the rate of activation is equals to rate of decay, growth reaches a maximum called *saturation activity*. There are two types of activation, namely (1) *(n, γ) reaction* and (2) *(n, p) reaction*. Examples of radionuclides produced by neutron activation are Co-60, P-32, and Cr-51. For example, ^{113}Xe is a reactor produced radionuclide, having half-life of 5.2 d, emits beta and low energy gamma rays of 81 keV. It is an inert gas, soluble in blood, used for lung ventilation imaging.

In (n, γ) reaction, target captures neutron, becomes radioactive and stay in an exited state. It goes to the ground state with emission of γ rays:

$$\,^{59}_{27}\text{Co} + \,^{1}_{0}\text{n} \rightarrow \,^{60}_{27}\text{Co} + \gamma$$

In (n, p) reaction, target nucleus captures neutron and ejects a proton instantly. This reaction finds application in the production of ^{32}P by fast neutron bombardment:

$$\,^{32}_{16}\text{S} + \,^{1}_{0}\text{n} \rightarrow \,^{32}_{15}\text{P} + \,^{1}_{1}\text{H}, \text{ followed by,}$$

$$\,^{32}_{15}\text{P} \rightarrow \,^{32}_{16}\text{S} + \,^{0}_{-1}\beta$$

The activated target nucleus is unstable and tends to have β *emission*. Though (n, γ) reaction is not carrier free, but carrier free products can be made by (n, p) reaction. Even with an intense neutron flux, only fraction of target area is activated ($1:10^6 - 10^9$), therefore specific activity of the radionuclide produced is low.

Accelerator Produced Radionuclides

Accelerators are used to accelerate charged particles such as *protons, deuterons, and alpha* particles to high energies of the order of 10–20 MeV. After acquiring high kinetic energy, the particle is used to bombard a target nucleus, to produce radionuclides. There are two types of accelerators, namely *(p, n) reaction and (d, n) reaction. Cyclotron, linear accelerator, and Van de Graaff generator* are used as accelerators. Cyclotron is most widely used to produce medical radioisotopes. Exclusive medical cyclotrons are available in hospitals to produce short lived radioisotopes such as *positron emitters*.

Cyclotron

Cyclotron is a device used to accelerate charged particle to acquire high kinetic energy. It is a circular accelerator, first developed by **Lawrence** (1930).

Principle: When a charged particle moves perpendicular to a magnetic field, it experiences *magnetic Lorentz force*. The period of motion of a charged particle is independent of its velocity under a uniform magnetic field.

Design: It consists of a *hollow metal cylinder* divided into two sections *D1* and *D2 (Dees)* in a semi-circular shape **(Fig. 2.14)**. They are kept separated and placed inside an evacuated chamber of pressure 10^{-3} Pa. An *ion source* is placed at the center, in the gap between two Dees. The Dees are connected

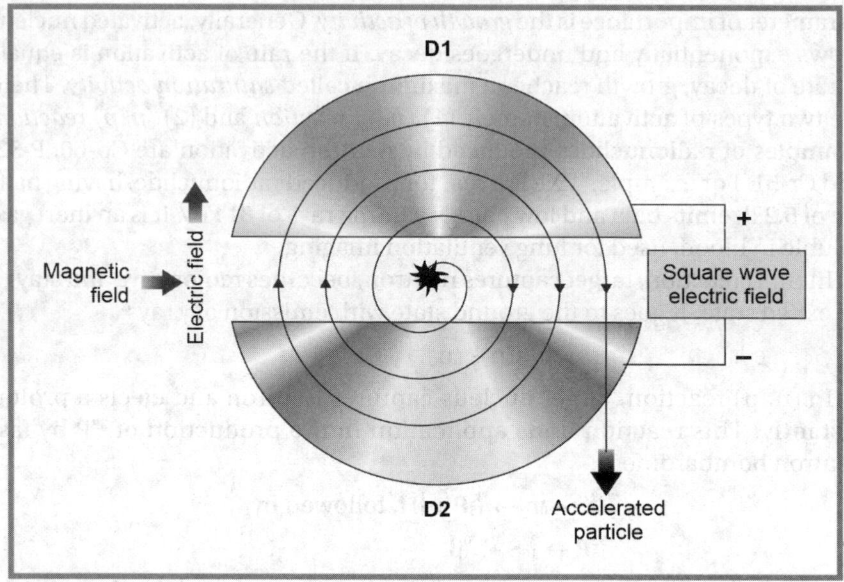

Fig. 2.14: Cyclotron principle of operation, the electric and magnetic field are perpendicular to each other.

to a high frequency alternating potential (oscillator) for electric supply (30 kV, 25–30 MHz). The whole apparatus is placed between pole pieces of a strong *electromagnet* that gives an uniform magnetic field. The direction of magnetic field (B) is normal to the plane of Dees and electric field.

Working: When a particle, say positive ion with charge, q and mass, m is emitted from an *ion source*, it is accelerated towards the Dee having a negative potential at that instant. The particle gains energy of about 30 keV and moves along a semi-circular path due to the magnetic field. By the time the particle arrives at the gap, polarity of Dee gets reversed, and particle is once again accelerated, and enters other Dee with greater velocity, describing a semicircle path of greater radius. Thus, particle describes a circular path of radius, r when its velocity is v, then magnetic Lorentz force provides the *centripetal force*:

$$Bqv = \frac{mv^2}{r} \text{ or } \frac{v}{r} = \frac{Bq}{m} = \text{constant}$$

where, *Bqv* is magnetic Lorentz force offered by the magnet, and $\frac{mv^2}{r}$ is *centripetal force* for circular motion and both are equal. It is also seen that $v \propto r$, which implies that an increase in velocity increases radius of circular path. Thus, particle moves several spiral paths of increasing radius. After spiraling several times within the Dees and acquiring large velocity (Kinetic energy), the particle reaches the outer orbit. The particle is extracted from cyclotron and directed onto an external target, e.g., O-18 is used as target for F-18 radioisotope production. The time taken (t) to describe a semicircle is given by:

$$t = \frac{\pi r}{v} = \frac{\pi r m}{Bqr} = \frac{\pi m}{Bq}, \text{ by substituting } v$$

It is seen that time (t) is independent of radius (r), and velocity (v) of the particle. *The period of motion of a charged particle is independent of velocity under an uniform magnetic field.* This is the basic principle of cyclotron. If is frequency of rotation, then:

$$2\pi f = \omega = \frac{v}{r} = \frac{Bq}{m} \text{ or } f = \frac{Bq}{2\pi m}, \text{ by above equation}$$

Since $\frac{Bq}{2\pi m}$ is a constant, the frequency of rotation is also a constant. Period of rotation $= 1/f = \frac{2\pi m}{Bq}$. RF oscillator is adjusted to satisfy this condition for a given magnetic field, B and ion charge, q. This means that particle frequency must be equal to electrical oscillator frequency. Kinetic energy of the particle is given by:

$$KE = \frac{1}{2} mv^2 = \frac{q^2 B^2 r^2}{2m}, \text{ by above equation}$$

Cyclotron can accelerate *protons, deuterons, and an alpha particles.* At high velocities, $\frac{Bq}{2\pi m}$ is not a constant, due to *relativistic mass variation* of particle. As velocity increases mass also increases. This means that frequency of rotation of the particle decreases, and particle takes longer time to complete its semi-circular path. It results in phase instability and particle will not arrive at the gap just when polarity reverses. However, this effect can be overcome by decreasing the frequency of an alternating voltage over short intervals to keep in step with accelerated particles. This is the principle of *synchrocyclotron or synchrotron.*

Medical Cyclotron

Nowadays dedicated medical cyclotrons are available for production of short-lived positron emitters, e.g., F-18 **(Fig. 2.15)**. They are mostly self-shielded proton accelerator type and much safer in a hospital environment. Self-shielding is provided by Boron water and Lead for neutron and gamma rays, respectively. Major components of medical cyclotron are magnet, ion system, extraction system, target, RF system, vacuum system, and subsystems like power supply, cooling system, gas distribution, hot lab, and quality control.

Hydrogen cyclotrons are available either with positive-ion or negative-ion acceleration facility. The most common type is negative-ion cyclotron (H⁻) having a proton and two electrons. In this magnetic field is increased with increasing radius by having special design of magnet called *hill and valley design.* This will provide an azimuthally varying magnetic field, so that relativistic mass variation is accounted. However, an increase of magnetic field makes particle to deviate from median plane in which it is revolving. Hence, optimal varying magnetic field is applied to keep particle in the gap as well as in the median plane.

An ion source system allows hydrogen gas to flow across *Tantalum cathodes*, where Hydrogen gets ionized and accepts one electron and become

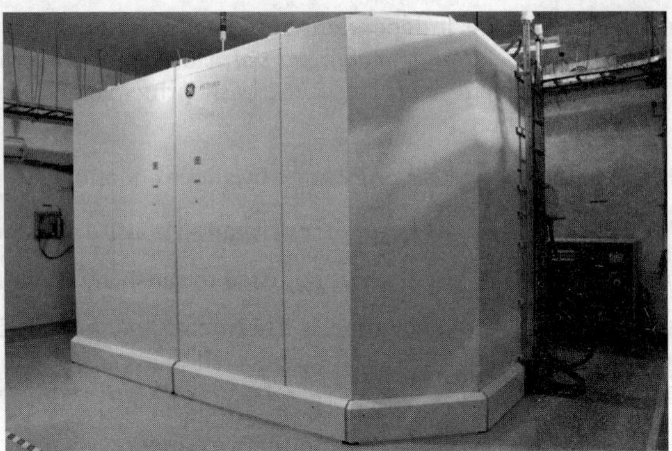

Fig. 2.15: Medical cyclotron facility.
(*Courtesy:* GE Healthcare)

negative ion. The ion source is mounted at the center of the cyclotron between the Dees. Two resonators with RF power system accelerate the particle under the influence of an azimuthally varying magnetic field. The Dees may be 2 or 4 and in the latter case, the particle is accelerated 8 times (one push and pull, for each gap). Vacuum (1.2×10^{-5} mbar) is required to avoid collision of accelerated particles and gas molecules as well as to insulate the Dees.

The extraction carousels use six Carbon foils, when it comes to an outer orbit it is passed through a *Carbon foil*, which removes two electrons. The ion become positive, the beam is extracted from the cyclotron and directed on to an *external target*. The target body is made up of Silver and has provision for liquid/gaseous target under Helium gas cooling. The target material of water enriched with ^{18}O is for ^{18}F production by (p, n) reaction [Fluoro-deoxy glucose (FDG), half-life 110 min]. The other positron emitters that can be produced in the medical cyclotron are ^{15}O, ^{13}N, ^{11}C. The cyclotron may produce 10 Ci activity in 2 hours under a beam current of 100 µA with particle energy of 16.5 MeV.

Negative-ion cyclotron extraction efficiency is about 100% and require less shielding. It is possible to extract two beams in the same cyclotron to hit two different targets. For this Carbon foil is positioned to face part of a beam, so that only portion of the beam is extracted to hit the first target. The remaining beam continues to orbit, will be extracted later with a second Carbon foil, to hit the second target. Thus, two radionuclides can be produced simultaneously. However, it requires much higher vacuum, compared to positive ion cyclotron.

In positive-ion cyclotron, the beam is deflected electro statistically by a plate with negative potential. Since electrostatic deflectors are inefficient, about 30% of beam current is lost during extraction. Hence, beam extraction efficiency of accelerator is lower.

Table 2.2: Cyclotron produced radionuclides.

Nuclide	Photons, keV	Reaction	Decay mode	Half-life
^{11}C	511	^{14}N(p, α)^{11}C	β^+, EC*	20.4 min
^{13}N	511	^{16}O(p, α)^{13}N	β^+	10 min
^{15}O	511	^{14}N(d, n)^{15}O	β^+	2 min
^{18}F	511	^{18}O(p, n)^{18}F	β^+, EC	110 min
^{67}Ga	93, 185, 300	^{68}Zn(p, 2n)^{67}Ga	EC	3.26 days
^{111}In	172, 247	^{109}Ag(α, 2n)^{111}In	EC	2.83 days
^{123}I	159	^{122}Te(d, n)^{123}I	EC	13.2 hr
^{201}Tl	68–80	^{201}Hg(d, 2n)^{201}Tl	EC	3.04 days

*EC = electron capture

(*Courtesy:* Simon R Cherry et al, 2012)

Cyclotron Produced Radionuclides

Cyclotron accelerators produce radionuclides by bombarding stable nuclei with high energy particles. Protons, deuterons, neutrons, and alpha particles are commonly used to produce radionuclides. Gallium-67 is an example of a widely used cyclotron-produced radionuclide. The production reaction is:

$$^{68}\text{Zn} + \text{p} \rightarrow {}^{67}\text{Ga} + 2\text{n}$$

where, Zn-68 is the target and a proton (p), accelerated to about 20 MeV, is the bombarding particle. Two neutrons are emitted during this reaction. Few cyclotrons produced radionuclides are given **Table 2.2**. ^{67}Ga is a cyclotron produced radionuclide, with half-life of 3.26 days, emits gamma rays of energies 93,185 and 300 keV, respectively. It is used as Gallium citrate to detect tumors and abscesses. ^{111}In is a cyclotron produced radionuclide, has a half-life of 2.83 days, emits gamma rays of 172 and 247 keV energies. It is used for *labeling white blood cells and platelets*, to detect abscess and thromboses. ^{201}Tl is a cyclotron produced radionuclide, has a half-life of 3.04 days, and emits X-rays of energy 60–80 keV. It is used as *thallous chloride* in myocardial perfusion imaging.

Radionuclide Generator

Radionuclide generator consists of a parent and daughter in a container. The daughter can be separated and extracted from the parent. Decay of parent replenishes daughter activity, so that repeated extraction is possible. A system for holding parent in such a way that the daughter can be easily separated for clinical use, is called a *radionuclide generator*. ^{81m}Kr is a generator produced inert gas, has half-life of 13 sec and emits gamma rays of 190 keV. It is inhaled with air for pulmonary ventilation study. ^{111m}In is a generator produced radionuclide, having a half-life of 100 m with gamma energy of 390 keV. It is often used as replacement to Indium-111. Various generators used in nuclear medicine are: (1) Mo-^{99m}Tc generator, (2) ^{68}Ga generator, (3) ^{113m}In generator, and (4) ^{87m}Sr generator. The most common generator is Mo-^{99m}Tc generator, which has wide application in clinical use.

Molybdenum- ^{99m}Tc Generator

Technetium-99m emits gamma energy of 140 keV with half-life 6 h and has 90% clinical use. It is obtained from Mo-99 on daily basis from the generator, which is a Lead shielded container **(Fig. 2.16)**. Its energy is suitable for easy absorption and collimation by a thin crystal with good spatial resolution. It can be easily labeled to get variety of radiopharmaceuticals. Its half-life and pure gamma emission help to inject large activity to patient, resulting in reduced noise in the image. Since its half-life is short, it is impossible to store it for a week time. This can be overcome by obtaining parent ^{99}Mo of longer half-life from which ^{99m}Tc is obtained continuously over a week.

Molybdenum-99 is produced by nuclear fission fragments of ^{235}U and is in the form of *Ammonium molybdenite* ($NH_4^+ MoO_4^-$) of half-life 67 h. When it is supplied to the hospitals, the Tc-99m activity has built up to a maximum, equal to the parent (Mo). ^{99m}Tc can be collected periodically depending upon the clinical use. Two types of generators are commercially available:

❑ Wet generator
❑ Dry generator

A wet generator contains saline all times, whereas saline must be added to dry generator whenever ^{99m}Tc is needed. Generator is shielded with *Lead or Tungsten* and supplied to hospitals with 37–740 GBq activity of ^{99}Mo. In dry generator, Ammonium molybdenite is loaded onto a porous alumina column which contains 5–10 g of *alumina resin* (Al_2O_3). *Ammonium molybdenite* easily pass through the porous and attached to alumina

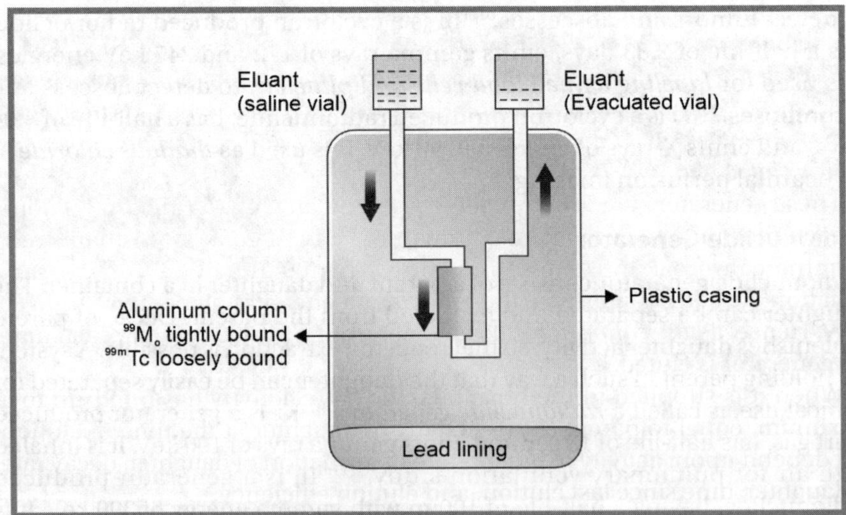

Fig. 2.16: Technetium generator.

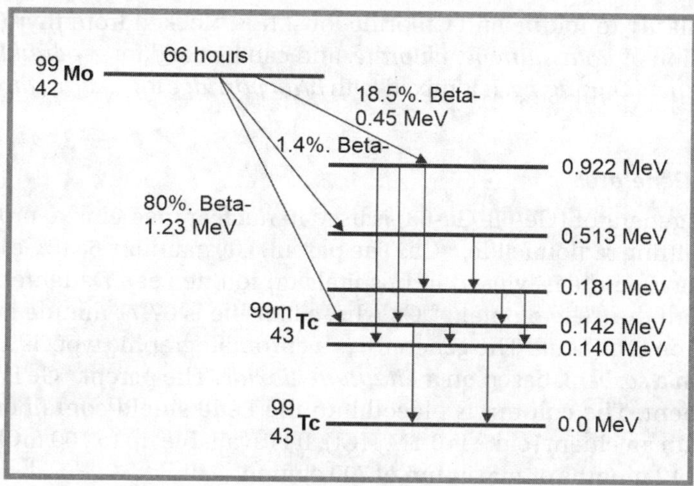

Fig. 2.17: Decay scheme of Molybdenum-99: beta minus decay.

molecules **(Fig. 2.17)**. Molybdenum-99 decays to ^{99m}Tc, which is easily separated from parent since ^{99m}Tc is less tightly bound than its parent. This process is called an *elusion*.

Sterile *isotonic* saline (0.9%) is passed through the column to remove Tc-99m. Chloride ions get exchanged with TcO_4^- ions only and produces *Sodium pertechnetate, Na$^+$* (^{99m} TcO_4^-). This process is called an *elusion* and takes only few minutes. This flows under pressure and is collected in sterile rubber caped vial. After elusion, the Tc-99m decays with half-life of 6 h.

^{99}Mo is not soluble in saline and hence remains in the column. After elusion, ^{99m}Tc activity grows and reaches maximum in about 24 hours. Now production rate of daughter and decay rate of parent are equal, and they are said to be in *transient equilibrium*. The end of the column is provided with a *milli-pore filter* to get required sterility by a bacteriostatic agent in the elute. Thus, sterile, pathogen free is *Technetium pertechnetate* (^{99m}TcO$_4^-$) is produced with high specific activity. It flows under pressure and is collected in sterile *rubber caped vial*.

These generators are usually called *cows* and an elution *(milking)* is done in each morning, to get maximal growth of ^{99m}Tc. If generator is damaged, alumina can break into the saline elute. This results in an unnecessary radiation dose to patient since the Mo gamma energy is higher (740 and 780 keV). Hence, a *dose calibrator* is used to determine Mo-99 content, each time the generator is eluted.

When it is supplied to the hospitals, the ^{99m}Tc activity has build-up to a maximum, equal to parent (Mo). Activity of daughter at the time of elution will depend upon, activity of parent, rate of formation of daughter, decay rate of daughter, time since last elution, and elution efficiency.

^{99m}Tc is used in clinical medicine as *Sodium pertechnetate-99m*, which is used for imaging tissues (e.g., thyroid, gastric mucosa, salivary glands), due its similarity to Iodine and Chloride ions. It is blocked from thyroid by administration of *Potassium per chlorate*, and can be used for *cerebral blood flow*, and *testicular imaging*. It is mixed with *bran porridge* for *gastric emptying studies*.

Gallium-68 Generator

Gallium-68 generator (Ge-68/Ga-68) is used in nuclear medicine to produce *positron* emitting radionuclide, ^{68}Ga. The parent, Germanium-68 (^{68}Ge) half-life is 271 days, and easily used in hospitals up to one year. Daughter, ^{68}Ga is eluted from the ^{68}Ge to obtain ^{68}Ga whose half-life is 67.71 minute hence, transportation is difficult. The generator is a chromatographic type, is a glass column with a *sorbent*, based on a *Titanium dioxide*. The parent ^{68}Ge is fixed on the sorbent. The column is placed into the Lead shield container and provided with an eluent (elute is 0.1M HCl). It is available up to 100 mCi with a self-life of 12 months or maximum of 700 elution.

^{68}Ga obtained from the generator is used for positron emission tomography (PET) studies for calibration, and labelling techniques. For example, ^{68}Ga-PSMA-11 is a novel PET agent to detect recurrent metastatic prostate cancer. It is used in combination with tracer kits for diagnosis of neuroendocrine tumors and prostate cancer. Imaging of prostate, restaging of cancer, recurrence of cancer and accessing therapeutic response are its important application. It offers low-cost solution for radiolabeling of biomolecules with Ga-68 in PET. Patients can be given large doses with low radiation doses.

RADIOPHARMACEUTICALS

A radionuclide that has desirable imaging properties can usually be used to make variety of *radiopharmaceuticals*. Generally, a radiopharmaceutical is formed by mixing the radionuclide with a compound to be labeled at room temperature. Of course, it may require additional *chemicals, sterile workstation, shielded syringes and a glove box*, in a room filled with sterile air and positive pressure. Radiopharmaceuticals should have desirable characteristics for nuclear imaging.

The physical half-life should be short, compatible to duration of preparation and injection, and objective of the study. It should decay to a stable daughter. It should emit mono energetic gamma rays (50–300 keV), for scatter elimination. Energy is high enough to exit the patient and low enough for easy collimation. Decay by an isomeric transition and electron capture is preferable. It should not have an alpha or beta particles or an *Auger electron* or very low energy photons. It is easily attached to a pharmaceutical at room temperature, but no effect on its metabolism. It should localize largely and quickly in the target of interest.

It should have low toxicity and is readily available at the hospital site. All radiopharmaceuticals should be pyrogen-free prior to injection. It can be filtered by a sterile filter of pore size 0.22 μm to remove organisms. Pharmaceutical-grade chemicals, sterile water, and sterilized equipment are recommended to minimize the pyrogen risk. Appropriate pH of the solution is vital.

It can be easily eliminated from the body with an effective half-life, on duration of examination. Hence, dynamic time course of the radiopharmaceutical in the body is important. Radiopharmaceutical's uptake may differ, it may be rapid or slow uptake. The biological half-life and the physical half-life determine the number of radioactive decays which will be observed in an organ. Generally, hours to days is required for significant uptake in the target tissue, blood vessels and an visualization of target. Hence, long half-life radionuclides are found useful for radiopharmaceutical labeling, compared to short lived ones.

Specific Activity

Specific activity is the activity per unit mass, expressed in MBq/µmol. It is determined by losses in specific activity that occurs during chemical synthesis of the radiopharmaceutical. Especially this is important in isotopes of elements that have high natural abundance. For example specific activity of ^{11}C is 3.5×10^8 MBq/µmol, whereas the specific activity of labeled ^{11}C radiopharmaceutical is $\approx 1 \times 10^5$ MBq/µmol. Generally, clinical radiopharmaceuticals have high specific activity, to have typical injection of micro-gram to nanogram quantities. Pharmacologic effects demand milligram level of material.

Radiochemical Purity

Chemical purity is the fraction of sample that is present in the desired chemical, and the desirable value is >99%. Radiopharmaceutical purity is fraction of radioactivity in the sample that is present in the sample in the desired chemical form. The desired purity is >95%. Impure radiopharmaceutical distributes differently in the body and adds background to the image of the desired compound.

Labeling Strategies

There are two ways of labeling, namely (1) small molecule, and (2) large biomolecule. Small molecule can be labeled by *direct substitution or by creating analogues*. In direct substitution, a stable atom in the molecule is replaced with a radioactive atom of the same element. Labeled compound will have the same biological properties of the unlabeled compound. For example, replacing a ^{12}C atom in glucose with a ^{11}C radioactive atom to create ^{11}C-*glucose*. The radiopharmaceutical undergoes same distribution and metabolism in the human body as unlabeled glucose.

Alternatively, an original compound is modified, referred as an analogue. The analogue permits use of radioactive isotopes of elements which are not widely found in nature. The biological properties of the molecule can be altered by changing uptake rate, clearance, or metabolism. For example, replacing the *hydroxyl group (OH)* on the second carbon in glucose with ^{18}F gives *Fluro-deoxy-glucose (FDG)*.

Table 2.3: ^{99m}Tc-labeled radiopharmaceuticals, prepared from cold kits.

Compound	Abbreviation	Application
^{99m}Tc-MDP	Methylene diphosphonate	Bone scan
^{99m}Tc-DMSA	2, 3-Dimercaptosuccinic acid	Renal scan
^{99m}Tc-DTPA	Diethylenetriaminepenta acetic acid	Renal function
^{99m}Tc-Sestamibi	2-Methoxy-2-methylpropyl isonitrile	Myocardial perfusion, breast cancer
^{99m}Tc-HMPAO	Hexamethylpropylene amine oxime	Cerebral perfusion
^{99m}Tc-HIDA	N-(2-6-dimethylphenol-carbamoylmethyl)-iminodiacetic acid	Hepatic function
^{99m}Tc-ECD	N, N'-1-2-ethylenediyl-bis-L-cysteine diethylester	Cerebral perfusion

(*Courtesy:* Simon R Cherry et al, 2012)

In the case of large biomolecule, the radioactive label is kept away from the biologically active site of the molecule. For example, *antibodies, peptides,* and *proteins* are labeled with different radionuclides with minimal effect on their biologic properties.

Technetium-99m Labeled Radiopharmaceutical

Commonly used pharmaceutical in nuclear medicine is ^{99m}Tc. It is easily prepared by injecting a known quantity of ^{99m}Tc pertechnetate in a sterile vial containing *lyophilized pharmaceutical.* The radiopharmaceutical complex is formed instantaneously and can be used for multiple doses over a period of several hours. Though ^{99m}Tc radiopharmaceutical is prepared easily at room temperature, the other products require multiple steps, but they are simple and have very high labeling efficiency.

Technetium generator produces Technetium pertechnetate (^{99m}TcO$_4^-$). Generator is provided with cold kits to prepare different ^{99m}Tc complexes. The content of the cold kit is mixed with ^{99m}TcO$_4^-$ to have multiple ^{99m}Tc complexes. Generally cold kit consists of *stannous chloride*, a reducing agent. It reduces the ^{99m}Tc to lower oxidation state, permitting it to bind to a complexing agent. Thus, ^{99m}Tc labeled radiopharmaceutical, targeted to different organ and different biologic process can be prepared. It can be done quickly and easily in a hospital setup **(Table 2.3)**.

Radionuclides Labeled with Positron Emitters

Positron emitting radionuclides like ^{11}C, ^{13}N and ^{15}O are replaced by direct substitution method **(Table 2.4)**. As a result, labeled compound with same biochemical properties of the original compound is obtained.^{18}F is substituted for Hydrogen to have its labeled analogue. FDG is commonly used since it is a glucose analogue. We know that glucose is used to produce an *adenosine triphosphate*, the energy source of the body. Disease patterns alter the

Table 2.4: Positron emitting radioisotopes and their clinical application.

Radio Nuclide	Half-life	Tracer	Application
O-15	2 min	Water	Cerebral blood flow
C-11	20 min	Methionine	Tumor protein synthesis
N-13	10 min	Ammonia	Myocardial blood flow
F-18	110 min	FDG	Glucose metabolism
Ga-68	68 min	DOTANOC	Neuro-endocrine imaging
Rb-82	72 sec	Rb-82	Myocardial perfusion

(*Courtesy:* Kuppusamy Thayalan, 2023)

energy demands of the cells in the body. FDG accumulates in the cells that is proportional to the metabolic rate of glucose. It is an important marker for *neurodegenerative decease, epilepsy, coronary artery disease* and *malignancy*. All the above radionuclides are short lived, hence require local cyclotron production and rapid synthesis techniques.

Localization of Radiopharmaceuticals

The radiopharmaceutical uptake in tissue is driven by one or more of the mechanisms: (1) active transport, (2) compartmental localization, (3) diffusion, (4) phagocytosis, (5) capillary blockade, and (6) cell sequestration.

Active transport involves cellular metabolic processes that expend energy to concentrate the radiopharmaceutical into a tissue against a concentration gradient above plasma levels, e.g., thyroid uptake scanning with *Iodine*. Compartmental localization refers to introduction of radiopharmaceutical into a well-defined anatomical compartment, e.g., *blood pool scanning* with human *serum, albumin, plasma, or red blood cells*. Diffusion is simply the free movement of substance from a region of high concentration to that of lower concentration, e.g., *bone scanning* with *pyrophosphates*. Cells of reticuloendothelial system are distributed in the *liver, spleen,* and *bone marrow*. These cells recognize small foreign substances in the blood and remove them by *phagocytosis*, e.g., *liver, spleen and bone marrow* scanning with *radiocolloids*. When particles slightly larger than RBC are injected intravenously, they become trapped in the marrow capillary beds, is called *capillary blockade*, e.g., *lung scanning with macroaggregate* (8–75 mm). In cell sequestration, red blood cells are withdrawn from the patient, labeled with ^{99m}Tc, heated in a boiling water bath for 30 minutes. When reinjected, the spleen's ability to recognize and remove the damaged RBC can be evaluated.

Quality Control

As a part of quality control, these pharmaceuticals are tested for their radionuclide purity, radiochemical purity, chemical purity, and sterility, before injected to the patient. Radionuclide purity is the presence of unwanted radionuclides in the sample and is periodically checked using a *well counter*. Radiochemical purity refers to chemical purity of an isotope and is checked by *thin-layer chromatography*. Chromatography separates compounds that are soluble in saline. Chemical impurity can occur due to temperature changes, presence of unwanted oxidizing or reducing agents, pH changes, or radiation damage to pharmaceuticals. This will reduce the uptake in the organ and increases the background activity, thereby degrading image quality. Radiochemical impurity also increases patient dose. Sterility means that the radiopharmaceutical is free of any microbial contamination. Even a sterile preparation may contain pyrogens, which may cause a reaction, if administrated to a patient. Hence, sterility and pyrogenicity tests should be performed before the an agent is administered to the patients.

BIBLIOGRAPHY

1. Cherry SR, Sorenson JA, and Phelps ME. Physics of Nuclear Medicine, Elsevier, Philadelphia; 2012.
2. Thayalan K. Basic Radiologic Physics, 2nd edn. Jaypee Brothers Medical Publishers (P) Ltd, New Delhi; 2017.
3. Thayalan K. The Physics of Radiation Oncology, Jaypee Brothers Medical Publishers (P) Ltd, New Delhi; 2023.

Production of X-rays

DISCOVERY OF X-RAYS

X-rays were discovered by the German physicist, **WC Roentgen** (1895). He was investigating conduction of electricity through gases in a glass tube at low pressure. During that he noticed that the positive electrode in the glass tube gave off invisible rays which made *Barium platinocyanide* fluorescent screen kept near the tube to glow (Fluorescence). The rays were highly penetrating, even fogged photographic plates and passed through black paper, and even thicker objects. They were not deflected by an electric and magnetic field. Therefore, Roentgen concluded that they were not charged particles. As their nature was not known he called them X-rays. Later, they were shown to be an electromagnetic radiation of short wavelength. Roentgen received the first physics *Nobel prize* for his discovery (1901).

Properties of X-rays

- X-rays are electromagnetic radiation of shorter wavelength (0.1–10 nm).
- They travel in straight line with velocity equal to light: 3×10^8 m/sec.
- X-rays are not deflected by an electric and magnetic fields.
- X-rays penetrate through substances that are opaque to visible light.
- X-rays produce fluorescence in materials like Calcium tungstate ($CaWO_4$), and Cesium iodide (CsI).
- X-rays affect photographic X-ray film or digital detector and form latent image.
- X-rays produce an ionization and excitation in a medium.
- X-rays produce chemical changes in certain substances.
- X-rays produce biological effects in living organisms. The cells can be either damaged partially or killed due to X-ray exposure.

Origin of X-rays

X-rays are produced when fast moving electrons are stopped by means of target material. The moving electrons possess kinetic energy. When electrons

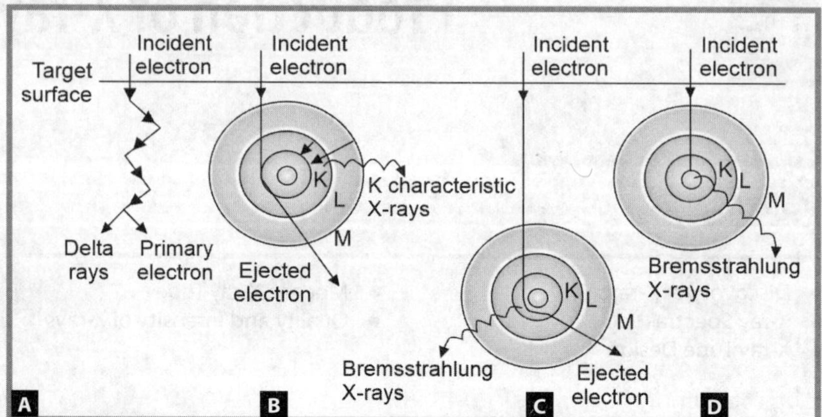

Figs. 3.1A to D: Interaction of electron with target atoms: (A) Ionization of target atoms; (B) Characteristic X-rays; (C) Interaction with nuclear field; (D) Interaction with nucleus.

are suddenly stopped, their kinetic energy is converted into heat and X-ray energy. This conversion is taking place at the target material which stops the electrons. Therefore, an electron interaction with target is the basis for X-ray production **(Figs. 3.1A to D)**. The electron interacts the target in four possible ways:

- ❑ Ionization of target atoms
- ❑ Production of characteristic X-rays
- ❑ Interaction with nuclear field
- ❑ Interaction with nucleus

Ionization of Target Atoms

Fast moving electrons enter the surface layer of the target and undergoes collisions **(Fig. 3.1A)**. In this process, an incident electron transfers sufficient energy and removes an electron from an atom, most likely in an outer orbit. This involves small energy transfer resulting in ionization of target atoms. The incident electron may undergo number of such collisions and each time its direction gets altered. A 100 keV electron may encounter 1,000 such interactions before coming to rest and most of its energy appears as heat in the target. The removed electron, known as a *secondary electron*, may have sufficient energy and produce further ionization with target atoms. They are less in number and produce their own track known as *delta rays*.

Production of Characteristic X-rays

This is an interaction between an incident electron and K-shell electron **(Fig. 3.1B)**. In this process, an incident electron directly hits the K-shell, transfers sufficient energy, and removes the K-shell electron. This is referred as an ionization in K-shell or inner orbit ionization. The vacancy in the K-shell is filled by an electron from outer shells like L and M by an electron transition.

During this transition, the difference in binding energies of the two shells is given out as X-ray photons. These photons are known as *characteristic X-rays* since they represent the shell and atomic number of the target material. The ejected electron may perform further interaction in other target atoms.

Interaction with Nuclear Field

The incident electron occasionally reaches nearer to nucleus of an atom in the target **(Fig. 3.1C)**. Since the electron is a negative particle, it is attracted by the positive nucleus. It is made to orbit partially around the nucleus, decelerates and goes out with reduced energy. The loss of energy appears in the form of X-ray photons, known as *Bremsstrahlung*. The energy of the X-ray photon depends on the degree to which an electron is decelerated by nuclear attraction. It depends on the distance between the nucleus and an interaction point. The interaction point, closer to the nucleus have maximum energy, whereas points away from the nucleus will have minimal energy. Thus, photon energy can take any value from zero to maximum. This process is unlikely at low electron energies, but dominant at high energies.

Interaction with Nucleus

The electron may hit the nucleus directly and is stopped completely in a single collision **(Fig. 3.1D)**. The entire electron energy appears as bremsstrahlung radiation. This type of interaction is very rare, but capable of giving high energy X-rays.

The event *A* or ionization of target atoms dominates (>99%) the electron interaction process and produce heat. The interaction of *B*, *C* and *D* are much rare in the diagnostic radiology range of energies, leading to lesser amount (< 1%) of X-ray production. Thus, X-ray tube is inefficient in the conversion of electron energy into X-rays but produces large amount of heat.

X-RAY SPECTRA

X-ray photons produced by an X-ray tube are heterogeneous in energy. There are two types of X-ray spectrum:
- Bremsstrahlung spectrum
- Characteristic X-ray spectrum

Bremsstrahlung spectrum consists of X-ray photons of all energies up to maximum in a continuous fashion, which is also known as *white radiation*, because of its similarity to white light. It is also referred as *continuous spectrum*. A characteristic spectrum consists of X-ray photons of few energies which is also called as *line spectrum*. The position of the characteristic radiation depends upon the atomic number of the target.

The intensity of the X-rays is plotted against X-ray photon energy in a graph **(Fig. 3.2)**. The area under the curve is proportional to total number of X-ray photons emitted. The highest X-ray energy is determined by the peak voltage (kVp) applied in the X-ray tube. The characteristic spectrum is superimposed

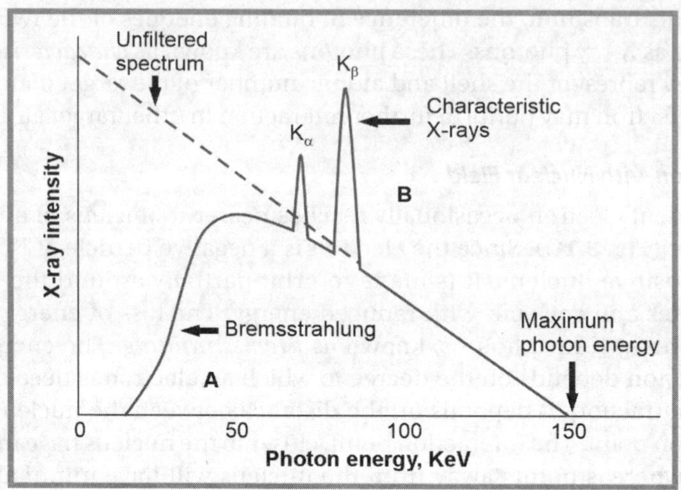

Fig. 3.2: X-ray spectrum: (A) Bremsstrahlung; (B) Characteristic spectrum.

on the bremsstrahlung spectrum. An unfiltered beam spectrum (theoretical) will be a straight line and mathematically given by **Kramer's equation**:

$$I_E = KZ\,(E_m - E)$$

where, I_E is the intensity of X-ray photons with energy E, Z is the atomic number of the target, E_m is the maximum X-ray photon energy, and K is a constant. The unfiltered X-ray spectrum looks like a ramp.

In practice, the X-ray beam is a filtered beam due to an inherent filtration and added filtration. The filtration hardens the beam by absorbing low energy X-rays up to 10 keV, which is evident by the bremsstrahlung spectrum. As photon energy increases the number of photons increases initially, later decreases linearly up to maximum photon energy. The X-ray spectrum is influenced by (1) applied voltage, (2) target material, (3) tube current, (4) exposure time, (5) bremsstrahlung process and (6) filtration. To specify the quality of X-rays, a rule of thumb is used, which states that an effective energy is about 1/3 to 1/2 of maximum X-ray energy.

Bremsstrahlung X-rays

Bremsstrahlung is a German word refers to braking radiation. It is a process of *radiative collision* between an electron and nuclear field in the target **(Fig. 3.3)**. The electrons between the cathode and an anode have potential energy that is equal to the product of their electrostatic charge. As the electrons accelerate, this potential energy is transformed into kinetic energy. The electron while passing near the nucleus may suffer a sudden deflection and an acceleration by the action of *Coulomb forces* of attraction. As a result, their velocity changes, the electron may lose their kinetic energy, in the form of *bremsstrahlung X-rays*. The electron may have one or more such interactions and this may result in partial or complete loss of energy.

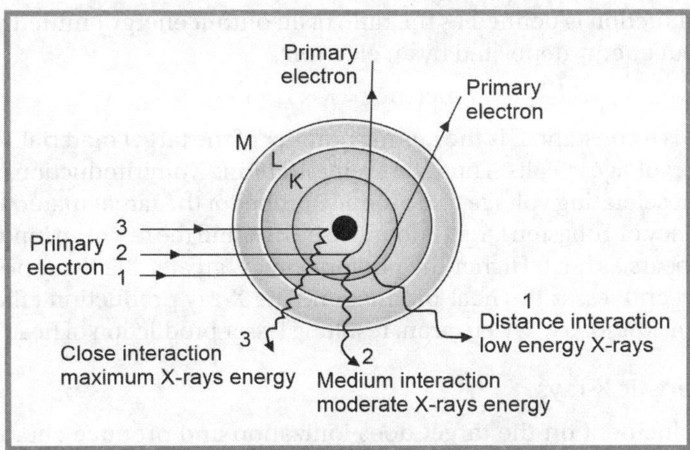

Fig. 3.3: Production of bremsstrahlung radiation.

Probability (P) of bremsstrahlung process is much low, about 1–5% and it is proportional to Z and kVp:

$$P \propto Z \times kV_p^2$$

in which kV_p is proportional to electron beam energy.

The amount of bremsstrahlung production is determined by the distance between the bombarding electron and nucleus. At very large distance, the Columbic force is weak, only low energy X-rays are created, but this process has higher probability to occur. When the electron is very close to the nucleus, Columbic force is strong, electron lose more kinetic energy, resulting production of high energy X-rays. But this process has lower probability to occur. When the electron is in the middle, the electron interaction is moderate, and the X-ray energy is also moderate. If the electron hits the nucleus directly, it loses all its kinetic energy, but the probability of this type of interaction is very low (5%). To conclude, low energy X-rays are produced in greater abundance compared to high energy X-rays.

Thus, the bremsstrahlung radiation will have all possible energy from zero to maximum. The maximum energy is determined by maximum kinetic energy of an incident electron. The direction of emission of bremsstrahlung photons depends on the energy of an incident electron. At electron energies below 100 keV, X-rays are emitted equally in all directions. As the kinetic energy of electron increases, the direction of X-ray emission becomes increasingly forward. In diagnostic radiology, it is technically advantages to obtain X-ray beam on the same side of the target, i.e., at 90° with respect to an electron beam direction.

In diagnostic X-ray tubes, thicker targets are used to stop entire electron beam. Hence, X-rays are produced in all directions around the target. Those X-rays that are produced in the forward direction will be absorbed by the target itself, remaining X-rays forms an useful beam. The term efficiency of

X-ray production is defined as the ratio of an output energy emitted as X-rays to an input energy deposited by an electron:

$$\text{Efficiency} = K \times Z \times kV_p$$

where, K is a constant, Z is the atomic number of the target material, kV_p is the peak tube voltage in volts. Thus, the bremsstrahlung X-ray production increases with an accelerating voltage and atomic number of the target material.

Efficiency of Tungsten target is found to be <1% and the rest of an input energy, >99% appears as heat. Higher the photon energy, greater the X-ray production efficiency and lesser the heat production. The X-ray production efficiency is more than 50% for a 6 MV electron, resulting lesser production of heat.

Characteristic X-rays

Electron incident on the target does ionization and produce characteristic X-rays. An electron with kinetic energy may interact with atoms of the target by ejecting an orbital electron from K-shell. As a result, there is a vacancy in the K-shell and the atom is said to be ionized. The original electron will have energy $E_o - E_{KE}$, where, E_{KE} is the kinetic energy given to the orbital electron. The outer orbital electrons like M or L orbit will move to fill the vacancy at the K-shell **(Fig. 3.4)**. In doing so, the difference in binding energy of the two shells is radiated as X-ray photons, which is referred as *characteristic radiation.* This will have only discrete energies. Since the binding energy difference is unique to an atom, the X-rays emitted are characteristics of that element. If the transition involved an electron from L-shell to K-shell of a Tungsten target, then the emitted photon will have energy (hv):

$$h\nu = E_K - E_L$$
$$= 69.5 \text{ keV} - 10.2 \text{ keV}$$
$$= 59.3 \text{ keV}$$

where, E_K and E_L are the binding energies of K and L-shells of Tungsten atom, respectively. The K-shell characteristic X-ray energies are slightly lower than

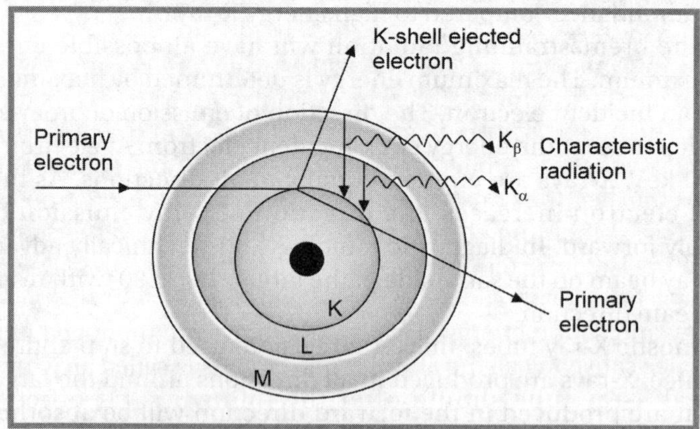

Fig. 3.4: Production of characteristic X-rays.

Table 3.1: K-shell characteristic X-rays (keV) and target material.

Transition	Tungsten, Z = 74	Molybdenum, Z = 42	Rhodium, Z = 45
$K_{\alpha 1}$	59.32	17.48	20.22
$K_{\alpha 2}$	57.98	17.37	20.07
$K_{\beta 1}$	67.24	19.61	22.72

(*Courtesy:* Jerrold T Bushberg et al, 2012)

the K-shell binding energy. Electron transition may be from an adjacent and non-adjacent shells.

Energy transitions are designated by the shell capturing the electron with a subscript of α or β. The subscript α refers to an adjacent shell transition, e.g., L to K transition is denoted as K_α X-rays. The subscript β refers to a non-adjacent shell transition, e.g., M to K transition is denoted as K_β X-rays. Thus, transition results in fine energy splitting of characteristic X-rays, due to subshells of the given orbit. Only K-characteristic X-rays are very important in diagnostic radiology ($K_{\alpha 1}$, $K_{\alpha 2}$ and $K_{\beta 1}$ transitions). The K-shell characteristic X-rays for various target atoms are given in **Table 3.1**.

The characteristic X-rays other than K-shell transitions are not important since they are entirely attenuated by tube window and filters. K characteristic X-rays are emitted only, if the incident electrons have energies greater than the binding energy of the K-shell electron. Hence, the kilovoltage applied must be greater than 69.5 keV for *Tungsten*, 20 keV for *Molybdenum*, and 23.2 keV for *Rhodium* targets, respectively which is called as *Threshold energy*. As the energy of an incident electron increases above the threshold energy, the percentage of characteristic X-rays also increases. A 100 kV X-ray spectrum consists of about only 10% characteristic X-rays.

X-RAY TUBE DESIGN

Production of X-ray requires the following: (1) electron source-Cathode, (2) target to stop the electrons-Anode, (3) high voltage supply to accelerate electrons-kV, (4) vacuum, and (5) tube insert-glass envelope.

Electron can be produced either by an ionization in gas or by thermionic emission. The electron source acts as a cathode and the target acts as an anode. A high voltage is applied between the cathode and anode. This voltage accelerates the electrons to a higher velocity, in turn the electron gains high kinetic energy. When the electrons are stopped by the target, the electron kinetic energy is converted into X-ray energy. This is analogy to applying a sudden break in a moving car or cycle, in which kinetic energy is converted into heat energy and sound energy. This is how X-rays are produced in the X-ray tube. A device satisfying all the above requirements is called an X-ray tube.

An ideal X-ray tube should offer the following: (1) efficient X-ray production, (2) efficient heat removal, (3) constant X-ray beam quality, and (4) consistent performance under different operating conditions. The tube

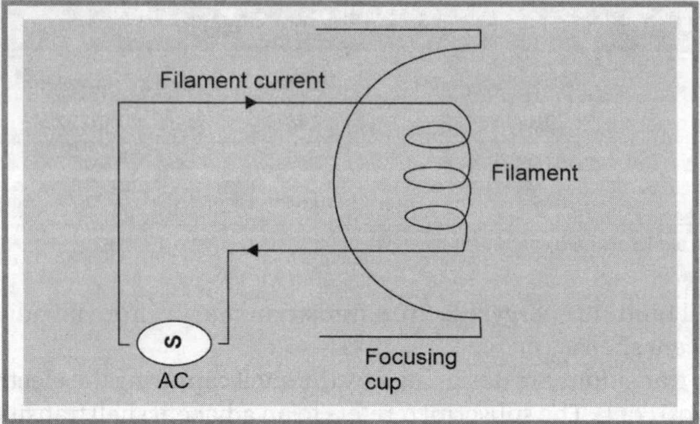

Fig. 3.5: Cathode assembly.

should be designed in such way that, it should withstand voltages from 20 to 150 kV and currents up to 1,000 mA. In radiography, tube current may vary from 100 to 1,000 mA, whereas in fluoroscopy, it is 1–10 mA. In addition, exposure time must be varied over a wider range.

Cathode

The cathode is made up of Tungsten wire in the form of helical filament, surrounded by a *focusing cup* (**Fig. 3.5**). Tungsten is used as filament material because of its (1) high melting point, (2) low vapor pressure, (3) good ductility (easily drawn into fine wire) and (4) low work function (4.5 eV). Tungsten exhibits thermionic emission well below its melting point. The Tungsten filament wire is about 0.2 mm in diameter, that is coiled to form vertical spiral about 0.2 cm in diameter and 1 cm in length. The coil format provides large surface area for electron emission.

The filament circuit supplies a voltage of 8–12 V and selectable filament current of 3–7 A. Electrical resistance to electron flow, heats the filament to very high temperature, releasing surface electron through thermionic emission process. The rate of emission depends on temperature, and it can be adjusted by filament current. A trace of Thorium in the filament not only increases the efficiency, but also prolongs the filament life.

If the applied voltage between an anode and cathode is low, the electrons form a cloud near the cathode, referred as *space charge*. Tube should overcome the space charge effect to produce X-rays efficiently.

Focusing Cup

Usually, filament is provided with a focusing cup which surrounds the filament to shape the electron beam. It is used to focus the electron on a small area on an anode. It also controls the width of an electron distribution and directs the electron towards the target. There are two ways by which the focusing cup is energized, namely (1) unbiased and (2) biased

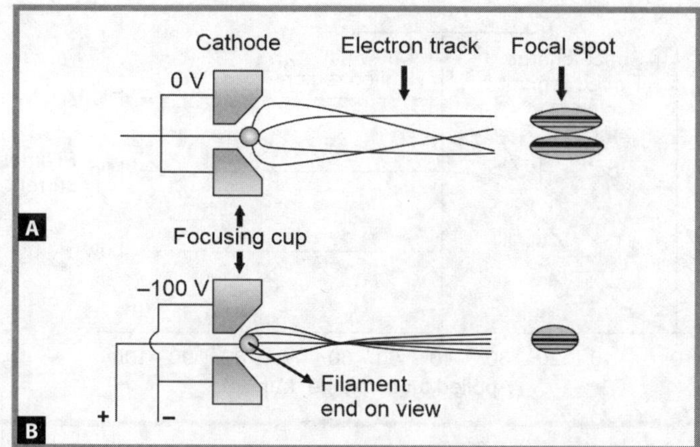

Figs. 3.6A and B: (A) Unbiased focusing cup potential is 0 V, relative to filament; (B) Biased focusing cup, potential is −100 V, relative to filament.

(Figs. 3.6A and B). If the focusing cup and the filament is given the same potential, it is called an unbiased X-ray tube. Its electron spread is wider and focal spot width is larger.

In a biased X-ray tube, an insulated focusing cup is used and is given more negative supply, −100 V than the filament. That is the filament and the focusing cup are given different voltages. It creates a tighter electric field around the electron, which reduces the electron spread and gives smaller focal spot width. Thus, focusing cup width determines focal spot width and filament length determines the focal spot length. This principle is used in *Grid controlled X-ray tubes.* In this, the focusing cup acts as third electrode and function as a switch to turn tube current ON and OFF. Though X-ray tube is energized, X-ray emission is stopped temporarily for clinical procedures.

Space Charge Effect

To understand an operation of an X-ray tube, it is essential to know how the tube current depends on tube voltage, for a given filament excitation **(Fig. 3.7)**. When the applied kV is zero or small, the electrons surrounding the filament forms a cloud, resulting in *space charge effect*. These electrons tend to repel electrons back into the filament hence, the tube current is very small. As kV increases (0 to 40 kV), the effect of space charge reduces gradually, and the tube current also increases. This is called *space charge limited region*. In this region, the tube current strongly dependent on applied kV, for a constant filament current.

Above 40 kV the space charge effect disappears, and the tube current is controlled by the filament current. This is called the *saturation or emission limited region*. In this region, the tube current undergoes little change with an increase in tube voltage. The tube current is 5 to 10 times lesser than the filament current in this region.

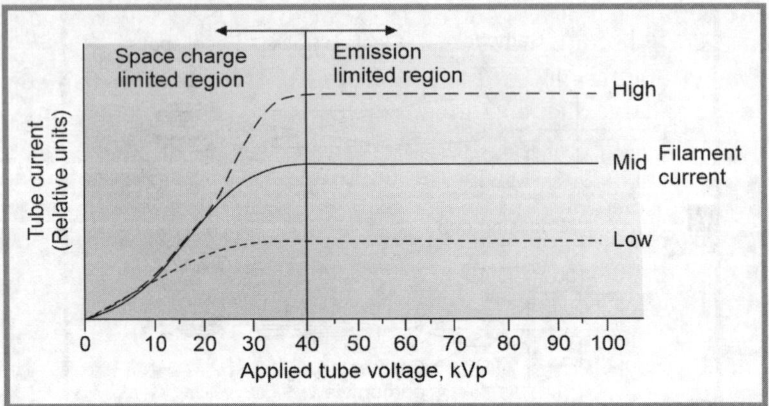

Fig. 3.7: Space charge effect.

Most of the X-ray tubes are operating in between the space charge region and an emission limited region. Thus, the tube current is determined by both kV and filament current. In the space charge limited region (<40 kV), the tube current is influenced only by the applied voltage. In the emission limited region (>40 kV), the tube current is controlled by the filament current, and it is independent of an applied voltage. To deliver the selected tube current, a space charge compensating circuit is used. This circuit also corrects the small increase in tube current, at higher applied voltage (>40 kV).

The above characteristics of the space charge effect curves depend upon many factors, namely (1) distance between anode-cathode, (2) configuration of focusing cup, (3) focal spot size, and (4) filament temperature. Particularly, the change of potential of the focusing cup, will drastically alter the curves.

Anode

The anode electrode contains a target which is maintained at a positive DC potential. The target material should possess the following properties, namely: (1) high melting point to withstand high temperature, (2) high atomic number to increase the X-ray production efficiency, (3) high thermal conductivity to dissipate heat quickly, (4) low vapor pressure at high temperature to prevent evaporation of target material, and (5) easily machined to make smooth surface.

Tungsten (W) is the metal widely used as target because of its high melting point, 3387°C and high atomic number, 74. However, its thermal conductivity is low (174 $Wm^{-1}K^{-1}$) and hence, Tungsten is embedded over a thick block of *Copper*. The thermal conductivity of Copper is 400 $Wm^{-1}K^{-1}$, so that the heat will be removed much quickly to the surrounding. The vapor pressure of Tungsten is 5,000 kPa, which is low by which it releases less vapor into the vacuum. In stationary anode design, the Tungsten is a square or rectangular plate of 2 or 3 mm thick, and dimension of greater than 1 mm. *Carbon* in the form of *graphite* is also used as target material. It provides increased radiating surface of anode. It is also a good radiator due to black, has low mass and high melting point.

However, rotating anode design employs disk of 75–200 mm diameter with *beveled edges*. Large diameter anodes are used in CT and fluoroscopy, which increases heat capacity and heat dissipation. However, they are prone for mechanical damage, which is prevented by making radial slots in the anode. The above type of anode is called *stress relieved anodes*.

Molybdenum has higher heat capacity than Tungsten, hence used as *anode stem* in rotating anode design. The anode tends to crack under severe stress caused by heating. Therefore, *Tungsten-Rhenium alloy* (90% Tungsten + 10% Rhenium) is always used, which makes the target tougher and reduces surface pitting. *Molybdenum* (Mo, Z = 42) and *Rhodium* (Rh, Z = 45) are commonly used as anode materials for mammographic X-ray tubes. These targets can give characteristic X-rays, suitable for soft tissue imaging and contrast studies.

Focal Spot Size

The area of target within which the electrons are absorbed, and X-rays are generated is called *focal spot or focal area*. If the focal area is very small, penumbra will be lesser, and the picture sharpness will be good, but heat removal is difficult. On the other hand, if the focal area is large, heat will be removed quickly, penumbra is larger, and the picture sharpness is bad (unsharpness). This can be compromised by careful design of the X-ray tube.

Usually, focal spot is defined in two ways namely: (1) actual focal spot, and (2) effective focal spot. The actual focal spot size is an area on the anode in which the electrons are bombarding. Effective focal spot size is the length and width of the emitted X-ray beam as projected down, along the central axis of the X-ray tube. The effective focal spot length is always smaller than an actual focal spot and they are related as follows:

$$\text{Effective focal length} = \text{Actual focal length} \times \sin \theta$$

where, θ is the *anode angle*. The focal spot size is usually expressed in terms of effective focal spot size, which varies from 0.3 to 2 mm square. The focal spot sizes of 0.3 mm, 0.6 mm, 1.0 mm, and 1.2 mm are commonly employed in radiology. The focal spot size has a major effect on *spatial resolution*, particularly when appreciable magnification of the object occurs. Focal spot size can be measured by using a *pinhole camera*, *slit camera* and *star pattern*. It is one of the quality assurance test for X-ray tube.

Line Focus Principle

X-ray tube requires a specialized focal area in the target, which is larger in size to spread heat easily and smaller in size to act as a point source. The point source reduces penumbra effect, resulting sharp images. Hence, the target of an X-ray tube is mounted at very steep angle (θ) with respect to the motion of the incident electrons. The X-rays will appear to come from a small focal area (effective focus), whereas the electrons are bombarding relatively in a larger focal area (actual focus). Therefore, heat is removed much quickly while preserving the image sharpness. This is known as *line focus principle* **(Fig. 3.8A)**.

Consider the electrons that are made to strike on a target of length, ab, width, cd and anode angle, θ, then:

$$\text{Effective focus} = \text{Actual focus} \times \text{sin of anode angle}$$
$$cd = ab \times \sin \theta$$

For example, if θ = 17° and ab = 3 mm, then

$$cd = 3 \text{ mm} \times \sin 17°$$
$$= 3 \text{ mm} \times 0.2924$$
$$= 0.877 \text{ mm} \approx 1 \text{ mm}$$

In such tubes, electrons bombard on a rectangular area of 3 mm × 1 mm, while the X-rays appear to come from an effective area of 1 mm × 1 mm. Now, the loading gain of the X-ray tube is given by the relation:

$$\text{Loading gain} = \frac{\text{Actual focal area}}{\text{Effective focal area}} = \frac{3 \text{ mm} \times 1 \text{ mm}}{1 \text{ mm} \times 1 \text{ mm}} = 3.0$$

If θ is made smaller, the loading gain may be increased but the angular width of the useful X-ray field is reduced.

Anode Angle

Anode angle is defined as the angle of target surface with respect to central ray in the X-ray field **(Fig. 3.8B)**. It has strong relationship with focal spot size and the usable X-ray field size. A small anode angle gives smaller effective focal spot, but its usable X-ray field is limited. Large anode angle gives larger usable X-ray field, but the effective focal spot is larger. To optimize the design, larger anode angle with small filament length is used. This will provide smaller effective focal size with wide field coverage.

The optimum choice of an anode angle depends on the clinical application. A small anode angle (7° to 9°) is useful for small field of view (FOV) imaging,

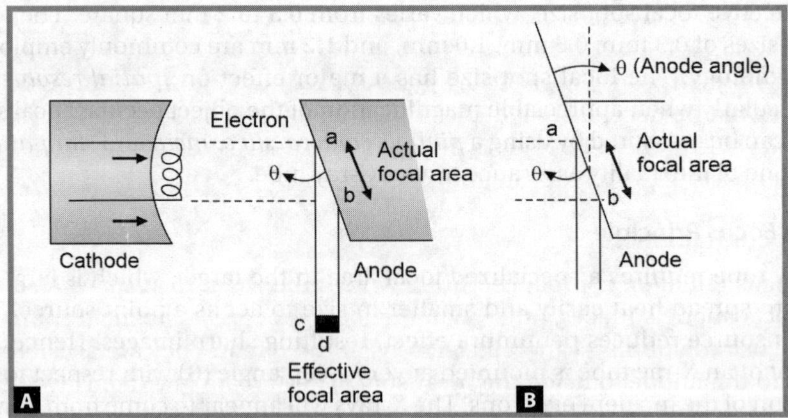

Figs. 3.8A and B: Line focus principle.

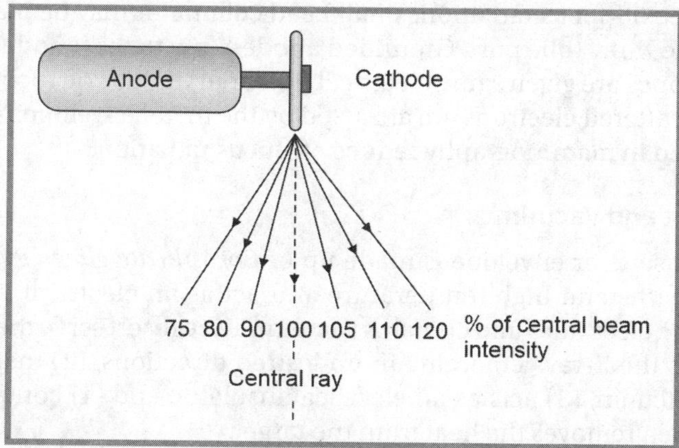

Fig. 3.9: Heel effect.

such as angiography, where the FOV is limited by an image intensifier. Larger anode angles are necessary for general radiography work to achieve larger FOV coverage at short focus to image distances (FID). Modern X-ray tubes are designed with an anode angle of 10–13° with focal spot sizes of 0.6–1.3 mm.

Heel Effect

Heel effect refers to reduced intensity of X-ray beam towards an anode side of the X-ray field **(Fig. 3.9)**. The X-ray photons that are emitted on the anode side of the field must pass through a greater thickness of an anode than those directed towards cathode side. This results in a reduced X-ray intensity on the anode side of the field. The expected intensity drop at the anode side is about 25%.

Magnitudes of the heel effect depends on: (1) anode angle, (2) focus to film distance (FFD), and (3) field size. The heel effect decreases with increase of anode angle but affects *image resolution* and *thermal rating*. The heel effect is less important at large FFD, because the film subtends a smaller beam angle. Collimation of useful field size will reduce heel effect but cannot be eliminated completely. To reduce heel effect, anode angle should be increased, and field size should be decreased. For better balance of the transmitted X-rays, the cathode side of the X-ray tube is oriented over thicker parts, and anode over thinner parts of the patient anatomy.

Off-focus Radiation

Off-focus radiation is produced by an X-ray tube when high speed electron interacts anode surfaces, other than the focal spot area. The main source of off-focus radiation is scattered electrons at the target. They are accelerated back to the anode, outside the focal spot. They create low intensity X-rays over the face of an anode. Off-focus radiation increases patient exposure, geometric blurring, and background fog, resulting poor image quality.

To reduce off-focus radiation, small Lead collimator may be placed much closer to the X-ray tube port. Grounded anode X-ray tubes (anode and metal tube envelopes are given same electrical potential) reduce off focus radiation since the scattered electrons are attracted by the metal envelope. X-ray tubes that are used in mammography reduce off-focus radiation.

Tube Insert and Vacuum

The tube inserts or envelope is made up of *Borosilicate glass (Pyrex)*. Pyrex glass can withstand high temperature and act as an electrical insulator. It supports the electrodes and contains vacuum. Tube insert serve the following, (1) absorbs the X-rays emerging in undesired directions, (2) maintains the required vacuum, (3) acts as an electrical insulator, and (4) contain cooling system which removes the heat from the target.

Glass is not an ideal insert for X-ray tubes since Tungsten vapor condenses and forms an electrically conducting thin layer at the bottom. This may lead to arcing and loss of vacuum due to puncture of glass. Glass is also susceptible to damage from electron bombardment. Hence, metal envelope has been developed with low attenuation *Beryllium window* (Z = 4), for X-ray transmission. However, metal may short circuit cathode and anode due to its conductivity. To eliminate this, *ceramic or glass* insulations are done at the end of the tube. This type of envelope is called *meta-ceramic or metal glass* design. A high vacuum is maintained between the anode and cathode. Vacuum is necessary to: (1) avoid collision between electrons and gas molecules, which gives rise to an ionization that reduces the kinetic energy of the electrons, (2) prevent oxidation of electrodes, and (3) acts as an electrical insulator.

The required vacuum is less than 10^{-5} mm Hg. The X-ray tube insert is enclosed in a sealed housing. The housing should dissipate heat quickly and it depends on the volume of oil that it contains. It should provide shielding for leakage radiation also.

X-ray Tube Housing

The tube housing supports, insulates, and protects the tube insert from an environment **(Fig. 3.10)**. The tube housing is internally shielded with Lead to attenuate X-rays emitted in other directions except through the window. The shield offers radiation protection, electrical protection, thermal protection, and physical protection.

Steel casing is lined with Lead to prevent radiation emerging in all directions. The *Perspex/Beryllium window* is convex upwards to reduce filtration of the X-ray beam by *oil*. To prevent an electrical shock, the shield is earthed. Wherever high-tension cables enter the shield, insulated sockets are used. The shield is filled with *mineral oil*, which act as an electrical insulator and prevents sparking across the insert.

The oil also acts as a cooling medium and expands at higher temperatures. The oil expansion activates *bellows* to operate a micro switch, so that further use of the tube is prevented. The oil expansion also helps to prevent entry

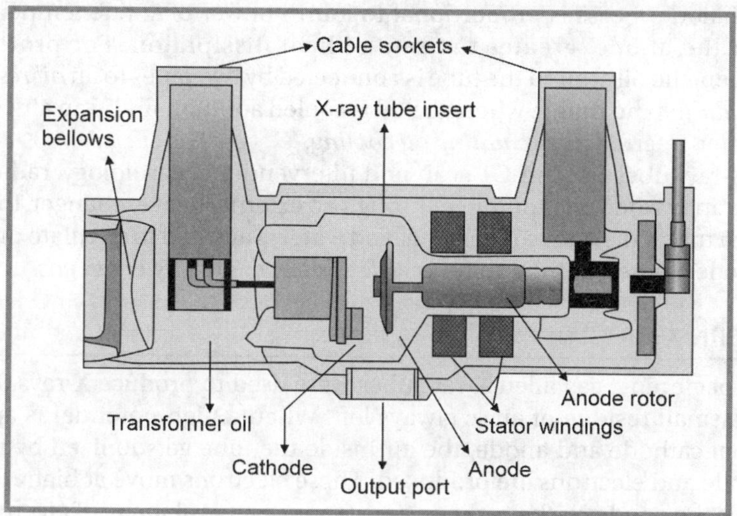

Fig. 3.10: X-ray tube and housing anatomy.

of air into the tube insert. The shield also protects the insert from an accidental damage caused by knocks and bumps.

The effectiveness of tube housing in limiting the leakage radiation must meet the specifications of the safety code-diagnostic radiology—Atomic Energy Regulatory Board (AERB). The leakage radiation measured at distance of 1 m from the source shall not exceed 115 mR (Air-Kerma or 0.1 mGy) in one hour, when the tube is operating at each of the ratings specified by the manufacturer.

X-ray Tube Cooling

In an X-ray tube, only <1% of the electrical power supplied is converted to X-rays. The remaining electrical power (>99%) is converted into heat. This large amount of heat may melt the target and therefore heat should be removed much quickly from the target. Hence, efficient cooling systems are necessary.

In general, targets are made by inserting a layer of Tungsten in *Copper block*, and X-ray tubes are usually enclosed in metal cases, which are filled with oil for insulation purpose. The heat produced on the focal area is conducted quickly into an anode disk, stored temporarily, later transferred to the insulating oil by radiation process. The insulating oil surrounds the glass envelope as well as Copper block, referred as *static oil cooling*. The heat taken up by the insulating oil is transferred to the housing (*metal case*) by convection process. In some designs, fan is used to assist the convection process and removes the heat from the housing.

In the case of rotating anode tube, Molybdenum neck is so long and prevents heat conduction to the rotor. If the anode assembly is coated black, it will promote heat dissipation by radiation process. The rate of heat dissipation by radiation process is proportional to fourth power of anode temperature. Hotter the anode, greater the rate of heat dissipation. For prolonged operation, the oil around the tube is connected by two pipes to an *oil reservoir* with *radiator* and pump, where the oil is cooled additionally by an air current and water, referred as *circulating oil cooling*.

In X-ray tubes used in CT scan and interventional cardiology/radiology-angiography work, oil is pumped through an external heat exchanger. In some modern tubes, the anode is earthed, and water is allowed to circulate through the anode. Sometimes the water is additionally cooled by *Freon gas.*

MODERN X-RAY TUBES

In the beginning, gas filled X-ray tubes were used to produce X-rays. In this tube, a small residue of air is always left. When a high potential is applied between cathode and anode, the air inside the tube gets ionized by a third electrode and electrons are produced. These electrons move at higher speed towards the anode by the cathode and produce an avalanche of electrons by collision with air molecules. Remaining positive ions are attracted towards cathode and release many more electrons by its impact. When the electron stream strikes the target, X-rays are emitted. They produce electrons by *ionization* of gas but had its own limitations.

Coolidge (1913) developed a prototype X-ray tube by using *thermionic emission* principle, to overcome the limitations of earlier X-ray tubes. When a Tungsten filament is heated by an electric current, electrons will be emitted from the filament. This is known as thermionic emission and the tubes are called *hot cathode tubes* or *electron tubes* which are operated at the saturation potential. The wavelength of the X-rays is controlled by altering the applied tube voltage. The tube current can be varied by altering the temperature of filament. Thus, the applied voltage and tube current are independent of each other, and can be controlled separately which is the advantage of this tube. Based on the Coolidge X-ray tube, several X-ray tubes have been designed referred as modern X-ray tubes. These tubes are divided in terms of design into:
❑ Stationary X-ray tube
❑ Rotating anode X-ray tube
❑ Grid-controlled X-ray tube

X-ray tubes are divided into low, medium, and high based on loading capability. Low loading anode tubes have anode of about 60 mm diameter and focal spot size of about 0.4–0.6 mm focal spot size, e.g., mammography imaging. General radiography uses medium loading tubes which has about 100 mm anode disc, and about 0.2–1.0 mm focal spot size. CT and DSA use high loading tubes and the corresponding values are 200 mm and 0.5–0.8 mm, respectively.

Stationary Anode X-ray Tube

The stationary anode X-ray tube consists of a *cathode* and an *anode* which are kept in an evacuated *glass envelope* **(Fig. 3.11)**. The cathode consists of a

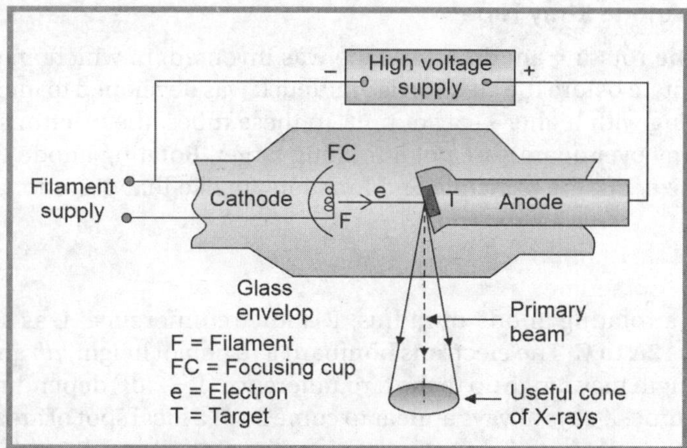

Fig. 3.11: Stationary anode X-ray tube.

Tungsten filament in the form of a coil placed in a shallow *focusing cup*. The filament is heated by passing an electric current through it from a low voltage supply.

The anode is made of *Copper block* in which a small *Tungsten* plate is embedded. The Tungsten plate serves as a target. The target is positioned on line focus principle, to increase the ratio of the actual focal area to the effective focal area. The anode angle is usually 15°–20°. A high voltage supply is applied between the cathode and anode to accelerate electrons. A vacuum of the order of 10^{-5} mm Hg is maintained in the tube.

When the filament is heated to white light, it emits electrons. The focusing cup *(Nickel)* produces a negative electric field that focuses the electron to the focal area. The focusing cup also protects the adjacent parts of the tube wall from damage by electron bombardment. If the anode is made positive with respective to filament, these electrons will be attracted to the anode. This will constitute an electron current around the circuit in anticlockwise direction. The tube current is measured by milli-ammeter (mA).

Since the space between anode and cathode is a high vacuum, the electrons do not collide with gas molecules in crossing the gap and acquire very high velocities. The electrons which are accelerated by the applied voltage possess high kinetic energy. When electrons are suddenly stopped at the target, X-rays are emitted in all directions. About one-half of these are absorbed in the target itself. The remaining portion emerges as a useful primary X-ray beam. During the production of X-rays, large amount of heat is produced in the target. Hence, suitable cooling system is provided to remove the heat much quickly.

Stationary anode tubes have a small target area that limits the heat dissipation, this limit the X-ray output, but they are small and light weight. Dental X-ray units *(intraoral and ortho-pan tomography)*, portable X-ray units, and portable fluoroscopy systems use stationary anode X-ray tubes.

Rotating Anode X-ray Tube

In 1933, the rotating anode X-ray tube was invented, in which an anode is made to rotate before the electron is emitted. It was developed to increase the heat loading with higher X-ray output. In these tubes, the electrons transfer their energy over a large area of a rotating target. Rotating anode tubes are larger in size, but the principle and function are like that of stationary X-ray tube.

Principle

Consider a rotating anode of radius, R and circumference, L as shown in **Figures 3.12A to C**. The electrons bombard a region of height, *ab* and width, *cd*. The length may range up to the circumference ($L = 2\pi R$) depending on the exposure time. X-rays always appear to come from a focal spot of area cd × cd.

Let us consider a stationary anode of an actual focal area 7.3 mm × 2 mm, and a rotating anode of radius, $R = 30$ mm and length 7.3 mm, then:

$$\text{Loading gain} = \frac{\text{Actual focal area of rotating anode X-ray tube}}{\text{Actual focal area of stationary X-ray tube}}$$

$$= \frac{2\pi \times 30 \times 7.3}{7.3 \times 2} = 94.2 \approx 100$$

Thus, the rotating anode X-ray tube helps to increase the loading to an extent of 100. This means that single rotating anode is equivalent to 100 independent stationary anode X-ray tubes. It is possible to design a rotating anode tube having an area up to 500 times more for electron interactions, compared to stationary anode tube. The construction of such a rotating anode is a remarkable technological development. The diameter of the Tungsten disk determines the total length of the target track, and obviously affects the maximum permissible loading of the anode.

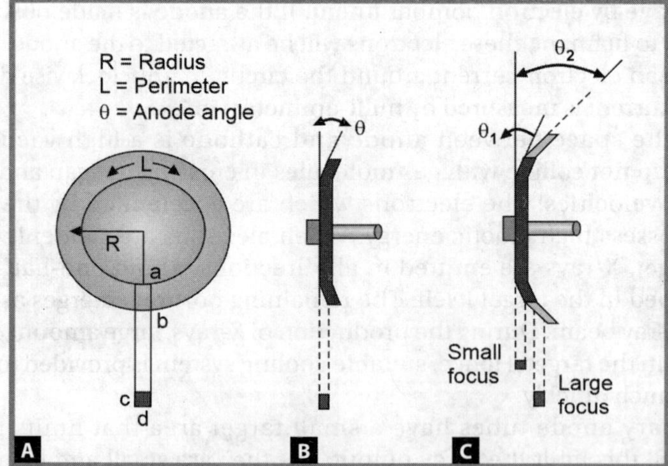

Figs. 3.12A to C: Rotating anode assembly (front and side view): (A) Rotating anode front view; (B) Single focus; (C) Double focus.

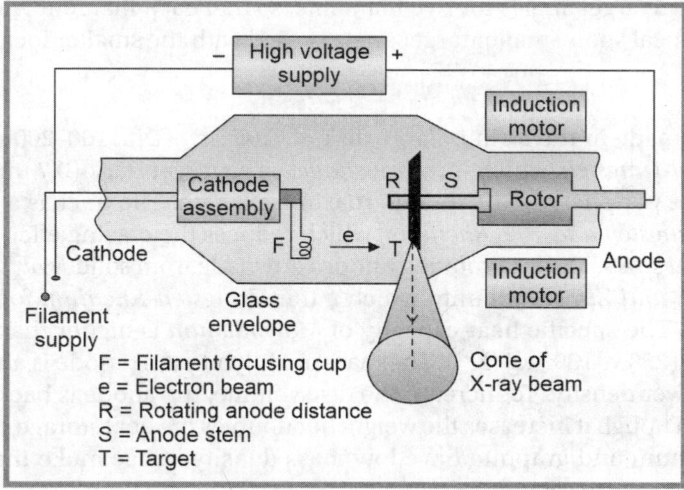

Fig. 3.13: Rotating anode X-ray tube.

Cathode

Rotating anode X-ray tube consists of a cathode and an anode which are kept in a *glass bulb* **(Fig. 3.13)**. The cathode is a *Tungsten filament* which is offset from the long axis of the X-ray tube to face the target near the periphery of the anode disk. Usually, rotating anode tubes are fitted with two filaments **(Fig. 3.14)**, one larger than the other set side by side in the cathode assembly. One filament is designed to focus electrons on a larger area of an anode, which require heavy tube loading. The other filament is used to focus the electrons on a smaller area of target. This type is used when high resolution is required. Both filaments should focus the electron on the same part of the anode, so that focal spot is at the same point for both modes of operation. Some tubes

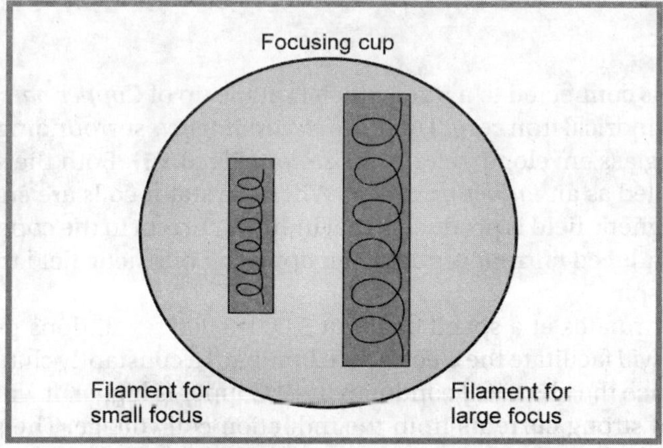

Fig. 3.14: Cathode with dual filament.

provide two target angles for two filaments, so that each filament will have a separate focal spot. Smaller target angle is used with the smaller focal spot.

Anode

Anode is made in the form of large disk of *Tungsten* (Dia. 100–200 mm), or an *alloy of Tungsten*, which is *saucer shaped*. The target track (0.7 mm thick) is near the periphery of the disk, to maximize length. The track is a mixture of *90% Tungsten and 10% Rhenium*, which reduces the crazing effect caused by *thermal stress*. Modern rotating anodes are made from solid *Molybdenum, Titanium, and Zirconium* onto which a thin *Tungsten-Rhenium* focal track is coated. The specific heat capacity of *Molybdenum* is higher than that of Tungsten (250 vs 130 J kg^{-1}K^{-1}). The mass of Molybdenum anode is also lower due its lower density. To increase the disc volume, the anode is backed with *graphite.* Though it increases the weight but doubles the heat storage capacity. Molybdenum and graphite have low mass density hence make the anode lighter and easy to rotate.

Some high output X-ray tubes have radial slots cut into the anode disc to reduce thermal stresses caused by repeated heating and cooling. Heavy duty X-ray tubes have *graphite layer (Carbon)* in the back of the anode disk. The anode disk has a *beveled edge*, and the angle of the bevel may vary from 6–20°. The bevel is used to achieve the line focus principle.

Anode Stem

The anode disk is mounted on a stem, which is attached to the *rotor*. The anode assembly rotates with the help of *bearings*. The stem is made of *Molybdenum*, which is having high melting point (2620°C) and poor heat conduction. The Molybdenum stem prevents the flow of heat from the Tungsten to the bearings of anode assembly, due its small cross section. Thus, the *bearings* are protected from heat, which may cause them to expand and bind. Higher the length of the stem, higher the inertia of the Tungsten disk, more will be the load on the bearings. Hence, it is desirable to keep the stem as short as possible.

Rotor

Anode disk is connected to a *rotor* which is made up of *Copper bars* arranged around a cylindrical iron core. There are *electromagnets* surrounding the rotor, outside the glass envelope, referred as *stator* **(Fig. 3.15)**. Both the stator and rotor are called as an *induction motor*. When the stator coils are energized, a rotating magnetic field is produced, that induces current in the copper bars of rotor. This induced current produces an opposing magnetic field that causes the rotor to spin.

The rotor rotates at a speed of about 3,000–9,000 revolutions per minute (rpm). This will facilitate the electrons to bombard a constantly changing area of target. Since the electrical conductivity of Copper is higher, it will facilitate induction of strong currents from the induction coil voltage. The surface of the rotor is blackened to enhance heat dissipation by radiation process. The

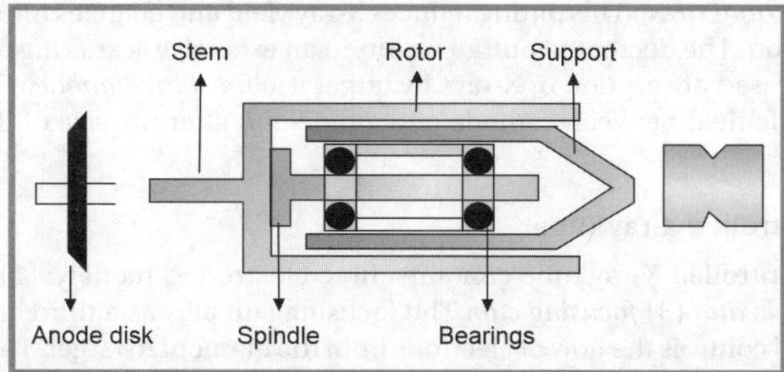

Fig. 3.15: Rotating anode X-ray tube and anode assembly inner view.

rotor support is made up of steel and positive high-tension supply is given at the end of rotor support outside the glass envelope.

Low speed rotor operates from 50 or 60 Hz power (single phase) and gives rotation of about 3,000 rpm. This speed is too slow for short exposure of the order of milli seconds. High speed rotor operates from 150 or 180 Hz power (3 phase) and gives a rotation speed of 10,000 rpm. As speed of rotation increases, the heat generated at the focus will be spread over a larger area on the anode. Modern X-ray tubes employ higher rotor speeds by increasing the frequency of stator supply with *frequency multiplying circuits*. The X-ray machines are designed so that the tube cannot be energized until the anode attains its full speed. This delay time (1 to 2 sec) is incorporated in the exposure switches. The power supplied to an induction coils produce *eddy current* which causes heating of the rotor.

Bearings

The anode assembly is rotated with the help of bearings, which are made of *steel ball races*. Bearings are in high vacuum environment and require special heat insensitive, *non-volatile lubricants*. The bearings are coated with *Lead or Silver* to act as *metallic lubricant*. Commonly available lubricants such as *oil and grease* cannot be used since they vaporize while heating and destroy the vacuum. Even dry lubricant like *graphite* would wear off as powder and destroy the vacuum.

When the X-ray unit is turned ON, the motor alone is energized first for a few seconds, until the rotor reaches its operating speed. Then, a high voltage is applied to the tube for a required exposure. After the exposure, the rotor is slowed down quickly by dynamic braking to avoid wear in bearings. Since the electrons are striking the whole circumference of the anode, no part of the anode attains very high temperature. The heat from the Tungsten disk is dissipated by radiating through vacuum to the wall of the X-ray tube, and then into the surrounding oil and tube housing.

The life of a rotating anode X-ray tube is limited, because of pitting due to continuous electron bombardment on an anode surface. These changes are due to *thermal stress*. This pitting reduces X-ray yield and changes the spectral distribution. The decreased output results in an excessive scattering of X-rays and increased absorption of X-rays by target itself. A *pitted anode* will affect the electric field between cathode and anode and alter the size of the focal spot.

Grid Controlled X-ray Tube

A grid-controlled X-ray tube contains three electrodes, namely: (1) *anode,* (2) *cathode and* (3) *focusing cup.* The focusing cup acts as a third electrode (grid) and controls the flow of electrons from the filament to target. The grid is electrically negative relative to filament. The voltage across the filament-grid produces an electric field along the path of an electron beam, that pushes the electrons even closer together. If large enough voltage is made, the tube current may be completely pinched OFF, and no electrons go from filament to target. The voltage applied between the focusing cup and filament acts like a switch to turn the tube current ON and OFF. Since the cup and filament are close together, the voltage necessary to cut OFF the tube current is not very large.

For example, a 0.3 mm focal spot tube operating at 105 kV requires about −1,500 V between the filament and focusing cup. This type of grid-controlled X-ray tubes are useful in some procedures involving rapid switching and short exposure times, e.g., Cini-angio-cardiography and pulsed fluoroscopy. These tubes are generally employed in interventional radiology and cardiology procedures.

QUALITY AND INTENSITY OF X-RAYS

Quality

The term quality describes the penetrating power of radiation and shape of the bremsstrahlung spectrum. Any change in kilovoltage will alter the spectrum shape as well as the efficiency. If radiation consists photons of single energy (mono-energy), then the quality can be described either by photon energy or wavelength. However, X-ray beam consists of many photon energies (heterogeneous) hence, its quality cannot be described by its photon energy. Therefore, the X-ray beam quality is usually specified by one of the following: (1) half-value layer, (2) applied voltage (kV), (3) filtration, and (4) effective photon energy.

Half-value Layer

The half-value layer (HVL) or half-value thickness (HVT) of a radiation beam is the required thickness of a material which reduces the beam intensity to one half. The half-value layer is always stated together with an applied voltage and filtration. *Aluminum* and *Copper* are the materials commonly used to specify HVL.

The HVL concept varies with beam homogeneity. In the case of a homogeneous beam, the first HVL reduces the beam intensity to half. The second HVL reduces the beam intensity further to ¼. It means that the first and second HVL are equal for a homogeneous beam. The X-ray beam is a continuous spectrum of non-homogeneous beam. It consists of both low and high energies. The low energy dominates and causes more in-homogeneity. The first HVL removes more low energy photons than the second HVL. Hence, the first and second HVL's are not equal. Since the first HVL removes only low energy photons, the useful beam is not affected much. The low energy photons are responsible for patient's skin dose. The second HVL affects the useful radiation energy photons, in turn the image contrast.

Usually, non-homogeneous beam can be expressed by equivalent energy. It is defined as the energy of mono-energetic beam which gives the same HVL as the non-homogeneous X-ray beam. To find the equivalent energy, one must know the μ of the X-ray beam:

$$\mu = \frac{0.693}{\text{HVL}}\ \text{cm}^{-1}$$

Using the linear attenuation co-efficient (μ) against photon energy graph of a homogeneous beam, one can find the equivalent energy of the X-ray beam.

Intensity

The term quantity refers to number of X-ray photons in the beam. Intensity is a measure of quantity of radiation. The intensity of a radiation beam is the energy flowing per unit area per unit time. It is equal to the number of photons in the beam multiplied by the energy of each photon. Terms like photon fluence, photon flux, energy fluence and energy flux are often used to describe X-ray beam intensity.

Photon fluence is the intensity per unit area and the photon flux is the photon fluence per second. Energy fluence is the product of photon fluence and photon energy. This is true for a mono-energetic beam. In the case of poly-energetic beam, the number of photons of each energy multiplied by its energy, and their sum gives the energy fluence. Energy fluence per unit time is called energy flux density or intensity of the beam. The energy flux density varies with Z, mA, and kV. Beam intensity is commonly measured in roentgens per minute (R/min) or air-kerma rate, and it is responsible for the degree of blackness (density) on the X-ray film.

The term exposure is often used in radiology, which is proportional to the energy fluence of the X-ray beam. It refers to both quality and quantity of the X-ray beam approximately.

Factors Affecting Quality and Intensity of X-ray Beam

X-ray production efficiency, quality, quantity, and intensity are affected by seven factors, namely: (1) applied voltage, (2) tube current, (3) filtration,

(4) target material, (5) exposure time, (6) generator waveform, and (7) distance.

Applied Voltage (kV)

Applied voltage affects both quality and intensity of X-rays. Energy of the photon emitted from the X-ray tube depends on electrons energy that bombards the target. The energy of the electrons in turn, is determined by peak kilo voltage applied. As applied voltage increases, the effective photon energy in the bremsstrahlung also increases. The maximum photon energy is proportional to peak value of an applied voltage. In addition, the X-ray production efficiency also related to applied voltage. The intensity increases with increase of applied voltage **(Figs. 3.16A and B)**. The amount of radiation produced increases as the square of the kilo voltage:

$$\text{Radiation exposure} \propto (kV)^2$$

Thus, increase in kV increases quality, quantity, and efficiency of X-ray production.

Tube Current (mA)

The number of X-rays produced depends on number of electrons that strike the target of the X-ray tube. The number of electrons depends directly on tube current (mA) used. Greater the mA, larger the electrons that are produced, resulting higher number of X-rays. The tube current affects only intensity but not the quality of X-rays. As the tube current increases, the intensity also increases:

$$\text{Intensity} \propto mA$$

Increase of applied voltage is compensated by reduction of tube current, which is required to maintain same exposure. The ratio of mAs varies with 5th power of kV ratio:

$$(kV_1/kV_2)^5 = mAs_2/mAs_1$$

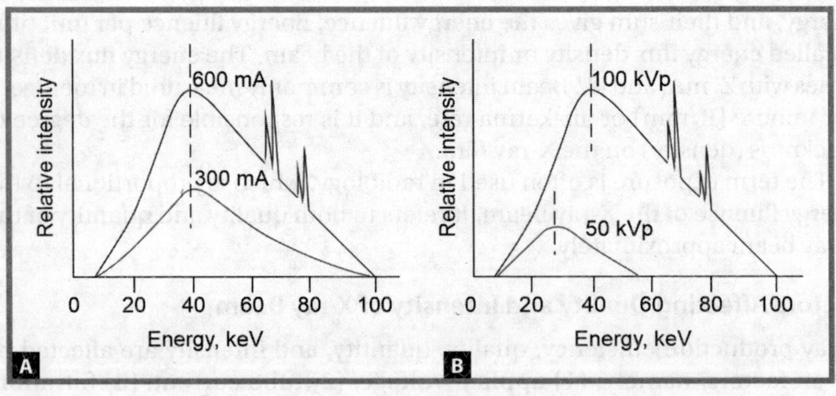

Figs. 3.16A and B: Effect of: (A) Tube current; (B) Kilo voltage on the X-ray spectra.

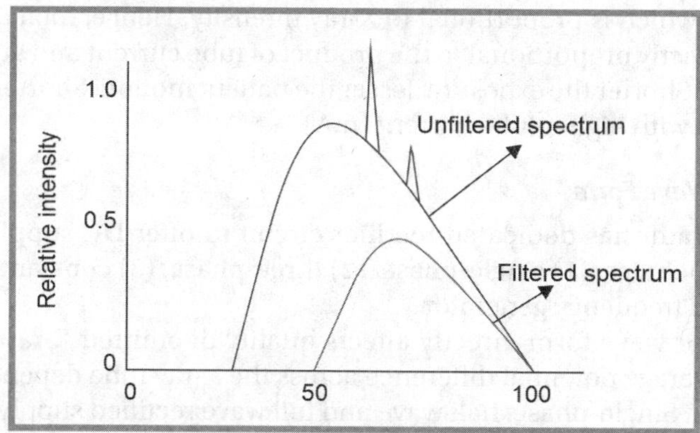

Fig. 3.17: Effect of filter on X-ray spectra.

Filtration

Filters are thin sheet of material (*Al, Cu, Mo*) which offer high attenuation for low energy photons. The purpose of using filter is to reduce patient exposure at skin level. Filters alter both quality and quantity of X-rays, by selectively removing low energy photons in the spectrum. This reduces the photon number (quantity) and shifts the average energy to higher values, by increasing beam quality. A filtered beam consists higher photon energies and is said to be hardened **(Fig. 3.17)**.

However, there are filters which can remove the high energy photons selectively, such filters are called *K-edge filters*. This concept is used in mammography to remove photon energy greater than 28 keV. Higher the filter thickness, lesser the patient's skin entrance dose. The required thickness of filter depends upon the kV and clinical application. Recommended filter should be used to have an optimal X-ray output. Checking the filter thickness is one of the quality assurance (QA) program for X-ray units.

Target Material (Z)

Atomic number of target material affects the intensity of the X-rays. The intensity increases with an increase of atomic number. X-ray production is more efficient, if higher the atomic number of target material. For example, *Tungsten* (Z = 74) would produce much more bremsstrahlung, than *Tin* (Z = 50), if both were used as target material under identical kV and mA.

The atomic number of target material also determines the energy (quality) of characteristic X-rays. Thus, atomic number of the target material determines the intensity of bremsstrahlung and quality of characteristic X-rays produced.

Exposure Time

Exposure time determines the length of X-ray production. It refers to beam ON time and directly proportional to an intensity of X-rays. Shorter exposure gives low intensity, whereas long exposure gives higher intensity. It is like mA of the

X-ray tube, which is proportional to X-ray intensity. Hence, total quantity of X-rays is directly proportional to the product of tube current and an exposure time (mAs). Shorter the exposure, lesser the patient motion. Shorter exposure always goes with higher tube current (mA).

Generator Wave Form

X-ray generator has dedicated rectifier circuit to offer DC supply. Type of generator includes: (1) single-phase, (2) three-phase, (3) constant potential, and (4) high frequency generator.

Generator wave form directly affects quality of emitted X-ray spectrum since the average potential difference across the X-ray tube depends on type of generator. Single-phase, half wave and full wave rectified supply offer only pulsating potential, resulting higher patient dose. A three-phase generator provides higher average applied voltage compared to that of single-phase. However, they are more expensive, has complex circuitry, and larger in size.

High frequency generator provides high frequency AC waveform up to 500–2,500 Hz. It is rectified and smoothened to provide a constant voltage supply. They provide accurate kV and mA with good reproducibility with high output. It not only gives constant potential but also improves image quality with lesser patient dose. They are much efficient and less costly.

Distance

The X-ray beam intensity decreases with distance from the target, because of divergence of the beam. The decrease in intensity is proportional to square of the distance from the target. The nonlinear fall-off intensity with distance is called an *inverse square law*. In general, if the distance from the X-ray source is changed from X to Y, then X-ray beam intensity changes by $(X/Y)^2$. If X = 1 m and Y = 2 m, then the intensity decreases by a factor of 4. Thus, doubling the distance from the X-ray source decreases the X-ray beam intensity by a factor of 4. If the distance is increased by a factor of 3, then the X-ray beam intensity decreases by a factor of 9, and so on. To summarize, the intensity (I) of X-ray radiation is given by the relation:

$$I \propto \frac{kV^2 \times mA \times Z}{d^2}$$

where, d is the distance between target and the point of measurement or source to image distance (SID).

Abdominal and pelvis X-rays are taken at 100 cm SID, whereas chest PA view is taken at 180 cm. This means that the former gives higher X-ray output, compared to chest PA view. Any imaging involving shorter SID, less than 100 cm, result in higher X-ray output, leading to greater amount of patient exposure, which is undesirable.

In practice, the X-ray intensity is usually referred as X-ray tube output and is measured in mR/mAs or μR/mAs, for a given kV. This means that the X-ray tube gives the intensity in milli or micro-roentgens, for unit mA tube current, for unit exposure time, s for a given kV. Usually, X-ray output ranges from 3 to

10 mR/mAs at 100 cm, for 70 kV setting. Measurement of X-ray output is one of the requirement of quality assurance program, which needs to be measured once in 2 years. This is very much required for e-LORA registration of X-ray units, as per present national regulations.

BIBLIOGRAPHY

1. Bushberg JT, Seibert J A, Leidholdt EM Jr, Boone JM. The Essential Physics of Medical Imaging, 3rd edn. Lippincott Williams and Wilkins, Philadelphia; 2012.
2. Thayalan K. Basic Radiological Physics, 2nd edn. Jaypee Brothers Medical Publishers (P) Ltd, New Delhi; 2017.
3. Thayalan K. The Physics of Radiation Oncology, Jaypee Brothers Medical Publishers (P) Ltd, New Delhi; 2023.

Radiation Interaction with Matter and Units

PHOTON INTERACTION

When X or γ radiation passes through a medium, they interact with atoms and molecules and does ionization and excitation. As a result, moving electrons are produced. Atoms and molecules absorb radiation energy and result in production of free radicals; *OH* and H**. These free radicals interact with biomolecules such as DNA and causes damage to cell, leading to *biological effects*. In addition, enough heat is also produced.

Electrons travel further in the medium, interact with other atoms, and produce ionization and excitation. As a result, energy is deposited on the cells, which are either damaged partially or completely. To conclude, the X or γ photon transfer energy to the electrons, in turn transfer the energy to the cells and produce biological effect. That is why X or γ photons are called as indirectly ionizing radiations (indirect action). Radiation also deposits energy directly on the DNA molecule and causes biological effect, which is known as *direct action*.

The above interaction is said to have wavelike and particle like properties. X and gamma rays interact with structures that are similar in size to their wavelength. Low energy photons tend to interact with atoms, medium energy to that of electrons, and high energy photons with that of nuclei. The above structural level interactions may be performed by five mechanisms:

❑ Coherent scattering
❑ Photoelectric absorption
❑ Compton scattering
❑ Pair production
❑ Photodisintegration.

Compton scattering, photoelectric absorption, and pair production are most important interactions in diagnostic radiology.

Coherent or Rayleigh Scattering

The photon interacts with electron of an atom and sets the atom in an excited state **(Fig. 4.1)**. The electric field of photon spends energy so that all the

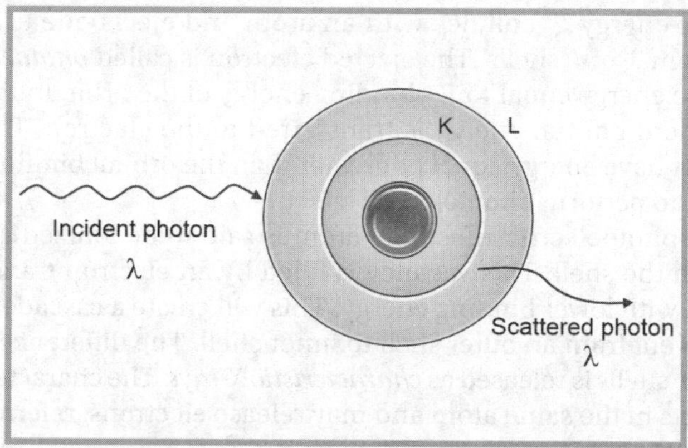

Fig. 4.1: Coherent scattering: The incident photon makes the atom to oscillates and the scattered photon goes in different direction with same wavelength.

electrons in atom oscillate in phase. The excited atom releases the excess energy as scattered X-ray with wavelength equal to the incident photon. The emitted radiation will have same energy of an incident photon, but the direction of the scattered photon is different to that of the incident photon.

Thus, in coherent scattering, the photon undergoes a change in direction without change in wavelength. In this process, no energy is transferred, no ionization occurs and mostly photons are scattered in the forward direction. In coherent scattering, no energy is converted into kinetic energy, and all are scattered. As photon energy increases, average scattering angle decreases. Its role in soft tissue is only about 5% above 70 keV photon energy. This interaction occurs mainly at low energy photons (15–30 keV), especially in mammography imaging.

Photoelectric Absorption

In the photoelectric absorption or effect (PE), photon transfers its full energy to an orbital electron and an electron is ejected from an atom **(Fig. 4.2)**.

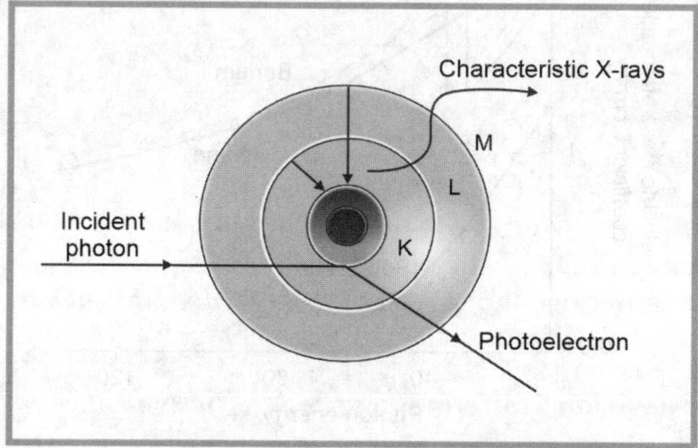

Fig. 4.2: Photoelectric effect.

A photon of energy E_o collides with an atom and ejects one of the bound electrons from K or L shells. The ejected electron is called *photoelectron* and it has kinetic energy equal to E_o–binding energy of the orbit. In this process, all the incident photon energy is transferred to the electron. The incident photon must have energy equal or greater than the orbital binding energy of an electron, to perform photoelectric effect.

After the photoelectric effect, the atom is said to be ionized and there is a vacancy in the shell. This vacancy is filled by an electron transition from higher orbit with lower binding energy. This will create a cascade of electron transition event from an outer shell to inner shell. The difference in binding energy of the shells is released as *characteristic X-rays*. The characteristic X-ray later interacts in the same atom and may release electrons, referred as *Auger electrons.*

The characteristics X-ray emission decreases in low Z material, hence it is rare in soft tissue imaging. The probability of photoelectric cross section per unit mass is proportional to $\dfrac{Z^3}{E_o^3}$, where, Z is atomic number and E_o is incident photon energy. As the X-ray photon energy increases, the subject contrast decreases. As the atomic number increases, the subject contrast increases, that is why Barium (Z = 56) and Iodine (Z = 53) are used as contrast agents.

Even though photoelectric effect decreases with an increase of energy, there are sharp discontinuity called *absorption edge* at some energy **(Fig. 4.3)**. The plot describes the relation between probability of photoelectric absorption and photon energy. As energy increases, photoelectric absorption decreases, then sudden raise in absorption is seen for some photon energy. At this photon energy the probability of photoelectric absorption is higher. This energy is called as an *absorption edge or K-edge* of that material, e.g., 33.2 keV of Iodine. Thus, tightly bound electron has more probability for photoelectric

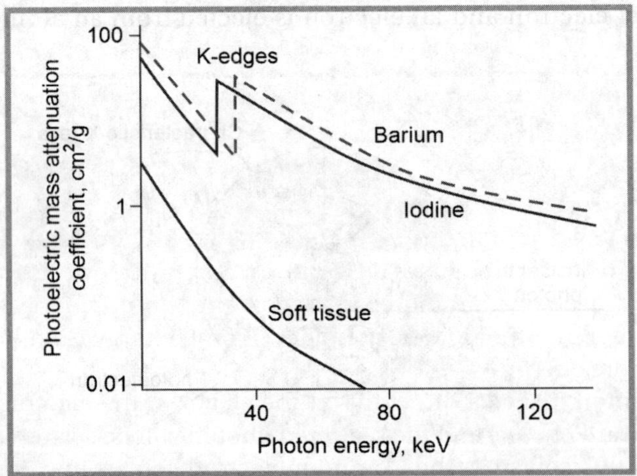

Fig. 4.3: Photoelectric absorption as a function of photon energy.

absorption and maximum absorption occurs when the photon has just sufficient energy to eject bound electrons.

Absorption edge of elements with photon energy increases with atomic number. For example, Iodine, Barium, and Lead absorption edges are 33.2, 37.4 and 88 keV, respectively, whereas H, C, N, and O has absorption edges in soft tissue well below <1 keV. Photoelectric effect absorption is much important in soft tissue imaging for photon energy < 50 keV. It will differentiate an attenuation between two tissues with slightly varying atomic number. This is called *differential absorption* and it plays a major role in diagnostic radiology.

In summary, photoelectric effect involves tightly bound electrons. The tightly bound electrons are mostly available in the K-shell hence, most photoelectric interactions occur at K-shell of an atom.

Compton Scattering

In compton scattering, photon interacts with a free or valance electron of an atom and gets scattered with partial energy **(Fig. 4.4).** The other part of energy is given to the valence electron, which is ejected from the atom. The ejected electron is called *Compton electron* which further loses energy by an ionization and excitation of atoms in the medium. The scattered photon further travels in the medium with or without interaction by Compton scattering or photoelectric absorption. It will have longer wavelength compared to an incident photon. The energy of an incident photon (E_0) is equal to the sum of the energy of the scattered photon (E_{sc}) and the kinetic energy (E_{e-}) of an ejected electron. Compton electron energy can be calculated by laws of conservation of energy and momentum as follows:

$$E_0 = E_{sc} + E_{e-}$$

$$E_{sc} = \frac{E_0}{1 + \alpha\,(1 - \cos\theta)}$$

$$E_{e-} = E_0 \frac{\alpha\,(1 - \cos\theta)}{1 + \alpha\,(1 - \cos\theta)}$$

$$\mathrm{Cos}\,\phi = (1 + \alpha)\,\tan\theta/2$$

where, θ is the angle of scattered photon.

$$\alpha = \frac{E_0}{m_0 c^2} = \frac{E_0}{0.511\ \text{meV}}$$

where, $m_0 c^2$ is rest mass energy of electron.

As the incident photon energy increases, both photons and electrons are scattered in forward direction. The fraction of energy transferred to scattered photon decreases with an increase of incident photon energy, for a given angle of scatter. In other words, at higher photon energy Compton electron will carry more energy.

If the photon makes a direct hit on the electron, the electron will travel straight forward $(\phi = 0^\circ)$ and the scattered photon will be scattered back with $\theta = 180^\circ$. In this collision, the Compton electron gets its maximum energy, while scattered photon goes with minimum energy.

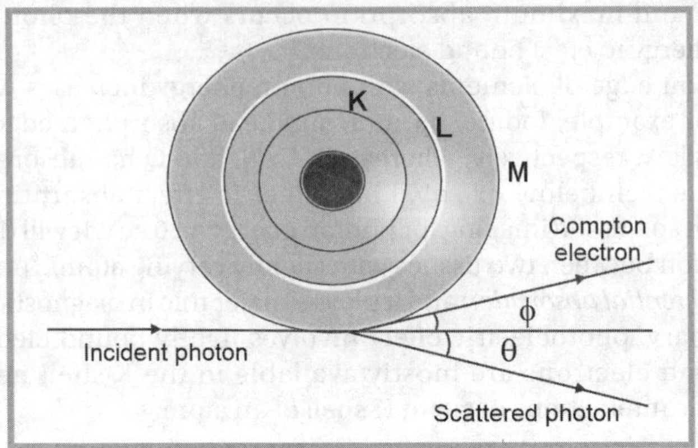

Fig. 4.4: Compton scattering.

$$E_{sc} = \frac{E_0}{1 + 2\alpha}$$

$$E_{e-} = E_0 \frac{2\alpha}{1 + 2\alpha}$$

If the photon makes a grazing hit with an electron, the Compton electron will be emitted at right angles ($\phi = 90°$) and the scattered photon will go in forward direction ($\theta = 0°$). In this collision, the electron receives minimal energy, and the scattered photon goes with maximal energy:

$$E_{sc} = E_0, \; E_{e-} = 0$$

Scattered photon may have maximum energy of 0.511 MeV and 0.255 MeV for its scatter angle of 90° and 180°, respectively. The Compton electron can go up to 90° only, whereas scattered photon can go up to 180°.

Compton scattering involves an interaction between a photon and a free electron, resulting ionization of atom. The incident photon energy is shared between scattered photon and an ejected electron. The probability of Compton scattering depends upon electron density (Number of electrons per gram × Density) in the medium. Except Hydrogen, the electron density is constant for tissues, and Compton mass attenuation coefficient is independent of atomic number (Z). Absence of neutron doubles electron density in Hydrogen. Hence, *hydrogenous material* has higher probability for Compton scattering. Compton interaction decreases with an increase of photon energy, it is $\propto 1/E_0$. The probability per unit volume is proportional to density of the material.

Compton scattering occurs in all energies in tissues, important in Diagnostic radiology, Nuclear Medicine and Radiation therapy. It is a predominant interaction in diagnostic energy range (100 keV to 10 MeV) in soft tissue. Scattered X-rays provide no useful information, reduces image contrast, and increases patient dose. In fluoroscopy, large amounts of radiation is scattered from patient and contributes to an occupational radiation exposure.

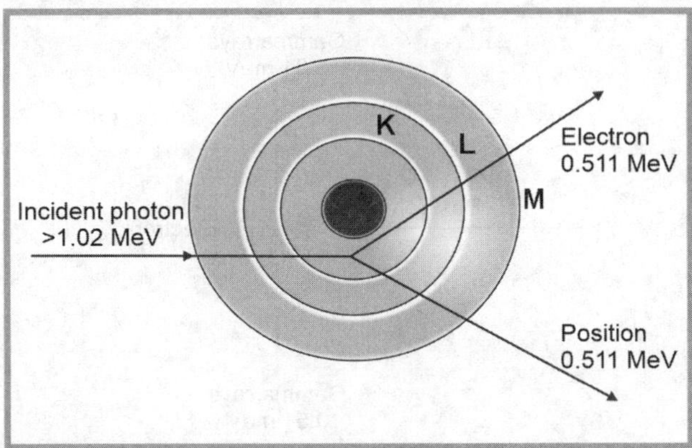

Fig. 4.5: Pair production.

Pair Production

When a photon having energy >1.02 MeV, passes near the nucleus of an atom, will be subjected to strong nuclear field **(Fig. 4.5)**. The photon interacts with an electric field of the nucleus and transfer energy to a positron and electron pair. This is known as *pair production* and each particle requires 0.511 MeV energy equal to its rest mass energy. The excess energy $(E_0 - 1.02$ MeV$)$ would be shared between positron and electron as kinetic energy. The particles are set in motion in forward direction with respect to an incident photon. The electron and positron lose their kinetic energy further by an ionization and excitation in the medium. This process is an example for conversion of energy into mass as predicted by **Einstein's** equation, $E = mc^2$.

In pair production, the interaction is between a photon and nuclear field. Pair production is a true absorption because all the energy of original photon is transformed. Threshold energy for pair production process is 1.02 MeV and its probability increases with an increase of photon energy. Thus, high energy photon is more easily stopped by pair production process, than low energy photon. This means that high energy beam is less penetrating than low energy beam if the attenuation is by pair production. This is the major difference compared with other interactions.

Probability of pair production depends on *Z^2 per atom, Z per electron* and *about Z per gram*. Its probability increases as logarithm of an incident photon energy, above threshold energy. It is more important for photons having energy > 5 MeV.

Positron Annihilation

The electron loses energy by an excitation and ionization and filling vacancy in the orbital shells. The positron travels in the medium and loses its energy by ionization, excitation, and bremsstrahlung process. At the end of its range, positron comes to rest and combines with a free electron from the surrounding and produces two gamma photons of each energy of 0.511 MeV.

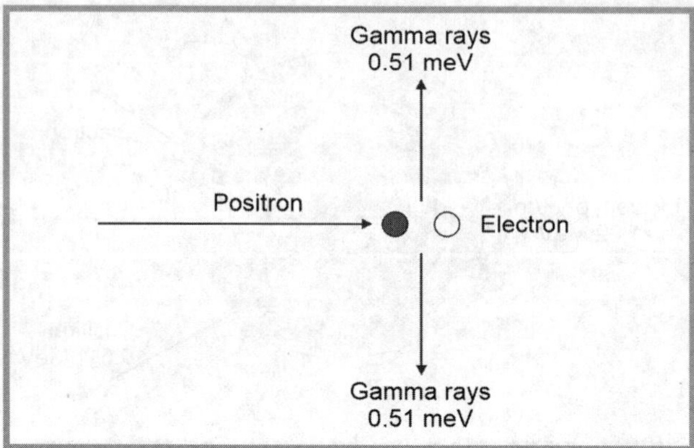

Fig. 4.6: Positron joins with an electron and undergoes annihilation with emission of two gamma photons of each energy of 0.51 MeV.

These two photons are ejected in opposite directions, to conserve momentum **(Fig. 4.6).** The combined mass (1.02 MeV) of two particles is converted into energy, and shared by two gamma photons. The above process is called *positron annihilation*. This is an example of conversion of mass into energy as per **Einstein's** hypothesis stated earlier, and forms the basis for *positron emission tomography (PET)*.

Apart from pair production, *triplet* production is also possible at high energies. When a photon having energy >2.04 MeV interacts with an electron, three particles will appear. They are positron and electron that is created and orbital electron. Threshold energy for triplet production is 2.04 MeV, it is twice the threshold energy of pair production. The triplet production is small, compared with pair production.

PARTICLE INTERACTION

Particle radiation includes alpha, beta, proton, electron, positron, neutron, and heavy nuclei. Heavy nuclei, alpha and protons are heavier particles compared to that of electrons and positrons. The behavior of heavy particles is different from lighter particles. However, both light and heavy charged particle have some common features. Neutron is an uncharged particle. Particle interaction is divided into:

❑ Heavy charged particle interactions, e.g., proton, alpha, heavy nuclei
❑ Light charged particle interactions, e.g., electron
❑ Neutron interaction

Ionization and Excitation

Charged particle collision mainly takes place in atoms and molecules of a medium. Particle is attracted to charges of opposite sign and repelled to charges of like sign. These forces of attraction and repulsion are called *Coulomb force interactions*. When a charged particle goes near the atom, it interacts with its electrical forces and may remove an electron from the orbit, referred as *ionization*.

The charged particle loses energy in the interaction, part of energy is used to overcome binding energy of an orbital electron. Remaining energy is given to the ejected secondary electron as kinetic energy. Hence, condition for ionization is that the particle energy should exceed the binding energy of an electron. During ionization, an electron and a positive atom pair is produced, which is said to be *ion pairs*. The energy required to produce one such an ion pair in air and soft tissue is 34 eV and 22 eV, respectively.

In the case of inner orbit electrons, an ionization is followed by emission of *characteristic X-rays and Auger electrons*. If the interaction takes place with outer orbit electrons, the above emissions are much smaller. However, ejected electron is capable of causing secondary ionization, and such electron is called *delta rays*. The delta rays may have sufficient energy to cause further ionization in the medium. A 10 keV electron may produce about 450 secondary electrons of energy of 10-7 eV. Majority of the charged particle interaction involves outer orbit electrons.

To a lesser degree the charged particle interacts with an inner orbital electron and moves the electron to higher orbits, which is called an *excitation*. The energy loss is lesser than that of an ionization energy loses. In an excitation, the particle transfers its energy to an orbital electron and the transferred energy should be less than the binding energy of an electron. The transferred energy will be spent as molecular vibrations, infrared emission, visible and ultraviolet radiation, etc.

The above loss of energy by an ionization and excitation is referred as *collational losses*. The ionization and excitation occur along the path of charged particle in a medium. The rate of energy loss is proportional to an electron density of the medium. The collisional energy loss depends on the ratio of Z of the medium and kinetic energy (E_{KE}) of the particle (Z/E_{KE}). About 70% of the charged particle's energy is spent via an ionization. As an electron energy decreases, the probability of an excitation increases.

Bremsstrahlung Process

If the charged particle overcomes the orbital electron cloud and reaches nearer the nucleus of an atom, an interaction between charged particle and nucleus takes place. In the case of heavy charged particles like proton or alpha, such nuclear reaction leads to production of radionuclides, e.g., proton can produce positron emitters such as ^{11}C, ^{13}N and ^{15}O in tissue. The condition is that the charged particle should have energy sufficient to overcome the Coulomb force and interacts with nuclei.

Alternatively, the nucleus can exert strong electrical force on the particle, and the particle may be deflected. Light charged particles like an electron undergoes similar action and get deflected. The deflected particle undergo deceleration and loses energy gradually, which is called *bremsstrahlung X-rays*. The bremsstrahlung may have energy from zero to maximum and forms a continuous spectrum.

Radiative Losses

Charged particle collision with nuclei of an atom is an inelastic collision results in bremsstrahlung, is called *radiative loss*. The probability of bremsstrahlung production depends on atomic number (Z) of the medium, mass (m), charge (q), and energy (E) of the particle as given below:

$$\text{Probability} \propto \frac{q^2 Z^2}{m^2 E^2}$$

Bremsstrahlung production depends on how the particle is closer to the nucleus. Particle closer to the nucleus radiates more energy in the direction perpendicular to the particle travel. Bremsstrahlung is more likely for light charged particle and it is negligible for heavy charged particle. Hence, the bremsstrahlung emission from alpha and proton particles is much low.

Ionization and excitation or collisional energy loss usually takes place in light Z material like tissue, whereas radiative energy loss happens in high Z medium. The ratio of radiative energy loss and collisional energy loss is expressed as follows:

$$\frac{\text{Radiative energy loss}}{\text{Collisional energy loss}} = \frac{E_{KE} \times Z}{82{,}000}$$

where, Z is an atomic number of the medium and E_{KE} is the kinetic energy of the particle. In the energy range of 10 keV–10 MeV, the ionization energy loss dominates over an excitation energy loss. If an electron with 75 keV energy interacts with a Tungsten target (Z = 74), then the above ratio = (75 × 72)/820,000 = 0.0065 = 0.65%. That is <1% energy appear as X-rays, whereas >99% appear as heat.

Neutron Interaction

Neutrons are uncharged particles, do not interact by Coulomb forces and prefer direct collisions. It interacts in three ways, namely:
- Elastic collision with nuclei
- Inelastic collision with nuclei
- Neutron capture

In an *elastic collision* the kinetic energy of neutron is redistributed between neutron and the nuclei, the energy is same before and after collision. This type of collision or scattering is called *neutron moderation*. Fast moving neutron prefer elastic collisions. The above principle is used in nuclear reactor to moderates neutrons hence, moderators are employed. In an *inelastic collision*, the neutron is absorbed by the medium with formation of compound nucleus, which is in an exited state and later releases neutron and gamma rays. This type of an interaction mostly happens to high energy neutron with heavier nuclei, referred as *neutron resonance scattering*. The elastic and an inelastic collision of neutron with an orbital electron is negligible.

Neutron capture is a similar process, but the compound nucleus emits gamma rays, e.g., ^{60}Co production. Slow moving or thermal electrons prefer this type of interaction. The probability for neutron capture is high for slow neutrons then fast neutrons and results in release of high energy. For example, if neutron is captured by Hydrogen, it is converted into deuterium (^{2}H) with emission of gamma rays of energy of 2.22 MeV.

Neutrons have small cross section, easily penetrates medium without interaction. Unlike charged particle, neutron has no range in the medium. The energy transfer depends on the direction of neutron and nuclei after collision. It follows the laws of conservation energy and momentum. Neutrons transfer their kinetic energy to the nuclei, and it depends on the size of recoil nuclei. The energy transfer is poor in high Z material, and they offer poor shielding for neutron. Maximum energy transfer occurs when the nuclei happen to interact with a proton, which is having same mass of neutron. In neutron-proton collision, the proton carries all the energy, and neutron is completely stooped. That is why Hydrogen rich material is used for neutron shielding. Hence, shielding materials for neutron is *water, paraffin wax, polyethylene, and plastic*, which are basically *hydrogenous* material. Though Lead is good shield for X-rays, it is poor towards neutron shielding.

Neutron interaction has no specific role in Nuclear medicine and Diagnostic radiology. Whenever neutron is used as therapy, the dose is deposited through protons. Since fat is rich in Hydrogen it absorbs more dose (20%) than soft tissue. Neutron mostly produce proton, neutron and gamma rays and its dosimetry is much complex.

ATTENUATION

When radiation travels in a medium it gets absorbed and scattered due to various interaction process as stated earlier. Either single interaction or combination of interactions help absorption and scattering in the medium. *Attenuation* is removal of photons from the beam, it is the product of an absorption and scattering. When a beam passes through an absorber, some photons are removed, and some are transmitted **(Fig. 4.7)**. Transmitted beam does not interact with an absorber and will have lesser number of photons.

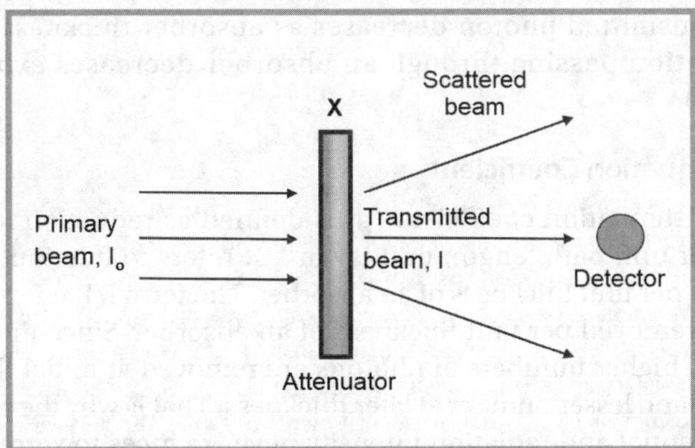

Fig. 4.7: Attenuation of radiation through an absorber of thickness x.

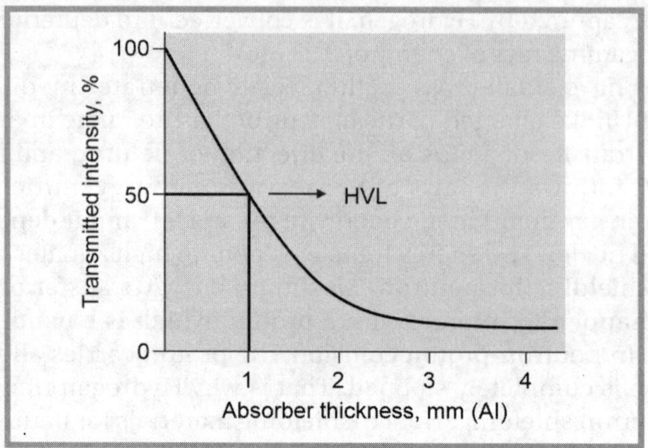

Fig. 4.8: Exponential attenuation of radiation and half-value layer.

Let N is number of incident photons and dN is number of photons removed in an absorber of thickness, dx, then:

$$dN = -\mu Ndx$$

$$\text{or } \frac{dN}{N} = -\mu dx$$

$$\text{or } \frac{dI}{I} = -\mu dx, \text{ if N is proportional I}$$

where, the I is intensity of the radiation having N number of photons. It means that if either N is doubled μ or is doubled, the chance of an interaction is also doubled. The above differential equation is solved and written, in terms of intensity:

$$I = I_o e^{-\mu x}$$

where, I is transmitted intensity of radiation, I_o is incident intensity on absorber, e is base of natural logarithm, and μ is linear attenuation coefficient of the absorber, and x is thickness of absorber. The minus sign indicates that number transmitted photon decreases as absorber thickness increases. Thus, radiation passing through an absorber decreases *exponentially* **(Figure 4.8)**.

Linear Attenuation Coefficient

The linear attenuation coefficient (μ) is defined as reduction in radiation intensity per unit path length, unit is cm^{-1}. It refers to fraction of photons that interact per unit thickness of an absorber. The term I/I_0 refers to fraction of photons removed per unit thickness of an absorber. Since the relation is logarithmic, higher numbers of photons are removed at initial thickness of an absorber and lesser number at later thickness. That is why the relationship is an exponential and radiation intensity never reduces to zero. The linear attenuation coefficient depends on photon energy and material density.

Worked Example–4.1

Calculate the linear attenuation coefficient of a material of thickness 1.8 mm, which reduces the intensity to 50%.

Here x = 1.8 mm, I/I_0 = ½ = 0.5, log 0.5 = 0.693

$$\mu = -(1/1.8) \times 0.693 = 0.38 \text{ cm}^{-1}$$

Note: $\mu = \dfrac{1}{x} \log \dfrac{I}{I_0}$

Narrow and Broad Beam Geometry

Radiation beam has both narrow and broad beam geometry. A narrow beam geometry is one which minimizes scattered radiation. On the other hand, broad beam geometry is one in which many scattered photons are recorded. A thick absorber is one in which the probability of photon interaction is >10%. A thick absorber with narrow and broad beam geometry is shown in **Fig. 4.9**.

In narrow beam geometry, scattered photons are not accounted by the detector. The detector receives only transmitted radiation through an attenuator and transmitted intensity consists only primary beam. The conditions for narrow beam geometry state that beam is well collimated with a narrow aperture at source. It will restrict probability of photon striking the wall and scattering towards the detector. Additional collimation at detector level will also improve arrangement. Absorber should be placed preferably midway between source and detector. Under these conditions, transmission of a monoenergetic beam obey the relation:

$$I = I_0 e^{-\mu x}$$

In the case of broad beam geometry, the beam is wider, not well collimated, and scattered photons are present always. Detector captures both transmitted primary and scattered radiation, and underestimate attenuation, resulting an increased HVL. Attenuation coefficient is not constant, it depends on thickness of absorber, its area, shape, photon energy and distance between

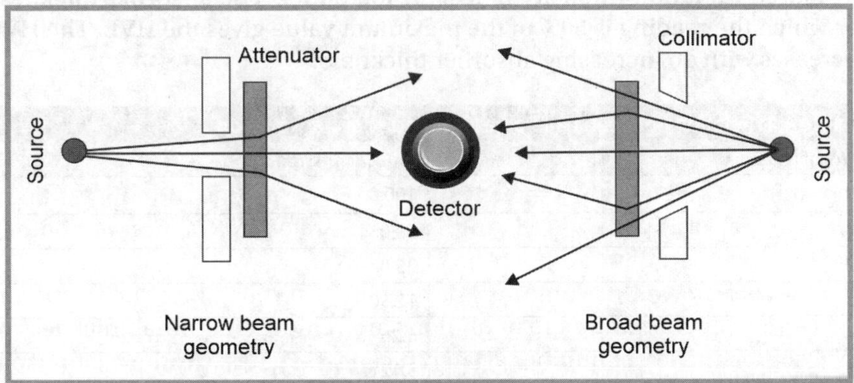

Fig. 4.9: Narrow and broad beam geometry: Broad beam geometry capture scattered radiation, underestimates attenuation and increases the HVL.

attenuator and detector. The attenuation curve is not an exponential in such cases. Increased transmissions in broad beam geometry relative to narrow beam geometry is called *build-up factor (B)*. If *T* is transmission factor for broad beam geometry, then:

$$T = B\,e^{-\mu x}$$

where, μ is linear attenuation coefficient, and x is thickness of absorber.

Shielding efficiency of a medium is good in narrow beam geometry and it is poor in broad beam geometry. In other words, narrow beam geometry requires lesser shielding thickness than broad beam geometry. Most of patient imaging conditions mimics broad beam geometry both in Diagnostic radiology and Nuclear medicine.

Half-value Layer

As stated earlier, *half-value layer (HVL)* is the thickness required to reduce radiation beam intensity to half of its original value. HVL is also referred as *half-value thickness (HVT)*. It is related to linear attenuation coefficient as:

$$HVL = \frac{0.693}{\mu}$$

HVL is constant for monoenergetic photons of narrow beam geometry. When an attenuator has *n* number of HVL thickness, then reduction of beam intensity is $(1/2)^n$. **Table 4.1** indicates decrease of radiation intensity with increasing HVLs (for heavily filtered X-ray beam). Average distance travelled by a photon in an absorber before encountering another interaction is called *mean free path* (X_m), it is related to HVL as:

$$X_m = \frac{HVL}{\ln 2} = 1.44 \times HVL$$

HVL can be measured under a narrow beam geometry by keeping the detector away from absorber. This is to detect only transmitted radiation and avoid scattered radiation. The radiation exposure is measured by varying absorber of different thickness. A graph is drawn between absorber thickness and measured radiation intensity in a semi-log paper. The absorber thickness for which the reading is 50% of the maximum value gives the HVL. The HVL increases with an increasing absorber thickness.

Table 4.1: Relation between half-value layer and % of transmission.

No. of HVLs	% Transmission
0	100.0
1	50.0
2	25.0
3	12.50
4	6.25
5	3.12
6	1.56

(*Courtesy:* Jerrold T Bushberg et al, 2012)

There is another term called *tenth value layer* (TVL) or *tenth value thickness* (TVT), which gives thickness of material that attenuates X-ray beam by 90%. This quantity is very useful in room shielding calculations for Diagnostic radiology and Nuclear medicine. The TVL and HVL is related as follows:

$$\text{TVL} = \frac{\ln 10}{\mu} = \frac{2.303}{0.693/\text{HVL}} = 3.32\,\text{HVL}$$

Worked Example–4.2

Calculate the HVL of X-ray beam, which passes through an absorber whose linear attenuation coefficient is 0.35 cm^{-1}.

$\mu = 0.35$ cm^{-1}

HVL $= 0.693/0.35 = 1.98$ cm

Worked Example–4.3

X-ray beam passes through an absorber of thickness 2 mm with transmission of 25%. Calculate the TVL of the beam.

Here x = 2 mm or 0.2 cm, $I/I_0 = 0.25$, **Note:** $\mu = \dfrac{1}{x}\log\dfrac{I}{I_0}$

$\mu = -\,(1/0.2) \times \log 0.25 = 3.01$ cm^{-1}

HVL $= 0.693/\mu$

$\quad\quad = 0.693/3.01 = 0.23$ cm,

and TVL $= 3.32 \times 0.23 = 0.76$ cm

Effective Energy

Attenuation coefficient varies with photon energy. Photon may be monoenergetic or polychromatic in nature. Linear attenuation coefficient is defined for monoenergetic beams of narrow beam geometry. There is difficulty in the application of this coefficient to polychromatic beams such as X-rays. Hence, an effective energy of a radiation is defined as the energy of monoenergetic beam that have same attenuation character. The effective energy thus obtained from monoenergetic beam data can be plotted vs HVL **(Fig. 4.10A).** It gives the relation between HVL and effective energy of orthovoltage beams. Since attenuation is based on μ, in turn μ is related to HVL, both can also be used to define an effective energy. If monoenergetic beam has same μ or HVL of radiation, then the effective energy of radiation is equal to that of monoenergetic beam.

Lead is often used as HVL material for megavoltage beams. However, it is not a good tool to define beam quality in that energy range. Low atomic number material like water is more sensitive than high Z material like Lead in the above energy range **(Fig. 4.10B).** Lead HVL increases initially and decreases as an energy increases beyond 20 MeV. This is due to mass attenuation coefficient of Lead which decreases initially, later increases as an energy increases. In the case of water, it continuously decreases with energy.

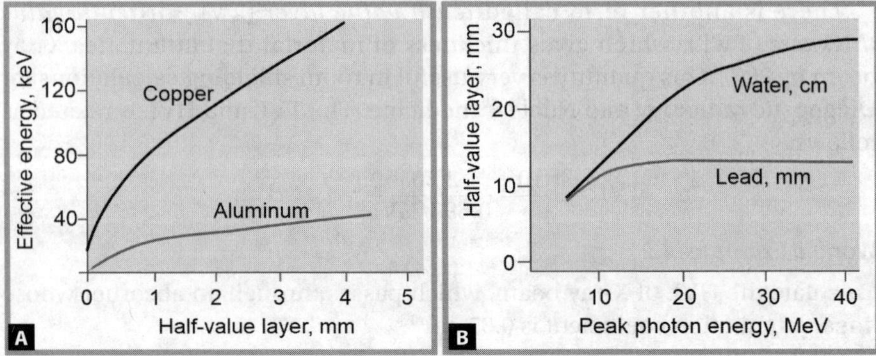

Figs. 4.10A and B: (A) Relation between effective energy and half-value layer, for orthovoltage beams, data obtained from the attenuation coefficients of monoenergetic beam; (B) Peak photon energy vs half-value layer for megavoltage beams relative to lead (mm) and water (cm).

Beam Hardening

Many radioisotopes or X-ray generator emit photons of more than one energy. Photon transmission curve of the source is equal to sum of exponentials of each photon energy. Transmission curve drops steeply at first due to removal of low energy components. Later, the curve flattens out due to greater penetration of high energy photons. Average energy of remaining photons increases with an increasing absorber thickness, which is called *beam hardening*.

While polychromatic X-ray beam passes through matter, low energy photons are removed. Hence, effective energy of the beam increases, resulting in *beam hardening effect*. The removal of low energy photons is beneficial, they are not contributing to an image formation, instead add patient dose. That is why X-ray tubes are provided with filters of specific thickness of Aluminum and Copper, which will harden the beam by increasing its effective energy. *Higher the filter thickness, greater is the beam hardening effect.* A heavily filtered beam increases penetrating power, in turn the half-value layer. Since diagnostic X-rays are heavily filtered beam, it is approximated to monochromatic X-rays.

In computed tomography, CT number is defined based on linear attenuation coefficient. Energy of X-ray beam also influences the CT number. Same tissue lying in front and back of the human body will experience different beam energy due to patient's attenuation. Hence, attenuation coefficient will vary at these points, resulting variation of CT numbers.

Similarly, different CT machines may give different CT numbers, due to variation of X-ray beam energy. Thus, beam hardening influences clinical imaging, resulting beam hardening artifacts.

Homogeneity coefficient is the ratio between first HVL and second HVL, which describes poly energetic nature of the beam. It is 0.5–0.7 for diagnostic X-rays and 1 for gamma rays, respectively.

Mass Attenuation Coefficient

Mass attenuation coefficient is obtained by dividing the linear attenuation coefficient by material density (ρ), symbol is μ/ρ, and unit is cm^2/g. Probability of attenuation depends on number of electrons per gram, whereas linear attenuation coefficient depends on density. Mass attenuation coefficient is independent of density, which fully depends on nature of material or atomic composition. It is used to quantify an attenuation of material, independent of their physical state. Product ρx is called *mass thickness,* expressed in g/cm^2. Additionally, there are an *electronic attenuation coefficient* ($_e\mu$) *and an atomic attenuation coefficient* ($_a\mu$), expressed in electrons/cm^2 and atoms/cm^2, respectively:

$$_e\mu = \frac{\mu}{\rho \times N_0}, \quad _a\mu = \frac{\mu \times Z}{\rho \times N_0}$$

where, N_0 is number of electrons per gram $= \dfrac{N_A \times Z}{A_W}$, Z is atomic number, ρ is density, N_A *is Avogadro's number* $= 6.02205 \times 10^{23}$, and A_W is atomic weight.

Mass Energy Transfer Coefficient

When a photon passes through a medium, it interacts with an electron and lose either partial or full energy. If it loses partial energy, it is scattered with remaining energy. The scattered photon again interacts with an electron and lose partial or full energy, and so on. Thus, part of photon energy is always transferred to an electron as kinetic energy. Energy transfer coefficient (μ_{tr}) defines partial energy transferred to an electron as kinetic energy per unit thickness of an absorber:

$$\mu_{tr} = \frac{\overline{E}_{tr}}{h\nu} \times \mu$$

where, $\overline{E}_{tr}$ is average energy transferred into kinetic energy of electron per interaction and $h\nu$ is photon energy. Mass energy transfer coefficient is μ_{tr}/ρ which is always lesser than mass attenuation coefficient.

Mass Energy Absorption Coefficient

Electron mostly loss their energy by an *inelastic collision* with an atomic electron. Few electrons interact with nuclear field and lose energy by *bremsstrahlung process,* which is radiated away. The bremsstrahlung energy loss is not included in the calculation of absorbed energy. If g is fraction of energy lost by bremsstrahlung process, then absorbed energy by collisional loss is $(1 - g)$. Energy absorption coefficient (μ_{en}) is the product of energy transfer coefficient and $(1 - g)$:

$$\mu_{en} = \mu_{tr}(1 - g)$$

By dividing the equation on both sides by ρ, the mass energy absorption coefficient and mass energy transfer coefficient is obtained:

$$\frac{\mu_{en}}{\rho} = \frac{\mu_{tr}}{\rho}(1 - g)$$

where, $\dfrac{\mu_{en}}{\rho}$ is mass energy absorption coefficient, and $\dfrac{\mu_{tr}}{\rho}$ is mass energy transfer coefficient. The mass energy absorption coefficient is always lesser than that of mass energy transfer coefficient. Electron interaction with low Z materials such as soft tissue results in loss of energy only by an ionization as collision, bremsstrahlung part is negligible. Hence, in diagnostic X-ray energy with low Z materials, both are almost equal, as bremsstrahlung loss is much small, i.e., $\mu_{en} = \mu_{tr}$. Bremsstrahlung is significant while particle of high kinetic energy travels in a high Z medium. Energy absorption coefficient is useful to predict biological effects in tissues during radiation therapy.

Total Attenuation Coefficients

Total attenuation coefficient in tissue for a given energy is the ability of tissue to remove photons from radiation beams. It is caused by photoelectric absorption coefficient (τ), Compton scattering coefficient (σ), and pair production coefficient (π). The total linear attenuation coefficient in tissue (μ_{tot}) is given the relation:

$$\mu_{tot} = \mu_{\tau} + \mu_{\sigma} + \mu_{\pi}$$

Coherent scattering is excluded since its contribution is negligible in medical applications. **Figure 4.11** shows individual and total mass attenuation coefficients for soft tissue as a function of energy. At low photon energy (<2 keV), the photoelectric process dominates attenuation in soft tissue. Total mass attenuation coefficient is higher at low energies, especially for high Z

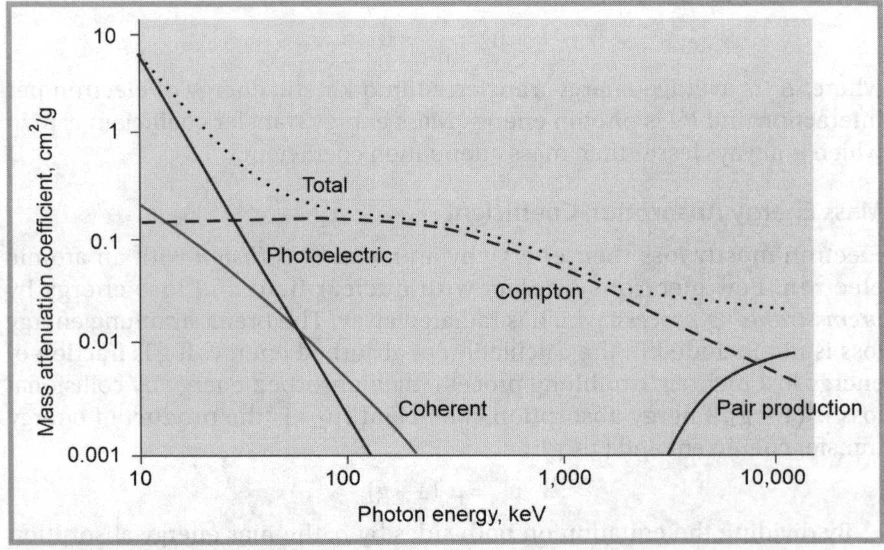

Fig. 4.11: Coherent, photoelectric, compton, pair production and total mass attenuation coefficient for soft tissue as function of photon energy.

materials. Photoelectric absorption is more important in high Z materials like bone, contrast medium, and intensifying screen. As energy increases photoelectric absorption decreases rapidly, until photon energies > electron binding energy. Afterwards, Compton scatter dominates the interaction process.

When the photon energy is about 1 MeV, total mass attenuation coefficient for high and low Z material do not differ greatly. This is due to Compton interaction which is independent of Z. Later, Compton interaction starts decreasing until pair production appears.

Compton scattering is present at all diagnostic X-ray range of energies, it is important in low Z materials (soft tissue) throughout energy range. Both photoelectric absorption and Compton scattering are equally important at 30 keV energy for air, water, and soft tissue, at 50 keV energy for bone, and at 300 keV energy for Iodine and Barium contrasts. The pair production is not very important in diagnostic radiology but is important in mega voltage radiotherapy. Thus, total attenuation coefficient decreases with increase of photon energy, and it is different for different materials **(Fig. 4.12)**. At low energy (100 keV), greater absorption is found between Lead, water, and air. At 1 MeV, the absorption is same for all the materials. However, the difference starts appearing after 10 MeV, due to pair production process.

In radiation therapy, an energy range is >1 MeV, probable interactions are Compton scattering and pair production. Compton interaction contributes more than the latter, and an absorption is equal both in bone and soft tissue. The bone absorption is slightly higher for beam energy >20 MeV. It is rare to

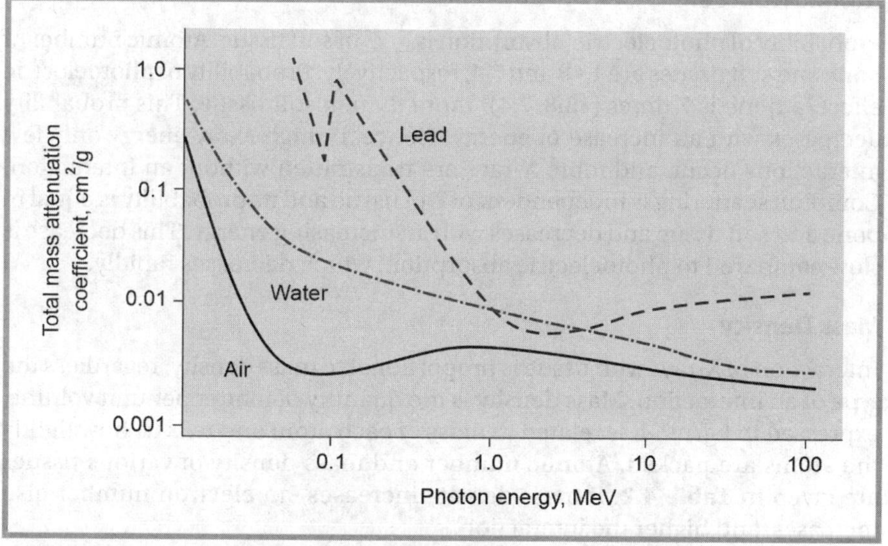

Fig. 4.12: Variation of mass attenuation coefficients with photon energy for lead, water, and air.

find in radiation therapy beams of >18 MeV in clinical use. The energy and the mode of dominant interactions are given below:

- ❑ 20–50 keV : Photoelectric absorption
- ❑ 60–90 keV : Photoelectric absorption and Compton scattering
- ❑ 200 keV–2 MeV : Compton scattering
- ❑ 5 MeV–10 MeV : Compton scattering and pair production
- ❑ 50 MeV–100 MeV : Pair production

RELATIVE IMPORTANCE OF INTERACTION IN TISSUE

Differential Absorption

When X-rays passes through tissue (1) it partly interacts with Compton scattering and photoelectric effect and (2) partly transmitted through body without interaction. Bone like anatomic structures are radio-opaque, and shows high absorption characteristics, resulting light areas (white) in radiographs. X-rays that are transmitted through the body without interaction, reaches detector resulting dark areas (black) in radiographs. Anatomical structures appear to be radiolucent to X-rays.

Hence, radiographic image is due to the difference between X-rays that are absorbed by interaction process and those transmitted without interaction. This difference is called *differential absorption*. Reduction of kV increases differential absorption and image contrast but increases patient dose due to higher mA. Scattered X-rays do not help image information, but it creates noise and degrades image quality. Hence, suitable techniques are used to reduce scatter.

Atomic Number

Probability of photoelectric absorption is $\propto Z^3$ of soft tissue. Atomic number of bone and soft tissues are 13.8 and 7.4, respectively. Probability of photoelectric effect in bone is 7 times $(13.8/7.4)^3$ more than in soft tissue. This probability decreases with an increase of energy. Hence, in high X-ray energy only few interactions occur, and more X-rays are transmitted without an interaction. Compton scattering is independent of Z of tissue and its probability is equal in bone and soft tissue and decreases with an increasing energy. This decrease is slow compared to photoelectric absorption, which decreases rapidly.

Mass Density

Interaction of X-rays with tissue is proportional to mass density, regardless the type of an interaction. Mass density is the quantity of matter per unit volume, expressed in kg/m^3. It is related to mass of each atom and tells us how tightly the atoms are packed. Atomic number and mass density of various tissues are given in **Table 4.2**. If mass density increases, an electron number also increases, and higher the interaction.

In addition to Z-based photoelectric effect, mass density also contributes to differential absorption. X-rays are absorbed and scattered two times

Table 4.2: Mass density of tissues and contrast media.

Substance	Effective atomic number, Z	Mass density, kg/m³
Lung	7.4	320
Fat	6.3	910
Soft tissue, muscle	7.4	1,000
Bone	13.8	1,850
Air	7.6	1.3
Barium	56	3,500
Iodine	53	4,930

(*Courtesy:* Stewart Carlyle Bushong et al, 2008)

(1,850/1,000 = 1.85) in bone than in soft tissue. The mass density helps in lungs imaging in radiography. For air and soft tissue, Z = 7.6 and 7.4, respectively, and atomic numbers are almost same. Lung is an air-filled soft tissue cavity, which can be imaged only by their difference in mass density (1.3 vs 1,000).

Contrast agents such as *Barium and Iodine* have high atomic number and high mass density, hence they are used with low kV techniques. However, use of high kV technique helps in visualizing the lumen of an organ. In this, X-ray penetrates contrast media, helps to outline the organ of interest.

Photon Energy

In diagnostic radiology, kilo voltage range is about 20–150 kV and effective photon energy ranges from 15 to 100 keV. Relative importance of interaction changes over this range. At low energy, photoelectric absorption is main cause of attenuation than Compton scatter. Hence, soft tissue and bone appear as *black and white* in X-ray film. The thickness of tissue is also important in an attenuation process. Thick layer of soft tissue and thin layer of bone may produce same amount of attenuation. However, use of low energy with photoelectric effect interaction can differentiate the above, by overcoming thickness effect.

In high energy, Compton scatter dominants and differentiation between soft tissue and bone reduces. Though Compton scatter depends upon density, tissue differentiation is still possible with use of high kV techniques. At low kV X-rays like mammography, about 75% of attenuation in soft tissues is due to photoelectric absorption. Compton scatter plays a minor role at this energy. At higher energy, photoelectric absorption accounts for 15–20% attenuation in soft tissues, and Compton plays a dominant role, e.g., chest radiography or gamma imaging.

RADIATION UNITS

Radiation units are necessary to express quantities of physical entities in a numerical scale for comparative purposes. Quantification of physical entities is normally done by estimating a measurable physical effect of the physical entity, e.g., heat is quantified based on expansion it produces in materials. The condition for quantification is the amount of physical entity and its effect should have a linear relationship. In radiological physics, the quantities of interest are:

❑ Amount of nuclear disintegration takes place per unit time.
❑ Ionizing photons present in a field.
❑ Energy transferred from radiation to tissue.
❑ Energy absorbed in tissue.
❑ Biological effectiveness of energy absorption.

In 1981, International commission on radiation units and measurements (ICRU) recommended units based on SI system as explained below.

Description of Photon Beams

A radiation beam can be described in terms of fluence (Φ), flux (φ), energy fluence (Ψ), and energy fluence rate (ψ). Fluence is number of photons or particles passing through a unit cross-sectional area, its unit is cm^{-2}:

$$\Phi = \frac{\text{Photons}}{\text{Area}} = \frac{dN}{da}$$

where, dN is number of photons incident on a sphere of cross-sectional area da. The fluence per unit area per unit time is called *flux or fluence rate* and its unit is $cm^{-2}s^{-1}$:

$$\varphi = \frac{\text{Photons}}{\text{Area} \times \text{Time}} = \frac{d\Phi}{dt}$$

Amount of energy passing through a unit cross-sectional area is called *energy fluence* and its unit is Jm^{-2}:

$$\Psi = \frac{\text{Photons}}{\text{Area}} \times \frac{\text{Energy}}{\text{Photons}} = \frac{dE_{fl}}{da}$$

where, dE_{fl} is sum of energies of all photons that enters a sphere of cross-sectional area da. For a monoenergetic photon beam, it is simply the product of fluence and photon energy. In poly energetic photon beam, number of photons of each energy is multiplied by its energy and their sum gives energy fluence. Energy fluence per unit time is called energy fluence rate (ψ) or intensity of the beam:

$$\psi = \frac{d\Psi}{dt}$$

Exposure

Exposure indicates the number of ionizing photons present in a field. The number of charged particles produced by an ionization is directly proportional to number of ionization events. Hence, ionizing photons are quantified based on total charge produced by them in a medium. Air is an universal medium to measure exposure. Average minimum energy necessary is about 34 eV, for photons to produce an ionization in an air.

Exposure is a measure of X and gamma ray photon flux and refers to radiation quantity measured in terms of an ionization in air per unit mass, in a small volume around a point. SI unit exposure is Coulomb/kg air. It is defined as that of quantity of X or gamma radiation that produces one Coulomb of charge of either sign in one kg of an air, at normal temperature and pressure (NTP). If Q is charge collected in an air mass of m, then exposure X is given by the relation:

$$X = \frac{Q}{m}$$

The old unit of exposure is *roentgen (R)*. One roentgen shall be the quantity of X or gamma radiation, such that the associated corpuscular emission per 0.001293 grams of air (1 cc of dry air at NTP), produces in an air, ions carrying 1 electrostatic unit (esu) of quantity of electricity of either sign. Roentgen is related to its SI unit:

$$1R = 2.58 \times 10^{-4} \text{ C/kg of air.}$$

In practice, milli-roentgen (mR) is used as unit: 1 mR = 1/1,000 roentgen (10^{-3} R).

Radiation monitors are usually calibrated in roentgen (R). It is used to measure X-ray output and radiological survey. The output of X-ray machine is often expressed in mR/mAs, e.g., a 75 kV X-ray unit with 2 mm Al filtration may give about 5–10 mR/mAs output at 100 cm distance. The measurement of exposure rate in air by an air-filled ion-chambers is easy, since effective atomic number of an air is equal to that of soft tissue. Thus, the measured exposure is proportional to the dose in soft tissue in diagnostic X-ray energy.

There are some difficulties in the unit of roentgen. Roentgen is defined only for X and gamma radiations in an air medium, and not suitable for human body measurements, because roentgen is not a unit of absorbed dose. It is a measure of charge and not directly related biological effects of radiation. Moreover, it can be used only up to energy of 3 MeV photon energy, since an electronic equilibrium is not established by higher range of electrons.

Kerma

Kerma stands for *Kinetic Energy Released in the Medium*. It is a measure of kinetic energy of uncharged particles (photons and neutrons) transferred to charged particles like electrons and protons, during their interaction with matter. Thus, kerma (K) describes an initial interaction of photon with an atom, and it is defined as sum of initial kinetic energy (E_{tr}) of all charged ionizing particles, liberated by photons in a material of mass (m):

$$K = \frac{E_{tr}}{m}$$

Kerma at a point is proportional to photon fluence, (Ψ) and can be written as:

$$K = \Psi \left(\frac{\overline{\mu}_{tr}}{\rho} \right)$$

It is known that: $\dfrac{\mu_{en}}{\rho} = \dfrac{\mu_{tr}}{\rho} (1 - g)$

or $\dfrac{\mu_{tr}}{\rho} = \dfrac{\mu_{en}}{\rho} \times \dfrac{1}{(1 - g)}$

Substituting this, $K = \Psi \left(\dfrac{\overline{\mu}_{en}}{\rho} \right) \times \dfrac{1}{(1 - \overline{g})}$

where, $\left(\dfrac{\overline{\mu}_{tr}}{\rho}\right)$ is mass energy transfer coefficient, $\overline{g}$ is average fraction of electron energy lost due to radiative process, and $\dfrac{\overline{\mu}_{en}}{\rho}$ is average mass energy absorption coefficient. The initial kinetic energy of electron is spent as inelastic collision as well as radiative process such as bremsstrahlung. Hence, kerma has two components:

❑ Energy expended by inelastic collisions (K^{col})
❑ Energy expended as radiative collision (K^{rad})

$$K^{col} = \Psi\left(\frac{\overline{\mu}_{en}}{\rho}\right)$$

$$K^{rad} = \Psi\left(\frac{\overline{\mu}_{en}}{\rho}\right)\left(\frac{\overline{g}}{(1-\overline{g})}\right)$$

By adding above two equations:

$$K = K^{col} + K^{rad} = \Psi\left(\frac{\overline{\mu}_{en}}{\rho}\right) \times \frac{1}{(1-\overline{g})}$$

where, Ψ is photon energy fluence.

The unit of kerma is joule per kilogram (J/kg) and the SI unit is gray (Gy) = 1 J/kg. The unit, Air-kerma is often used to measure X-ray machine output and X-ray tube leakage.

Exposure and Kerma

Exposure is defined in terms of charge collected in unit mass. If energy involved in collected charge is known, then exposure and kerma can be related. Since exposure is equivalent to kerma due to collision in air, K^{col} can be used to relate the exposure (X). Average energy required $\left(\dfrac{\overline{W}}{e}\right)$ to produce unit charge of ionization = 33.97 eV in air. If K^{col} is energy spent in air, then exposure (X):

$$X = (K^{col})_{air} \times \left(\frac{e}{\overline{W}}\right)_{air}$$

$$= \Psi_{air}\left(\frac{\overline{\mu}_{en}}{\rho}\right)_{air} \times \left(\frac{e}{\overline{W}}\right)_{air}$$

Absorbed Dose

Initial kinetic energy transferred to a charged particle is absorbed in tissue as absorbed dose. In this, some part of kinetic energy appears as bremsstrahlung X-rays and delta rays, which escape small volumes of tissues (**Fig. 4.13**). The initial kinetic energy minus energy that appears as bremsstrahlung X-rays is the true absorbed dose. Hence, absorbed dose refers to amount of energy absorbed per unit mass of medium. This is independent of radiation type and medium. It is defined as an energy absorption of one joule per kg of medium, and the SI unit is gray (Gy):

$$1\ Gy = 1\ J/kg$$

If E is mean energy absorbed in a medium of mass m, then absorbed dose (D):

$$D = \frac{E}{m}$$

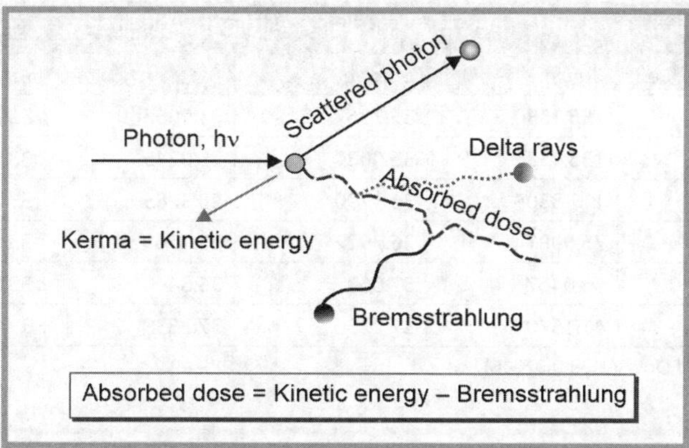

Fig. 4.13: Transfer of kinetic energy to the charged particles from the photon in the medium. Radiation energy is scattered, absorbed, and appear as bremsstrahlung and delta rays.

The special unit of absorbed dose is *rad* (r), which stands for *radiation absorbed dose*; 1 rad = 100 ergs/gram. The unit rad is related to gray as 1 Gy = 100 rad. In practice, milligray (mGy), centigray (cGy) and microgray (μGy) are used as units:

$$1 \text{ mGy} = 1/1{,}000 \text{ Gray } (10^{-3} \text{ Gy})$$

$$1 \text{ cGy} = 1/100 \text{ Gray } (10^{-2} \text{ Gy})$$

$$1 \text{ μGy} = 1/1{,}000 \text{ mGy } (10^{-6} \text{ Gy})$$

Since 1 Gy = 100 rad, 1 mGy = 100 mrad, and 1 μGy = 100 μrad

The units rad or gray is defined based on the energy delivered in the medium, hence they are suitable to describe a biological effect of radiation. It is used to quantify the patient radiation dose in Gy, in Diagnostic radiology, Radiotherapy, and Radiobiology. Absorbed dose is the energy spent over a path length whereas kerma is the energy transformed at a point.

Absorbed Dose and Exposure

The absorbed dose (D) in air is related to the exposure (X) as follows:

$$D = f \times X$$

where, *f* is *roentgen-to-rad conversion factor*. In diagnostic X-ray energies, the f-factor for an air, muscle and other soft tissue is close to 1 **(Table 4.3)**. The variation of roentgen-rad conversion factor with photon energy is given in **Figure 4.14**.

Conversion of Exposure from Dose in Air

Let *D* is the dose in air in Gy and *X* is the exposure in C/kg, then radiation exposure of 1 roentgen is given by:

$$1 \text{ Roentgen } (X) = 2.58 \times 10^{-4} \text{ C/kg}$$

Table 4.3: f-Factors for bone, muscle, fat and air over diagnostic energy range, m²/kg.

Photon energy, keV	Bone	Muscle	Fat	Air
40	156.1530	35.7362	21.9666	33.8500
50	136.4581	36.0081	25.0245	33.8500
60	111.3309	36.3290	28.3285	33.8500
80	75.0981	36.7922	33.1569	33.8500
100	56.0467	37.0627	35.5440	33.8500
150	41.1540	37.2296	37.2839	33.8500

(*Courtesy:* David J Dowsett et al, 2006)

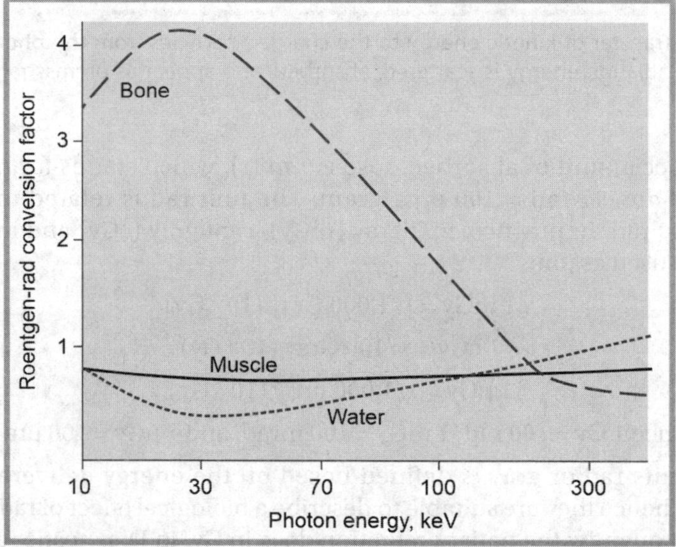

Fig. 4.14: Roentgen-rad conversion factor with photon energy.

The average energy deposited in air per ion pair is 33.97 J/C, and the total energy associated with 1 roentgen exposure is:

$$1 \text{ Roentgen (X)} = 33.97 \text{ J/C} \times 2.58 \times 10^{-4} \text{ C/kg}$$

$$= 0.00876 \text{ J/kg}$$
$$= 0.00876 \text{ Gy (since 1 Gy = 1 J/kg)}$$
$$= \text{dose in air (D)}$$
$$\text{Dose in air (D)} = 0.00876 \text{ Gy/Roentgen}$$

Thus, dose in air is equal to 0.00876 Gy per roentgen or 8.76 mGy per roentgen. Based on the above, the following relations may be used between dose and the exposure:

$$\text{Dose in air (mGy)} = 8.76 \times \text{Exposure (R)}$$
$$\text{Dose in air (µGy)} = 8.76 \times \text{Exposure (mR)}$$

Absorbed Dose in Air

When a photon beam travels in a medium, under charged particle equilibrium exists then the absorbed dose is equal to collision kerma, if bremsstrahlung is negligible:

$$D_{air} = \left(K^{col}\right)_{air} = X \times \frac{\overline{W}}{e}$$
$$= 0.876 \times \left(\frac{rad}{R}\right) \times X(R)$$

BIBLIOGRAPHY

1. Bushberg JT, Seibert J A, Leidholdt EM Jr, Boone JM. The Essential Physics of Medical Imaging, 3rd ed. Lippincott Williams and Wilkins, Philadelphia; 2012.
2. Bushong SC. Radiologic Science for Technologists, 9th edn. Mosby-Elsevier, 2008.
3. Dowsett DJ, Kenny PA, and Johnston RE: The Physics of Diagnostic Imaging, 2nd edn. New York: Hodder Arnold; 2006.
4. Khan FM. The Physics of Radiation Therapy, Lippincott Williams and Wilkins; 2003.
5. Thayalan K. Basic Radiological Physics, 2nd edn. Jaypee Brothers Medical Publishers (P) Ltd, New Delhi; 2017.

Radiation Detection and Measurements

PRINCIPLES OF RADIATION DETECTION

Ionization

Radiation exposure causes an ionization in matter which involves removal of electrons from neutral atoms or molecules, resulting in positive and negative ions. The positive and negative ions are called *ion pairs*, which can be collected by applying an electric field, that gives rise to *current or pulse.* Total charge collected is proportional to radiation intensity. *Ionization chamber, proportional counter, Geiger-Muller counter, and semiconductor detector* fall under this category. Gaseous and solid media are used in their detector design.

Photographic Effect

Ionizing radiation affects photographic film and alters its density, in turn forms latent image. The film is processed, and its optical density is measured by a densitometer. The degree of blackness is related to an intensity of radiation exposure. It can be quantified in terms of an *optical density (OD)*, which is proportional to radiation intensity. This type of dose evaluation is called *film dosimetry*, and it can be performed either with *radiographic film or radiochromic film.*

Luminescence

This is a process in which radiation excites atoms of a material and its energy is converted into an ultraviolet or visible light flash. The light flashes can be detected by a *photomultiplier tube (PMT) or photodiode,* which gives an electrical signal. The electrical signal is proportional to an incident radiation intensity. Detectors making use of the above principle are called *scintillators*, e.g., *NaI.*

Thermoluminescence

Radiation imparts energy to certain crystalline materials, which can store this energy for a long time, e.g., *Lithium fluoride, Calcium sulphate, etc.* The energy thus stored can be later released in the form of light or luminescence by heating these materials. Quantity of light released is proportional to radiation intensity. It can be measured and correlated to radiation dose. The devices based on the above effect are called *thermoluminescent dosimeter (TLD)*. Instead heat, laser can be used to stimulate luminance, referred as an *optically stimulated luminescence (OSL)*, e.g., AlO_2.

Chemical Effects

Ionizing radiation can cause chemical changes, e.g., oxidation of ferrous sulphate to ferric sulphate, which is principle of *Fricke dosimeter*. The concentration of ferric ions can be measured to correlate the energy absorbed or radiation dose delivered. Radiation can also cause color changes in certain plastics. Such color changes can also be measured and correlated to radiation dose. Such a systems are called *chemical dosimeters*.

Biological Effects

Radiation exposure alters lymphocytes magnitude and cause aberrations in chromosomes. Exposed individual's blood can be analyzed for chromosomal aberrations, e.g., *dicentric and ring formation*. The aberration score is a measure of radiation and is called *biological dosimetry*. This dosimetry is used during accident exposures, when no other information is available to assess individual's radiation exposure.

TYPES OF DETECTORS

Radiation detectors are classified by type of information they produce. Detectors that indicate number of interactions that occur are called *counters*, e.g., *GM counter*. Detectors giving information about energy distribution of incident radiation is called scintillation detector or *spectrometer, e.g., NaI.* Detectors indicating net amount of energy dissipated in the detector by multiple interactions are called *dosimeter.*

Radiation detectors produce an electrical signal following each interaction. The electrical signal passes through a series of an electronic circuit, for signal amplification, signal processing or data storage. The detector and its electronic circuit are called the detection system. There are two ways by which the circuitry may process signal, namely, (1) *pulse mode* and (2) *current mode.*

In pulse mode, signal from an each interaction is processed individually. In current mode, electrical signals from individual interactions are averaged together, forming a net current signal. GM detectors are operated in pulse mode, whereas ion chambers and scintillation detectors are operated in current mode.

Detectors operating under current mode never retain the interaction rate and energy deposited by an individual interaction. Charge collected from an interaction is proportional to energy deposited by the interaction. Total average electrical current measured is proportional to dose rate of the radiation. Current mode measurements are preferred in high interaction rates, for which there is no *dead time* losses. CT detector, flat panel detector used in fluoroscopy and an ion chamber in radiotherapy are operated in current mode.

Detector efficiency is a measure of its ability to detect radiation. It is the product of two terms, namely (1) *geometric efficiency,* and (2) *intrinsic efficiency.* Geometric efficiency is defined as ratio of photons reaching detector to number of photons emitted by source. Intrinsic efficiency is defined as ratio of number of photons detected to number of photons reaching the detector. It is often called as *quantum detection efficiency (QDE)* and it depends on *atomic number, density, thickness of the detector, and energy of radiation.* The detector efficiency varies from 0-1. All radiation detectors are broadly classified as:

❑ Gas-filled chamber detectors
❑ Solid-state detectors
❑ Biological dosimeter
❑ Chemical dosimeters

However, first three detectors have more application in diagnostic radiology.

GAS-FILLED DETECTORS

Gas-filled detector has volume of gas in between two electrodes, in which a voltage is applied. When exposed to radiation, the gas gets ionized and ion pairs are formed. Positive ion moves towards negative electrode and negative ion moves towards positive electrode. The electron travels through the circuit and reaches the cathode and recombines with positive ions. This forms an electrical current which can be measured by a meter.

There are three types of gas-filled detectors, namely, (1) ionization chamber, (2) proportional counter, and (3) Geiger-Muller (GM) counter. These detectors are classified based on the applied voltage. **Figure 5.1** shows detector current for various applied voltages between the electrodes. When the voltage is zero, the ion pairs produced by radiation recombine and no current flows through the circuit. If a small voltage is applied, current starts flowing through the circuit. As the voltage increases further, the current also increases, reducing the recombination of charges. This region is called *recombination region* of the curve.

As voltage is increased further no increase in current is observed and a saturation is reached. This is represented by a plateau in the graph stating that all the liberated charges are collected. This region is called an *ionization chamber region,* and ionization chambers operate in this region.

If the applied voltage is increased further, the current also increases further and the region is called *proportional region.* In this region, an electron travels

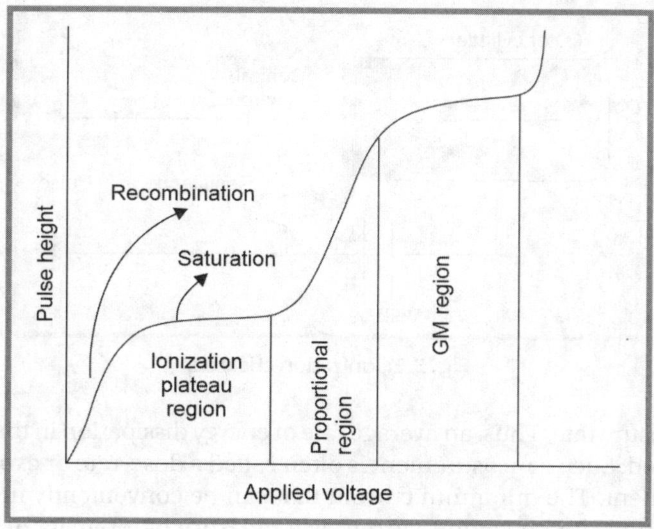

Fig. 5.1: Gas-filled detector: Relation between applied voltage and pulse height.

with high kinetic energy and cause additional ionization, releasing more electrons. This is called *gas multiplication*, which amplifies the detector current. The amplification increases as voltage increases. In this region, the charge collected is proportional to amount of energy deposited in the gas medium.

After the proportional region, the amount of charge collected is the same, regardless of energy deposited. This region is called *GM region*, in which the gas multiplication spread the entire length of the detector. GM counters cannot differentiate energy of radiation. If the voltage is increased further, discharge takes place in the detector, and it should not be operated further.

Ionization Chamber

An ionization chamber usually consists of an outer cylinder coated inside with *graphite* to make it conducting and a central electrode insulated from the chamber wall **(Fig. 5.2).** The cylinder is filled with either an air or with suitable gas for radiation interaction and detection. Air requires 34 eV to produce one ion pair, and a 100 keV photon can create about 3000 ion pairs.

When the chamber is exposed to radiation, ion pairs are formed and are collected by the electrodes. The flow of ions through the circuit, create an current signal. The amplitude of the signal depends upon number of ion pairs formed and independent of applied voltage. The amount of signal obtained from single interaction is very small and require amplification. Therefore, ion chambers are used in current mode, not in pulses mode. They are free from dead time loses and operated with wide range of voltages.

If the chamber is filled with air and an effective atomic number of the wall material is equal to air, then the amount of current produced is proportional

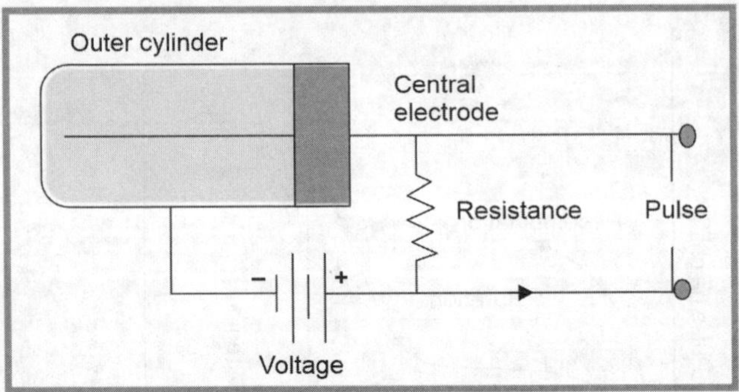

Fig. 5.2: Ionization chamber.

to an exposure rate. Thus, an average rate of energy dissipation in the chamber is measured. Such a measurement is often called a dose-rate or exposure rate measurement. The minimum current that can be conveniently measured is about 10^{-14}A. The ionization current is a measure of intensity of radiation. Such chambers are used as survey meters and dosimeters in radiology. However, their intrinsic efficiency is low because of lower air density.

Instead of air, high atomic number gases, *Argon (Z = 18) or Xenon (Z = 54)* and pressurizing gases can be used, to increase the sensitivity towards x and gamma rays. Such chambers are used in an isotope calibrator and CT scans as detectors. The advantages of an ion chamber are, walls can be made tissue equivalent, all type of radiation can be measured and can be calibrated to any energy. The disadvantage includes small signal current which requires high amplification and restricted sensitivity.

Proportional Counter

In ionization chamber, the applied voltage collects only electrons emitted by direct action of radiation. In the case of proportional counter, not only the electrons produced by direct action, but also secondary electrons are collected to generate electric signal. It is proportional to the energy of an incident radiation as name suggests. They can be operated either in pulse mode as counters or spectrometers.

Proportional counter is a specially designed co-axial cylinder filled with specific gas medium, operated with higher voltages (1000 V). In general, noble gases such as *Argon* and *Xenon* are used. The gas medium should allow easy migration of free electrons. Gas pressure increases density and gives higher *quantum detection efficiency*. Operating voltage varies with nature of gas medium. The design should optimize gas amplification factor. It should address the amount of amplification and an uniformity of amplification within the chamber.

When radiation interacts a gas medium an initial ionization takes place and ion-pairs are produced. About 34 eV energy is required to produce one ion-pair. The higher electric field applied across the electrodes accelerate the electrons towards anode with high kinetic energy. Electrons collide with neutral gas atoms and causes additional ionization, resulting ion-pairs and so on. This cascade process is called *Towsend avalanche or gas amplification factor*. It increases with increase of an applied voltage as shown in **Figure 5.1**. Thus, gas amplification factor of 10^6 can be obtained.

The electrons accelerated between two collisions must acquire sufficient energy to ionize another neutral gas atom. This means that the electron must acquire energy greater than an ionization potential of the gas atom in one mean free path. The electric field required to initiate secondary ionization is the order of several kV/cm. The electrons reach a critical distance from the anode where the avalanche takes place. This distance is equal to a few mean free path and is closer to the anode.

Detectors operating in this mode are called *proportional counters*. This means that the ionization caused by the incident radiation is multiplied by the gas amplification factor. In other words, the total charge produced is equal to number of ionizations multiplied by an amplification factor. Since, the mobility of electrons and positive ions vary, when the electrons reach a finite distance, the positive ions hardly moved to a negligible distance. The positive ion sheath near the anode reduces the electric field and unable to register another avalanche event. Once the positive ion sheath moves to a critical distance from the anode, next avalanche event is recorded. The voltage pulse at the anode reaches a maximum rapidly and falls slowly. It depends on the mobility of positive charges and time constant of the input circuit of preamplifier. The time during which the counter is unable to respond to another ionizing event is called the *resolving time.*

The electrical signal/pulse produced by the proportional counter per an ionization event is much larger than an ionization chamber. Hence, they are suitable for counting or detecting an individual radiation interaction. The number of electrons collected at the anode, or the pulse height is proportional to an initial ionization. The pulse height depends on linear energy transfer (LET) of an ionizing radiation. Since, an electric pulse is proportional to the amount of deposited energy, it can be used for energy sensitive counting. It can differentiate different energies based on an electrical pulse. However, they are inefficient detectors for high energy X and gamma rays.

Proportional counters are rarely used in medicine but have wider application in health physics research and industry, for measuring α and β particles. It is useful to study alpha and beta particles and analyze their energy spectrum. Alpha particles can be detected at lower voltage than beta particle of low LET. Proportional counters provide a large surface area and serve as detector in CT scan (*Xenon* gas). Its atomic number is high and kept under high pressure, to have greater photoelectric absorption. Proportional counters are superior then an ionization chamber since its output is quite high. It is superior to GM counters since it analyzes spectra, and has smaller resolving time.

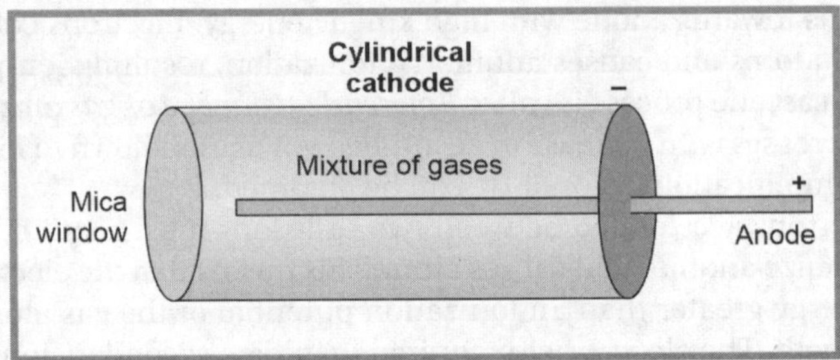

Fig. 5.3: Geiger–Muller tube.

Geiger Counter

The Geiger–Muller (GM) counter consists of a cylindrical cathode with a fine wire anode along its axis **(Fig. 5.3)**. Cathode serves as outer electrode, made by *metal or metallic film* sprayed on inside of a *glass or plastic* tube. A high voltage of 500–1500 V is applied across the chamber. It is filled with a special mixture of gases *(Argon + quenching gas)* at a pressure of about 10 cm of Hg. It is available in two types:

- ❑ End window or thin window (0.1 Al or SS)
- ❑ Windowless (0.01 mm mica).

Former is used for penetrating radiation whereas the later is used for nonpenetrating radiation. Thin window counters are often provided with *pancake type detectors*. Their entrance is provided with removable covers.

Function

When X or gamma ray passes through a gas medium it produces an initial ionization, resulting an ion-pairs. The ion-pairs are accelerated towards respective electrodes. Since the electrons are accelerated towards the anode by a strong electric field, they gain energy and does further ionization in the gas medium, releasing more electrons. This is known as *primary avalanche* of gas or amplification. Accelerating electron can also cause an excitation in the gas medium. The excited molecule returns to ground state within 10^{-9} sec and release visible light and ultraviolet. They interact with cathode and emits electrons by *photoelectric absorption* process. These electrons give *secondary avalanche* in the gas medium while moving towards anode. Both primary and secondary avalanche is called *secondary ion cascade or avalanche ionization*. It becomes more dominant and the initial ionization slowly fads away. It determines pulse size unchanged by energy of the particles. Thus, a huge amplification of the order of 10^{10} is obtained as signal. The ionization current passing through the circuit generates a voltage spike (pulse or signal). It is amplified electronically (5–50 V) and passed to the counter. GM counter can be connected to a loudspeaker for audible sound.

The Geiger counter is operated at a higher applied voltage and the characteristic curve gas four regions, namely *threshold voltage, knee, plateau, and spontaneous discharge region.* Plateau region is about 150–200 voltage long and independent of the applied voltage. It is usual to operate the counter at a voltage midway along the plateau. Operating voltage of the plateau region is about 1/3 of the distance from the knee to the spontaneous discharge region.

GM counter has higher efficiency for charged particles and records every particle separately. However, beta particle cannot penetrate the window. Hence, it is provided with a window, which is opened for beta particle and low energy photon detection. They are inefficient towards X and gamma rays, <1%. It cannot detect neutron and uncharged particles. GM counter voltage pulse size is independent of radiation energy, e.g., 1 keV and 5 keV ionizing radiation gives same size pulse. Hence, they cannot be used as spectrometer to detect energy and as dose rate meter.

Dead Time

GM counters suffer from dead time and recovery time losses. The electron and positive ions differ in mass and velocity. By the time an electron reaches the anode, the positive ion hardly moved at all from the anode. Hence, the potential near the central electrode is lowered and a hose of slow-moving positive ion sheath is formed. This terminates the avalanche process, and no further pulse is possible unless the ion sheath reaches a critical distance. Time during which subsequent an ionizing event cannot produce pulse is called *dead time or pulse resolving time of the detector.* Time during which the pulse height build-up to the threshold value is called *recovery time:*

Resolving time = Dead Time + Recovery time

GM dead time ranges from 50 μs–200 μs, whereas dead time of other detectors is < few μs.

Application

GM counter is rugged, simple, and inexpensive. It detects alpha, beta and gamma radiations. It response to an individual photons, beta particle or single disintegration of atoms. They are used to detect low level radioactive contamination. The particle is counted as counts per minute (CPM), whereas radioactivity is measured in μSv/hr or mR/hr. It can be used as *survey meter as well as contamination monitor.* It is ten times sensitive than an ion chamber and more sensitive in diagnostic radiology energy range. Portable GM counter may be paralyzed in a very high radiation field, and it is seldom used for an accurate reading. Quenching chemicals easily disintegrates, hence life span of GM counter is limited.

SOLID-STATE DETECTORS

Radiographic Film Dosimeter

Radiographic film consists of four layers, namely *base, adhesive layer, emulsion, and overcoat* (**Fig. 5.4A**). The emulsion is the main component of

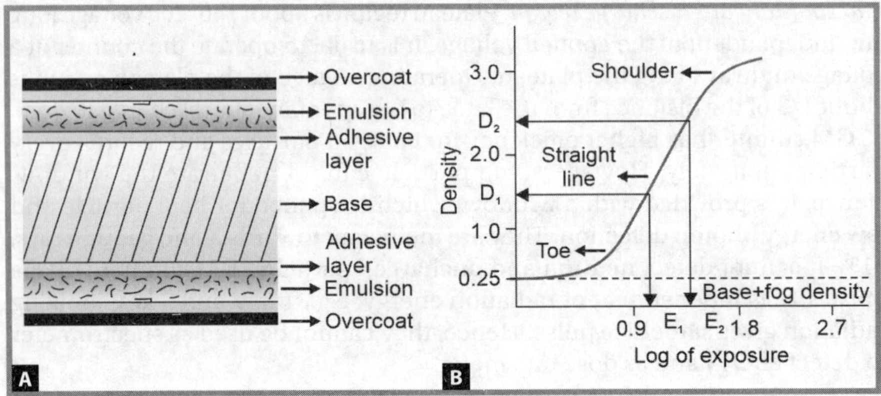

Figs. 5.4A and B: (A) Radiographic film cross-section; (B) Characteristics curve of the radiographic film.

film that contains *Silver bromide (Ag Br) crystals*. Usually, Ag Br and Ag I are mixed in the ratio 98% and 2% and used in the crystal. Ag Br crystals are either in tabular or cubic grain size of 0.1 μm thickness. Silver bromide is made by dissolving Silver in *nitric acid* and mixed with *Potassium bromide*. Lattice structure of atoms in the crystal has imperfections, which provide sensitivity centers for latent image formation. Ag Br crystals are spread over *gelatin* in an uniform manner, forms emulsion of 3–5 μm thickness. It is arranged as a single unit consisting *of base, adhesive layer, emulsion, and overcoat.*

The base gives structural support to film, and it is flexible, fracture resistant, and easy to handle without kinking. Adhesive layer is a thin coat that binds emulsion with base and provides integrity to film during processing. The overcoat protects emulsion from scratches, pressure, contamination, and handling damages. In radiographic film, emulsion is coated on both sides and such a film is called *double side coated film.*

When film is exposed to an ionizing radiation Silver bromide gets ionized as Ag^+ and Br^-, and Bromine is split into Br plus e^-. Thus, Bromine provide secondary electrons, which migrates to sensitivity centers. Silver atoms, Ag^+ also move to sensitivity center and get attached with e^- and become neutral Ag. Neutral Silver atoms are black and form latent image, which is proportional to radiation intensity. In a dark room, film is processed; developed, rinsed, fixed, washed, and dried. Metallic Silver is made visible and unexposed Ag Br are removed from the film.

Blackness of film is evaluated by using an optical densitometer. The densitometer consists of a standard *light source, aperture, and a light detector*. While the film is exposed, transmitted light from film is measured and an optical density is obtained. The optical density (OD) of film is given by the relation:

$$OD = \log_{10}\left(\frac{I_0}{I_t}\right)$$

where, I_0 is light intensity measured without film and I_t is light transmitted through film, $\left(\dfrac{I_0}{I_t}\right)$ is inverse of transmittance (T), which is measured by a densitometer. If the densitometer is calibrated with known optical density, it gives direct reading of an optical density. Using the **Hurter** and **Driffield** (H and D) characteristic curve of the film, radiation exposure can be obtained **(Fig. 5.4B)**. The H and D curve is drawn between log of radiation exposure and an optical density that gives characteristic response of the film. The curve has *base plus fag, linear and shoulder* regions. Generally, an optical density is measured at the linear part of characteristic curve.

Commercial films are available from *Kodak, Dupont, Agfa and kodak,* which are individually packed in a light proof and airtight covers and directly used with slab phantoms in day light. Care should be taken to avoid air bubbles within airtight cover. To overcome this, film is pierced with pin at one side and slap phantom is pressed over it from other side to remove air. Thus, pin prick can be used as an identification mark for film orientation.

Limitation of film includes change in processing conditions, inter film emulsion differences, and formation of artifacts. Hence, film is not recommended for absolute dosimetry. However, it can be used for checking an optical and radiation field congruence, field flatness and symmetry, and radiation distribution. Since film contains high Z active material, it overresponse to low energy X-ray photons.

Thermoluminescent Dosimeter

Thermoluminescence is a property of certain phosphors, in which irradiated crystal absorbs energy and later release the energy as luminescence while it is heated. The amount of luminescence is proportional to absorbed radiation dose. This phenomenon is known as *thermo luminescence* and the system is called *thermoluminescent dosimeter (TLD).*

Solid crystals possess allowed energy bands such as *valency, conduction, and forbidden* energy bands. The valency energy band is ground state and conduction band is high energy state. At room temperature, conduction band is empty, the electrons are in the valency band or in an equilibrium. The gap between valency and conduction band is having number of traps that are caused by defects in the crystal (caused by impurities). When TLD dosimeter is exposed to radiation, electrons in the valency band receive sufficient energy and move from valence band to conduction band **(Fig. 5.5).** The excited electrons form a trap in meta stable state just below the conduction band. The traps may be shallow, active, deep electron, and deep hole traps, respectively. Correspondingly holes are formed in valency band due to an electron vacancy. Number of electrons in the meta stable trap is proportional to radiation exposure. Thus, it stores absorbed radiation energy in the crystal lattice.

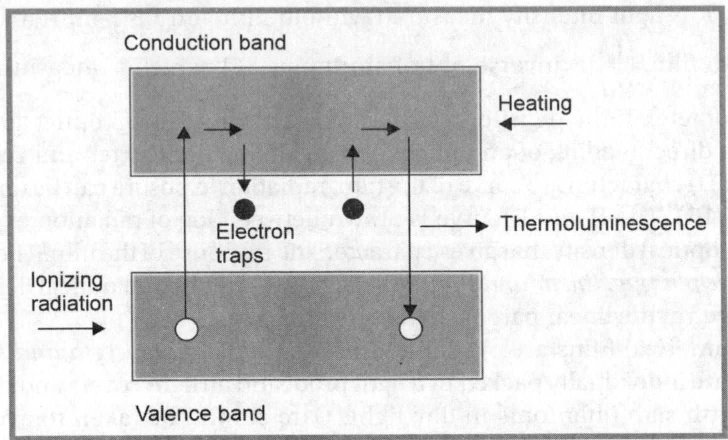

Fig. 5.5: Principle and function of TLD phosphor during irradiation and heating.

TLD Reader

After radiation exposure, dose measurements are made by using a TLD reader **(Fig. 5.6)**. The reader has *heater, photomultiplier tube (PMT), amplifier, and a recorder*. TLD dosimeter is placed in the heater *cup or planchet,* where it is heated (300°C) for a reproducible heating cycle. Temperature is measured by welding a *thermocouple* to the *planchet*. While heating, electrons in the meta stable state absorbs energy from heat and returns to their valency state (ground state) with emission of light and recombine with holes. The amount of light emission depends on temperature and number of trapped electrons. This phenomenon is called *thermoluminescence* (TL). Emitted light is detected by a photomultiplier tube (PMT), which converts light into an electrical signal. PMT signal is then amplified and measured by a recorder.

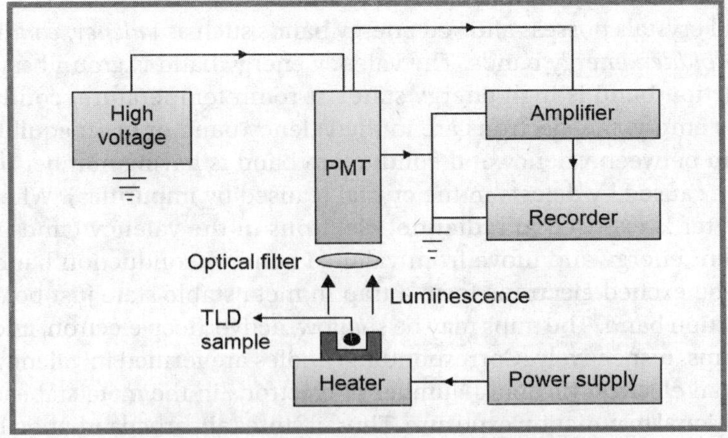

Fig. 5.6: Thermoluminescent dosimeter reader.

The reader is calibrated in terms of milli roentgen (mR) or milli sievert (mSv), so that the reader displays direct dose estimation.

Glow Curve

TLD response is defined as TL output per unit Gy absorbed dose by the phosphor. TL response varies with temperature or duration of heating. If temperature is kept constant, then TL response varies with time. If a linear temperature ramp is applied, TL signal shows number of peaks at specific temperatures, corresponding to traps of different energy levels. A plot drawn between TL response and heating time, is referred as *glow curve*. As temperature increases, electrons leaving the trap increases, in turn TL response also increases, it reaches a maximum and falls to zero. TL *thermogram* can be obtained by plotting an emitted light vs phosphor temperature.

The reading cycle of TLD is divided into *preheating, signal integration and annealing,* In the preheating, dosimeter is heated for few seconds at constant temperature to remove all low temperature signals. During signal integration, temperature is raised to a maximum. Finally, the dosimeter is *annealed* in a dedicated heating *oven* to remove all remaining signals. Now the dosimeter has been reset to zero and can be reused again.

Dedicated *annealing oven* is one in which various levels of temperature can be set. A typical annealing cycle consists of 400°C for 1 h, followed by 80°C for 24 h. However, it varies with phosphor material. Annealing process releases all residual energy stored from earlier exposure or confirms that all electrons in the metastable state is released. After annealing, the peaks in the glow curve disappear and curve becomes stable and predictable.

TLD Phosphors

Phosphors suitable for thermoluminescence are *Lithium fluoride (LiF: Mg, Ti, LiF: Mg, Cu, P)* and *Lithium borate ($Li_2B_4O_7$: Mn)* which are tissue equivalent. Materials having high sensitivity, but not tissue equivalent are *Calcium sulfate ($CaSO_4$: Dy), Aluminum oxide (Al_2O_3:C),* and *Calcium fluoride (CaF_2:MN).* LiF: Mg, Ti (TLD 100) phosphor is most widely used which has wide dose response over 10 μSv–1000 Sv and has less than 10% fading per year. Its effective atomic number (Z = 8.2) is close to that of tissue (Z = 7.4) with an accuracy of ±2%. If dimensions of the dosimeter are equal to an electron range, an *electronic equilibrium exists*, then ratio of absorbed doses of TLD and muscle is equal to their *mass stopping power ratio.* This ratio is constant over an electron energies of 10 keV–20 MeV. LiF: Mg, Ti (TLD 100) is useful for clinical dosimetry in radiology and research applications, which has a detection threshold of 0.1 μGy. However, it shows *supra linearity* at high doses, which requires corrections. $CaSO_4$:Dy is used as TLD material in India for personnel monitoring. It is not tissue equivalent (Z = 15.3), has wide range of dose response from 0.1 mSv–100 Sv with an accuracy of ±10%.

Influencing Factors

Number of factors influence TLD response that include *fading, dose, mass, energy, background signal, reproducibility*, etc. Decrease in TLD response in between irradiation and readout is called fading. *Thermal fading* can be overcome by preheating but cannot be eliminated fully. *An optical fading* can be avoided by wrapping dosimeter in an opaque envelope while keeping in area illuminated with an incandescent light. Dose response curve of TLD has *linear, supra linear, sublinear and saturation* regions. The dose measurements should be performed at the linear part of the curve. Hence, *dose response curve* must be established for a given TL material and reader. TL response is linear for doses up to 1 Gy, and it requires correction for higher doses. Since, TLD response is proportional to mass, samples of equal mass should be used.

In high energy photon beams, TLD should be used with build-up caps to achieve an electronic equilibrium. The build-up cap must be made of tissue equivalent material. For photon energies < 300 keV, thin TLDs are used without build-up caps, e.g., *Lithium borate*. However, TLD measurements should be compared with that of calibrated ion chamber readings. Background signal arises from an unirradiated samples due to *PMT dark current, background luminescence and residual signal* from previous irradiation. Reproducibility depends on quality of TLD material which needs to be tested randomly by irradiating the batch of known radiation.

Nowadays, computer controlled TLD readers are available to analyze *TLD chips, ribbons, powder, discs, pellets, rods, and micro cubes*. They display digital glow curve and temperature profile. They can handle one or more planchets at a time either with manual drawer or computer controlled, drawer function. Programmable annealing oven is also available along with the system. TLD finds application in patient and phantom dosimetry, in-vivo measurements, treatment verification QA, total body irradiation, build-up region dose distribution, brachytherapy, personnel monitoring, and dosimetry audit. However, dosimeters need pre-calibration, and corrections for energy, fading and non-linearity response.

Scintillation Detector

Radiation interacts with a crystal medium and does an ionization and excitation. Recombination or re-excitation releases thermal energy as molecular vibrations in liquid and gases or lattice vibrations in crystals. There are certain materials that emit visible or ultraviolet light during such process. They are called as *scintillators* and detectors made with such *scintillators* are called *scintillation detector*. There are two types of scintillators:

❑ Inorganic scintillator
❑ Organic scintillator

In both cases, the amount of light emission is proportional to the amount of energy deposited in the scintillator. The light emission is so small, it is about 100–1,000 photons per gamma ray of energy 70–511 keV. Hence, the signal needs to be amplified, hence all scintillation detectors are provided with

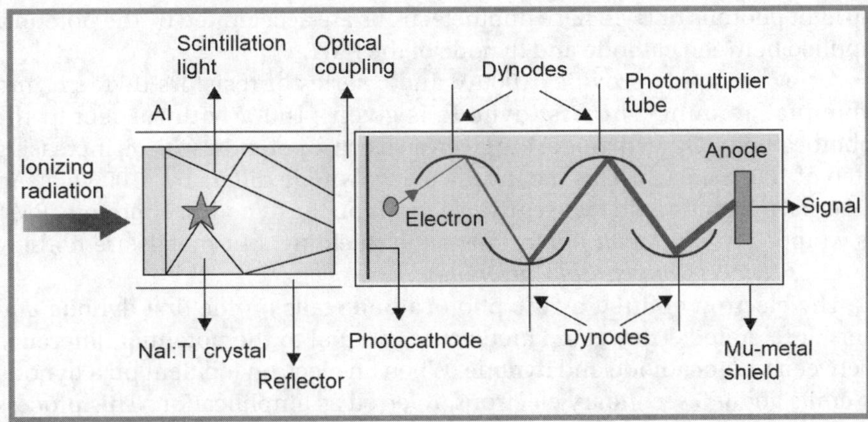

Fig. 5.7: Scintillation detector with photomultiplier tube.

photomultiplier tubes (PMT). The PMT not only collects the light and converts into an electric signal but also amplifies that signal. The electric signal is proportional to the light emission, in turn proportional to an incident energy of the radiation. The light emission increases with an incident radiation energy. A scintillation detector consists of the following **(Fig. 5.7)**:

❏ Scintillator crystal
❏ Photomultiplier tube or photodiode
❏ Electrical circuit to record the pulse

The scintillator crystal and the photomultiplier are coupled together by an optical material to minimize photon reflection losses. When a photon interacts with the crystal, the electrons are raised to an excited state. The excited electrons return to the lower energy state with emission of visible and UV light. This is called *luminescence* and each luminescence event has its own decay constant. That means that light emission takes some time to cease out which is called as *afterglow*. The crystal is surrounded by *Magnesium oxide* powder (reflective material) to prevent light losses. These photons are radiated in all directions. The *Magnesium oxide* layer reflects the photons towards the window side only.

Photomultiplier Tube

PMT is an electronic device which is an evacuated and sealed glass envelope (1–7.5 m diameter). It consists of:

❏ Photocathode inside the glass window
❏ Series of dynodes (10–12)
❏ Anode

Its front entrance is coated with *Cesium antimony (CsSb)* which serves as photocathode. Its conversion efficiency decides the quantum detection efficiency of the detector. The photocathode receives low energy light photons and ejects number of photoelectrons. Generally, 1–3 electrons are emitted per

10 light photons or UV. These photoelectrons are accelerated by the potential applied between cathode and dynode of the PMT.

A power supply provides 1000 V and a series of resistors divide it into an equal amount. The first dynode is given +100 V with respect to the photocathode. Other dynodes are given an electric potential with an increasing step of 100 volt each. This means that each dynode differs by +100 volts. An external magnetic field focuses the electrons on the dynodes. Therefore, PMT is wrapped in *mu-metal foil* for magnetic shielding. Mu-metals are nothing but *Iron, Nickel Copper and Chromium*.

The electron emitted by the photocathode falls on the first dynode and gets accelerated. They gain kinetic energy equal to the potential difference between photocathode and dynode. When an electron incident on a dynode it emits about 5 secondary electrons, referred as amplification. This process continues in second dynode and so on. For example, a PMT with 10 dynodes of 5 amplification each may give multiplication of 10^5. Electrons are attracted towards anode to give the final voltage pulse. This multiplication factor depends on photoelectron energy, and the voltage difference between the dynode and photocathode.

Finally, the PMT produces a voltage pulse in an output condenser, which is coupled to an external pulse amplifying circuit. Thus, the initial energy of a single ionizing particle, is transformed into a single voltage pulse. The whole system is enclosed in a light tight box to eliminate effects other than those due to an incident ionizing radiation.

The number of electrons ejected from the photocathode is proportional to the amount of light that reaches it. The amount of light in turn proportional to an energy absorbed from the photon beam by the crystal. Thus, the size of the pulse that emerges from the anode is proportional to the energy of an incident photon in the crystal. Hence, this detector can be used to distinguish between photons of different energy. Due to statistical variations within the crystal and PMT, there is a spread of pulses about the peak value.

Scintillation detectors are operated in pulse mode as spectrometer, where the afterglow is less important, and an electronic circuit will identify the individual interaction. If it is operated in current mode, an individual interaction cannot be identified.

Inorganic Scintillators

Inorganic crystal's structure gives the scintillation property and are basically solids. The atoms and molecules do not scintillate. Pure inorganic crystals emit light only in liquid Nitrogen temperature. Hence, these crystals are added with impurity or activators, which are responsible for the scintillation effects at room temperature, e.g., NaI:Tl and CsI:Na. Energy resolution is based on crystal characteristics.

Some of the crystal characteristics are conversion efficiency, matching-light emission and spectral sensitivity of PMT/Photodiode, decay time of excited state, transparent material-light, high Z-High detection efficiency, and rugged, unaffected by moisture, and inexpensive.

Table 5.1: Radiological scintillators.

Material	Density, g/cm²	Atomic Number	Conversion efficiency, %	Decay constant, μs	Afterglow, ms, %
NaI:Tl	3.67	11,53	100	0.25	0.3–5
$Bi_4Ge_3O_{12}$	7.13	83,32,8	12–14	0.30	0.005
CsI: Na	4.51	55,53	85	0.63	–
$CdWO_4$	7.9	48,74,8	40	14	0.1
$CaWO_4$	6.12	20,74,8	14–18	0.9–2.0	–
$CGd_2O_2S:Tb$	7.34	64,8,16	–	560	–

(*Courtesy:* Jerrold T Bushberg et al, 2012)

Scintillation crystals are the oldest, *Barium platinocyanide* was used during X-ray discovery by WC Roentgen. Film-screen radiography used *CaWO₄* for many years as intensifying screens in cassettes. It is replaced by rare earth phosphors, e.g., G*adolinium oxysulfide: Terbium. Cesium iodide: thallium* is used in thin film transistor (TFT) technology in digital radiography. Fluoroscopy uses *CsI: Na, ZnCds: Ag,* as an input and output phosphor in an image intensifier tube (IIT).

In CT scans, scintillator coupled with photodiode is used. Since, the X-ray flux is very high, it requires current mode operation, to avoid dead time loses. High resolution CT scan operating with subsecond, requires crystals with less after glow. *Cadmium tungstate and Gadolinium ceramics* are commonly employed as scintillators in such CT machines. **Table 5.1** summarizes the various scintillators used in radiology and their physical properties.

Sodium iodide (NaI:Tl) is used in all nuclear medicine applications. It is used in Gamma camera, thyroid probe, and gamma well counter, under pulse mode operation. It has high density (Iodine Z = 53) and provides high photoelectric absorption probability for X and gamma rays. It has very high conversion efficiency (13%) and emits light promptly with a decay constant of 230 ns, resulting high energy resolution. It is possible to manufacture large crystals of size about 59 cm long × 44.5 cm wide × 0.95 cm thick. However, they are fragile and hygroscopic and require tight *hematic sealing*.

Positron emission tomography (PET) uses thicker crystals of high density and high atomic number (Z). *Bismuth germinate, BGO ($Bi_4Ge_3O_{12}$)* is used as detector in PET scanners. The high atomic number (Bismuth, Z = 83) and high density, provide high intrinsic efficiency for positron gammas with a decay constant of 300 ns. The other PET detectors are *Lutetium oxyorthosilicate, LSO (Lu_2SiO_4O), Lutetium- yttrium oxyorthosilicate, LYSO ($Lu_xY_{2-x}SiO_4O$), and Gadolinium oxyorthosilicate, GSO (Gd_2SiO_4O)*. **Table 5.2** summarizes the physical properties of various scintillators used in nuclear medicine.

Table 5.2: Physical properties of various scintillators used in nuclear medicine.

Property	NaI:Tl	BGO	LSO:Ce	GSO:Ce	CsI:Tl	LuAP:Ce	LaBr:Ce
Density, g/cm²	3.67	7.13	7.4	6.71	4.51	8.34	5.3
Effective Z	50	73	66	59	54	65	-
Decay time, ns	230	300	40	60	1000	18	35
Photon yield/keV	38	8	20–30	12–15	52	12	61
Refractive index	1.85	2.15	1.82	1.85	1.80	1.97	1.9
Hygroscopic	Y	N	N	N	little	N	Y
Peak emission, nm	415	480	420	430	540	365	358

(*Courtesy:* Simon R Cherry et al, 2012)

Photodiode

Photodiode is a light sensitive semiconductor device that converts light into an electrical signal, e.g., *Si photodiode*. It is always used with a scintillator. The diode detects the light emitted from the scintillator. It is connected in reverse bias voltage and no current flows in the circuit. When photodiode is exposed to light, an ionization take place and charge is produced, resulting an electrical current. This current is proportional to amount of an incident light on the photodiode. It does not provide amplification as PMT does and its signal involves noise.

Photodiodes are smaller in size, cheaper and gives higher quantum detection efficiency of 60–80%. Nowadays *avalanche photodiode detectors (APD)* operated with much high internal electric field are available. The electrons gain energy in between collision and create secondary ionization, which gives a gain of 100–1000 as PMTs. However, it requires low noise electronics. APDs can be operated in Geiger mode with higher voltage. It gives much large signal, which is independent of an incident radiation energy. Scintillators with photodiodes are used in an indirect digital radiography as thin film transistor (TFT). It is also used in fluoroscopy as direct and an indirect flat panel systems, instead of an image intensifier tube. Photodiodes with $CdWO_4$ is used in CT scan as detector.

Organic Scintillator

Organic scintillator works based on molecular excitation which is one of its inherent property. Radiation excites the molecule, during deexcitation and visible light is released. It is available as *plastic and liquid scintillator* detectors. Liquid scintillation detector consists of *solvent, primary solute, secondary solute, and additives*. The scintillator (solute) is dissolved in a solvent in a glass or plastic vial. The radioactive material is added to the mixture and placed in between a pair of PMT. Commonly used solvent is *diisopropyl naphthalene (DIN)* and *phenylxylyl ethane (PXE)*, which absorbs most of the radiation energy. Primary solute absorbs energy from the solvent and emits light. Commonly used scintillator is *p-bis(omethylstyryl) benzene*

(MSB) and *2,5-diphenyloxazole (PPO)*. Secondary solute absorbs the light and remits photons of longer wavelength, to match the PMT response. Additives are added to improve efficiency of energy transfer from solvent to solute.

Liquid organic scintillators are suitable for low energy X-rays, γ-rays and nonpenetrating radiations. It also useful in assay of radioactivity specimens such as samples of blood and urine. It is widely used in ^{3}H and ^{14}C measurements. It is inefficient detector for penetrating radiation such as X and γ-rays and suffers from *quenching effects*. Quenching is the reduction of light output from the sample. Types of quenching includes chemical quenching, colour quenching, and dilution quenching. It can be minimized by dissolving oxygen purged by ultrasound or adding hydrogen peroxide, etc. Nowadays quench correction methods are available.

Semiconductor Detector

Semiconductor detectors are analogue of gas-filled detectors and works based on an ionization principle. It is an active radiation detector since immediate readout is possible. Detector materials have density more than 2,000–5,000 times compared to gases. Hence, they have higher stopping power, works much efficiently in X-ray and gamma ray energy range. Semiconductors are temperature dependent and gets damaged by an ionizing radiation over period. This changes its radiation sensitivity over ageing. They are relatively cheaper and available in variety of forms.

Semiconductors are crystalline materials whose conductivity falls in between a conductor and an insulator. Commonly used semiconductors are:

❑ Silicon (Si)
❑ Germanium (Ge)

Generally, they are poor conductors, when dopped with impurities they can be made as conductors. Impurities of en electron donor gives *n-type semiconductor*. Impurities of an electron acceptor atoms gives *p-type semiconductor*. Impuritie disturbs the crystal matrix so that an electron traps are formed. These traps are helpful to collect electrons after an ionization. The zone between the two is called *p-n junction or depleted region*. This region is a sensitive volume, in analogy with volume of gas in an ionization chamber and acts as barrier for current flow. Generally, semiconductor diode (PN Junction diode) is used as detectors with reverse bias voltage supply **(Fig. 5.8)**.

Function

When a semiconductor diode is exposed to X and gamma rays, an ionization and excitation are produced. Low energy electrons (valence band) in the depletion region are excited and raised to high energy state (conduction band). Absence of an electron creates a hole which is said to be positive. Hole moves towards p-type semiconductor and an electron moves towards n-type semiconductor. This produces a momentary current flow in the circuit and forms an voltage signal. It can be collected by an external circuit. The amount of energy required to create an electron-hole pair is 3–5 eV, compared to that

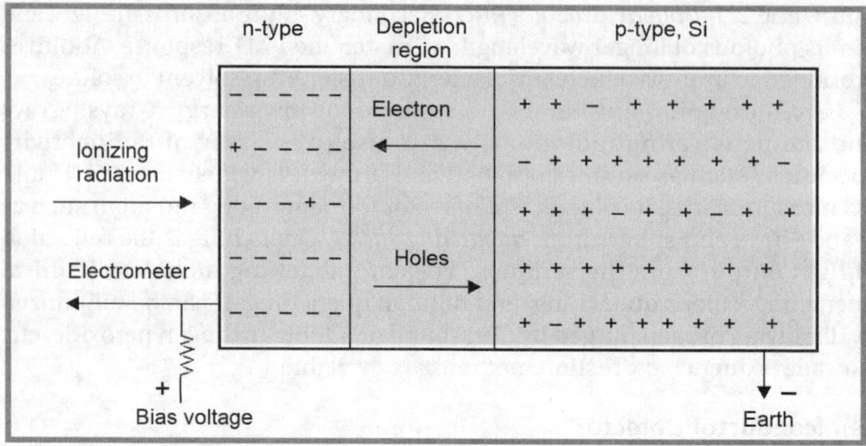

Fig. 5.8: Semiconductor detector: Silicon p-n junction diode made up of thin n-type material and single crystal of p-type silicon.

34 eV for ionization chambers. Hence, their electrical signal is 10 times larger than that of an ion chambers.

Semiconductor diode can be operated in two modes, namely with bias and without bias. In the former, resistance of the diode is a measure of intensity of radiation. The current is measured as a function of bias voltage. In the later, the voltage generated by the detector is proportional to radiation intensity. The charge collected from the diode is a measure of dose. The amount of charge generated per interaction is proportional to an energy deposited in the detector. Hence, the semiconductor behaves like a parallel plate ion chamber. That means that the size of the voltage pulse is proportional to the energy deposited in the detector. The voltage pulse is larger than an ion chamber and its amplitude is photon sensitive. The pulse raise time is shorter, since an electron, hole move rapidly. Hence, they can be used as spectrometers.

Semiconductor detector pulse is narrower than that of an ion chamber and hence energy resolution is better compared to an ion chamber and scintillation detector. The efficiency is 100% and its response is linear with exposure. It is independent of radiation type, and the absorption of energy at the entry window is smaller. Larger detectors of volume 100 cm^3 or more can be made for spectroscopic measurements. They can be made in small sizes and capable of measuring from 1 µGy to 16 Gy. Its dose rate response is linear from 5 µGyh^{-1} to 3 Gyh^{-1} and can be calibrated better than 5%. It is stable over wide temperature range (– 20 to + 80°C) and not hygroscopic. Since, the effective atomic number of Silicon is different from air, it is not tissue equivalent.

Semiconductor detectors are used in kV meter, digital pocket dosimeter (*Silicon*), and gamma ray spectrometry (*Germanium*). They can also be used as photodetectors (Si) in flat panel detectors in computed radiography. *Amorphous selenium (a-Se)* coupled with thin film transistor (TFT) is used in digital radiography. Photodiodes are semiconductor detectors which converts light into an electrical current. They are used along with scintillation detectors in CT scans. *Cadmium telluride (CdTe) and Cadmium zinc telluride (CZT)* crystals are used in nuclear medicine as detectors. Silicon diodes and metal oxide semiconductors-field effect transistors (MOSFET) are used in patient dosimetry.

BIOLOGICAL DOSIMETER

Biodosimetry is one of the method of measuring radiation absorbed dose in human. There are several physical and chemical methods that are available for the estimation of radiation absorbed dose in human, especially in radiation workers. Other methods are not very much useful under an accidental radiation exposure due to their nonavailability and partial body exposure. Hence, under an accidental condition it is the biological dosimeter that plays an important role in an estimation of radiation absorbed dose, as this method uses the biological sample such as blood, obtained from an exposed individual.

During radiation accident, various organs of the body receive radiation damage and they show different effect based on severity of damage. At cellular level, it is understood that any cell will suffer chromosomal damage. For biological dosimetry purpose, the cell to be assayed should be matured with a long residence time in the body and should be easily obtained from the body. Small lymphocyte present in the blood is highly suitable for this purpose. The cells in G_0 stage or resting phase of the cell cycle, neither divide or preparing to divide. The cell is only performing maintenance and its other functions. Hence, it is ideal to collect these cells for dicentric assay.

Chromosomal Aberration Analysis

Chromosome aberration occurs spontaneously. Radiation induced chromosome aberrations in human lymphocytes can be used to quantify radiation exposure during radiation accidents. The extent of genetic damage depends on cell type, number and kind of genes deleted, and either somatic or germ cell. *Chromosomal aberration analysis (CAA)* is based on measurement of frequency of dicentric chromosome. Blood sample is collected within few weeks of whole-body irradiation from an exposed individual and culture the lymphocytes in growth medium containing antibiotics and *phytohemagglutinin (PHA)* for 48 hours at 37°C. The PHA is added to stimulate cells to divide, and after 45 hours, *colcemide* is added to arrest the cells at metaphase.

At 48 hours the culture is centrifuged, and the cells are suspended in 0.075M Potassium chloride (KCl) for 10 minutes to provide *hypotonic treatment*. The cells are then resuspended in *fixative methanol: acetic acid (3:1)*. Cells are washed again with the above fixative and slides are prepared and stained with *fluorescence dye and Giemsa*. The cells are then scored for chromosomal aberration analysis. Cells having aberrations such as *dicentrics and rings* are carefully noted. For biological dosimetry purpose, several hundred cells are scored to get right estimation of dose. The scoring is studied with a standard dose response curve, to estimate radiation dose.

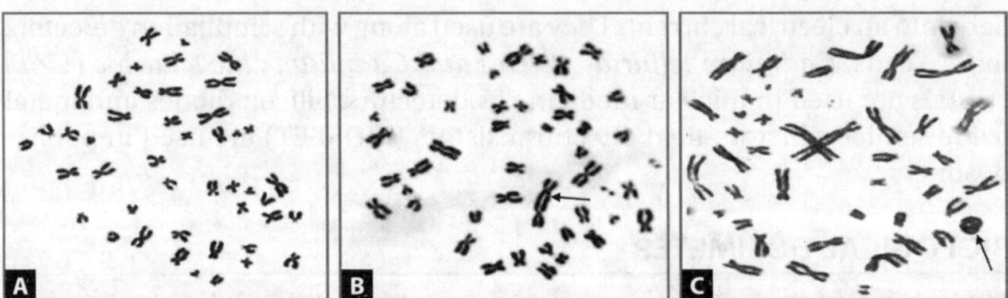

Figs. 5.9A to C: (A) Normal metaphase chromosome obtained from human peripheral blood lymphocytes; (B) Metaphase chromosome with a dicentrics (arrow) obtained from human peripheral blood lymphocytes exposed to gamma radiation; (C) Metaphase chromosome with a ring (arrow) obtained from human peripheral blood lymphocytes exposed to gamma radiation.

Dose-response Curve

It is important that the laboratory carrying out the biological dosimetry work must construct its own *dose-response curve*. The dose-response curve is prepared by exposing *in vitro* blood samples from normal persons with different radiation doses. The aberration per cell for each dose is scored. Then a graph is fitted between absorbed dose (Gy) and aberrations per cell in X and Y axis, respectively. The frequency of chromosome aberration is a linear quadratic function of dose for low LET radiation. Regarding to biological indicators, although various methods are available, the gold standard for estimation of radiation dose is chromosomal aberration technique by way of measuring the frequency of dicentric chromosome. **Figures 5.9A to C** shows the spread of chromosome as seen under the microscope.

The lowest dose that can be detected by the above method is 0.25 Gy, and 0.4 Gy for an acute and chronic radiation exposure, respectively. Chromosome aberrations are unstable and may be lost from the blood over time. The life span of a lymphocyte is only 150 days and hence, the dicentric yield decreases after a month or year of radiation exposure. This is useful and most sensitive technique during over exposures or suspected exposures in personnel monitoring, but it should be done within 6 months. The stable reciprocal translocations can be measured by *fluorescence in situ hybridization (FISH)*. In this, chromosome is labeled with chromosome specific fluorescent DNA probes. Then translocations can be viewed under the microscope. Since, reciprocal translocation exists for longer time, the Fluorescence In Situ Hybridization (FISH) method is most suited for delayed investigations.

CLINICAL DOSIMETERS

Ionization Chambers

Farmer (1955) designed an ion chamber, based on thimble chamber concept for measuring radiations. It looks like a thimble of a sewing machine. It has an air equivalent wall so that the volume of air is small **(Fig. 5.10)**. Later it was

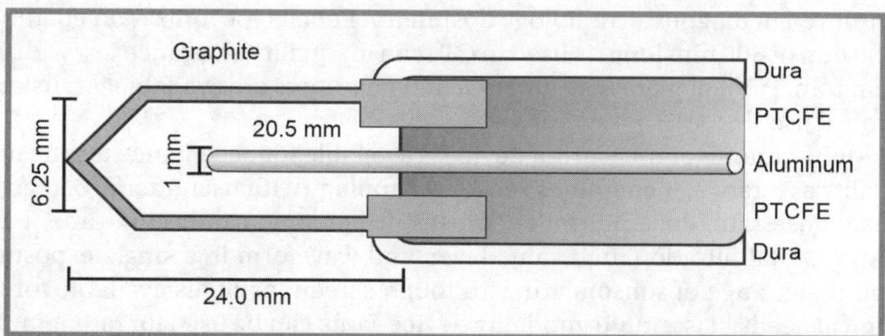

Fig. 5.10: Former type ionization chamber cross-section with air volume of 0.6 cc.

modified by **Aird and Farmer** for better efficiency and reproducibility with a stem leakage is about 0.4%. Farmer chamber consists of three electrodes:
- ❑ Central electrode
- ❑ Thimble wall
- ❑ Guard electrode

The *central electrode* is made up of Aluminum of 1 mm diameter, which collects the charge and provides current to the electrometer. The thimble wall or an outer electrode is made of *graphite* with a thickness range of 0.04–0.089 g/cm^2. Instead of *graphite, plastic (Polymethyl Methacrylate, PMMA), nylon, air or tissue equivalent plastic* can also be used.

The central electrode is insulated with *poly trichloro fluoroethylene (PTCFE)*, wrapped over by a cylindrical conducting guard electrode. The *guard electrode* is used to prevent leakage current from central electrode and defines the ion collecting volume. It is provided with second insulation, which isolates the guard from the outer electrode. Both the central electrode and guard are given same positive potential of about 300 V, whereas the *thimble wall* is at ground potential. The central electrode can be operated with negative voltage also, provided the polarity effect is minimum. It is connected to an electrometer for current/charge measurement. Generally, **Baldwin-Farmer** electrometer is used for measurements.

Chambers are provided with build-up cap made up of *acrylic* material for in air measurements. This will provide charged particle equilibrium during in air measurements. However, build-up cap is not used during in phantom measurements. When the chamber is used in water phantom, a thin waterproof sheath is used around the chamber. They can measure photon of energy up to 30–50 MV and electron energy of 6–50 MeV, respectively.

Several models of Farmer type chambers are available commercially, e.g., *PTW, Capintec, Wellhofer, Nuclear enterprise,* etc. Their central electrode and wall material composition is different. Chambers are semi-flex type, suitable for water phantom measurements. They have a short stem for mounting with flexible connection cable.

Typical chamber volume is 0.6 cm^3, provided without and with waterproof designs. Shallow-free ionization chambers of volume 6 cm^3 and 75 cm^3 are employed in diagnostic radiology dosimetry. Pencil type ionization chamber (100 mm or 300 mm long) is used in CT scan for quality assurance test with CT phantom. Parallel plate and spherical ion chambers are available for distinct clinical use.

Multi-parameter measuring device is available for acceptance testing and quality assurance. It combines sensor technology with user interface. It gives dose, dose rate, dose per pulse, pulses, frequency, irradiation time, tube voltage, total filtration, half value layer, and waveform in a single exposure. Complete range of sensors are with touch screen facility is available for all clinical needs. It is a multi-modality device same can be used for radiography and fluoroscopy. It is direction independent with built in memory.

Pocket Dosimeter

Pocket dosimeter is an ion chamber with a quartz fiber suspended with in an air-filled chamber, on a wire frame **(Fig. 5.11A)**. It has a built-in capacitance which can be charged by an external potential (charger). The positive charge is placed on the wire frame, by means of the charger. The *quartz fiber* is bent away from the frame due to columbic repulsion. This can be visible through an optical lens system upon which an exposure scale is superimposed.

The dosimeter should be fully charged prior to their use, so that an initial reading of the dosimeter is set at zero **(Fig. 5.11B)**. When exposed to ionizing radiation, ion pairs are produced in air. These ion pairs partially neutralize the positive charge, reducing the columbic repulsion and allowing the fiber to move. Hence, the quartz fiber moves closer to the wire frame that can be seen as down range excursion of the hair line fiber on an exposure scale *(graticule)*. The movement of the quartz fiber is proportional to the radiation exposure, which is measured in roentgen (R). The roentgen is the unit of exposure = 2.58×10^{-4} C/kg. The dose in air can be calculated from an exposure, where 1R exposure is equal to 8.76 mGy or 0.876 rad in air.

The dosimeter is available in different ranges varying from 0–200 mR, 0–500 mR, 0–5R, 0–20 R, 0–200 R, and 0–600 R, for measurement of X and gamma rays. It can detect photon energies from 20 keV–2 MeV. For personnel monitoring, smallest range of 0–200 mR is generally used. The accuracy of the pocket dosimeter is about ±10%. Pocket dosimeters are small and easy to use and do not provide permanent record. Sudden mechanical shock may result in wrong reading. Hence, these dosimeters should be handled with care so to indicate reliable reading of the doses received.

These dosimeters are available both in analog and digital types. The dose measurement range of digital pocket dosimeter is 10 µSv to 100 mSv. Presently, semiconductor (Si) diode-based electronic pocket dosimeters with digital display are available. They have an audio alarm, low weight, slim design, good energy, and polar response, with reliable readings, matching to TLD badges. They make loud bleep sounds for every 15 to 30 minutes on background. The sound become more frequent as dose rate increases and becomes continuous sound at high radiation fields. They can make loud audible signal and blinking

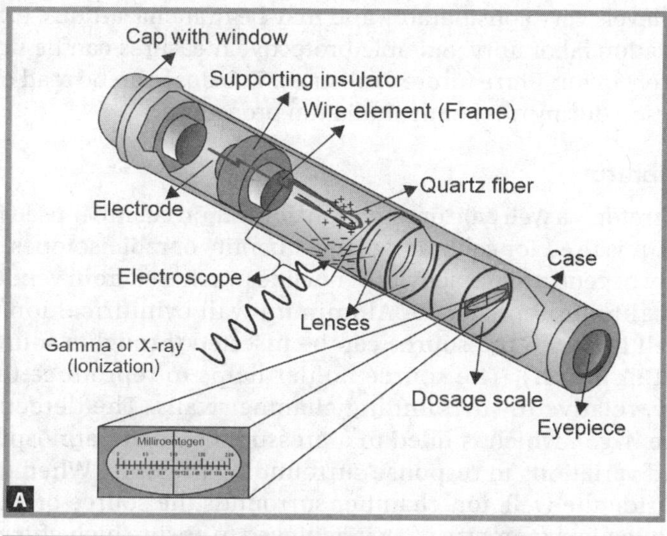

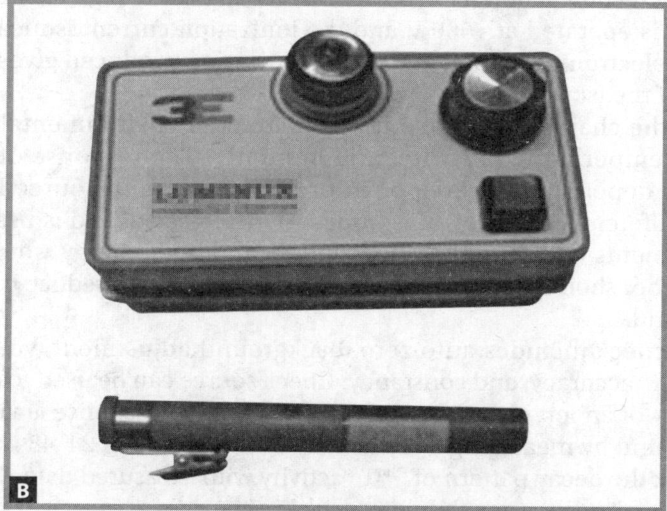

Figs. 5.11A and B: (A) Pocket dosimeter; (B) Charger.
(*Courtesy:* Meditronix corporation)

display if either the dose rate or accumulated dose exceed the set limits. The energy range of these dosimeters are 35 keV to 3 MeV and are available in mR and µSv display.

The main advantage of pocket dosimeter lies in its ability to provide instant-on the spot check of radiation dose received by a personnel. Film and TLD will not show an accumulated exposure immediately. In addition to the regular film badges, the radiation doses received by the radiation worker can be assessed by wearing a pocket dosimeter, which gives an instantaneous radiation exposure. This is very useful in nonroutine work, in which the radiation levels vary considerably and may be quite hazardous, e.g., cardiac catheterization laboratory. Suitable protective measures can be undertaken immediately to minimize future exposures. The dose can be read off directly by the person during or after the radiation procedure.

Dose Calibrator

Dose calibrator is a well type or re-entrant ionization chamber used in nuclear medicine. It is used for calibrating large quantity of radioisotopes. It verifies the activity of generator or activity of nuclide purchased from vendors.

Dose calibrator consists of Aluminum wall cylindrical ion chamber with a well in which the source can be inserted through a source holder **(Figs. 5.12A and B).** The source holder helps to reproduce the source geometry, relative to surrounding chamber walls. The detecting gas is ultra-pure *Argon* which is filled to a pressure of 5 or 12 atmosphere. This is to avoid variations in response surrounding pressure. When the source is kept inside the well, ion chamber surrounds the source on all sides so that the detection geometry of 4π is achieved to ensure high efficiency. The chamber is operated at +500 V and the ionization current is measured by using an electrometer. Total amount of ionization produced gives the total activity of the isotope.

Once the chamber is sealed it is free from an environmental changes such as temperature, pressure, and humidity. The response of the well chamber depends on source position in the well and source length. It cannot differentiate energy of isotopes. Hence, Lead shield is used during measurements to differentiate low energy and high energy isotopes. The ion chamber should be shielded with 2 inches of Lead to reduce the natural background.

Daily check includes auto zero, background adjustment, voltage test, data check, accuracy, and constancy. Check source can be used to check the constancy of an ion chamber. Linearity of chamber response is vital which can be found by measuring ^{99m}Tc activity over a period of 24–48 hours. One can check the decay pattern of ^{99m}Tc activity with measured data. The linear response of the calibrator should be within ±2%.

Nowadays, dose calibrator comes with menu driven 8-inch color VGA touch screen display. It displays radionuclide, activity, unit of measure, count rate values, and calibration number. It is provided with software upgrade and printer capability via USB. Maximum measurable activity is 6/20 Ci of ^{18}F with a resolution of 0.1 µCi and accuracy of 2%. It has built in dose calibration, quality control and self-diagnostics. It has 80 nuclides symbols and half-lives in memory. Response time is within 2 sec and 4–16 sec for low activity samples.

Dose-area Product Meter

Ionization chambers can be used to measure radiation intensity and field area simultaneously, while the beam is ON **(Fig. 5.13).** It is basically a flat

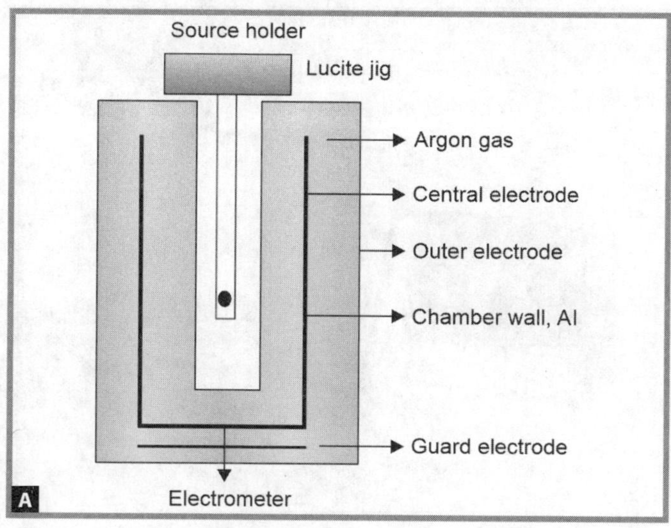

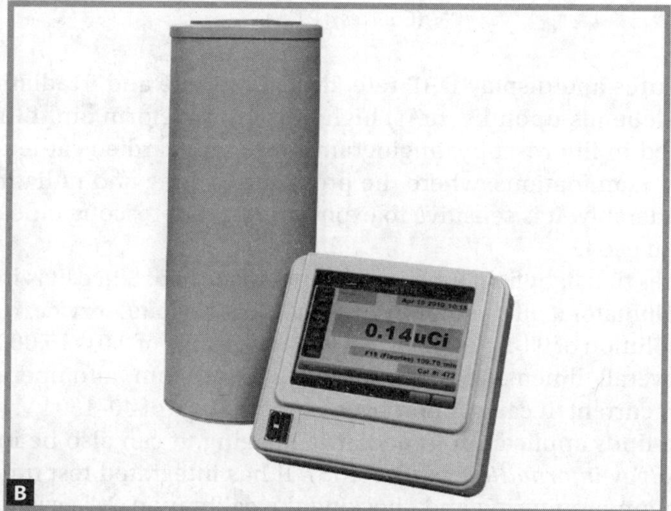

Figs. 5.12A and B: (A) Design of well type isotope calibrator used for radioisotope activity calibration in nuclear medicine; (B) Commercial model. (*Courtesy:* Meditronix corporation)

transparent ionization chamber fitted over the collimator of the X-ray unit. Usually, technologist or radiologist decides field area for each patient. It indicates that how much patient area is exposed with a given radiation dose. Hence, assessment of radiation hazards and associated biological effect is made easy. Air is used as medium hence the attenuation is much lesser. As it measures air dose and radiation field area, it gives the dose area product (DAP), hence the name dose-area product meter:

$$\text{Dose-area product} = \text{Dose} \times \text{area} \ (cGy.cm^2 \text{ or } \mu Gy.m^2)$$

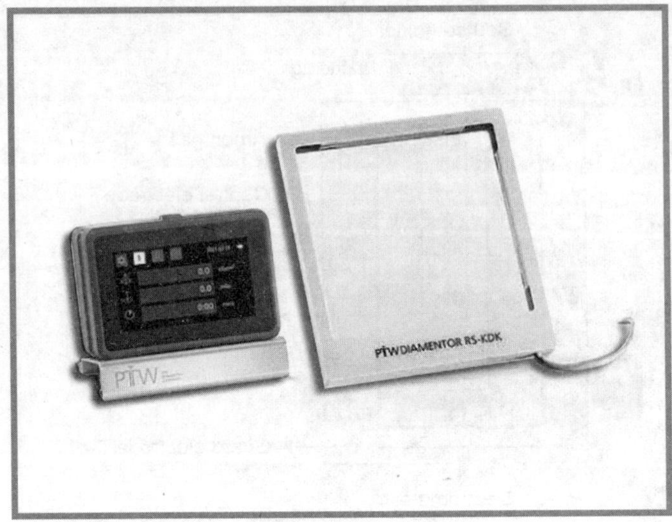

Fig. 5.13: Commercial dose-area product (DAP) meter design.
(*Courtesy:* PTW)

It measures and display DAP rate, dose, dose rate and irradiation time, but dose depends upon kV, mAs, high tension waveform and filtration. It is employed in fluoroscopy, angiogram, DSA, and cardiac catheterization laboratory examinations, where the procedure is long and radiation levels vary considerably. It is sensitive to exposure rate, fluoroscopy time and area of the beam used.

It ensures that light field functions are not disturbed. Since, it is integrated into the collimator it offers smooth and day to day hospital service. It provides higher resolution of 0.01 μGym^2 over a DAP rate range of 0.01–15,000 $\mu Gym^2/$sec. The overall dimension is about $164 \times 209 \times 10$ mm^3 and operated with 24 V direct current. It can support over a tube voltage of 40–150 kV. Its higher resolution finds application in pediatric imaging. It can also be integrated with *radiology information system (RIS)*. It has integrated test function for fast operation monitoring and checking the calibration. It is available with flexible cable of 25 m with dual ionization chamber and printer. However, the DAP meter will not record the source to patient distance, magnification mode, changes in the kV etc., which also influences the patient dose. DAP meter is also called as *Roentgen-area product (RAP) meter*.

RADIATION SURVEY METERS

The assessment of radiation levels at different locations in the vicinity of radiation installation is known as *area monitoring or radiation survey*. These measurements will give an idea about the radiation status of the installation. Based on measurements taken, one could confirm the adequacy or inadequacy of the existing radiation protection status. In case, if the radiation levels are found to be higher than the permissible levels, suitable remedial measures can be taken. Hence, the objective of the above measurement is to ensure radiation safety and minimize personnel exposure. An ideal monitor should have an uniform response to X and gamma radiation over the range of 15 keV to 3 meV. It should cover a wide range of exposure rates from 0.25 mR/h to a few 10 R/h. It should be able to assess beta radiation levels and be operable with battery cells.

Instruments used for the above purposes are called radiation survey meters and area monitors. In general, any survey meter/area monitor should consist of two main parts, namely, a device which detect the radiation, and a display system to measure the radiation. These instruments differ from each other in the medium in which the response takes place and in the method by which the response is detected and quantified. Types of survey meters are:

❏ Ionization chamber survey meter
❏ Geiger–Muller (GM) survey meter
❏ Scintillation detector survey meter
❏ Neutron survey meter

Selection of a particular detector depends on variety of factors like type of radiation, quantity to be measured, response of detector for the energy, etc. They can be used as portable radiation survey meters, capable of measuring radiation in mR/h or μSv/h. They are available in the form of vehicle mounted radiation meters, zone monitors, and doorway mounted meters, etc.

Ionization Chamber Survey Meter

Ionization chambers for low level X-ray monitoring (exposure/exposure rate) are fabricated out of air-equivalent materials (*bakelite, tufnol*) and they can be used over a wide range of energies from 7 keV to 2 MeV. A typical survey meter consists of a 500 cc chamber connected to a battery operated electrometer and can measure exposure rates from few mR/h to about 10 R/h (**Fig. 5.14A**). Some of these are provided with an end window of thin *mylar film* for beta radiation detection.

Ionization survey meters are used whenever an accurate measurement are required. They approximate the condition under which the roentgen is defined. It is used to check X-ray machine output, monitoring radionuclide therapy patients, and survey radioactive material packages. Ion chambers are influenced by changes in temperature, pressure, photon energy and exposure rate. These limitations are less important in medical applications (5% loss of exposure rate at 10 R/h).

Ion chambers are capable of monitoring higher radiation exposure rate levels, and available in different ranges: 0–5 mR/h, 0–50 mR/h, 0–500 mR/h, 0–5 R/h, and 0–50 R/h. They response slowly (8–2 sec) to rapidly changing exposure rate hence, needs warm up and stabilization before measurements are made.

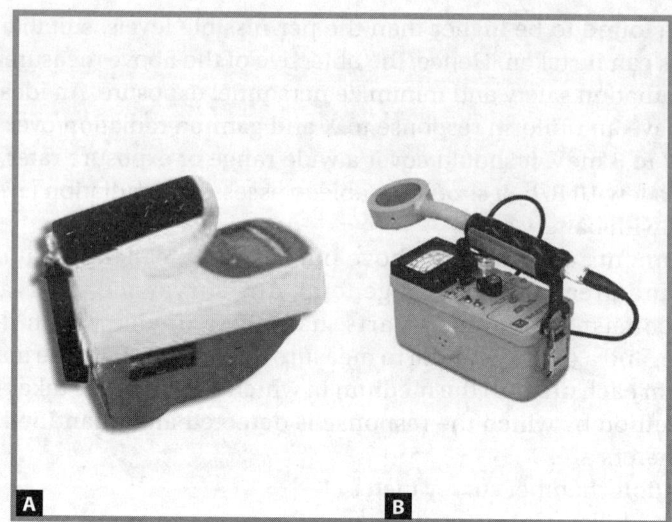

Figs. 5.14A and B: Survey meters: (A) Ion chamber survey meter; (B) GM type survey meter. (*Courtesy:* Meditronix corporation)

Nowadays, survey meters are provided with a lot of special features like auto-ranging and autozeroing, optional beta slide, simultaneous measurement of dose and dose rate, operated by two 9 volts alkaline batteries, check source, communications interface with windows based excel add-in for data logging, programmable flashing LCD display and audible alarm with dose equivalent energy response (SI units).

GM Survey Meter

GM type instruments are very sensitive and useful for monitoring of low-level radiation. Since electronic amplification is not necessary, the electronic circuit of GM is very simple, compared to that of an ionization chamber **(Fig. 5.14B).** This feature makes the GM type instruments rugged and less costly. GM counters used for radiation monitoring generally use a mixture of gases (*Argon, Neon, and Chlorine/Bromine*). It detects the presence and provides a semi-quantitative estimate of the radiation field magnitude. It provides measurements in counts per minute (cpm). It also provides an approximate measurement of mR/h, since it does not reproduce the conditions under which exposure is defined. However, the relationship between cpm and mR/h is a complicated function of photon energy.

GM counters for X-ray and gamma rays monitoring use *Copper or Chromium cathodes* for better efficiency. The primary photons interact with the cathode materials to produce secondary electrons. Since, GM meters are pulsed in nature, they should be used only in X-ray units that emits continuous X-rays. They should not be used in X-ray units, that emits pulsed X-rays (e.g., linear accelerators).

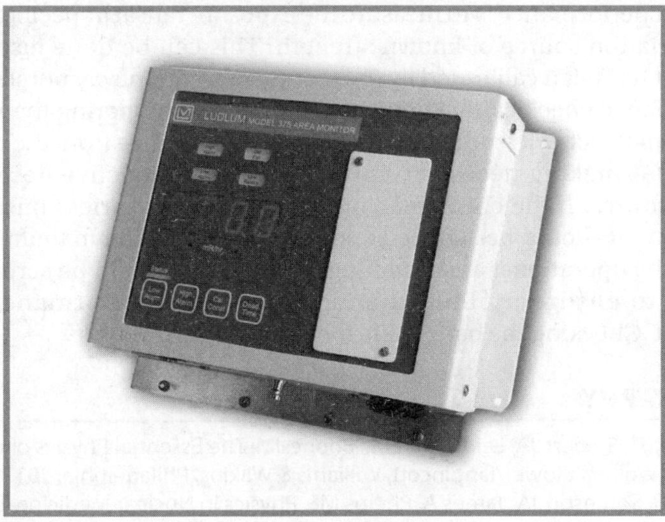

Fig. 5.15: Zone monitor used for area monitoring in Iodine-131 therapy wards at nuclear medicine.
(*Courtesy:* Meditronix corporation)

GM type meters are mainly used as radioactive contamination monitor with thin window (1.5–2 mg/cm^2), with large surface area. It will respond to alpha (>3 MeV), beta (>45 keV), X and gamma ray (>6 keV) radiations. GM detector is sensitive to particle radiation, but relatively insensitive to gamma radiations. It is suitable to measure natural background radiation which is about 50–100 cpm. It is mainly used in nuclear medicine for low level contamination surveys. GM type area monitors are used in nuclear medicine in Iodine–131 therapy wards **(Fig. 5.15).** GM counters have long dead time (100 μsec) and result in 20% loss at 100,000 cpm measurements. They should not be used in high level radiation fields or when accurate exposure rates are required.

Though GM survey meters often display with mR/h, it is not a true exposure rate, but a good approximation. Hence, an ionization chamber survey meters are preferred for accurate radiation survey. Geiger counters are available in different forms, namely, flat, thin window counters (*pancake*) and are suitable for radioactive contamination and low-level radiation survey. It has peak sensitivity at the diagnostic energy range hence, it can be used for leakage measurements.

Calibration and Maintenance of Radiation Monitoring Instruments

Radiation monitoring instrument must be purchased along with calibration certificate and kept in good working condition. It should be further calibrated from an authorized calibration laboratory. They should be periodically checked to confirm that reliable readings are indicated. They should also be checked after any servicing or repairs. The simplest method of checking the instrument performance is to measure the exposure rate at a specific distance from a radiation source of known strength. This can be done just after an instrument has been calibrated by the manufacturer or newly purchased.

Performance check can be done at any time, by comparing the recorded reading with the check reading made at the same distance from the radiation source, after making necessary corrections for radioactive decay of the radiation source. If the check reading after correction varies considerably, the instrument should be serviced and recalibrated by the manufacturer. In addition, the operational and handling instructions should be scrupulously observed to ensure prolonged and trouble-free performance of the instrument. Checking the battery life frequently is also vital.

BIBLIOGRAPHY

- Bushberg JT, Seibert JA, Leidholdt EM, Boone JM. The Essential Physics of medical imaging, Wolters Kluwer/Lippincott, Williams & Wilkins, Philadelphia; 2012.
- Cherry SR, Sorenson JA, James A, Phelps ME. Physics in Nuclear Medicine, Elsevier, Philadelphia; 2012.
- Metcalfe P, Kron T, Hoban P. The Physics of Radiotherapy X-rays and Electrons, Medical Physics Publishing, Madison; 2007.
- Thayalan K. Basic Radiological Physics, 2nd edn. Jaypee Brothers Medical Publishers (P) Ltd, New Delhi; 2017.
- Thayalan K. The Physics of Radiation Oncology, Jaypee Brothers Medical Publishers (P), New Delhi; 2023.

Screen-Film Radiography

RADIOGRAPHY

Radiography is a medical investigation in diagnostic radiology in which X-rays are used to produce a shadow picture of a patient. This will enable us to visualize an internal structure of a patient. It is the first imaging modality in medicine to obtain two-dimensional image of patient's anatomy by using a X-ray film or digital detector **(Fig. 6.1A).** It is used in variety of diagnosis, starting from bone imaging to chest radiography. In a radiography technique, the radiation from a X-ray tube is transmitted through patient's body, and then reaches the film/digital detector. After processing the film, a radiograph is obtained which is a negative image. The production of good radiological image requires a number of accessories such as (1) beam restrictor and collimator, (2) filter, (3) grid, (4) cassette, (5) an intensifying screen, and (6) X-ray film or digital detector, in addition to a X-ray unit. The principle of the above accessories will be discussed in the following topics.

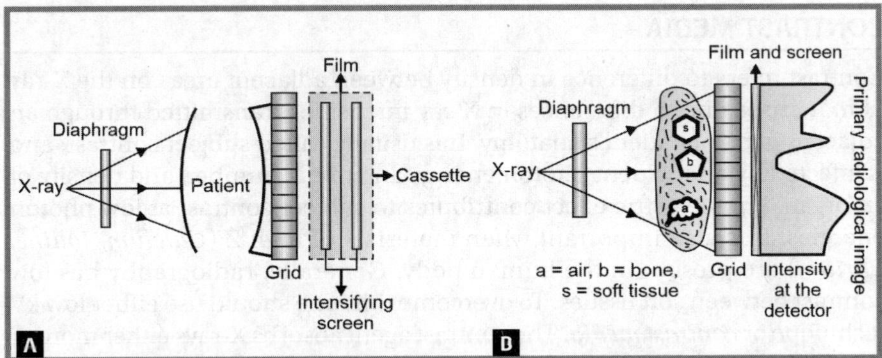

Figs. 6.1A and B: (A) Radiography principle; (B) Primary radiological image.

Table 6.1: Physical characteristics of air, fat, water, soft tissue, and bone.

Medium	Effective atomic number (Z)	Density g/cm³	Electron per gram × 10²³	Electron density × 10²³	Linear attenuation coefficient @50 keV
Air	7.6	0.00129	3.00	0.0038	0.000029
Fat	6.3	0.91	3.34	3.04	0.193
Water	7.42	1.00	3.34	3.34	0.214
Soft tissue	7.22	1.04	3.36	3.40	0.214
Compact bone	13.8	1.85	3.19	5.91	0.573

(*Courtesy:* Jerrold T Bushberg et al, 2012)

Primary Radiological Image

Human body is heterogeneous. It is mainly made up of air, fat, water, soft tissue and bone of differing density and atomic number **(Table 6.1)**. When X-rays pass through body, it gets attenuated differentially by different tissues, and results in variation of transmitted radiation. This variation is referred to as primary radiological image **(Fig. 6.1B)**. Since the eye is insensitive to X-rays, the above image is converted into visible image either by using a X-ray film or fluorescent screen or digital detector.

The beam that emerges from the patient contains primary and scattered radiation. Only the primary beam contains useful information of patient. Hence, the scattered radiation must be removed, before reaching the film. In the diagnostic range, the X-ray interacts mostly by photoelectric effect, which is proportional to Z^3. The Compton interaction is minimum and mostly with low Z materials. Overall, photoelectric effect dominates over Compton scattering at this energy level. Hence, bone, soft tissue and fat will offer differential attenuation to X-rays. As a result, the transmitted radiation comes out of these organs will also have variation. Thus, bone, soft tissue, and fat can be distinguished from one another.

CONTRAST MEDIA

Contrast refers to difference in density between adjacent areas on the X-ray film. It arises due to differences in X-ray intensities transmitted through an adjacent parts of patient's anatomy. It is usually called subject contrast, and is affected by an incident photon energy, an atomic number, and density of an organ. Photoelectric effect contributes to subject contrast at low photon energies. It is also important when materials of high Z (*Calcium, Iodine, Barium*) are present in the human body. Generally, radiography has low contrast between soft tissues. To overcome this, one should use either low kV technique or *contrast media.* The contrast agent absorbs X-rays either more or less than the surrounding tissues. They are necessary to visualize many organs in the body with much detail.

Contrast agents are used to improve subject contrast, they are basically *radiopaque media*. They have high atomic number to maximize photoelectric absorption. They are compounds of one or more elements. Their absorption edge should be just below the transmitted X-ray spectrum. The type of contrast agents used are:

❑ Air
❑ Iodine compounds
❑ Barium compounds

Air has negligible density compared to tissues and absorbs very little X-rays. Hence, air cavities can be easily distinguished from other body tissues. However, its role is limited due to the arrival of CT and MRI. It is used only in double contrast Barium enema examinations.

Iodine (Z = 53, K-edge = 33 keV) is also an excellent contrast agent. It can be injected intravenously to improve subject contrast. Barium is administered as a contrast agent due to its high Z (56) and physical density. Its K-edge is 37 keV, which matches the photon energies used in fluoroscopy. Organs filled with Barium or Iodine absorbs X-rays very strongly relative to surrounding and transmits very little radiation, thereby improving subject contrast. The characteristic radiation from Iodine and Barium are energetic, leave the patient and reaches the detector. In angiography, a vessel under an investigation is injected with contrast media. Initially an ionic Iodine is used, it is replaced by non-ionic contrast media now a days. It has low a concentration of ions and reduce physiologic problems and reactions.

BEAM RESTRICTORS AND COLLIMATORS

X-ray beam restrictor is a device that is attached to the X-ray tube housing, to regulate the size and shape of X-ray beam **(Figs. 6.2A and B).** They can be classified into three categories, namely:

❑ Aperture diaphragm
❑ Cones and cylinder
❑ Collimator

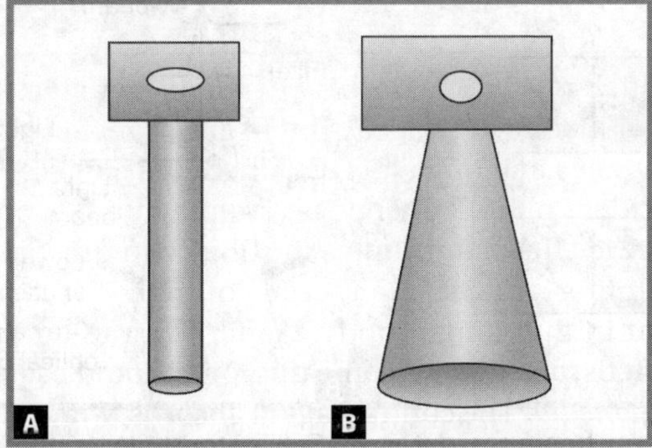

Figs. 6.2A and B: X-ray beam restrictors: (A) Cylinder; (B) Cone.

Aperture diaphragms consist of a sheet of *Lead* with a hole in the center. The size of the hole determines the size and shape of X-ray beam. It is simple and the aperture can be altered to any size and shape. The disadvantage of an aperture diaphragm is that it produces large penumbra. The penumbra can be reduced by keeping aperture diaphragm far away from the X-ray target. Aperture diaphragms are used in *dental radiography* with rectangular collimation. In addition, it is used in *trauma* and *chest radiography.*

The use of cones and cylinders will reduce penumbra considerably. Both have an extended metal structures that restrict the useful circular beam to required size. The position and size of the distal end determines the field size. If the X-ray source, cone, and film are not aligned properly, then one side of the film may not be exposed, which is called *cone cutting.* Cone is an ideal beam restrictor, but the flare of the cone should be greater than the flare of the X-ray beam. These systems provide only limited number of field sizes. Cone is used in *sinus radiography* which restricts scattered to radiation large extent.

The collimator is the best X-ray beam restrictor. It defines the size and shape of the X-ray field that emerges from the X-ray tube. The collimator assembly is attached to tube housing at the tube port. It consists of two sets of Lead *shutters*, which can be moved independently. Each shutter consists of four or more Lead plates of 3 mm Lead thickness, which can absorb X-rays completely, to provide a well-defined X-ray field. When the shutters are closed, they meet at the center of the X-ray field.

The collimator also has a *light* and *mirror* arrangement, to illuminate the X-ray field. The light bulb is positioned laterally, and the mirror is mounted in the path of the X-ray beam at an angle 45° **(Figs. 6.3A and B).** The target and the light bulb should be kept at an equal distance from the center of the mirror. The collimator provides a variety of rectangular X-ray field size, and the light beam shows the center of the X-ray field. The light field and radiation field should match exactly with each other, referred as field *congruence.* The

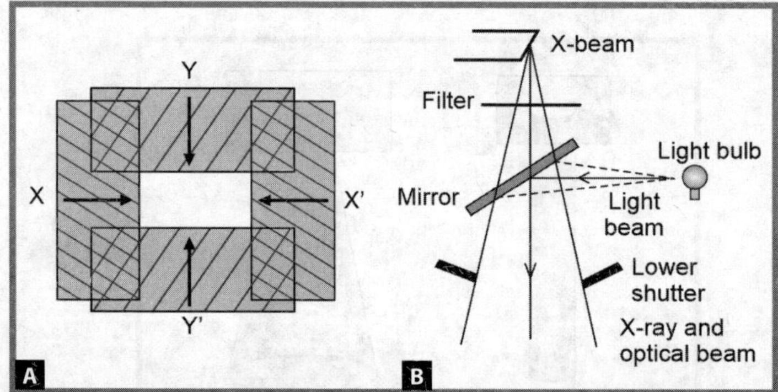

Figs. 6.3A and B: X-ray beam restrictor: (A) Collimator shutters; (B) Light and mirror arrangement to create radiation and an optical field coincidence.

variation must be within 4% of SID. The alignment of light beam and X-ray beam should be checked periodically. A well collimated beam covers lesser area of the patient and gives less patient dose. It also generates less scatter radiation, which improves image quality.

Collimators that automatically limit the X-ray field size to the useful area of the detector is also available, referred to as *positive beam limitation* (PBL) collimators. A sensor in the cassette holder, adjust the collimator opening, equal to the cassette dimensions. Thus, PBL collimators limit the irradiated volume and reduce the patient dose.

FILTERS

A filter is a metallic sheet introduced in the path of X-rays, to reduce patient dose **(Fig. 6.4)**. Diagnostic X-rays consist of both low energy and high energy X-rays. When X-rays pass through a patient, only high energy X-rays penetrate through the patient and form radiological image. The low energy X-rays are absorbed only in first few centimeters of tissue, in turn increase radiation dose. Introduction of filter absorbs these low energy X-rays and reduce patient dose. This process of removing low energy X-rays by introducing metallic sheets is called *filtration*. Filtration has two components namely:

❑ Inherent filtration
❑ Added filtration

Total filtration = Inherent filtration + Added filtration

Filtration resulting from the absorption of X-rays by X-ray tube and its housing is called an *inherent filtration*. This usually varies between 0.5 mm and 1.0 mm of Al equivalent. Added filtration results from additional absorbers placed in the path of the X-ray beam:

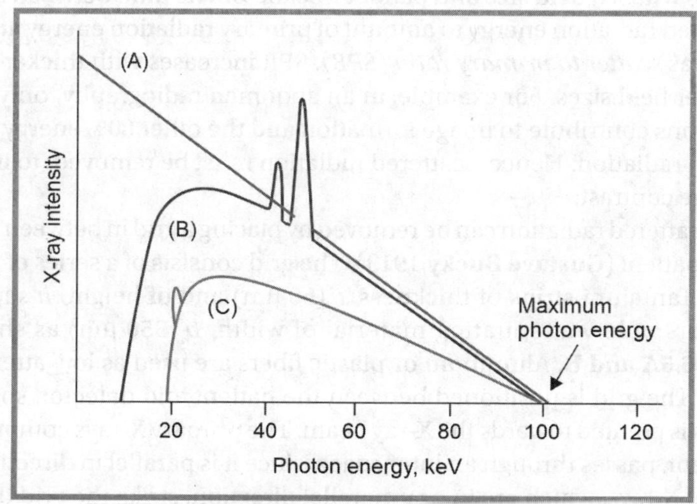

Fig. 6.4: Effect of filter: (A) Unfiltered spectrum; (B) Filtered spectrum with inherent filter; (C) Filtered spectrum with an added filter.

Al and Cu are the materials usually used as filters in diagnostic radiology. The thickness of added filter varies from 1.0 mm to 1.5 mm of Aluminum (Al). Al (Z = 13) is an excellent filter material for low energy X-rays. *Copper (Z = 29)* is a better filter for high energy X-rays. A compound filter consists of two or more layers of different metals like Cu + Al. The layers are arranged in such a way that the high Z layer always faces the X-ray tube.

Heavy metal filters (Gd, Ho) are also used in general radiography. These filters make use of K-edge absorption, and offer an increased absorption of X-rays, while imaging with contrast agents. They enhance contrast for Iodine and Barium, reduce patient dose and increase tube loading. The recommended beam filtration for radiography is follows:

❑ 1.5 mm Al below 70 kV
❑ 2.0 mm Al between 70 and 100 kV
❑ 2.5 mm Al above 100 kV

X-ray units with proper filters reduce patient dose significantly, up to 80%. Filters are simple and inexpensive. Though filters reduce the intensity of X-ray beam significantly, it does not affect the maximum energy of X-ray beam spectrum.

GRID

When a beam of X-ray passes through the patient, it is partly absorbed and scattered. The partly absorbed primary beam gets transmitted and gives a partly useful shadow in the film. The scattered radiation will tend to spoil the shadow. Scattered radiation contributes a constant background fog to the image in the film. This will increase noise in the image. Scattered radiation increases with kV, field size and patient thickness. The ratio between amount of scattered radiation energy to amount of primary radiation energy at a point is called as *scatter to primary ratio (SPR)*. SPR increases with thicker patient and larger field sizes. For example, in an abdomen radiography, only 20% of the photons contribute to image formation and the other 80% energy goes as scattered radiation. Hence, scattered radiation must be removed, to increase the image contrast.

The scattered radiation can be removed by placing a grid in between the film and the patient (**Gustave Bucky**, 1913). The grid consists of a series of parallel Lead or Tantalum strips of thickness, *c* (50 μm) and of height, *h* separated by spacers of low attenuating material of width, *b* (350 μm) as shown in **Figures 6.5A and B**. Aluminum or plastic fibers are used as low attenuating spacers. The grid is positioned between the patient and detector, so that its long axis is pointed towards the X-ray beam. The primary X-rays coming out of the patient, passes through an inter space, since it is parallel in direction. The scattered X-rays, which are in non-parallel direction, strike the grid bars and get absorbed. The ratio of the primary transmission to scatter transmission of a grid is called the *selectivity*.

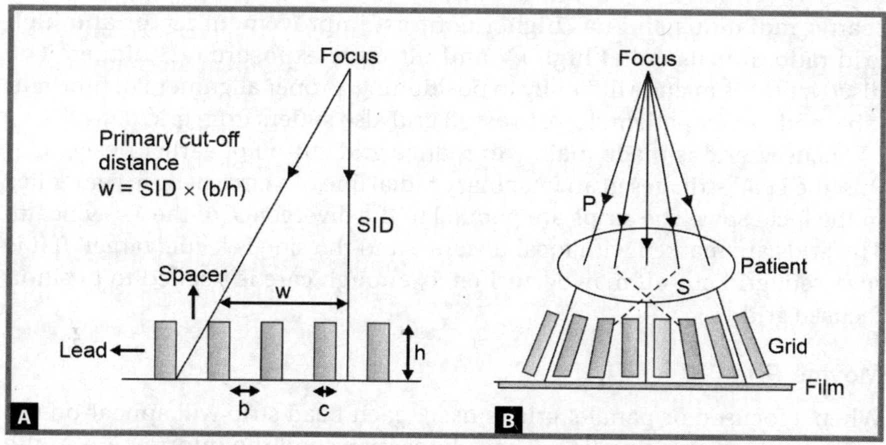

Figs. 6.5A and B: Grid: (A) Grid design; (B) Principle of grid.

Grid Ratio

The ability of the grid to discriminate against scattered radiation is measured by grid ratio, which is defined as the ratio of height (h) to width (b) of the spacer between the Lead strips:

$$\text{Grid ratio} = \frac{h}{b}$$

As the grid ratio increases, the grid removes more scatter radiations. The strip line density is $1/(b+c)$ lines per unit length. Typical grid ratio ranges from 4:1 to 16:1 and strip line densities are 25–60 lines per cm.

The performance of a grid can be understood by *contrast improvement factor*. It is ratio between image contrast with grid and image contrast without grid at 100 kV. Higher grid ratio provides higher contrast improvement factor. However, it increases patient dose, as it employs higher exposure techniques. *Bucky factor* is another parameter which is related to patient dose. It is the ratio between patient dose with grid and patient dose without grid. Bucky factor increases with increase of kV and grid ratio.

Types of Grid

Grids may be classified as (1) parallel grid, (2) crossed grid, (3) focused grid, and (4) moving grid. In a parallel grid, the Lead strips are parallel to each other in their longitudinal axis. Most of the X-ray tables are provided with linear grids. It is easy to design but has the property of *grid cut-off*. This means that the attenuation of primary radiation is greater at the edges, and it can be a partial or complete cut-off. The distance of grid cut-off may be estimated from the ratio between source to image distance (SID) and grid ratio.

Crossed grid is made up of Lead strips that are parallel to long axis and short axis of the grid. Usually, it is designed with two parallel grids, that are perpendicular each other. The grid ratio of crossed grids is equal to the sum of the ratios of the two parallel grids. Crossed grids are efficient in removing scatter radiations and has higher contrast improvement factor and high grid ratio. It is useful at high kV and tilt-table exposure techniques. The disadvantages include difficulty in positioning, proper alignment of tube and table and higher patient dose. Crossed grid also suffers from grid cut-off.

Focused grid is made mainly to reduce grid cut-off of earlier designs. In this, the Lead strip lies in an imaginary radial line of a circle whose center lies in the focal spot. The strips are parallel to the divergence of the X-ray beam. The grids are marked with focal distance and the side is facing target. If it is reversed, grid cut-off may occur hence, enough care is needed to position focused grid.

Moving Grid

When a focused or parallel grid is used, each Lead strip will appear on the radiograph as very fine line. These lines may spoil the information in the film. However, these lines may be removed by moving the grid during the radiographic exposure. This is the principle of *Potter-Bucky grid* (**Hollis E. Potter, 1920**). Generally, focused grids are used as moving grids. The grid may be made to move continuously in one direction. The grid motion is timed by the exposure control of X-ray machine. It starts moving just before the X-rays are turned ON and continues to move even after the exposure is OFF. The traveling period of grid should be greater than an exposure time.

There are two types of moving grids, namely, *(1) reciprocating grid and (2) oscillating grid.* The reciprocating grid is driven by a motor and the grid moves back and forth several times, during exposure. The distance traveled may be 2 cm. In the oscillating type, the grid is kept in a frame, which has 2–3 cm clearance on all sides. An electromagnet pulls and releases the grid before the exposure. The grid oscillates in circular path about the frame and comes to rest after 20–30 seconds. Moving grids increases distance between patient and film, resulting in magnification, cassette motion and *image blur*. However, the motion blur is undetectable hence used widely.

The use of grid increases exposure because it will absorb some of the primary radiation. To reduce exposures, grids with smaller ratios are preferred. Low ratio grids such as 8:1 is used with energies up to 90 kV. High-ratio grids such as 12:1 is preferred for high energy radiation. In mammography, grid ratio of 4:1 or 5:1 is used. These grids produce films with better contrast and increased patient dose. Grids are generally used for body parts >12 cm thick or techniques >70 kV. It can produce artifacts when improperly aligned. Grid is not preferred in pediatric imaging since it increases patient's radiation dose.

Air-gap Technique

Air-gap technique is an alternative method of eliminating scatter radiation with large radiographic fields. When a X-ray beam passes through the patient, it gets scattered in all directions. The intensity of scatter radiation is maximum at the patient's surface and decreases rapidly at an increasing distance from the surface. If sufficient gap is allowed between the patient and film, scattered photons will not reach the film, e.g., *lateral neck radiograph*.

Higher focus to film distance is used with an air-gap technique, to maintain image sharpness. Hence, it requires greater exposure factors compared to grid, but the patient exposures are generally low. Air-gap technique also introduce magnification. It is most effective when the point of scatter exists closer to the film. Air-gap techniques are used in neuroradiography and mammography.

CASSETTE

A cassette is a light proof rigid holder that contains screens and film **(Fig. 6.6)**. Cassettes are usually hinged (latches) on one side and can be opened from the other side. The side which is having the latches is the back side and other side facing the patient is called front side. The front side is made of material of low atomic number, like *plastic or Carbon fiber*. This is to maximize the transmission with low attenuation. *Carbon fiber* (Z = 6) absorbs only 50% of X-rays compared to *Aluminum*. Cassette with Carbon fiber can be operated with low radiographic techniques, resulting in lesser patient dose. The back side is usually made of heavy metals (*Lead*), having high atomic number, to minimize back scatter radiation.

There is a small window at the back side, to provide patient ID. Patient information can be given in the form of flash card; later, it is exposed to ID camera. The ID camera optically exposes the window and record the image of flash card. Inside the cassette, there are two permanently mounted *intensifying screens*, called front and back screens. The X-ray film is loaded between the two screens. The screens may have different thickness or equal thickness.

Compressive materials, such as radiolucent plastic foam is kept in between the back screen and the cassette cover. The compressive material maintains good screen-film contact when the film is loaded. Good physical contact between film and screen is necessary, to avoid artifacts and to have good image quality. X-rays, by passing the back screen get back scattered

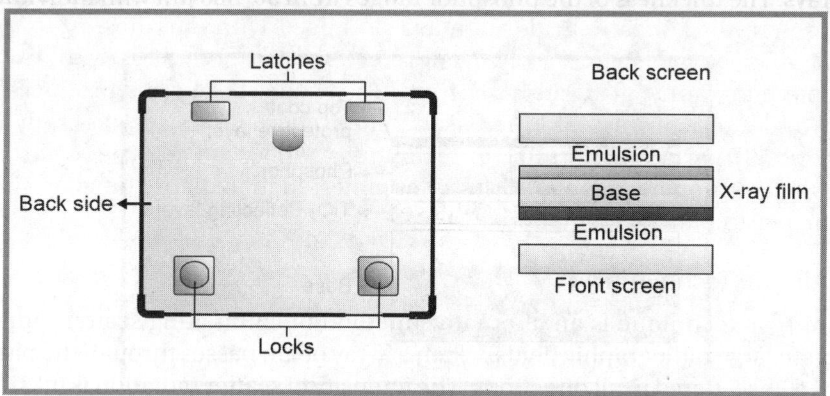

Fig. 6.6: X-ray cassette.

and reaches the film, which results in an image fog. The film loading and unloading into the cassette is done at the darkroom. Cassettes are available in different sizes, namely 8 × 10, 10 × 12, 14 × 14 and 14 ×17, in inches.

INTENSIFYING SCREEN

Film is insensitive to X-rays and requires a higher number of X-rays to produce an image, which increases patient dose. To avoid this, intensifying screens are used in cassettes in medical imaging. They absorb X-ray photons and emit more visible light or an ultraviolet, for which the X-ray film is more sensitive. The light or UV exposes the film and gives the final image, which will improve efficiency of radiographic imaging, with lesser patient dose. Thus, the intensifying screens amplify the effect of an image formation. Generally, intensifying screen consists of four layers, namely, (1) base, (2) reflecting layer, (3) phosphor, and (4) protective coating **(Fig. 6.7)**.

Structure of Screen
Base

The base is made of polyester with 1 mm thick. It serves as a mechanical support on which the reflecting layer, phosphor and protective layers are mounted. The base material should be moisture free, resistance to radiation damage and discoloration, chemically inert, and flexible.

Reflecting Layer

The reflecting layer is made up of white substance such as *Titanium dioxide (TiO_2) or Magnesium oxide*. It is a shiny material of thickness 25 µm, which reflects light towards the phosphor and makes light emission isotropic. Thus, the reflective layer increases the efficiency of intensifying screen, by doubling the number of light photons.

Phosphor

The phosphor is a crystal of inorganic salts, which emits light when exposed to X-rays. The thickness of the phosphor ranges from 50–300 µm with individual

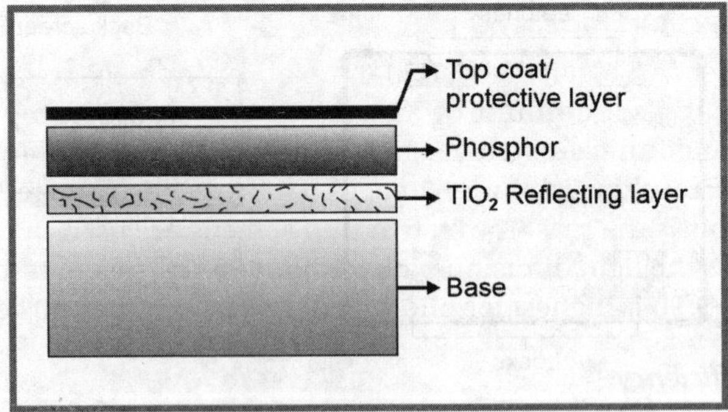

Fig. 6.7: Intensifying screen.

crystal size of 5–15 µm. The commonly used phosphors are *Calcium tungstate (CaWO₄), Zinc cadmium sulfide, Cesium iodide and Barium strontium sulfate.* The phosphor should have high atomic number, high conversion efficiency, spectral matching and less after glow. It should not be affected by heat, humidity, and environmental factors.

In recent times, rare earth phosphors (Z = 57–71) such as *Gadolinium oxysulfide (Gd₂O₂S:Tb), Lanthanum oxysulfide (La₂O₂S:Tb), Lanthanum oxybromide (LaOBr) and Yttrium tantalate (YTaO₄)* are used as screen phosphors. They can be manufactured with speed range of 200–1200. They have suitable K-shell absorption edges over diagnostic photon energy of 35–70 keV. Their absorption and conversion efficiency are high. The spectral emission of rare earth phosphors is discrete and is centered at 540 nm. Therefore, green sensitive film must be used with these phosphors. These phosphors reduce patient dose since it requires lower radiographic techniques. They also have less thermal stress and require lesser room shielding, as radiation levels are low. Though *Cesium iodide (CsI)* is used in fluoroscopy and digital radiography, it is moisture sensitive and fragile. Hence, it is not used in screen-film radiography.

Protective Coating

Protective coating (10–20 µm) is transparent to light and is facing the X-ray film. It is resistant to abrasion and damage caused by handling. It also prevents formation of static electricity and provides a surface for cleaning. The total thickness of the intensifying screen is about 1.15–1.3 mm.

When X-ray passes through the front screen, the phosphor absorbs X-rays and emits light in all directions. The reflecting layer reflects the light towards the film, so that no photon is lost. Some portion of the X-rays that are bypassing the X-ray film is absorbed and converted into light by the back screen. Thus, an intensifying screen converts large amount of X-ray photons (95%) into light photons of blue or green wavelength. Since, the X-ray film is sensitive to blue or green light, it absorbs the entire light and gives the image.

Screen Characteristics

Quantum Detection Efficiency

Quantum detection efficiency (QDE) or an absorption efficiency of a screen is the ratio between amount of X-rays absorbed and amount of X-rays incident. Though thicker screens give higher QDE, they suffer with lateral light diffusion, resulting in blurred images. Thicker screen also reduces spatial resolution. This is the reason why two thin screens are used in radiography, which reduces the light diffusion path without loss of spatial resolution. The QDE of Gd₂O₂S:Tb is highest for photon energy greater than 50 keV.

Conversion Efficiency

Conversion efficiency of a phosphor is the ratio between an amount of light emitted and X-ray absorbed. The overall efficiency of screen-film system is the product of absorption efficiency and conversion efficiency. It depends upon intrinsic conversion efficiency of the phosphor. It is 5% for *Calcium tungstate* and 15% for $Gd_2O_2S:Tb$ with green light emission of wavelength 545 nm. Presence of light absorbing dye reduces the conversion efficiency.

Speed

Speed of a screen is inversely related to an exposure (1/R) required to produce a given density. As speed increases, an exposure required decreases. Screens are generally classified as fast, medium, and slow speed screens. High speed screens (1200) are thicker and provide less spatial resolution with less patient exposure. Slow speed screens (100) are thinner but have better spatial resolution. The rare earth screens are faster, because they have a higher absorption efficiency and higher conversion efficiency, at the mean X-ray energy used.

Patient exposure is decreased greatly when intensifying screens are used. The reduction in patient exposure is measured by a term called *intensification factor*. The intensification factor is the ratio of X-ray exposure needed to produce a given density (optical density of 1) on a film without screen and with screen:

$$\text{Intensification Factor} = \frac{\text{X–ray exposure to produce certain density without screen}}{\text{X–ray exposure to produce same density with screen}}$$

It is a measure of speed of a screen. The usual intensification factors are 30–50. The $Gd_2O_2S:Tb$ screen gives an intensification factor of 50, over the diagnostic X-ray energy range.

Noise

Noise appears on the radiograph as speckled background. It occurs when fast screens and high kV techniques are used. Screen with higher conversion efficiency, increases noise. However, an increase in absorption efficiency will not affect noise. Increase of conversion efficiency, enhances quantum mottle, resulting higher noise. This may occur in very fast screens, with grainy and mottled image. *Rare earth screens* are 2 times faster than *Calcium tungstate*, which do not increase noise significantly.

Spatial Resolution

Spatial resolution refers to ability of a radiography system to differentiate two adjacent structures. It is expressed in line pairs per mm (lp/mm). If this number is higher, better the spatial resolution and smaller the object that can be imaged. Screens have lower spatial resolution compared to direct exposure film. The spatial resolution is 7 lp/mm for fast screens, 15 lp/mm for fine-detail screen, and 50 lp/mm for direct exposure film. Human eye can resolve 10 lp/mm. When the film is used with screens, the light interacts with film by larger area, which is the cause for reduction in spatial resolution. Smaller crystals and thinner phosphor layer always improve spatial resolution.

Handling of Screen

Screen must be handled with care. Any foreign material on the screen, such as paper, blood, scratches, hair, dust, and stains will block light photons and produce area of under exposure, leading to an artifact and image degradation. The film should not be made to slide into the cassette, while loading. Its sharp edge may scratch the screen. It should be removed by tilting the cassette, so that the film fell on the technologist hand. Finger, nails should not be used to take the film from the cassette. The cassette should not be kept open in the darkroom. The screen may be cleaned periodically (monthly) with a solution containing *anti-static compounds or soap and water*. It should be rinsed and dried after every cleaning. Film-screens should have good contact, and this must be checked periodically with a help of a wire mesh.

X-RAY FILM STRUCTURE

The transmitted X-rays from the patient should be converted into visible image, to the human eye for interpretation. The device that does the job is called an *image receptor*. The image receptors are X-ray films, fluorescent screens, and solid-state devices. Medical X-ray film is used for capturing, displaying, and storing radiographic images. X-ray film consists of:

❏ Base
❏ Adhesive layer
❏ Emulsion
❏ Overcoat

The emulsion is coated on both sides hence, it is called double side emulsion film **(Fig. 6.8)**.

Base

Base gives a rigid support on which an emulsion is coated. It is transparent for viewing the radiograph clearly. It should be flexible, fracture resistant, and easy to handle without kinking. The base should have dimensional stability, so that it should not produce an image distortion. It should have an uniform

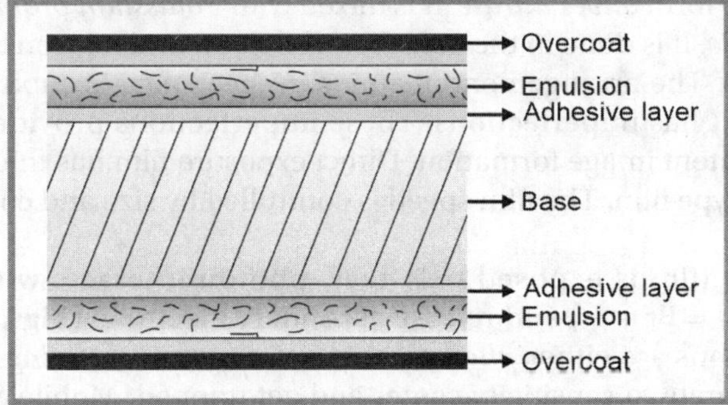

Fig. 6.8: X-ray film and its composition.

lucency and transparent to light. It should be inert, so that the sensitometry properties of the emulsion are not affected.

Initially, glass and *Cellulose nitrate* were used as bases. Later (1920), the base *Cellulose triacetate (CTA) and Polyester (1960)* are being introduced. The Polyester is made from *polyethylene terephthalate resin*. Polyester base is resistant to warping from age, stronger with higher dimensional stability. It is thinner in size (175 µm) and easy to transport in automatic film processor.

The X-ray film base is usually added with a dye, so that the film looks like blue. These films are called *blue tinted*, which reduces eye strain and fatigue. It gives pleasing appearance to intermediate densities in an image and increases the diagnostic accuracy.

Adhesive Layer

Adhesive layer (substratum) lies in between the base and emulsion, in the form of thin coat. It uniformly binds the emulsion to the base. Substratum contains solvents which can etch the base and provides anchorage for the emulsion to be coated on it subsequently. Usually, monolayer *Gelatin* is used as substratum. It also helps to maintain proper contact between an emulsion and base and provide integrity during film processing.

Emulsion

The emulsion (3–5 µm thick) is coated over an adhesive layer. Emulsion consists of *Gelatin and Silver halide crystal* in an uniform manner. Gelatin is transparent to light and porous to chemicals. It gives support for Silver halide, by holding them properly. Among the halides, *Silver bromide* (98%) and *Silver iodide* (2%) is used as crystal in the film. These halides are flat and have high atomic numbers; *Bromide (Z =35), Silver (Z=47), and Iodide (Z=53)*, compared to Gelatin (Z = 7). The halide crystals are available in tabular, cubic, octahedral, polyhedral, or irregular grain shapes. *Tabular grain* shape (thickness 0.1 µm) is commonly used in radiography. In addition, emulsion layer contains additives like chemical sensitizers, wetting agents, anti-foggants, hardeners etc., which gives quality to the film.

The crystal is formed in dark as follows: The metallic silver is dissolved in *Nitric acid,* to form *Silver nitrate*. It is mixed with *Potassium bromide*, to form *Silver bromide*. It is done in the presence of Gelatin under given temperature and pressure. The arrangement of atoms in the crystal is cubic and lattice structure that has imperfections. These imperfections provide sensitivity centers, for latent image formation. Direct exposure film has thicker crystals than screen type film. The film speed is controlled by size and concentration of the crystal.

When the film is exposed to X-rays, photon interacts with *Bromine* (photon + Br⁻ = Br + e⁻) and release secondary electrons **(Figs. 6.9A to F)**. The interactions are either *photoelectric or Compton scattering* type. These electrons migrate to sensitivity center and get trapped. Mobile *Silver* atoms (Ag⁺) are attracted to the sensitivity centers, where they combine with

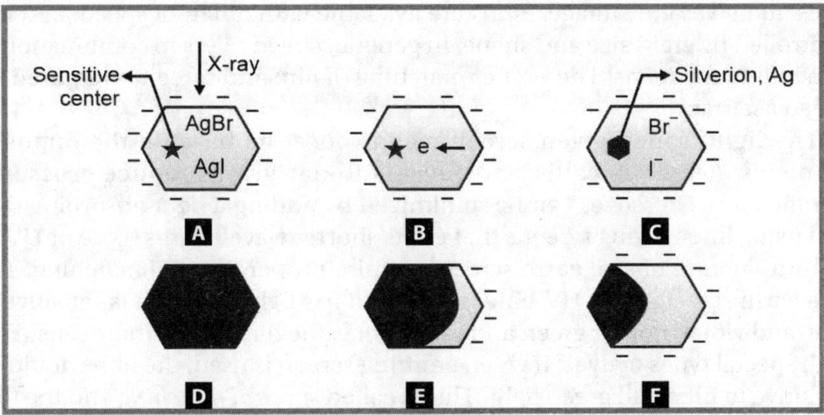

Figs. 6.9A to F: Latent image formation: (A) X-ray exposure provide electrons; (B) Electrons moves to the sensitive center; (C) Mobile silver atoms move to the sensitivity center combine with electron and forms latent image; (D) Process repeated, latent image widens; (E) Additional silver formation during processing; (F) Final metallic silver image.

electrons and become metallic silver ($Ag^+ + e^- = Ag$). Metallic Silver atoms give latent image, which is invisible. Basically, the Bromine and Iodine are present at the surface, whereas Silver is inside the crystal. Mostly electrons are provided by Bromine and Iodine atoms, resulting in collapse of crystal structure. As a result, Bromine and Iodine are free to move to the Gelatin area. No more ionic force is acting in the crystal.

Overcoat

Gelatin is covered by a layer called an over coat or topcoat. It protects the light sensitive emulsion from scratches, pressure, contamination, and handling damages.

Types of Film

X-ray film is double side coated, that is above said layers are coated on both sides of the film. It provides better density and contrast with less exposure. It also reduces curling of film. Film is classified as (1) screen type film, (2) direct exposure or non-screen type, (3) dental film, (4) mammography film, and (5) laser printer film. Films are available in variety of sizes. The most common sizes are 7 × 7, 8 × 10, 10 × 12, 14 × 14 and 14 × 17 (in inches).

Screen Type Film

Screen-film is a double side coated film with double the speed of single side emulsion film. Hence, it is more sensitive to light and faster. Its selection depends on contrast, speed, spectral matching, crossover, and safe light. It is available with low and high contrast levels and multiple latitudes. High contrast film contains an uniform and smaller size grains and produces black and white image. Low contrast film has large grains with wide range of sizes and gives grey image. Films are available with different speed, and it is controlled by grain size and shape. In general, speed refers to combination of film and two screens. The proper matching of film and screen is required for speed accuracy.

The light from a given screen may expose the base on the opposite emulsion, which is called *crossover*. Tabular grains reduce crossover significantly. Crossover can be minimized by adding a light absorbing dye, and using intensifying screens that emits shorter wavelengths (blue or UV).

Introduction of rare earth screens require proper spectral matching. The rare earth screens emit UV, blue, green, and red light. The film is sensitive to blue and violet, not for green and red. Hence, the film is spectrally sensitized with special types of dyes. If green emitting screen is used, the film should be sensitive to blue and green light. This is called *spectral matching* and the film is called *green sensitive film or orthochromatic film*. If there is mismatching, it will reduce the speed and give higher patient dose. In the case of screen type film, the reciprocity law fails.

Direct Exposure/Nonscreen Film

The emulsion of a direct exposure film is thicker and consists of high concentration of AgBr crystals, with single side emulsion. They are mainly used to image thinner body parts, such as hands, feet, etc. It employs higher radiographic techniques and involves increased radiation dose to the patient. It is rarely used today in medical imaging. Nonscreen type has thicker emulsion and requires long exposure. It is sensitive to direct action of X-rays. It is 4 times faster than screen type film. Reciprocity law hold good in direct exposure films.

Dental Films

Dental films are direct exposure films used in an intraoral and extraoral examinations. Intraoral film has double side emulsion and available in 5.7×7.6, 3.1×4.1, and 2.2×3.5 sizes (cm). These films are made with an outer wrapper by a water-proof paper or plastic **(Figs. 6.10A to D)**. It is sealed to prevent an *ingress of saliva*. The side facing the X-ray has either a pebbled or a smooth surface in white. Reverse side is made of two colors to avoid wrong placement of film in mouth. A black paper on either side of the film protects from light, saliva, and damage by fingers. There is a *Lead foil* on the back side of the film to prevent back scatter and tissue dose. Lead sheet contains an embossed pattern to ensure correct placement. It is used for *periapical, bitewing, and occlusal* radiographs.

Extraoral films are available either with nonscreen or screen. Screen type film is also used in dental radiography for panoramic view, oblique view, skull view, etc.

Mammography Film

Mammography film is a single side emulsion type orthochromatic film, always used with single intensifying screen at the back side. It has two emulsion

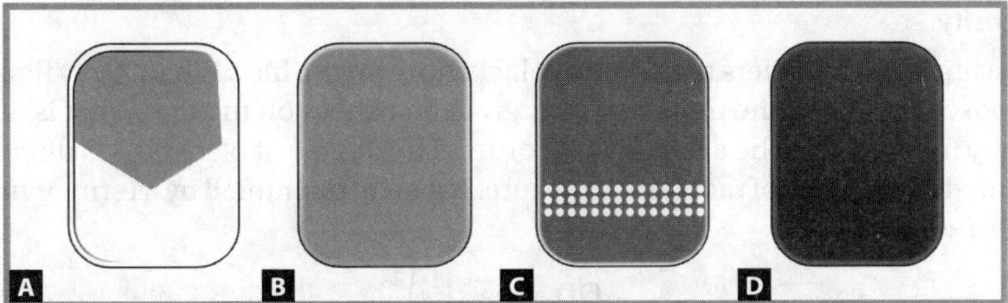

Figs. 6.10A to D: Dental film: (A) Outer wrapper; (B) Film; (C) Lead foil sheet; (D) Protective black paper.

layers on one side of the film. The first layer provides high contrast in *breast parenchyma* with an improved visualization. The second layer provides maximum density to visualize radio dense breast. It gives increased gradient and high dynamic range.

Currently, green emitting *Terbium-doped Gadolinium oxysulfide screens* with green sensitive film is used. It gives superior image quality with 40% reduction of dose. Surface of the film base opposite the screen is coated with a light absorbing dye, to reduce reflection of light from the screen. The above coating is called an *antihalation coating* and the effect is called *halation*. This coating is removed during processing, to improve the image viewing.

Laser Printer Film

Laser printer films are used in computed tomography, digital radiography, etc., to print digital images. Basically, they are not X-ray films though it is used in radiology. It consists of laser camera with *Helium-Neon laser* with emission of red light (632 nm). Digital image information required for one film is stored in memory through an interface. This modulates a laser beam via an *acoustic-optical modulator* in terms of brightness and grey levels. Intensity of the beam is controlled by a digital value of the input signal. A *lens system* is used to focus the laser beam onto a mirror which moves the laser beam from side to side across the film. At a time one line of information is printed that contains 3500–54100 pixels. The film moves vertically to print another line. Thus, laser beam writes the image on the film in *raster fashion.*

The film is a single side emulsion, fine grain *Polyester-based Silver halide film.* Laser wavelength and film matching is much vital. *He-Neon laser* requires film, that have sensitivity at 632 nm. Different types of lasers are under use and offer consistent image quality. It is also available with multiple film sizes and multiple image formats per film. Laser images are superior but susceptible to dust, vibration, and artifacts.

Characteristics of X-ray Film

Characteristics of X-ray film can be discussed in terms of (1) density, (2) characteristic curve, (3) speed, (4) latitude, (5) contrast, and (6) an emulsion absorption.

Density

The term density refers to degree of blackening on the film. When X-ray film is exposed to X-rays, the metallic Silver gives blackness on the film. That is why X-ray film is said to be a negative recorder. The degree of blackness is directly related to intensity of radiation exposure. It can be quantified by a term *optical density (OD)*:

$$OD = \log_{10}\left(\frac{I_o}{I_t}\right)$$

where, $\left(\frac{I_o}{I_t}\right)$ is the inverse of transmittance (T), which is measured by a *densitometer*. If I_o is light intensity measured without film and I_t is light transmitted through the film, then $T = \frac{I_t}{I_o}$. The useful range of density in diagnostic radiology is 0.25–2.0. As OD increases the transmittance decreases.

Characteristic Curve

The relation between radiation exposure and an optical density is plotted as a curve, known as the characteristic curve or *H and D curve*, named after **Hurter and Driffield** (1890). The film density is plotted on the vertical axis and log of film exposure on the horizontal axis. The curve has *sigmoid shape* and has three portions, called *toe, straight line and shoulder* as shown in **Figure 6.11.** The toe is the low exposure region, and the shoulder is the high exposure region of the curve. Base plus fog level is the film blackening in the absence of any radiation exposure and typically ranges from 0.1 to 0.25 OD units. It refers to background fogging and tinting (blue) of base. The maximum film density ranges from 2.5 to 3.0 OD units.

All radiographic techniques should produce a density in the straight-line portion. The contrast is related to slope of the linear portion of the curve. Higher the slope, higher is the image contrast. The parameter which describes the contrast of film is called an *average gradient*. It is the slope of straight line, connecting two given points in the characteristic curve:

$$\text{Average gradient} = \frac{D_2 - D_1}{\log_{10}(E_2 - E_1)}$$

where, D_2 and D_1 are the optical densities on the straight-line portion of the curve, resulting from log of exposure E_2 and E_1. The average gradient value ranges from 2.5 to 3.5. The gradient is the mean slope between two specified densities. A high gradient refers to higher radiographic contrast of the film.

Reciprocity Law

Reciprocity law states that an optical density (OD) produced on a radiograph is proportional only to total energy imported to the X-ray film and independent of exposure time. That means, whether it is short or long exposure, the OD will be the same, if the given mAs is constant. This can be given as E = It, where *E* is exposure, *I* is intensity, and *t* is time. This means that *E* is a constant whatever

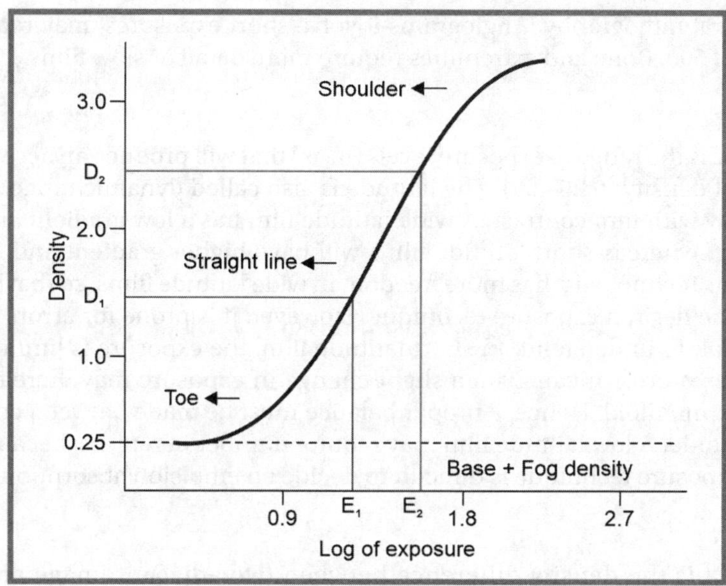

Fig. 6.11: Characteristic curve of X-ray film.

the combination of I and t. It is true only for direct exposure of films, not true for screen-film systems.

In the case of screen-film combination very long or very short exposure time results in density values that are less than the expected. This means that use of very high mA and short exposure time, or very low mA and long exposure time, will not give the same density. This is known as *reciprocity law failure* as stated by **Abney**. Reciprocity law failure is significant at < 0.1 msec or >2 sec of exposure time. The OD is lesser at such low and high exposure times. The reciprocity law is very important for special procedures, e.g., *angiography (short exposure) and mammography (long exposure)*. Different films have different reciprocity characteristics.

Speed

The speed refers to sensitivity of the film-screen combination. Fast film requires lesser radiation exposure to achieve a given film density and slow film requires more radiation exposure. There are two types of speed in use, one is an *absolute speed* and the other is *relative speed*. The absolute speed of a film is defined as the reciprocal of exposure in roentgens (1/R) that required to produce a density of 1.0 above base plus fog density. It is determined from the H and D curve and used only in performance evaluation.

Relative speed is a measure compared with a standard film screen combination. For example, *Calcium tungstate* screen–film combination is called *par speed* and given a value of 100. Another combination of film-screen having twice the speed of Calcium tungstate is given the speed of 200. In this way, the *rare earth screen* combination is given speed of 400, which is used in general radiography. Angiograms involve short exposures, may require a speed of 600. Bone and extremities require more detail or slow films.

Latitude

Latitude is the range of exposure levels (mAs) that will produce an acceptable range of density (0.25–2.0). The latitude is also called dynamic range, varies inversely with film contrast. A wide latitude film has a low gradient and low contrast, whereas short latitude films will have higher gradient and higher contrast. Technologist has more freedom in wide latitude films, so that he can select the desired exposure technique. However, it is prone for errors which is difficult to understand. In short latitude film, the exposure is limited and becomes more critical. Even a slight change in exposure may increase the contrast manifold. Hence, a proper balance must be made between contrast and latitude. A low latitude film may require number of retakes, because the exact exposure technique is difficult to decide an emulsion absorption.

Contrast

Contrast is the density difference between two adjacent image areas in a radiograph. Film contrast tells us how the film responds to different exposure, and it depends on characteristics curve, film density, screen or nonscreen exposure and film processing. It is determined by the slope of the characteristic curve. Film gamma is the maximum slope of the characteristic curve. Double emulsion film provides greater contrast than single emulsion film. High contrast single emulsion films are used in mammography.

Emulsion Absorption

Silver halide grains in the film must absorb the light emitted by an intensifying screen. This depends upon the wavelength of emitted light. Generally, Silver bromide absorbs ultraviolet, violet, and blue lights. It is possible to extend this to green color by coating with a special dye, referred to an *ortho film*. A film coated with a dye which absorbs red light is called *pan film*.

Film Handling, Packing and Storage

X-ray film is a delicate material should be handled carefully. It should be handled always by its edges with clean and dry hands. One should avoid touching the film surface by fingernails, scissors, knives, and screw drivers. Sharp edges like fingernails may produce artifacts. Film should not be bend, crease, or rough handled. In the dark room all white light must be switched off and handled only under the safe light. It should be exposed to *safe light* for a period equal to unload a film from cassette. Films left out for too long under the safe light will fog. Improper safe light illumination is a cause of film fog. Excessive examination of film under the safe light causes an *aerial fog*. Rule of thumb is that the film is safe if a 15 W bulb kept at 3 m distance is used for 1 minute. The loading bench must be earthed, to avoid static charges that build-up in the cassette while opening.

Films are supplied in boxes of 50 or 100 sheets. The packing may be by an *interleaved or noninterleaved* method with chemically treated paper. An expiry date is given on the box, which is the self-life of the film. Film should not be used after an expiry date, usually 6 months. Aged films may have loss of speed, contrast with an increased amount of fog. Film should be stored vertically on its edges. If so, the film will not stick to one another, less likely to warp, and have less pressure artifacts. The storage is made in such a way that oldest film should be used first. Film may be purchased monthly, so that the storage may not exceed more than 30 days.

X-ray film is sensitive to temperature and humidity, at high temperature the film will be spoiled before expiry. Higher temperature and humidity (60%) may cause *fog* and reduce image contrast. Hence, it should be stored at cool places, at 20°C both day and night. It is also pressure sensitive and should be kept always in *upright position*, vertically on its edges like keeping books in shelfs. The film will not stick to each other and less likely to wrap.

Film is sensitive to light and should be stored and handled in dark. Exposure to low level light may increase the fog. Hence, a well-sealed darkroom and a light proof *storage bin* is a must. Ionizing radiations may fog the film and reduce contrast. Film is more sensitive after an exposure than before. In the first exposure, the optical density is raised above the toe. Successive exposure may cause higher optical density. Hence, it should not be stored near radioactive substance and nuclear medicine areas.

X-RAY FILM PROCESSING

After X-ray exposure film has both exposed Silver ions and unexposed AgBr crystals. Exposed Silver ions in the film consists of latent image which is not visible. Only fewer Silver ions are converted into metallic Silver. During film processing all the exposed Silver ions are converted into metallic Silver so that the Silver become black and made visible. Thus, film processing converts the latent image into visible radiographic image. Film processing involves a series of procedures **(Fig. 6.12)**:

❑ Developing
❑ Rinsing
❑ Fixing
❑ Washing
❑ Drying

Developing

Development is a chemical process that converts an invisible latent image into visible metallic Silver image. The solution used for this purpose is called *developer* which is an alkaline solution. The developer converts the exposed Silver ion into metallic Silver, by reduction process ($Ag^+ + e^- = Ag$). The developer provides electrons to the sensitivity centers and makes the Silver atom neutral. Negative Bromine ions move into the developer, and an unexposed AgBr is unaffected by the developer.

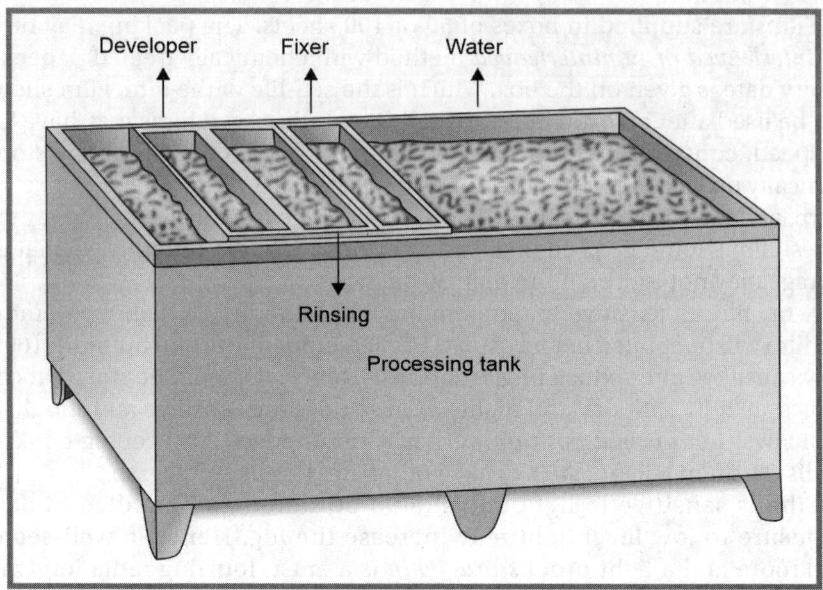

Fig. 6.12: Manual X-ray film processer consists of developing, rinsing, fixing and washing tanks.

A developer solution is a reducing agent, contains *developing agent, activator, restrainer, preservative, solvent. Hydroquinone plus phenidone or metol* are used as developing agents. Hydroquinone is slow acting and is responsible for high contrast black shades. Phenidone acts rapidly and produces lighter gray shades. It controls the toe of the curve whereas hydroquinone controls the shoulder part of the characteristic curve.

Activator maintains alkalinity which adjust the Hydrogen ion concentration (pH) of the developer. It softens the Gelatin, open the pores of the film, and allows the developer to perform its work. It also serves as a buffer to control Hydrogen ions liberated during development. Common activators are *Sodium carbonate, Sodium hydroxide, Potassium carbonate and Sodium metaborate. Potassium bromide* is used as restrainer, which restricts the action of the developing agent only to those exposed AgBr crystals. It is an antifog agent, which decreases the fog by protecting the unexposed crystals. Fog is a development of unexposed silver halide grains, that do not contain the latent image. It also decreases the rate of development of latent image to a lesser degree. Thus, it improves radiographic contrast by reducing fog.

Sodium sulfite or *Potassium sulfite* is used as preservative. It controls the oxidation of the developing agent, by absorbing oxygen in an air. Hydroquinone is prone to aerial oxidation, its life is increased by the preservative. Preservative controls proper development rate and maintains balance among developer components. Oxidation products of developing agents decompose the alkaline solution and form colored materials that can stain the emulsion. The preservative dissolves these oxidation products and form colorless *sulfonates.*

Solvent dissolves the chemicals and helps for their ionization. It also aids softening of Gelatin emulsion. *Water* is used as solvent to dissolve all the chemicals. It is a soft water, otherwise salts in the chemicals may react with chemicals, resulting precipitates. Water softener like *Calgon* can be added to the developer.

Development depends on crystal size, developer concentration, development time, and temperature. Manufacturer recommended concentration, time and temperature must be employed to get an optimal contrast, speed, and fog. Otherwise, it will reduce image quality. Usually, 4–5 minutes is enough for X-ray film development. Rapid developer requires about 3 minutes at 68°F temperature.

Rinsing

Developed film contains chemicals like un-oxidized developing agents and oxidation products. Gelatin contains black metallic Silver and an unexposed, undeveloped AgBr crystals. Hence, film requires rinsing to remove soluble chemicals and oxidation products. Rinsing also partially stops the reaction of the developer and neutralizes the alkalinity of the residual developer. Thus, it reduces fog formation. If rinsing is not sufficient, developer may go to the fixer solution resulting *dichromatic fog and brown staining* of the film. It shortens the life of fixer solution and destroys its hardening action.

Rinsing is done with water bath for 30 sec. Acid rinse bath may be prepared by adding 2 liters of 28% acetic acid to 1 gallon of water. After proper rinsing, water is added to make it 5 gallons *(1 gallon = 4.55 liters)*. It helps to extend the life of the fixer solution. Water and acid mixed bath can also be used. Rinsing is not necessary in an automatic film processor, where the transport rollers squeeze the film and wipe out residual developer.

Fixing

Fixing is the process of making an image permanent without fading. The solution that does the job is called *fixer*. It removes an unexposed Silver halides without damaging the image, hardens the Gelatin emulsion, and stops residual development. The fixing solution consists of *activator, fixing agent, hardener, preservative, and solvent.*

Acetic or Sulfuric acid is used as an activator, which neutralizes the alkalinity of the residual developer on the film and stops its action. It provides suitable medium for the fixer and hardener to act, prevents stain formation.

Sodium thiosulfate or Ammonium thiosulfate salts (Hypo) are used as fixing agents. Its function is to change the residual, unexposed, undeveloped AgBr crystals into soluble slats, without damaging the Silver image. It dissolves the unexposed, undeveloped Silver halides, leaving the developed metallic Silver in the exposed areas of the film. Sodium thiosulfate reacts with AgBr and form Sodium bromide + Sodium salts of *argento-di-thiosulphuric acid.* Excess hypo known as hypo retention, may cause oxidation and make image discolor (brown), over a period. Improper fixing makes the radiographs nearly opaque and black. Silver combines with hypo and forms *Silver sulfide*, which appear *yellowish brown.*

Developed film may absorbs moisture and get swelled, hence requires hardening of the emulsion. *Potassium alum, Chromium alum and Aluminum chloride are* used as hardener. It hardens the Gelatin emulsion, thereby protecting it from physical injuries. When an undeveloped Silver bromide is removed from the film, the emulsion starts shrinking. The hardener enhances the shrinking process and makes the emulsion too hard. Now, it is suitable for transport through washing and drying. Hardener pH is very vital it should be about 4.5–4.9 for Potassium alum. Hardener makes drying quicker, protects from an external injury and use of higher temperature.

Developer may mix with fixer solution and may cause chemical imbalance. Preservative protects the fixing agent from decomposition. *Sodium sulfite* is used as preservative, which maintains the chemical balance by keeping the pH level (4.0–5.0). It also helps the film and prevents residual developer. Insufficient rinsing can be addressed by adding a week acid and stabilizer (*Sodium metabisulfite)* in the fixer solution.

Fixing time may be 1–4 minutes that depends on an age of the fixer and number of proceed films. A fixer is said to be exhausted if the fixing time is > 10 minutes. Film should not be exposed during fixing and the optimum temperature is 18–24°C. *Water* is used as solvent to mix the chemicals.

Used fixer solution contains Silver and it should not be disposed directly into the drainage, since it can cause ecological damage. Silver is a declining natural source and costly and contain 1 g of *Silver* per liter. The fixer solution should be collected in a container for Silver recovery. Various method of Silver recovery is available. After Silver recovery only the solution is disposed into the swage.

Washing

After fixing, the film must be washed with water, to remove fixing-bath chemicals, especially hypo. Otherwise, it will discolor and fade, black Silver change into to *brown Silver sulfide*, resulting *yellow brown stain*. Incomplete washing permits the *hypo-retention*, which may cause image fading, and make the film brown with age. *Silver sulfite* and other salts from the fixer may deposit on the film surface, make is difficult to view the radiographs. Film is washed with running water for about 20 minutes at 20°C. While film is immersed in *water, thiosulfates* are removed by diffusion process. When the water has an equal amount of *thiosulfate* diffusion stops. Hence, water needs replacement often, alternatively running water is the best option. Single tank washing and two- stage cascade system of washing is available.

Drying

The final step in processing is drying the radiograph. After washing, film is wet and prone to damage. The film may be dried in dust free open-air area, where the temperature is less than 35°C. Film should not be removed from the hangers, until the drying is complete. The speed of drying depends on the quantity of evaporated water from an emulsion. Hot-air drying cabinets are used, which is equipped with a fan and heating element to flow hot air over both surfaces. Other wetting agents are *Photo-flo and Alcohol* which are used after wash that decrease drying time. Photo-flo minimizes water marks or streaks formed during development, and reduces surface tension of water, so that water drain rapidly from the film surface. Alcohol is used in emergency, after washing, the film is put in an alcohol tray for 2 minutes at 70° F. It replaces water from the pores of the emulsion, finally the film is dried.

Influence of Development Time and Temperature

Development is a chemical process, which depends on both temperature and time. Development time is proportional to the Silver deposits, as time increases Silver deposit also increases or vice versa. Time of development depends on emulsion and thickness of the film.

Temperature change affects the chemical reactions. A good *thermometer* is essential, and an optimal temperature is 20–22°C. Higher temperature increases reduction of Silver and enhance the number of Silver grains or vice versa at lower temperature. Hence, an optimum time and temperature is required. At higher temperature, >24°C the emulsion become so soft, and produce chemical fog. To overcome this, development time must be decreased. One quarter (1/4) of development time is decreased for 1C° raise of temperature.

At low temperature film is underdeveloped. If temperature is <16°C, the action of *hydroquinone* ceases and the resulting radiograph lacks contrast and density. This can be overcome by increasing the developer time. To achieve good development, 1/4 minute of development is increased for 1°C of temperature decrease.

In manual development, radiographic exposure is based on 5-minute development at 29°C. Processing of films on the above basis is called *time–temperature development*.

Replenisher

During developing, loss of developer happens since each film goes with some residual developer. This loss needs to be replenished. Hence, replenisher is used to restore the concentration of developer chemical to the original value. It also compensates the reduction in alkalinity and overcomes the accumulation of Bromide. Replenisher contains higher concentration of *hydroquinone, metal, and alkali.* One gallon (4.55 liters) of replenisher should be added for every 40 numbers of 14″ × 17″ films or their equivalent area. In properly replenished developer, one can develop 125 films of size 14″ × 17″ per gallon of solution.

Replenisher should never be added to the developer while the film is developing. If it is added, steaks of high density will be produced. The developer solution should be discarded if the volume of added replenisher is equal to 3–4 times original volume of developer. Unused developer if any, over a period 3 months must also be discarded.

Darkroom

Darkroom is an X-ray film processing room, and it is located adjacent to the X-ray room. It must have sufficient space, about 10' × 10' × 10' (cubic feet). The walls of the darkroom must be thick enough (23/35 cm) to protect against ionizing radiation. The common wall will have a *hatch (pass box)* to pass cassettes to the dark room. Pass box has two light-tight, X-ray proof doors, which are revolving on vertical axis. It is designed in such a way that no light from the X-ray room can penetrate the dark room. It is divided into two compartments; one is passing the loaded cassette to the X-ray room and the other is retuning the exposed cassette to the dark room. Floor should be durable, easily cleaned, not slippery and resistant to staining and corrosive substances. Windows should be avoided, and air-conditioning is an ideal choice. Darkroom consists of **(Fig. 6.13):**
❏ Dry side
❏ Wet side
❏ Safe light

The entrance of the darkroom must be light tight and are provided with interlocked doors. Types of door entrances are (1) double door entrance, (2) labyrinth or maze entrance, and (3) revolving door entrance.

Inside walls of the darkroom are light colored not with black color which gives depressive mood. A glassy cream or white paint is good for walls which reflects the light adequately. Alternatively, glazed tile walls can be used which is easy for washing. A good quality modern emulsion paint is used for ceiling. Floor should be nonpores, stain resistant, and not slippery type. Hard rubber

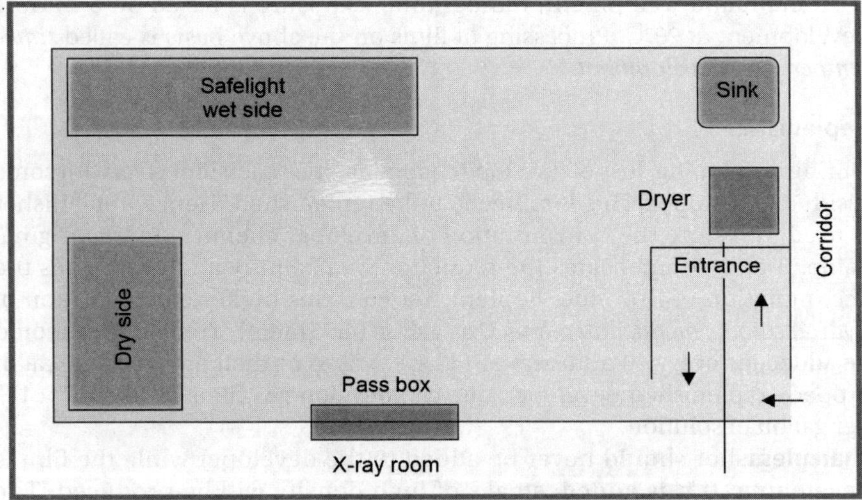

Fig. 6.13: Darkroom for X-ray film processing and its compartments.

or rubber sheet is preferred for floor, but they should be fastened with water-proof adhesives.

The work area of the darkroom is divided as *dry side and wet side.* The dry side is provided with loading bench which is covered with a sheet of *fiberboard linoleum or plastic material.* Required dimension is 2.5 m × 0.6 m per operator to handle 3–4 large cassettes. The height is 0.9 m mounted on a plinth with toe space at the bottom. Dry bench should have set of *pigeonholes* for unopened boxes, light-tight, folding sectional box for films with an electrical safety device, storage for cassettes, and closed wastepaper basket. It is also provided with drawers to keep *scissors, clips, writing and marking material, rubber stamps, safelight/filters, thermometer, etc.* Film hanger should be suspended over the center of the dry bench. They should be placed on special hooks attached to the side wall of the dry bench.

Wet side consists of *processing chemicals, two stirring paddlers, thermometer, stop clock and processing tanks.* Processing tanks are placed in an order: developing tank, rinsing tank, fixing bath, and washing tank. They are placed next to each other and forms a large built-in unit. All tanks are made up of stainless steel or plastic. The space between the film and the bottom of the bath must be 0.8 inches. Upper edge of the film is 1 inch below the bath's upper level. This will support to develops 4 films at a time. To prevent electrical shock, all metallic objects are earthed.

Safelight

Darkroom is illuminated by a safelight which keeps the film unexposed or does not fog films, and it can be either *direct or an indirect safelight.* X-tray films are sensitive to only blue, green and UV light, hence *red or brown or olive-green light* is preferred for safe lighting. Usually, red lamps of < 25 watts are used as safe lights in an indirect lighting. The lamp directs the light towards ceiling which reflects the light back into the room. One indirect light for every 6.5 m² ceiling area, at a height of 2.1 m above the floor level is sufficient for good illumination. They should be fitted with good filters.

In the case of direct safelight, <15 W bulb is used at a distance 1.5 m. Working distance between the safelight and film should not be less than 1.2 m. For a blue sensitive film, an amber light (550 nm) is used. It will fog the green sensitive film. Green sensitive film needs red filter of 660 nm. The red filter can be used for both blue and green sensitive film. The effectiveness of the safelight is tested periodically.

GEOMETRIC FACTORS

Image quality is affected by number geometric factors, namely (1) sharpness, (2) magnification, (3) distortion, and (4) focal spot blur.

Sharpness

Image sharpness is an ability of a X-ray film or screen-film combination to define an edge. Due to light diffusion in the screen, the screen-film system may fail to record a sharp edge. This is known as image *unsharpness (blur)*. A system may have ability to record sharp images but fails to resolve fine details. In contrast, images with unsharp edges may reveal fine details. Thus, sharpness and resolution are different, but interrelated. Unsharpness may be classified as follows:

❑ Geometric unsharpness
❑ Absorption unsharpness
❑ Detector unsharpness
❑ Motion unsharpness

The geometric unsharpness arises from focal spot size. The X-rays coming slightly from different locations in the focal spot, produces blurred margin at the edge of an object. This is called *penumbra*, which results in loss of sharpness, known as *focal spot blur*. Penumbra is a region at the beam edges, having variable intensity that decreases from beam center to outside. The penumbra width increases with increase of focal spot size.

In contact radiography, the focal spot blur is zero. This increases with increasing focal spot size and it is minimum in an extremity radiography. Focal spot blur increases with magnification. Therefore, small focal spot size (0.1 mm) is always recommended for magnification radiography. Such a set-up will not only reduce penumbra but also an image blur. It has an additional benefit of better visibility of *micro-calcifications*.

Absorption unsharpness arises if the patient does not have object that have sharp edges. This is due to gradual change of X-ray absorption towards the edges of an object. It produces a poorly defined margin in an image. This unsharpness increases for round and an oval anatomy, e.g., *coronary angiogram*.

Detector blur is due to screens used in screen-film radiography. Screen unsharpness is caused by light diffusion in the intensifying screen. Thick screens have greater light diffusion, whereas thin screens have lesser light diffusion. Thicker screen (>0.4 mm) produces lateral light diffusion, resulting in blurred images. The screen blur increases with separation of film from the screen. Screen blur decreases with an increase of resolution, crystal size, and contrast, but has limited value in assessing system performance.

Patient motion introduces unsharpness into the radiograph, which is called *motion blur*, e.g., heart motion. Movement of focal spot during exposure can also cause motion artifacts. This can be minimized by increasing mA and decreasing exposure time. Shorter exposure always reduces motion unsharpness. Use of faster screen also decreases motion unsharpness. Immobilization devices and compression paddle (mammography) can be used to reduce motion blur. There is no motion blur in magnification radiography. The total unsharpness (U_T) of an image is given as follows:

$$U_T = \sqrt{U_g^2 + U_a^2 + U_d^2 + U_m^2}$$

where, U_g^2 = geometric unsharpness, U_a^2 = absorption un-sharpness, U_d^2 = detector unsharpness, and U_m^2 = motion unsharpness.

Magnification

All radiographic images are magnified, and the magnification factor (MF) is the ratio between an image size and object size. It means that all images are larger than their object size. Magnification is desired in some procedures, especially in magnification radiography. Majority of radiography examination gives minimum magnification. Instead of measuring an object and an image size, distance ratio is used:

$$MF = SID/SOD$$

where, *SID* is the source to image distance and *SOD* is the source to object distance.

When the object is closer to the source, the magnification is larger. When the object moves away from the source, magnification decreases. This is true for objects positioned in the central beam as well as lateral to the central beam, for a given SID. To minimize magnification, one can have large SID by keeping an object very close to the receptor as much as possible. For chest radiography, the SID is about 180 cm, and the magnification is almost unity. In abdomen radiography, the SID is 100 cm, and the MF is about 1.1. Lesser the magnification means lesser the image blur and higher the resolution.

Distortion

Distortion is the result of an unequal magnification of different parts of an object. It may be caused by an object thickness, object position and object shape. Thick objects produce more distortion than thin objects.

Patient with irregular anatomy may contribute to distortion in a radiograph. If an object plane and an imaging plane are not parallel then distortion occurs, due to positioning. The distortion is minimal for an object that is positioned at the center. Object that is positioned lateral to the center may have severe distortion. The objects that are lateral may have an unequal magnification than that at the center. The angle of inclination of an object also influences the degree of distortion.

Focal Spot Blur

Focal spot (F) of an X-ray tube is not a point and have a dimension (0.6–1.8 mm), which produce penumbra at the edge of a field. Penumbra is a region at the edges, where radiation intensity decreases laterally. It causes blurred region at the edges of a field in a radiograph, which is called focal spot blur (f):

$$f = F(MF-1)$$

where, *MF* is the magnification factor.

The focal spot blur increases with large focal spot size and higher magnification. It is small on the anode side and large on the cathode side, due to *Heel effect*. To reduce blur, smaller focal spot size and lesser magnification should be used. To have lesser magnification, the patient–film distance is reduced by keeping them close to each other.

IMAGE QUALITY

Radiographic image quality refers to visibility of a given anatomy and an accuracy of its structural lines that is recorded. It should represent an anatomy accurately and be visualized well for further interpretation. A good image should have maximum spatial resolution and minimum distortion. High-quality images are required to make an accurate diagnosis. Radiographic image quality depends on:

- ❏ Brightness
- ❏ Contrast
- ❏ Spatial resolution
- ❏ Noise
- ❏ Detective quantum efficiency

Brightness

Brightness is an amount of luminescence or light emission in the radiograph. Density is the degree of blackness on the processed film. A radiograph must have an optimal brightness or density to view an anatomical details. High brightness goes with reduced density or voice-versa. An optimal brightness and density depend on kV, mA, and s which has direct impact in screen-film radiography, but little in digital radiography.

Contrast

The term contrast refers to difference in density between adjacent areas on the radiograph. The contrast includes (1) subject contrast, (2) film contrast, and (3) fog and scatter. The product of subject and film contrast gives the radiographic contrast.

Subject contrast is the difference in X-ray intensities transmitted through different parts of a patient. It depends on patient thickness, tissue mass density, an effective atomic number, shape of subject, and photon energy (kV). Thicker and thinner body part attenuates radiation differently and varies the transmitted X-rays. If the tissue absorbs fewer X-rays, called positive contrast result in dark images, e.g., lung. Negative contrast objects absorb more X-rays, appear white, e.g., bone. The subject contrast is proportional to relative number of transmitted X-rays. Tissues of equal thickness, having different mass density contribute to subject contrast. Photoelectric absorption varies with an effective atomic number. If the adjacent tissue's effective atomic number is different, they contribute subject contrast.

Contrast media such as *Barium (Z = 56), and Iodine (Z = 53)* will enhance subject contrast. Higher the atomic number/density of the tissue, greater the attenuation. In addition, *Air (negative contrast) and Carbon dioxide (angiography)* are used as contrast agents. Chest radiographs have more natural contrast than others in human body due to presence of bone, fat, and lung.

Shape of anatomy, which coincides with X-ray beam increases subject contrast. Shapes that have change in thickness for X-ray path may reduce subject contrast. X-ray beam quality affects subject contrast. High kV gives lower subject contrast, whereas low kV gives higher subject contrast. CT scan with high voltage reduces subject contrast. However, low voltage with *Iodinated contrast agents* will improve subject contrast.

Film contrast is the difference in film density of a lesion, compared to an adjacent tissue. It depends on film density and how film amplifies the subject contrast. Film contrast tells us how the film responds to difference in exposure. An under exposed film have low densities (0.5 OD), results in lower contrast. Overexposed films have higher density (>2 OD) but gives poor image contrast. The desired optical density is about 1.5. This can be achieved by selecting correct image receptor. The film contrast depends on characteristic curve, film density, screen or nonscreen exposure, and film processing.

Slope of the characteristic curve determines the film contrast. Correct gradient is 2 for radiography and >3 for mammography. High gradient films are generally said to be high contrast films. Double emulsion film will produce greater contrast compared to single emulsion film. Film latitude is inversely proportional to film gradient, low latitude films offer higher gradient, in turn higher contrast. In this, air-kerma values are narrow, use of high kV will give better subject contrast. Wide latitude films offer lower gradient and lower contrast. Since the air-kerma values are wider, use of low kV gives higher subject contrast. Mammography uses low latitude films with breast compression.

Fog and scatter produce an unwanted film density, which lowers final radiographic contrast. Base + fog, represents the toe of the characteristic curve. Base refers to density of film base, base + fog is an inherent blackness without any radiation exposure and it should not exceed >0.2OD. It increases with contaminated developer, an improper film storage, higher temperature, long developing time, and high-speed films. Scatter radiation arises from Compton scattering and it increases with patient thickness, field size and photon energy. Use of grid and good collimation may reduce scatter radiation.

Resolution

Resolution is the ability to image two closely placed small objects, as two independent images. There are three types of resolution, namely (1) spatial resolution, (2) contrast resolution, and (3) temporal resolution.

Spatial resolution refers to ability of an imaging system to record an object in the two special dimensions (X, Y) of an image. In other words, it is the ability to resolve a small high contrast objects and record its image, e.g., bone-soft tissue interface. An image of higher spatial resolution said to have sharp and distinct image. On the other hand, lower spatial resolution images are said to be *blurred*. Spatial resolution of our human eye is 200 μm, this is the smallest object we can able see with our eye. Human eye can visualize black shades on light background since it has higher contrast. However, radiological images are made with gray shades whose contrast is lesser. Human eye cannot see < 200 μm sizes and require higher object size.

Spatial resolution is measured in spatial frequency, not by an object size. Spatial frequency refers to line pair (lp) that is a black line on white background **(Fig. 6.14A)**. One lp consists of a line and an interspace of equal width. It is expressed in lp per millimeter (*lp/mm*). It is analogy to a sound wave (sine) having frequency in cycles/mm. Objects of an image that are separated by small distance (mm), possess high spatial frequency, like sound waves. Spatial resolution depends on focal spot size, detector blur and patient motion.

If D is the size of the object, then spatial frequency (F) = 1/2D. For example, if an object size is 0.5 mm, then spatial frequency:

$$F = \frac{1}{2 \times 0.5} = 1\ lp/mm$$

The human eye can resolve about 5 *lp/mm* at a viewing distance of 25 cm. If the spatial frequency is 5 *lp/mm* one can see 10 objects in 1mm. Then the size of an object is 1/10 = 0.1 mm. Spatial resolution of screen/film radiography is 5–10 lp/mm, whereas it is 4 lp/mm for digital radiography.

Contrast resolution is the ability to distinguish an anatomical structure of similar subject contrast, e.g., *liver-spleen*. It is an ability to differentiate many shades of gray from black to white. Digital radiography has better contrast resolution than screen-film radiography. In general, film-screen radiography has an excellent spatial resolution, whereas CT has superior contrast resolution.

Temporal resolution is an ability of an imaging system to localize an object in time, from frame to frame and follow its movement. Temporal resolution is high for fluoroscopy.

Spatial resolution is measured by (1) point-spread function (PSF), (2) line-spread function (LSF), (3) edge-spread function (ESF), and (4) modulation transfer function (MTF).

Point-spread Function

The image produced for a single point object is called PSF, e.g., imaging a Lead sheet that has tiny hole (10 μm) or performing CT scan of a wire, kept perpendicular to the slice plane. Then, an image profile is measured by a densitometer, that gives the PSF **(Fig. 6.14B).** The point appears blurred

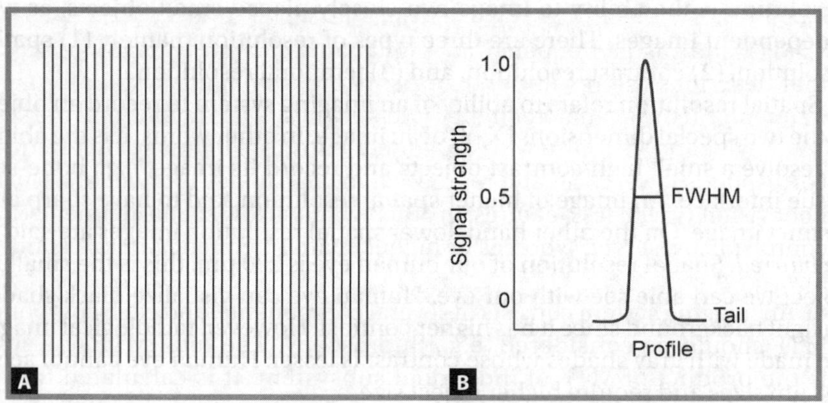

Figs. 6.14A and B: (A) Line pair; (B) Point-spread function (PSF).

because of focal spot, motion, and detector size. The dimension of the profile is measured at half width, which is called *full width half maximum (FWHM)*. If the separation of two-point sources is greater than the FWHM, they can be resolved. The presence of scatter radiation will broaden the FWHM, with an extended tails, which creates image blur or an unsharpness.

Line-spread Function and Edge-spread Function

Though PSF describes the response of an imaging system, it represents a discrete point on an image surface, and it is not suitable for system like screen-film, involving fixed area. Hence, functions like LSF and ESF are recommended. LSF describes the response of an imaging system to a linear stimulus. It is an image of a narrow line source, and its width (FWHM) is a measure of blur. In this, imaging is done with a slit (10 μm, Platinum), then 90° image profile is measured, by a densitometer. This can be measured for both vertical and horizontal axis.

Similarly, edge-spread function (ESF) is measured in fluoroscopy by using a sharp edge. Wide LSF refers to poor spatial resolution, whereas narrow LSF refers good resolution. Narrow LSF up to 1 mm can be measured by bar a phantom which consists of parallel Lead bars of thickness 0.5 mm. Wide LSF can be measured by FWHM, e.g., Nuclear medicine. FWHM and spatial resolution are related as follows:

$$FWHM = \frac{1}{2 \times LSF}$$

Modulation Transfer Function

Modulation transfer function (MTF) is a ratio of recorded signal frequency to an original signal frequency. It is the ratio of an output to input modulation as a function of spatial frequency. An ideal image is one that appears exactly as an object, that is MTF always 1. In clinical practice, there is no such an ideal imaging system and the MTF is always <1. The output is always less than 100% due to blur offered by focal spot, motion, and detector size:

$$MTF = \frac{Recorded\ signal}{Available\ signal}$$

MTF and spatial frequency are plotted in a curve **(Fig. 6.15).** It is a curve that describes the resolution capability of an imaging system for a given frequency. If the spatial frequency is lesser, the MTF is higher, and the system will have good visibility with an added features. Higher spatial frequency corresponds lower MTF, and reproduction of an image is difficult. It will have poor visibility with less features. In other words, at low spatial frequency image contrast is preserved whereas at higher spatial frequency image contrast is low.

An imaging system consists of several components, and each component's MTF should be considered, e.g., fluoroscopy. The total MTF of a system is the product of MTF of individual subsystem. It is calculated from the measurements of LSF. Thus, MTF is a useful to quantify the resolution of each

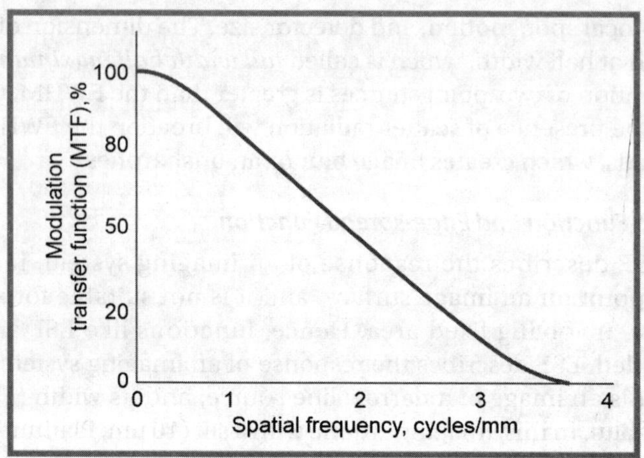

Fig. 6.15: Resolution capability of an imaging system: Spatial frequency vs MTF of the system.

component in an imaging system. In day-to-day practice, measurement of spatial resolution is done by using *star phantom* in radiography and *line pair phantom* in computed tomography.

Noise

Radiographic *noise* or *mottle* is a random fluctuation of film density about a mean value, following an uniform exposure. Noise degrades an image quality and limits the ability to visualize low-contrast objects or lesions. Radiographic noise is divided into: (1) quantum noise, and (2) screen-film noise.

Quantum noise is due to random variations of X-ray photons, incident on the detector which gives grainy appearance. It depends on the concentration of X-ray photons. It can be reduced by increasing number X-ray photons reaching the detector. This will make an invisible lesion into visible, but contrast is unchanged. Quantum noise is most important source of noise in radiography. The adjacent areas of the film receive photons that differ from the mean value, which contribute to quantum noise. The number of X-ray photons required to produce an image is about 10^5 per mm^2, whereas light photography uses 10^9 photons of per mm^2 hence, the noise is very low in the later.

Screen-film noise is further divided into: (1) screen noise, (2) film noise, and (3) quantum noise. The screen noise is caused by nonuniformities in screen construction (grain size) but usually negligible in modern screens. Film noise is caused by grain structure of emulsions, which has very little concern in radiography. Quantum noise is a major contributor in screen-film noise. It is created by the statistical fluctuations in the number of photons (quanta) per unit area, absorbed by an intensifying screen. To increase the screen-film speed, thicker screens are recommended. Such screens are called *fast screen* and absorb same number of X-rays as that of thinner screen. An image noise of thicker screen remains the same in such a system.

If N is the mean number of X-rays recorded by a pixel in a detector, then noise $(\sigma) = \sqrt{N}$, where σ is the *standard deviation*, which indicates photon fluctuation. Usually, Poisson statistics is used to quantify quantum noise. In these statistics, the mean (N) is equal to variance (σ^2). The relative noise, or coefficient of variation (COV) $= \sigma/N$. As the number of photons (N) increases, the relative noise decreases. As per statistics, 68% of the regions may contain within one standard deviation (σ). Similarly, 95% and 99% of the region may lie within 2σ and 3σ, respectively. The inverse of the relative noise is called *signal-to-noise ratio (SNR)*:

$$\text{SNR} = N/\sigma = N/\sqrt{N} = \sqrt{N}$$

To increase SNR, the number of photons (N) reaching the detector must be increased. As photon number increases, the relative standard deviation decreases, and the noise is reduced. If the X-ray tube emits 100 photons, the standard deviation is 10, and the relative standard deviation is 10%. If the number of photons is increased to 10,000, the standard deviation is 100 and the relative standard deviation is only 1%. This will reduce an image noise, but it increases patient dose. Hence, optimal balance of SNR and radiation dose is a must. The detector does not detect all the incident photons. The screen-film system detects only 60% of an incident X-ray photons.

To quantify noise, *Wiener spectrum* (WS) is used. It is a measure of total noise recorded by the film. Later, the film is scanned by a microdensitometer and density fluctuations are analyzed. The spectrum plots the noise of the system as a function of frequency content. Low and high frequency noise can easily be identified. The acceptable frequency range is 0.2–1 lp/mm. The Wiener spectrum can be related to MTF, photon number (N) and film gamma (G) as follows:

$$\text{WS} = \frac{G^2}{N} \times \text{MTF}^2$$

Fluoroscopy system uses an image intensifier tube with TV system or flat panel systems. Few number of X-ray photons are used to form a single image frame in fluoroscopy, compared to radiography. Hence, quantum noise is greater in fluoroscopy, 10% more compared with radiography. In mammography, number of incident photons (air-kerma) vary drastically hence, its image is less noisy than a fluoroscopy image.

Detective Quantum Efficiency

Radiological image quality evaluated by above parameters are not adequate to evaluate the performance of an imaging system. Generally, an imaging system is made up of several subcomponents and the signal-to-noise ratio

(SNR) is not the same at various stages of the subcomponents. X-rays are poly-energetic in nature and an effective energy is always employed. Hence, the X-ray spectrum incident on the detector is an effective quantum efficiency type. In the case of digital setup, an image is post-processed to improve image quality. This may lead to an increased noise in an image, which will alter an output signal-to-noise ratio (output SNR). Hence, an output SNR is different from an input signal-noise ratio (input SNR).

Hence, there is need for a single parameter to address the above issues. The detective quantum efficiency (DQE) is such a parameter, which comprehensively evaluate the performance of an imaging system. It is expressed in terms of ratio of the SNR:

$$DQE = \frac{\text{Output SNR}^2}{\text{Input SNR}^2}$$

It describes the imaging system's accuracy of response towards radiation. It replaces resolution, MTF, contrast, and mottle and addresses the subcomponents of an imaging system. The DQE of film is maximum over an optical density of 1 and 2. Therefore, film processing is very much critical to achieve the above density. In screen-film system, thin screen phosphor is used to improve resolution. This will increase noise resulting in low output SNR, thereby reducing DQE. Hence, an optimal balance is required between resolution and noise. The screen-film system can detect even a small anatomy of the order of 130 µm.

In fluoroscopy, usually the noise levels are higher, since smaller number of photons is making the image. DQE relates an input screen absorption efficiency and its X-ray-to-light conversion efficiency, to obtain SNR figure. Dynamic range is decided by an electronic noise and video camera. The DQE measurement considers the number of photons reaching an input window, absorbed by an input screen and photons forming an image. DQE is better in digital radiography relative to screen-film radiography, and it is 50–70% for fluoroscopy.

Optimal Quality Image

Quality radiographic images can be produced with proper patient preparation, selection of an imaging modality and correct exposure techniques. Patient anatomy should be placed closer to the receptor/film. An axis of the anatomy should lie parallel to the receptor plane. The central X-ray beam should pass through the center of an anatomical region. If multiple anatomy is to be imaged with equal magnification, then all the anatomical structures must be positioned at an equal distance from the film. The patient must be immobilized to avoid motion blur. Motion blur can be reduced by the following:

❑ Short exposure time
❑ Instructing the patient

❏ Higher source to image distance (SID)
❏ Short object to image distance

Selection of exposure technique plays an important role in obtaining a good quality image. The exposure time should be always shorter to reduce motion blur and improve an image quality. High frequency generator provides short exposure time than single phase generator.

The kV controls radiographic contrast since it influences both quantity and quality of X-rays. As kV increases, higher number of X-rays are transmitted through the patient. Compton interaction also increases, differential absorption is reduced, resulting reduction of subject contrast. The scatter radiation that reaches the film is higher, which increases noise in an image, resulting loss of contrast. As the contrast is low, the latitude is larger and the margin of error is increased. Hence, high kV reduces contrast, and the only advantage is the reduction of patient dose with wide latitude of exposures.

Tube current, mA controls an optical density in the film since it influences quantity of X-rays. As mA increases, the number of X-rays reaching the film also increases, resulting in higher optical density. The radiographic noise is lower, but patient dose is higher. Too low mA and high mA shift an optical density away from the straight-line portion of the characteristic curve. Thus, it indirectly affects the radiographic contrast. Therefore, use of high kV with minimum mA and short exposure time is recommended to obtain a good quality radiograph.

Imaging System Performance

Diagnostic performance of an imaging system must be good. That means the system should maximize *true positive* and *true negative* results. True positive are positive test results in patients, who have the disease. True negative are negative results in patients, who have no disease. In a similar way, *false positive* refers to positive results for patients with no disease and *false negative* for negative results for patients with disease.

Imaging system should have *sensitivity and specificity*. The former is an ability to detect a disease, also called true positive fraction. A most sensitive system will have low false negative results. Specificity is an ability of the system to identify absence of disease, also called true negative fraction. This type of system should have low false-positive results. To compare the performance of an imaging system, *receiver operating characteristic curve (ROC)* is employed. It is a curve drawn between the sensitivity in Y-axis and specificity in X-axis. The area under the curve is a measure of performance of an imaging system **(Fig. 6.16)**

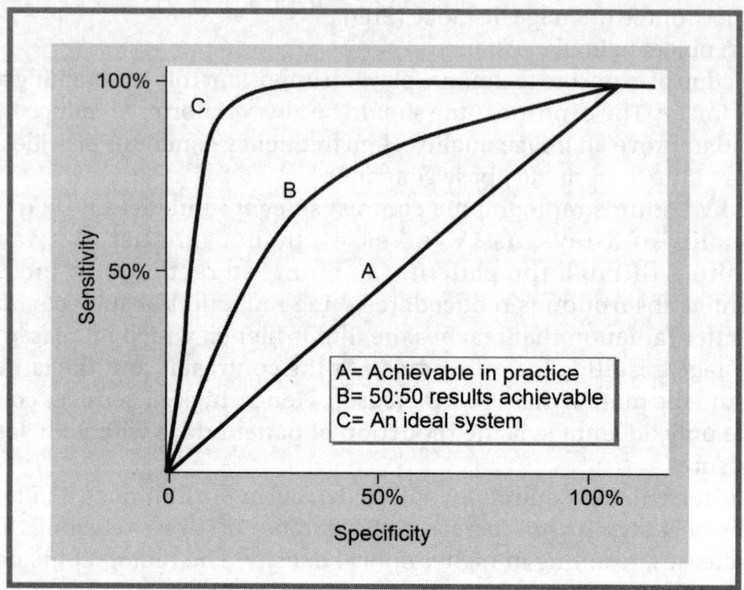

Fig. 6.16: Receiver operating characteristic curve of an imaging system.

BIBLIOGRAPHY

1. Bushberg JT, Seibert JA, Leidholdt EM, Boone JM. The Essential Physics of Medical Imaging, 3rd edn. Lippincott Williams and Wilkins; 2012.
2. Thayalan K. Basic Radiological Physics, 2nd edn. Jaypee Brothers Medical Publishers (P) Ltd, New Delhi; 2017
3. Thayalan K. Medical X-ray Film Processing, 2nd edn. Jaypee Brothers Medical Publishers (P) Ltd, New Delhi; 2021

Computed Radiography and Digital Radiography

BINARY AND DECIMAL NUMBERS

Screen-film devices are replaced by receptors that can produce digital images. Basically, both computed radiography and digital radiography can produce digital images. The advantages of digital images are: (1) data can be stored and transferred, (2) postprocessing is possible, (3) display of images on a computer monitor, and (5) use of picture archiving communication systems (PACS) for tele-radiology, etc.

Digital system uses binary numbers, for which the base is 2 and has two digits, namely, 0, 1. Generally, decimal numbers are used which has a base of 10 and uses digits 0 to 9. In a binary, value of a digit, the position of a digit is 2 times higher than it is in right. In a decimal number, value of a digit in a position is 10 times higher than it is in right. Decimal point is allowed in decimal system, whereas it is not allowed in binary. For example, the value of a binary number 10 is:

$$(1 \times 2^1) + (0 \times 2^0) = 2$$

Similarly, one can convert any binary number into a decimal number by raising powers of 2 in a series and then adding them **(Table 7.1)**

Digital memory and storage uses the term *bit, bytes, and words*. A bit is a small portion of a disk or tap that can be magnetized for data storage. Bits are grouped in bytes and words and 1 byte (B) is equal to 8 bits. The number of bits in a word may be 16, or 32 or 64, depending upon the computer system. Various digital units under use are:

❑ 1 kilobyte (KB)	$= 2^{10} = 1024$ bytes	
❑ 1 Megabyte (MB)	$= 2^{20} = 10,48,576$ bytes	$= 1024$ kB
❑ 1 Gigabyte (GB)	$= 2^{30} = 1,07,37,41,824$ bytes	$= 1024$ MB
❑ 1 Terabyte (TB)	$= 2^{40} = 10,99,51,16,27,776$ bytes	$= 1024$ GB

Table 7.1: Binary and equivalent decimal numbers.

Binary number	Decimal number
0	0
1	1
10	2
11	3
100	4
101	5
110	6
111	7
1000	8
1001	9
1010	10

The image is divided into number of matrix elements called *pixels*. Each pixel is assigned a value, related to signal intensity. The value stored in the pixel is in binary format and the maximum value that is stored is called *bit depth*. A pixel having a high value represents *dark grey shade*, whereas pixel of low value represents *white-grey shade*. This is analogy with film, where high dose gives dark shade and low dose gives white shade. A single bit can store either black or white, like an electrical switch, which can be switched ON or OFF. In general, computer memory and storage use many bits and each bit have two states, namely, 0 or 1. Similarly 2 bits may have 4 possible states, 3 bits have 8 states and so on.

In general, if there are N bits then the possible states are 2^N, e.g., 8 bits may have 2^8 states that is equal to 258 grey shades. However, radiography involves large field size with a resolution of about 10 lp/mm, to provide an optimal contrast. Therefore, it requires higher bit depth of 8, 12 and 16, respectively. For example, 16 bits depth can provide 65,536 numbers of grey shades. That is why digital radiography needs large storage space in the range of 4–32 MB, which is very much higher compared to computed tomography (CT) scanner.

COMPUTER BASICS

A typical computer has the following components: (1) central processing unit (CPU), (2) memory, (3) data entry, and (4) export device. Computer memory stores various bit values, either in *random access memory (RAM) or read only memory (ROM)*. RAM is a temporary memory, whereas ROM is a permanent memory. CPU instructions are stored in the ROM. In addition, there are buffer and cache memories. The former is used in video display, and the later performs as a buffer in between RAM and memory disk. Basically, computers are operated with software systems, which can store files.

Table 7.2: Computer input, output, and data storage devices.

Input devices	Output devices	Data storage devices
Mouse	Monitor (LED, LCD, CRT)	Hand drive
Keyboard	Printer	CD-ROM
Joystick	Projector	DVD-ROM
Light pen	Plotter	Flash media
Track ball	Audio speaker	Thumb drive
Touch screen	Headphone	Memory stick
Scanner	–	iPOD
Digitizer	–	Digital camera
Microphone	–	

An operating system is a software, which acts as an interface between an user and computer hardware. Such operating systems are as follows: *Windows (Microsoft), Mac OS, iOS (Apple), UNIX, Android OS (Goggle), and VMS (Main frame computer).* Computer programs are written using the following languages: *C, C++, COBOL, FORTRON, Java, Java script, Python, and Pascal.* Computer employs lot of peripheral devices in the form of an input device, an output device and data storage devices **(Table 7.2).**

Computer is connected via co-axial cable, telephone lines, magnetic tape transfer, microwave, and fibre-optics. A *modem* is used to transfer data through telephone lines. Cable modem is used to transfer data in cable television lines. The data transfer rate (per second) is called *Baud rate*. Network concept is used to connect modem computers, e.g., *Ethernet.*

Digital Systems and Image Format

An ideal digital radiography system should have the following: (1) physical design should have compatible size with screen-film cassette, (2) immediate readout facility, (3) robust and less costly, (4) high quantum efficiency with low radiation dose for an image capture, (5) spatial and contrast resolution like film, (6) wide dynamic range, and (7) DICOM compatible. Presently, these systems are employed in the form of (1) computed radiography (CR), (2) charge-coupled detector (CCD), and (3) digital radiography (DR). Digital radiography further divided into an indirect conversion X-ray detection system and direct conversion X-ray detection system **(Fig. 7.1).**

A digital image is divided into number of rows and columns, called *matrix.* The matrix sizes are 128 × 128 (Gamma camera), 256 × 256 (MRI), 512 × 512 (CT, US), 1024 × 1024 (DSA), 2560 × 2048 (CR, DR) and 4096 × 6144 (Mammography). The smallest element in a matrix is called *pixel.* It stands for *picture element* in 2D image format which is seen on a TV monitor or in a hard copy print out. Voxel stands for *volume element,* it represents a discreate value in 3D patient anatomy. Hence, a pixel (2D) in the monitor represents an voxel (3D) on the patient. A pixel size is the ratio of *field of view* (FOV) and

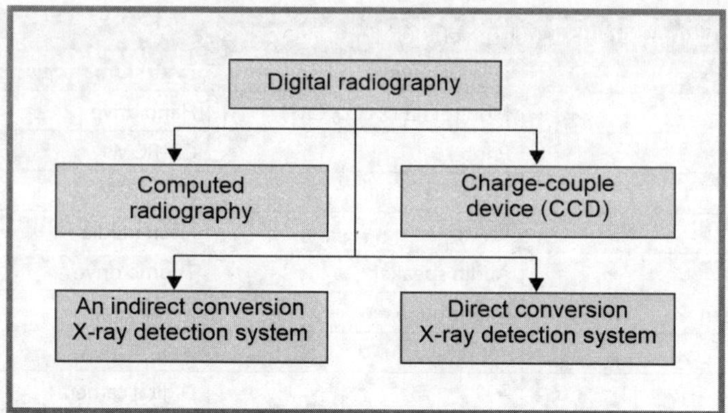

Fig. 7.1: Different path of getting digital radiography images.

matrix size. Typical pixel sizes used in diagnostic radiology ranges from 0.5–1 mm. As the matrix size increases or FOV decreases, the pixel size decreases. Smaller pixel size is always preferred for better resolution.

DIGITAL DETECTOR SYSTEMS

Digital systems use the following detectors, to produce radiological image:
- Gas detector
- Solid state detector

Gas detectors are basically ionization chamber that contains air or special gases. When exposed to X-rays, ion pairs are produced in the gas. These ion pairs are collected by applying an electric field between the electrodes. Thus, measurement of an ionization current creates an electrical signal. The total charge collected is proportional to radiation intensity. Detectors in an imaging system use gases of high atomic number (Z) at high pressure, e.g., *Xenon (Z = 54).*

Solid state detector consists of an inner and outer energy bands such as *valance and conduction bands.* When the detector is exposed to X-rays, valance band electrons absorb energy by Compton and photoelectric process. These electrons move to conduction band and form electron traps, just below the conduction band. In some phosphor, the electrons return to the ground state instantaneously, with emission of light. Some phosphors require light/heat stimulation to return the electrons to the ground state with emission of light. Such an emission of light is called *luminescence.* Solid state detectors come in the following category: (1) photostimulable phosphor detector, (2) scintillator detector, and (3) photoconductor detector. These detectors are explained in details in later paragraphs.

Photostimulable Phosphor

Photostimulable phosphor (PSP) is basically a crystal with an impurity, e.g., *Barium fluoro bromide (BaFbr).* If exposed to an ionizing radiation, electrons move from an valance band to conduction band and form traps below the conduction band. It requires red laser light as stimulant to return the trapped electrons to the valence state. As a result, blue light is emitted, which can be measured by a *photomultiplier tube (PMT)*. The detected light intensity is proportional to an incident radiation intensity. This principle is used in imaging plates, in computed radiography. These plates are exposed to intense white light to erase remaining electrons, so that it can be reused again.

Scintillator

In the case of scintillator, the radiation excites atoms of the phosphor and emits light flashes instantly, e.g., NaI. It can be detected by a PMT or photodiode, which gives an electrical signal. The detected electrical signal is proportional to an incident radiation intensity. *Gadolinium oxysulfide* (GOS) and *Cesium iodide* (CsI) are used as scintillators in digital imaging.

Photoconductor

Photoconductor is a solid-state device, e.g., *Selenium* ($Z = 34$). When the detector is exposed to X-rays, energy is deposited, and the detector emits electrons directly. The produced electron charge is collected by applying voltage across the photoconductor as signal. Collected electric charge signal is proportional to an incident X-ray intensity. Since Selenium absorption is very poor, *Lead iodide* and *Mercury iodide* are used now a days.

COMPUTED RADIOGRAPHY

Computed radiography (CR) is a form of digital radiography, introduced by *Fuji film* (1983). It records an latent image in a *photostimulable phosphor (PSP)*-containing an *imaging plate (IP)* through a laser light stimulation. In screen-film radiography, the intensifying screens emit light after an exposure whereas CR uses trapped electrons in high energy metastable state to form an image. Both can form latent image and can be used in any X-ray unit. CR has two parts, one is the phosphor which work on *photostimulable luminescence (PSL) principle, and the other is CR reader.* They store the latent image of the X-ray attenuation pattern in an imaging plate and readout the stored image.

When the patient is imaged, the transmitted X-ray attenuation pattern is stored in an imaging plate as latent image. A laser *raster scanning* is used to readout the stored imaging information through photostimulable luminescence. The amount of luminescence is proportional to radiation exposure. The luminescence signal is converted into electric signals by the photomultiplier tube (PMT). An analog-to-digital converter is used to generate high quality images. The imaging plate is reused after removing the residual energy in the plate by an intense light.

Basically, it is an energy transfer mechanism inside the photostimulated phosphor. The electron-hole pair combination in situ is proportional to the absorbed radiation energy of the host lattice.

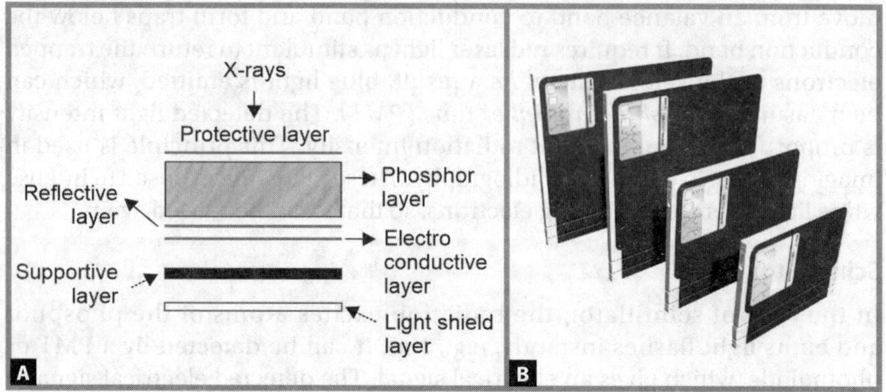

Figs. 7.2A and B: (A) Cross-section of an imaging plate; (B) Commercial CR cassette of different sizes.
(*Courtesy:* M/s Agfa Healthcare India Pvt Ltd)

Imaging Plate

Imaging plate replaces an intensifying screen and X-ray film (**Fig. 7.2A**). PSP can be made as flexible screen, which is enclosed in a rugged cassette and is called an *imaging plate (0.5 mm).* In the imaging plate, the PSP particles are randomly present throughout the binder, and it can be handled like a screen-film cassette. *Protective layers* on both sides avoids scratching and ensure durability. *Phosphor layer* is made with a *polymer binder*. An *electro conductive layer* prevents the degrading of image quality by static electricity. The supportive layer in the middle gives mechanical strength to the plate. The *light shield layer* with Lead backing blocks the back scattered radiation.

IP cassettes are available in various sizes, namely 14 × 17 inches, 14 × 14 inches, 10 × 12 inches, and 8 × 10 inches with a pixel range of 200 × 200 – 100 × 100 μm. It is available in variety for general radiography, mammography, etc. The matrix sizes available are 1760 × 2140 for normal resolution and 2000 × 2510 for high resolution. The spatial frequency is 2–3 lp/mm for standard radiographic work and 10 lp/mm for mammography work. Commercial CR cassettes made of photostimulable phosphors are shown in **Figure 7.2B.**

Photostimulable Phosphor

Photostimulable phosphor (PSP) used in CR must fulfill three conditions, namely, (1) emission of phosphor should overlap the maximum quantum efficiency wavelength of the photomultiplier, (2) exhibit fast response to the laser scanning and (3) no significant signal deterioration for at least 6 hours. However, it is rare to find such phosphors.

Commonly used phosphor is *Barium fluorohalides with europium: BaFBr: Eu²⁺ or BaFI: Eu²⁺ or BaI: Eu²⁺* . The *Europium* is called an activator, and it is present in small quantity, which is responsible for the PSL property. It is like a sensitivity center in a film emulsion. The atomic numbers of BaFBr are 56, 9 and 35 with K-shell binding energy of 37, 5 and 12 keV, respectively. $RbBr:Tl^+$ and $CsBr:Eu^{2+}$ can also be used as phosphors due to their easy preparation and form of needle like structure array but exhibit quick latent image loss. Commercially available material are $BaFBr:Eu^{2+}$ and $CsBr:Eu^{2+}$. The trace element-activator, Eu^{2+} is dopped to replace Ba^{2+} ions in the crystal to have luminescent centers. Such a doping alters not only the structure but also the physical properties of the phosphor. $BaFBr: Eu^{2+}$ shows efficient X-ray absorption over 35–50 keV energy due to its K-edge absorption of Barium. At higher energy, >50 keV, GOS:Tb and CsI:Tl phosphors gives better performance, hence they are used in flat panel X-ray detection systems.

Since metastable electrons represents the image, these phosphors are called *storage phosphor screens (SPS)*. Photostimulable phosphor (PSP) particles are small, 3-10 µm, randomly present and offer excessive scattering, resulting white appearance of SPS. The SPS can be made with linear phosphor which increase absorption of X-rays and restricts the spread of stimulated emission. It is stable and protected electro statistically.

Mechanism of Luminescence

When a phosphor is exposed to radiation, the X-rays interact with halide ions mostly by Compton and photoelectric with outer shell electrons. Valency electrons absorb energy and goes to conduction band, and store radiation energy as trapped electrons at the high energy metastable state, representing the latent image. Thus, it creates halide ion vacancy and interstitials which excites the electrons to metastable state.

For example, the divalent Europium atoms (Eu^{+2}) get oxidized into trivalent Eu^{+3} with release of electrons in the valence band **(Fig. 7.3)**. These electrons move from the valence band to conduction band, later they are trapped at the F-centers in the *forbidden zone*. The electrons can stay in these centers for longer period. Thus, billions of electrons are trapped in the F-centers. The number of electrons per unit area is proportional to an absorbed radiation energy:

$$X\text{-ray} + Eu^{+2} = Eu^{+3} + e^-$$

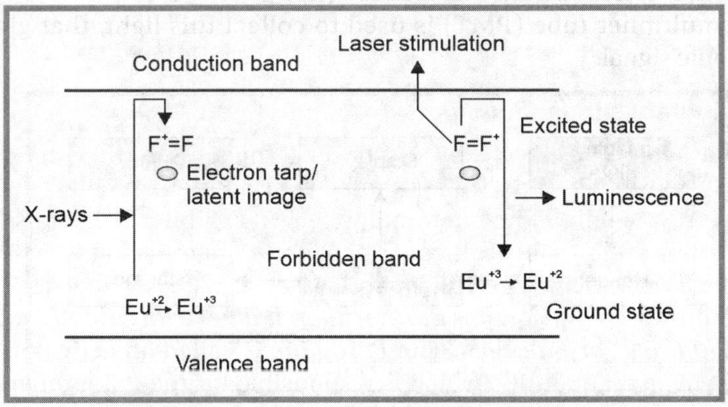

Fig. 7.3: Principle of photostimulable phosphor, Eu = Europium.

Over time, 50% of these electrons return to the ground state on their own immediately. It results in gradual deterioration of the stored energy. Exposing the phosphor to a red laser light laser source, force the carriers trapped in the defect center to absorb enough energy from stimulation light to overcome the energy barrier. The electrons reach the conduction band, where they become mobile again. They move to the valence band, with an emission of *blue-green light* or light-stimulated luminescence. The electron recombines with Eu^{+3} and is converted into Eu^{+2}.

The blue-green light energy is greater than that of laser light energy. That is why, it is called *photostimulable phosphor* which is used in an imaging plate technology. Hence, an imaging plate (IP) is read within 8 hours, otherwise latent image may fade, resulting in CR signal loss.

The IP will not give up all its trapped electrons in the first stage of laser light. It retains some number of trapped electrons. If the residual latent image is there it gives *ghosting cloud appearance* during its reuse. Hence, it is to be exposed to white *light source (fluorescent lamp)*, which moves all the trapped electrons to the valence band, thus emptying the F centers. Now, the imaging plate can be used for another radiation exposure or patient. PSP is sensitive to background radiation and likely to get fogged.

Phosphor Reader

Computed radiography system consists of (1) imaging plates of various sizes, (2) reader, (3) computer, and (4) printer in addition to X-ray unit **(Fig. 7.4)**. The imaging plate is used instead of screen-film cassette. It can be re-used again and again by erasing old image data. The computer offers image processing, storage, and image display facility. The following is the procedure involved in computed radiography:

❑ CR cassette is exposed to X-ray beam.
❑ Cassette is inserted into the reader.
❑ Imaging plate is removed from the cassette.
❑ Plate is scanned by He–Ne laser beam (633 nm), and blue-green or UV, light (390 nm) is released from that location (X, Y).
❑ Photomultiplier tube (PMT) is used to collect this light, that gives an electronic signal.

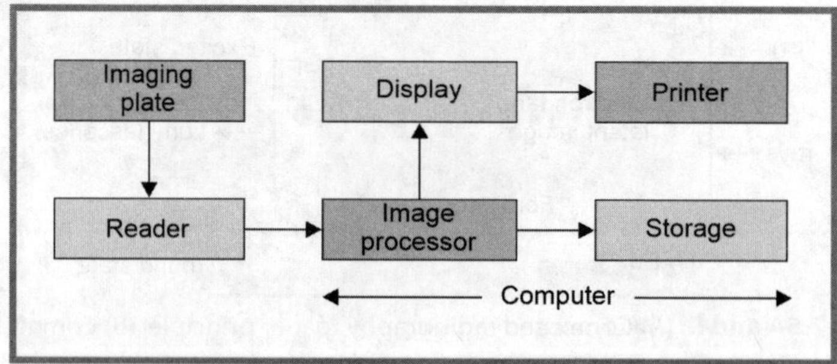

Fig. 7.4: Block diagram of computed radiography system.

❑ Electronic signal is digitized and stored in memory.
❑ The plate is exposed to bright white light, to erase the residual energy, for another use.

The reader is most critical part of CR imaging system. It consists of (1) entry system for an imaging plate, (2) laser light source, and (3) photomultiplier tube (PMT) as shown in **Figures 7.5A and B.** After radiation exposure, the CR cassette is inserted into the reader, where an imaging plate is removed

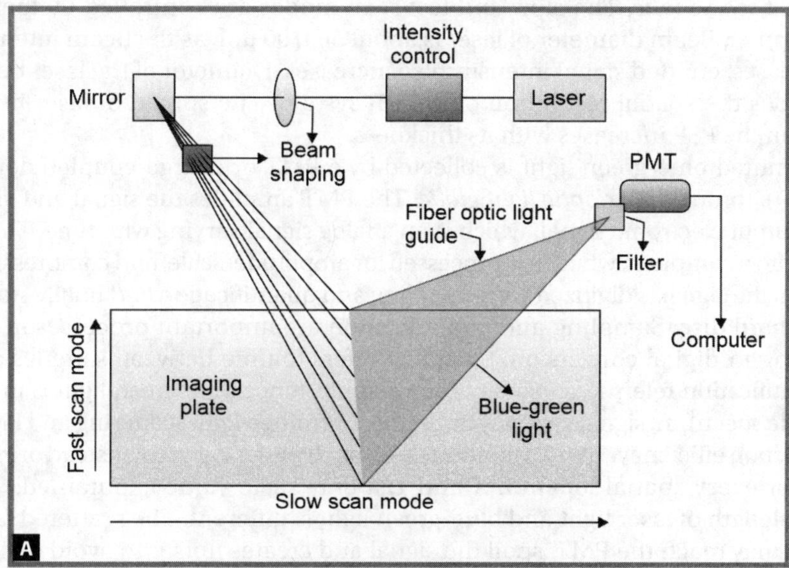

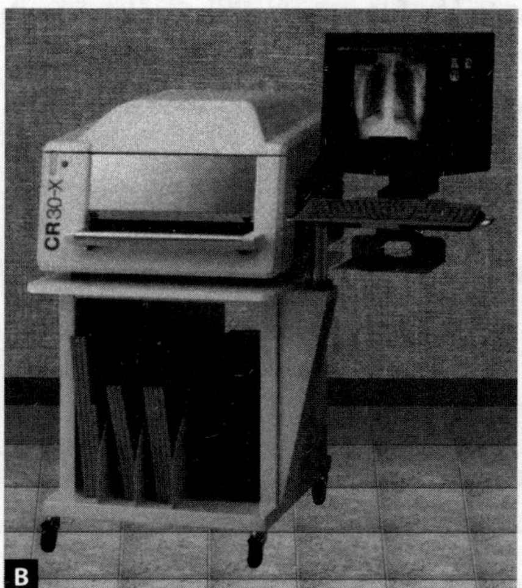

Figs. 7.5A and B: (A) Computed radiography reader principle; (B) Commercial computed radiography system.
(*Courtesy:* M/s Agfa Healthcare India Pvt Ltd)

and fitted to a drive mechanism. The drive mechanism moves the plate with constant velocity along the Y-axis. This is usually done with slow motion and is called *slow scan mode.*

A rotating and multifaceted mirror reflects the red light from a laser light source (He–Ne laser, 633 nm). This light is deflected back and forth across a phosphor plate in the horizontal X-direction, which releases visible, blue-green light of 390 nm **(Fig. 7.6).** This means that the trapped energy due to radiation exposure is released from that spatial location (X, Y). This is done in *fast scan mode.* The slow and fast scan modes are controlled by the CR computer. Beam diameter of laser is about 50–100 µm, as the beam intensity increases, emitted signal intensity also increases. Diameter of the laser beam decides the spatial resolution of the CR system. The spread of laser beam within the PSP increases with its thickness.

Emitted blue-green light is collected by a PMT or charge-coupled device (CCD), through *fiber optic light guide.* The PMT amplifies the signal and gives an output electronic signal, which is an analog signal varying with time. This is fed into a computer, where it is processed for amplitude, scale, and compression. Then, the signal is digitized with sampling and quantification and finally stored in a hard disc. Sampling and quantification are important processes in the analog-to-digital conversion. Sampling refers to time between samples and quantification refers to a value of each sample. Since blue-green light is in the visible spectrum, signal loss may occur due to emitted light scattering and PMTs collection efficiency. Hence photodiode is much preferred in CR instead of PMT.

For every spatial location X and Y, a gray scale value is obtained. The wavelength of laser light and blue-green light is different. The scattered laser light may reach the PMT, spoil the signal and creates noise. To avoid this, an *optical filter* is mounted in front of the PMT. This filter attenuates the scattered laser light and transmits the blue-green light emitted by the phosphor, thereby increasing the signal-noise ratio.

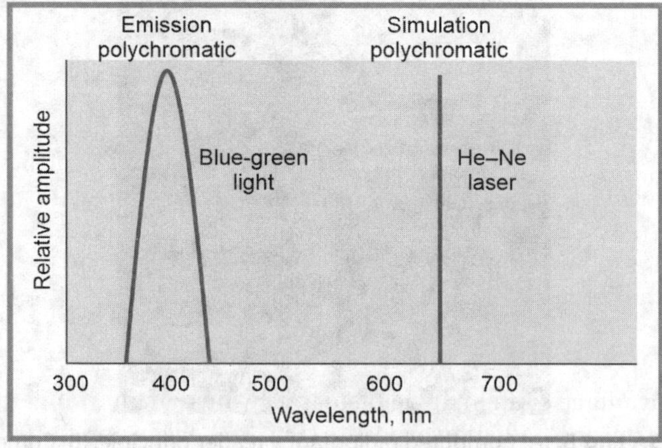

Fig. 7.6: Computed radiography spectrum: Plot of wavelength vs relative intensity of simulation and emission light.

In some other systems, the cassette is inserted vertically, and an imaging plate is withdrawn downwards, during which it is scanned by a horizontal laser. In this, the imaging plate is not completely removed from the cassette, which avoid roller damage. The laser scanning is done right angle to the grid lines, which also avoid aliasing artifacts.

The laser beam size is very important, and it should be kept less than 100 μm at the mirror level. The laser beam shape, size, speed, and intensity must be kept constant at an imaging plate level. This is achieved by means of a beam shaping devices. A reader can process about 70 cassettes in one hour.

Image Display

The digital image is shown in the computer monitor for further postprocessing. In a CR system, an image capture, storage and an image display are independent functions. In the case of screen-film system, all the above functions are coupled together. Each image pixel is assigned a location with a grey scale value. The image can be brought to the required brightness level. To do this, *window level and window width* can be adjusted by the user. The window level refers to center value of the window width, which control an image brightness. Window width refers to range of grey scale value, which controls an image contrast. Proper window width and level achieves good brightness and an image contrast. Lesser is the window width, higher the image contrast.

In the postprocessing, one can manipulate digital image data. To achieve this, tools such as *histogram equalization, low–pass spatial filter, unsharp masking, background and energy subtractions* are employed. Histogram equalization eliminates black and white pixels, since their contribution is little. This will facilitate to expand the display range. To reduce noise in an image, low-pass filter is used. In this, portion of an averaged value of the surrounding pixels is added to each pixel. Unsharp masking tool is used to subtract the smoothened version from an original. It can be added later, to resemble the original. To reduce scattered radiation, background subtraction is used, which improves an image contrast.

Energy subtraction is used, where low and high kV images are obtained for a given anatomy. For example, in chest radiography bone can be subtracted, to clearly view lung and soft tissues. Alternatively, soft tissue can be filtered, to view bones clearly. This will differentiate calcified and noncalcified lung nodules. Nowadays, *computer-aided detection (CAD)* along with an artificial intelligence (AI) are used to make the diagnosis. After postprocessing, an image is fed into a laser printer for making a hard copy. The principle and function of the printer is explained in the next chapter.

Image Characteristics

The main advantage of an imaging plate is its wide dynamic range, and it has wide latitude towards radiation exposure **(Fig. 7.7).** It can accept 100 radiation intensities of either low or high. Usually, screen-film system requires a radiation intensity of 5 μGy for an optimal image. The technologist has freedom to

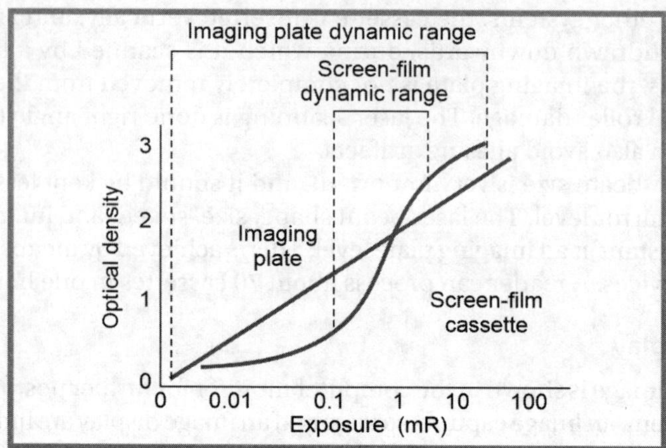

Fig. 7.7: Comparison of dynamic range of computed radiography—imaging plate and screen-film systems.

select his exposure techniques (kV, mAs) in computed radiography. However, technologist cannot understand his error since it is adjusted in an image postprocessing. Retake rate is lesser compared to screen-film radiography.

An image produced with low radiation exposure involve higher quantum noise, whereas an image produced with high radiation exposure involves low quantum noise but involves higher patient dose. The main source of noise is the scatter radiation. The drive mechanism, laser and computer devices also contribute to noise in an image.

Computed radiography systems are faster compared to 400 speed screen-film system. Hence, images can be produced with lower patient dose. In screen-film radiography, kV controls contrast and mA control an optical density. This concept is no more valid in computed radiography because CR image contrast is constant, irrespective of an exposure technique. Therefore, high kV and lower mAs can be used to produce CR images, which reduce patient dose further.

Spatial resolution of CR system is less (3.5–5.5 lp/mm) compared to screen-film systems (5–10 lp/mm) and it is preferred in portable radiography. It is very difficult to access detector dose and some vendors offer *detector dose indicator (DDI facility)*. Hence, these systems require an elaborate quality assurance.

CHARGE-COUPLED DEVICE

Charge-coupled devices (CCD) is made from *metal-oxide semiconductor capacitors as a light-sensitive sensor* for recording images. Charge-coupled device (CCD) forms an image from visible light. It is usually used with an intensifying screen and an image intensifier tubes. Basically, CCD chip is an integrated circuit, made up of *Amorphous Silicon* **(Fig. 7.8).** Its surface is edged with pixel electronics, e.g., 2.5 × 2.5 cm CCD may contain 1024 × 1024 pixels on its surface. The *Silicon* surface is photoconductive, if it is

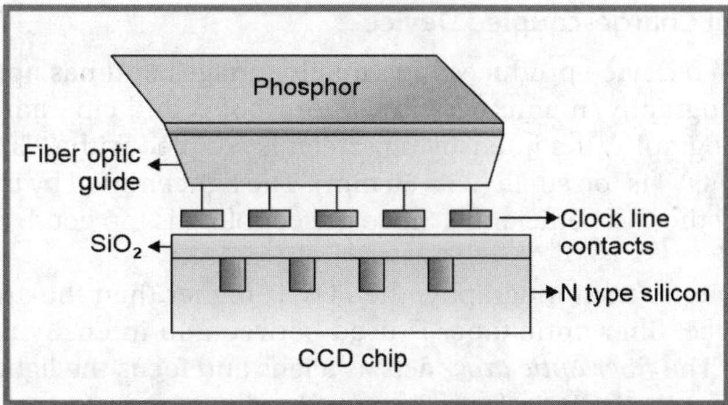

Fig. 7.8: Design of charge-coupled device (CCD).

exposed to visible light, electrons are liberated that build-up in the pixel. Higher the light intensity, higher the number of liberated electrons. The electrons are kept in the pixel by an electronic barriers on each side of the pixel. Thus, each pixel act as a capacitor and the collected charge is proportional to light.

Electronic charge in each pixel is readout along column wise. The electron in each pixel is shifted to another pixel, by adjusting the voltage barriers of an each pixel **(Fig. 7.9).** Thus, the charge pocket in one column moves in an unison and finally reaches a pixel at the bottom row. The bottom row is readout pixel by pixel and the charge is shifted to the readout electronics, which produces an electronic signal. This signal is digitized by an analog-to-digital converter (ADC) and the digital signal is used to construct an image matrix with bit depth of 8–12.

Similarly, next column is read pixel by pixel and charges are shifted to the bottom row that gives another signal. This process is repeated until all the pixels in the detector system are readout completely. The readout is faster and it is at the rate of 30 frames per second. The CCD geometry is uniform and distortion free. It has wide dynamic range with low electronic noise.

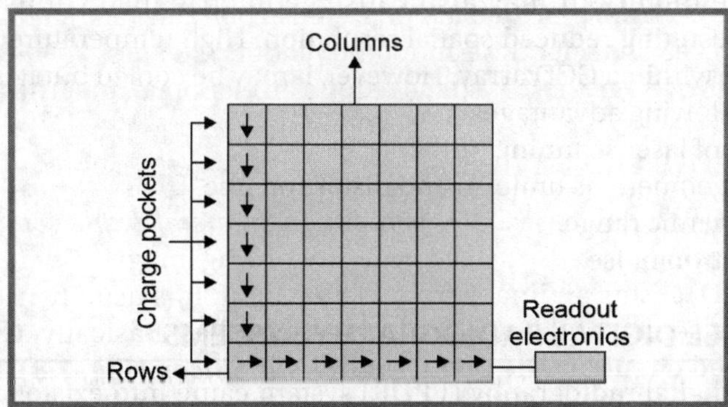

Fig. 7.9: Movement of charge pockets column by column through the bottom row.

Application of Charge-coupled Device

Charge-coupled device produces high quality images and has application in dental radiography, mammography, fluoroscopy, and cineradiography. In dental radiography, the intensifying screen is coupled with CCD and the field of view (FOV) is too small (25 × 50 mm). The light emitted by the screen is collected by the CCD efficiently. Since the coupling is too good, only little light is wasted.

In digital biopsy mammography, the FOV is higher than the area of the CCD and hence, fiber optic taper is used between an intensifying screen and the CCD. The *fiber optic taper* acts as a lens and focus the light emitted by the screen on the CCD surface. The input and output surface of the fiber optic taper is 50 × 50 mm and 25 × 25 mm, respectively. The loss of light is not significant in this system.

Since CCD has fixed a dimension, it is usually smaller than an imaging area. Hence, fiber optic guide is needed to taper the radiation beam and address the demagnification factor. It is suitable for dental and mammography where the radiation field is small. In chest radiography, the FOV is larger (35 × 43 cm) than the CCD surface and the amount of light lost is higher (99.7%). The amount of light lost is proportional to the *demagnification factor* required to couple an input area to an output area. As lesser number of photons are used to construct an image, a secondary *quantum sink* will occur. This will increase image noise and reduce image quality. This will also result in higher radiation dose to the patient. Hence, CCD is not used in chest radiography.

Large Area CCD

Large number of CCDs coupled to have an array for large scale detection. The luminescence from the scintillator is directed towards the CCD array by using an *optical lens system*. The detector base is a glass substrate on to which light sensitive a-Si with thin-film transiter is embedded in the form of pixels. The charges are readout to form the final image.

The optical lens system may reduce the number of photons reaching the CCD array. It will reduce the quantum efficiency with high noise resulting poor image quality. It may also cause geometric distortions and light scattering resulting reduced spatial resolution. High temperature can rise of signal noise within a CCD array. However, it may be cooled but it is costlier. CCD has following advantages:

❏ No need of laser scanning.
❏ Camera geometry is uniform and distortion free.
❏ Wide dynamic range.
❏ Low electron noise.

FLAT-PANEL DIGITAL RADIOGRAPHY SYSTEMS

Flat-panel digital radiography (FPDR) system came into existence in 1990, it converts an incident X-ray photons into an electric charge and read an image by using photoelectric conversion arrays. Its readout time is faster relative to computed radiography. Low-dose, real-time X-ray imaging uses flat-panel detectors. It includes chest X-rays, dental X-rays, mammography, and extremity X-rays. It also finds application in an industrial radiography and X-ray security scanners in railway stations and airports.

FPDR is made as large area flat panel with solid state detectors and an integrated with *thin-film transistor (TFT)* readout and having fast access with best image quality. It should have higher spatial resolution, contrast resolution and dose efficiency. In general, they are available in two configurations:
❑ Indirect conversion X-ray detection system
❑ Direct conversion X-ray detection system

In an indirect systems, the X-rays are converted into light by a phosphor and then an light is converted into an electric signal. In direct systems, the X-rays are converted directly into an electric signal **(Figs. 7.10A and B).** The difference between an indirect and direct digital radiography systems are given in **Table 7.3**.

Indirect Conversion X-ray Deduction System

Indirect conversion X-ray detection system is a large area flat-panel system. It converts X-ray photons into electrical charges and readout the image using photoelectric conversion arrays. It displays faster readout time relative to computed radiography.

Indirect conversion system consists of a (1) scintillation phosphor, (2) amorphous Silicon (a-Si) photodiode, and (3) thin-film transistor (TFT)

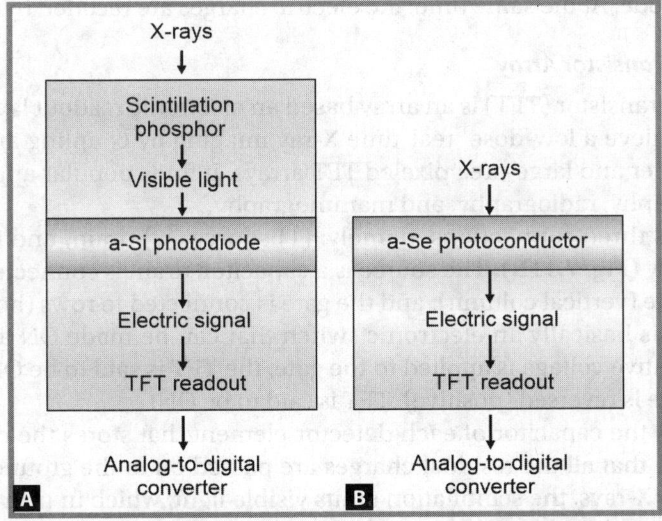

Figs. 7.10A and B: Principle of digital radiography: (A) Indirect; (B) Direct conversion flat panel systems. (TFT: thin-film transistor; a-Si: amorphous Silicon; a-Se: amorphous Selenium).

Table 7.3: Comparison of an indirect and direct conversion digital radiography systems.

S. No.	*Indirect conversion digital radiography system*	*Direct conversion digital radiography system*
1.	Silicon phosphor is used: Z = 14	Selenium phosphor is used: Z = 34
2.	X-ray is converted into light then electron signal	X-ray is directly converted into electron signal
3.	Phosphor is thinner	Phosphor is thicker
4.	Causes blur due to light spread	No blurring due to electron travel
5.	Fill factor is lower	Fill factor is higher
6.	Contrast resolution is poor	Contrast resolution is higher
7.	Limited detector size	Large area plate can be made

arrays **(Fig. 7.11A).** The scintillation crystal used is either *CsI: Tl or Gd$_2$O$_2$S: Tb,* which converts an incident X-ray photons into visible luminescence. It works like an intensifying screen in a cassette. It is made up of thin-film of scintillator on the top for X-ray conversion, pixelated Amorphous Silicon (a-Si) photodiode arrays adjacent to scintillators and a TFT array.

Topmost component is the scintillation phosphor, followed by Amorphous Silicon which is a fluid that can be painted on a given surface. The entire assembly is put in a protective enclosure with external cable connections. There is no need of fiber optic guide as in the case of CCD for image demagnification.

When exposed to X-rays, X-ray photons are converted into visible light by scintillators and subsequently converted into an electric charge by the photocathode. At the same time, the electric charges are recoded by the TFT.

Thin-film Transistor Array

Thin-film transistor (TFT) is an array based an electronic readout layer. They able to achieve a low-dose, real-time X-ray imaging by coupling an energy transfer layer and large-area pixeled TFT arrays. It finds popular application in angiography, radiography, and mammography.

TFT has three connections, namely: (1) source, (2) drain, and (3) gate, respectively **(Fig. 7.11B).** The source is a capacitor, drain is connected to the readout line (vertical column), and the gate is connected to rows (horizontal line). TFT is basically an electronic switch that can be made ON and OFF. When negative voltage is applied to the gate, the TFT is said to be OFF, if the gate voltage is reversed (positive), TFT is said to be ON.

Initially, the capacitor of each detector element that stores the charge is earthed, so that all the residual charges are passed on to the ground. When exposed to X-rays, the scintillation emits visible light, which in turn exposes the light sensitive photodiode (a-Si). The photodiode releases electrons, so that charge build-up in each detector element, which is stored by the capacitor. Later, the charge in each detector element is readout by an electronics.

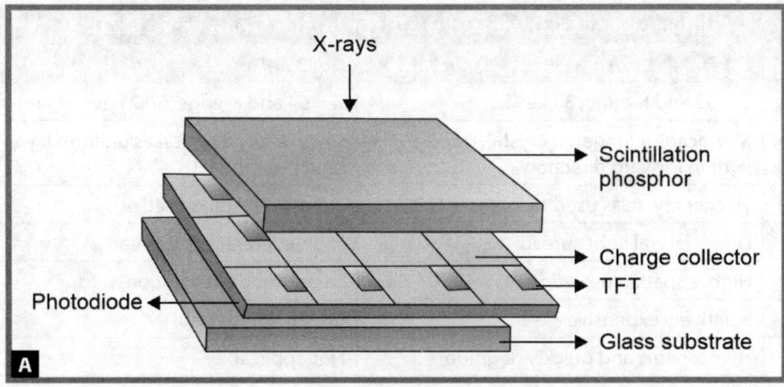

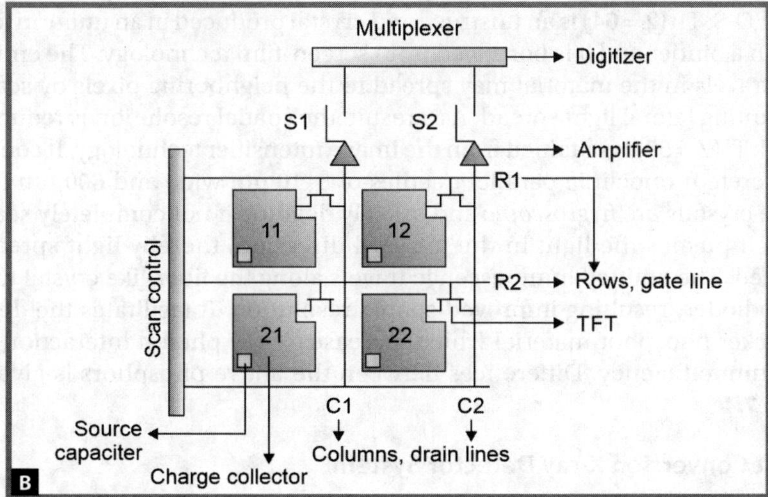

Figs. 7.11A and B: (A) Indirect conversion X-ray detection (Flat panel) system; (B) The thin-film transistor (TFT) readout process by scan control.

During the X-ray exposure, negative voltage is applied to the *gate* and all the transistor switches are in OFF position. The charge accumulated in each detector element is stored in the *capacitor*. During the readout process, positive voltage is applied to the gate, such a way one row at a time. Thus, the switches of detector elements in a row are made ON. This will connect vertical wires C1, C2, to the digitizer through switches S1, and S2. *Multiplexer* select the column sequentially (one column at a time) and the charge is amplified and allowed to move to the digitizer. Thus, the gate selects a row and multiplexer selects a column and the charge in each detector element is readout sequentially. Finally, the signal is digitized and stored for image analysis.

Phosphor Materials

The commonly used scintillators are: (1) Terbium-doped Gadolinium oxysulfide ($Gd_2O_2S:Tb$), known as GOS and (2) Thallium-doped cesium iodide (CsI:Tl).

Table 7.4: Comparison of CsI:Tl with Gd_2O_2S:Tb phosphor (Thayalan K, 2021).

S. No.	CsI:Tl	Gd_2O_2S: Tb
1.	Z = 55 and K-edge: 33 keV	Z = 64 and K-edge: 50.2 keV
2.	Monoclinic elongated crystal, through light in forward direction	Unstructured crystal as uniform layer, held in a binder
3.	Thicker crystal is used to increase DQE	Thinner crystal is used
4.	Lesser lateral light spread	Higher lateral light spread
5.	Higher spatial resolution	Lesser spatial resolution
6.	Relatively expensive	Cheaper and robust
7.	Hygroscopic and quickly degrade	Not applicable

Gd_2O_2S: Tb (Z = 64) is an unstructured crystal produced in an uniform layer, held in a binder and it is borrowed from screen-film technology. The emitted light travels in the material may spread to the neighboring pixels by scatter, accounting lateral light spread. As a result, the spatial resolution is reduced.

CsI: Tl (Z = 55) is obtained from the image intensifier technology. It consists of discrete monoclinic parallel needles of 5–10 μm wide and 600 μm long. These crystals are *hygroscopic* and quickly degrade if not completely sealed. Since it pushes the light in the forward direction, thereby light spread is reduced. The emitted luminescence travels along the fiber-like crystal to the photodiodes, resulting improved spatial resolution. It facilitates the design of thicker phosphor material which increases X-ray photon interaction and quantum efficiency. Differences between the above phosphors is given in **Table 7.4**.

Direct Conversion X-ray Detector System

Direct conversion X-ray detection systems are designed by depositing a layer of X-ray sensitized material onto pixelated TFT arrays **(Fig. 7.12)**. It directly converts the X-ray photons into an electrical charges that is allowed to transfer into TFT arrays. Commonly used X-ray photoconductor material is *Amorphous Selenium (a-Se, Z = 34)*, which is fabricated by an evaporation at high temperature.

When it is exposed to X-rays, it absorbs the X-ray energy and convert into charge carriers which is proportional to incident X-rays. The hole-electron pair generated in the photoconductor travels along the filed lines parallel with limited lateral diffusion. This is due the application of an electric field in the a-Se. Holes can be collected by bias electrode and electrons by collection electrodes. The charges are stored on the storage capacitor and later readout by TFT. Each pixel is separated by the field-shaping in the a-Se layer, resulting high quality images.

There is no an intermediate material like scintillation phosphor which converts X-rays into light, as in the case of an indirect conversion X-ray detection system. Since Selenium is in amorphous form, large area plates

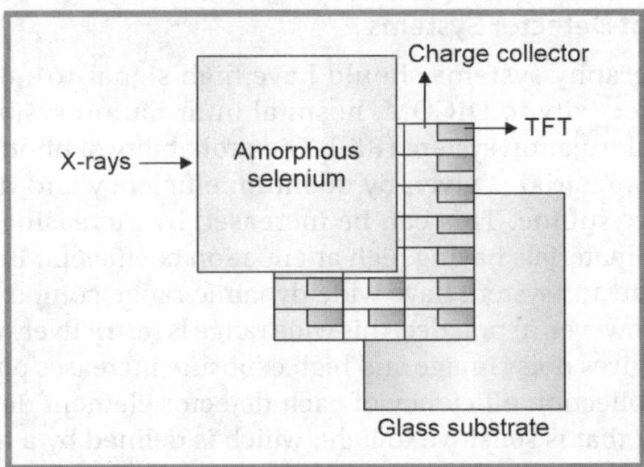

Fig. 7.12: Direct conversion X-ray detection (Flat panel) system.

can be made by *vapor deposition*, which is cost effective and is a reproducible technology. It has good X-ray detection properties and high spatial resolution. Selenium is also photoconductor, and it alters its electrical conductivity, when exposed to X-rays. The altered electrical signal is proportional to an intensity of X-rays.

Initially, 5 kV bias voltage is applied to the surface of the Selenium. Later, when it is exposed to X-rays, it emits electrons, which discharge part of the applied voltage. The amount of discharge is proportional to the radiation intensity, resulting in latent charge image. These charges are stored in the capacitor, and the pattern of charge is readout by scan control lines, like that of an indirect digital radiography system. Finally, the signal is amplified, digitized for image analysis. Selenium is susceptible to humidity and temperature variations and requires protection from environment. The differences between computed radiography and digital radiography is given in **Table 7.5**.

S. No.	*Computed radiography*	*Digital radiography*
1.	*Versatility*: Single cassette is used both for table and stand bucky	Require two separate detectors for table and stand bucky
2.	*Flexibility*: Oblique view and bed side X-ray is possible	Do not have the same flexibility
3.	Single CR system can support multiple X-ray units	Each room requires independent DR system
4.	No need for X-ray equipment modification	X-ray equipment need replacement
5.	DQE is about 30%	DQE is about 65%
6.	Throughput is lower	Throughput is higher
7.	Available at lower cost	Relatively expensive

Table 7.5: Comparison of computed radiography and digital radiography systems.

Comparison of Detector Systems

Digital radiography systems should have high signal-to-noise ratio and provide connectivity to DICOM, hospital information system (HIS) and radiological information system (RIS). The probability of photon interaction with detector material is given by quantum efficiency and it is higher for gadolinium oxysulfide. This can be increased by increasing the detector thickness and materials having high attenuation coefficient. Both direct and an indirect detector system have wide dynamic range compared to screen-film system. However, in practice, this wide range is restrictively used, because low exposure gives noisy image and high exposure increases patient dose.

The light collection efficiency of each detector element depends on the fractional area that is sensitive to light, which is defined by a term fill factor as follows:

$$\text{Fill factor} = \frac{\text{Light sensitive area in the detector}}{\text{Area of the detector element}}$$

In digital radiography, the detector is occupied by conductors, capacitors and TFT, and only partial area of the detector is sensitive to X-rays **(Fig. 7.13A)**. Hence, the fill factor is always less than 100% and it depends on individual detector system. The fill factor is higher for direct a-Se system compared to an indirect detection digital radiography systems.

Small detector element gives higher spatial resolution but reduces fill factor. As the light sensitive area increases fill factor also increases **(Fig. 7.13B)**. Low fill factor reduces the signal-to-noise ratio, resulting in poor contrast resolution. Hence, there is tradeoff between spatial resolution and contrast resolution for a given detector. The specifications of various detector materials are given in **Table 7.6**.

Portable Flat Panel Cassette

Nowadays, mobile digital radiography X-ray machines are used with portable flat panel cassettes, which can be inserted into a standard bucky tray cabinet or a CR system. Initially, these cassettes are wired to X-ray generator, for an image acquisition. Of late, wireless detectors with full field *automatic exposure*

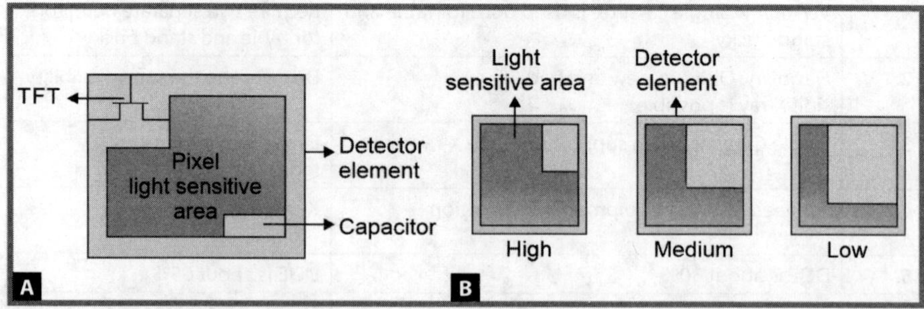

Figs. 7.13A and B: (A) Fill factor is the ratio of the light sensitive area to detector element; (B) Fill factor—as light sensitive area decreases the fill factor decreases.

Table 7.6: Specifications of DR detector materials.

Parameter	$Gd_2O_2S:Tb$	CsI:Tl	a-Se
Active area	22.5 cm × 28.7 cm	43 cm × 43 cm	35 cm × 43 cm
Thickness	500 µm	550–600 µm	500–1000 µm
Element array	2256 × 2878	2688 × 2688	2560 × 3072
Pixel pitch	100 µm	143 µm	1000 µm
Element pitch	140 µm	173 µm	139 × 139 µm
Fill factor	52%	68%	86–100%
Spatial resolution	5 lp/mm	3.5 lp/mm	3.6 lp/mm
Pixel depth	12 bit	12 bit	14 bit
Display time	3 s	10 s	7 s
Effective Z	64	55	34
Density, kgm^{-3}	7440	4510	4500
Sensitivity	13	19	50
k-edge, keV	50.2	33	12.6

(*Courtesy:* David J Dowsett et al, 2006)

detection (AED) technology is available **(Fig. 7.14).** Cassettes are made available with active area of 10" × 12" to 11" × 17", pixel area of 2816 × 2816 and pixel pitch of 154 µm. It provides large area coverage and unrestricted time windows. It is precalibrated and user friendly and known as direct digital. These cassettes are provided with handle with drop protection and smooth nonporous surface. It is light weight and has durability and long lifetime.

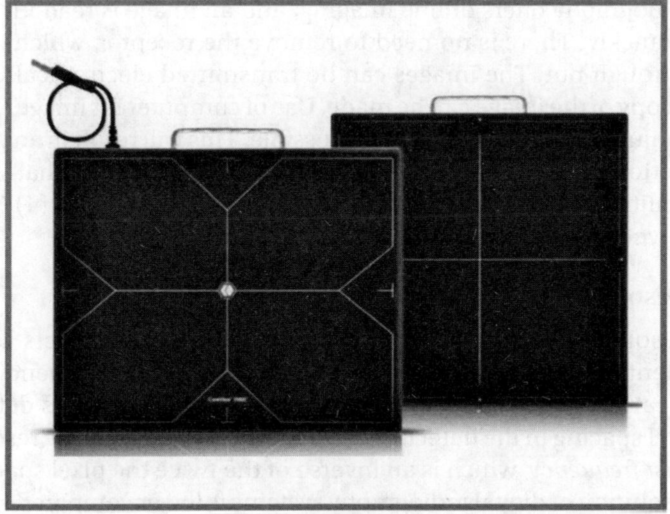

Fig. 7.14: A commercial portable flat panel detector.
(*Courtesy:* M/s CareRay Digital Medical Technology Co Ltd, China)

They basically use either CsI: Tl or Gd_2O_2S: Tb (GOS) crystals for making the detector. The CsI crystals are grown in a controlled condition and deposited directly on flat panels and sealed with a *hermetic packing*. It is made with water resistant *Al-alloy or Magnesium alloy frame, combined with Carbon fiber and impact absorbing rubber edging.* CsI gives excellent image quality, fast image availability with significant dose reduction. On the other hand, GOS detectors are cost-effective with an excellent image quality.

It can transfer an image data within few seconds with high transmission rate. It is also provided with battery support (up to 8 hrs), which can offer more than 1000 shots with 10 sec interval between shots. These images can be stored, and captured image is validated immediately. Option of retrieving old images, stored previously is also available.

Cassette holder is also available for easy positioning. These holders can be rotated up to 180/360 degree, or any angle from the floor level to 180 cm. They do have the provision to insert DR cassette with grid. It has wide application in general radiography, pediatric radiography, extremities, and special examinations. It can also be effectively used in NICU, OT and emergency imaging.

These cassettes have the following advantages, consistent image quality, reduced radiation dose, faster image formation, same size as a film or a CR cassette, DICOM complaint, low noise, high modulation transfer function (MTF), high detective quantum efficiency (DQE), easy patient positioning, increased workflow, easy to clean and dis-infect, excellent contrast detail, exam dependent, and consistent image quality.

DIGITAL IMAGE QUALITY

Digital radiography offers online imaging, and an image is readout from the receptor quickly. There is no need to remove the receptor, which increases patient through put. The images can be transmitted electronically, and an identical copy of the image can be made. Use of computer for image archiving, and postadjustment of contrast is also possible. This will result in an improved interpretation and improved diagnosis. The various factors that influence image quality are (1) spatial resolution, (2) contrast, (3) noise, (4) MTF, and (5) detective quantum efficiency.

Spatial Resolution

Spatial resolution is an ability to resolve two adjacent objects as two an independent images. It is generally denoted by lp/ mm in frequency domain as stated earlier. In digital radiography, the spatial resolution is determined by the pixel spacing in the detector. The frequency that limits the resolution is the *Nyquist frequency*, which is an inverse of the twice the pixel spacing. The spatial resolution of digital radiography systems is lower compared to screen-film system. However, they have better contrast resolution than screen-film system. The spatial resolution of digital radiography (DR) is 4 lp/mm whereas it is 10–15 lp/mm for screen-film radiography. This is the maximum limitation of DR, due to its pixel size. However, spatial frequency and an object size are interlinked. If the spatial frequency is 4 lp/mm, one can see 8 objects in 1 mm, including the interface. Then, the size of the object is 1/8 mm = 0.125 mm, which is minimum object size to be recorded in digital radiography.

Sampling Frequency

In the case of digital system, sampling frequency determines the spatial resolution. Sampling frequency is the number of samples per mm, which is determined by the matrix size. A matrix size of 100 × 100 covering an anatomical length of 10 mm, gives 100 samples in 10 mm or 10 samples in 1 mm. This means that each pixel will contribute one sample. If the matrix size is doubled, pixel size reduces to half, and the sampling frequency is doubled. The sampling frequency is related to the spatial resolution as follows:

$$\text{Spatial resolution} = \frac{1}{2} \times \text{Sample frequency or pixel spacing}$$

If the sampling frequency is 10 per mm, then the spatial resolution is 5 lp/mm. Such a system can resolve 5 line-pairs of black and white (grey shade). The maximum resolution that can be obtained in an imaging system is called *Nyquist frequency*.

Nyquist Frequency

Consider a detector of pixel width d mm, from center to center. If two pixels (2d, if d is the pixel size) covers a full cycle of a signal (both maxima and minima), then the period is $2d$ mm. The spatial frequency = 1/period = 1/2d, which is called *Nyquist frequency*. This gives an upper limit to detect images, in terms of spatial frequency. If the signal frequency is greater, the detector will not record the signal. The signal is said to be aliased and the event is called an *aliasing*. This may lead to an improper reconstruction of an image from an original. Aliasing may cause wraparound images, called an *aliasing artifact*. Thus, Nyquist frequency sets an upper limitation to the spatial resolution.

Digital Radiography Resolution

Spatial resolution is an ability to differentiate adjacent details in an object and its related sharpness. It is related to pixel size and matrix size. It can be measured by using a narrow slit, a sharp-edged object and a bar test phantom.

Digital radiography employs a matrix size of 2000 × 2500 over an anatomical dimension of 350 × 430 mm, and the sampling frequency is about 6 per mm. The limiting spatial resolution is ½ × 6 = 3 lp/mm. The above said example is a high resolution (HR) plate and is digitized to 10 bits. Standard resolution (ST) plates are available with 1760 × 2140 matrix size and digitized to 10 bits. Chest radiography employs a matrix size of 3584 × 4096. These are 12 bits depth matrix with a resolution of 5–10 pixels per mm.

Imaging plate have wide latitude and dynamic range. Its dynamic range is linear, and it can accept very low to high radiation exposures. The actual dynamic range is 1:10,000 compared to 1:1000 for screen-film system. Imaging plate does not have speed limitation and the speed concept is no more valid here. However, it is rated that the speed of an imaging plate lies in the range of 20–2000.

In flat panel system, the spatial resolution depends on pixel spacing in the detector. Nyquist frequency decides the limiting spatial resolution. The MTF of the direct flat panel system is high enough to view minute diagnostic details. Hence, a-Selenium based direct conversion flat panel detector exhibits better spatial resolution. The factors that influence the spatial resolution are, focal spot size, magnification, phantom scattering, patient motion, aperture size, and spatial sampling interval between measurement and lateral scattering effects of X-rays. The first four factors are an extrinsic and the last two are an intrinsic in nature.

Contrast

Contrast refers to relative brightness of two positions in an X-ray image. It is measured by the characteristic exposure curve of an imaging system. Contrast is described by the dynamic range of the X-ray detector. In a digital system, contrast is an ability to differentiate many shades of grey from black to white. Digital radiography has better wider and linear dynamic range, compared to screen-film radiography. It is described by the parameter, greyscale or dynamic range.

Dynamic range of an imaging system is the number of grey shades that it can reproduce. In screen-film radiography, an optical density range is 0–3, which represents a dynamic range of 1,000. However, one can visualize only 30 shades of grey, due to the limitation of human eye.

On the other hand, in digital radiography, the dynamic range is 14 bits capacity corresponding to 214 = 16,384 shades of grey. Here, the dynamic range is described by the pixel size and bit capacity. The dynamic range of computed tomography (CT) and magnetic resonance imaging (MRI) is of the order of 212, whereas it is 216 for mammography.

However, human eye cannot visualize all the grayscales. To overcome this, postprocessing of an image is done with *window width* and *window level*. This will enable us to expand any part of the 16,384 grayscales into white to black. Thus, DR offers about 4–5 times more response than screen-film radiography, for a given exposure technique. One can also visualize all the grayscales by an image postprocessing process. This is clinically beneficial, especially in soft tissue imaging.

The digital radiography offers better low contrast resolution than screen-film. However, they suffer from inferior spatial resolution. The contrast resolution is limited by noise or signal-to-noise ratio (SNR). The signal represents the number of X-rays that forms the anatomy. This depends on the difference between the X-rays transmitted to the detector and the X-rays absorbed within the patient.

Noise

Noise originates from various sources, from collection to capture elements. Noise arises from scatter radiation and detector system. It is an variation of signals in an X-ray image from an uniform object. Wiener spectrum is used to measure noise variation of an X-ray image.

Noise limits the ability to view a lesion or pathology in a digital image and it may appear as grainy or mottled. Noise in an image quality depends on quantum efficiency of the phosphor, charge collection by the capacitor and noise free readout of the stored signal. The indirect detector system uses light that undergoes scatter, resulting in reduction of signal-to-noise ratio. One should always look for high SNR, to preserve contrast resolution. This will satisfy ALARA principle of radiation safety.

The noise in the PSP imaging plate arises from the following ways: *(1) quantum noise, (2) light photon noise, and (3) fixed noise.*

An acceptable quantum noise is obtained up to 100 µGy, which is ensured in an imaging plate design. This is not true at higher doses, beyond 100 µGy. Quantum noise can be reduced by reducing the thickness of the protective layer of the phosphor. The light photon noise arises from the photomultiplier tube (PMT). It is due to fluctuations of photoelectrons at the PMT. Hence, PMT should have high photoelectric conversion efficiency. Fixed noise arises in the form of structural, imaging plate, laser, analog circuit, and ADC quantization noises. Structural noise dominates over others, and it can be reduced by having reduced grain size.

In digital radiography or flat panel system, noise arises from the following: (1) quantum efficiency of the phosphor, (2) capacitor charge collection, and (3) readout. In an indirect detection digital radiography, X-rays are converted into light and later as electron charge signal. The light photon undergoes scatter before reaching the TFT and reduces SNR. However, this is avoided in the direct conversion digital radiography system. Digital fluoroscopy exposure techniques are like an image intensifier tube system. Frame averaging is the concept used here to reduce noise.

Modulation Transfer Function

Spatial resolution can be measured by the modulation transfer function (MTF). It converts an object contrast values into contrast intensity levels of a X-ray image. MTF of direct conversion flat panel X-ray detector is higher than an indirect conversion X-ray detector.

The indirect detector system suffers due to light scattering, and there is trade-off between X-ray absorption and MTF. Thinner scintillation crystal gives high MTF but reduces X-ray absorption. Thicker crystal increases X-ray absorption but reduces the MTF, due to an increase of light scatter. In the case of direct conversion system, the thickness can be increased, so that X-ray absorption can be increased without loss of MTF. The MTF of the direct conversion X-ray detection system is high, up to the Nyquist frequency **(Fig. 7.15).** Higher Nyquist frequency and MTF facilitates visualization of finer diagnostic details.

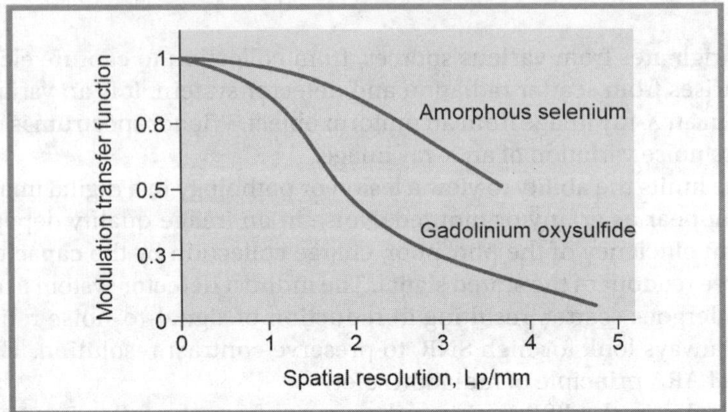

Fig. 7.15: MTF for direct and indirect conversion X-ray detector systems as a function of spatial resolution.

Detective Quantum Efficiency

Detective quantum efficiency (DQE) is a standard measure of evaluating an image quality in radiography. It is the best parameter to evaluate performance of an imaging system. It access an efficiency of a X-ray imaging detector towards X-ray photons. It accounts signal-to-noise ratio (SNR) and the system noise of the system in a combined way. It indicates the performance of the X-ray imaging detector in terms of X-ray imaging quality and the radiation dose. It also provides a measure of SNR for various subcomponents of the imaging system.

DQE can be measured by using a *Am-241 radioactive source*, which is equivalent to 120 kV X-rays. To measure an output, *photometer* with time constant circuit is used. The integration time should match the human eye. DQE is dose dependent and always stated with radiation dose. It varies with kV and radiation exposure. DQE influences the patient dose, and it depends on an input SNR. Higher the DQE, better an image quality. The expected DQE is about 100, that means an input and output SNR should be the same. No such an imaging system is available as on date, and DQE is always < 100%, due to an inefficiency in an incident X-ray detection, and internal source of noise.

In computed radiography, DQE evaluates the sensitivity and image quality. It serves as an index and addresses resolution, contrast, and mottle. The CR system's DQE is better than the screen-film at low spatial frequency (<2 lp/ mm), where the X-ray exposure levels are 10–25 µGy **(Fig. 7.16A)**. At higher special frequency (>2 lp/mm), it falls rapidly, due to noise from various sources. The limiting spatial resolution of the CR system is 5 lp/ mm, whereas it is 10–15 lp/mm, for screen-film system.

In the case flat panel system, the probability of photon interaction with the detector plays a vital role. It depends on linear attenuation coefficient

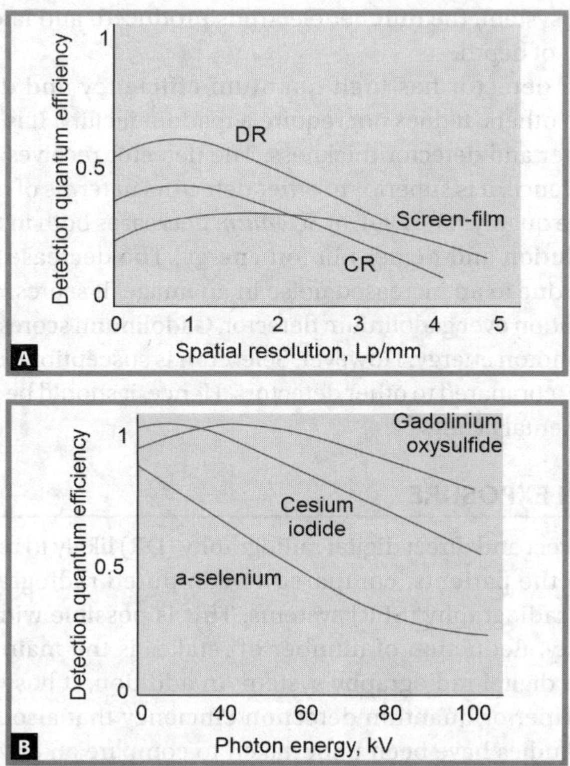

Figs. 7.16A and B: (A) Variation of DQE against spatial resolution, for DR, screen-film, and CR system; (B) Detective quantum efficiency of various imaging phosphors against photon energy.

(μ) and thickness of detector material and photon energy. The DQE is increased by increasing the quantum efficiency. That means that DQE is increased by increasing the detector thickness and having high μ value. The DQE is higher for *Gadolinium oxysulfide* over the photon energy of 40–100 kV **(Fig. 7.16B).** The drop in DQE is greater at higher energy, and greater for selenium.

Overall, DQE is higher at low photon energy, and it decreases with an increase of photon energy, after the K-edge. DQE of a CR system is about < 30 % at 0.5 lp/mm whereas it is 15% for screen-film system. DQE of flat panel system is 45–50% at 0.5 lp/mm. DQE differs between an indirect and direct conversion X-ray detection system. DQE of a-Se is higher (50%) compared to CsI and Gd_2O_2S. The various factors that affect the DQE are, noise, readout, dynamic range, and quantum efficiency.

In an indirect system, the X-ray interaction depth at the scintillator decides the brightness and lateral spread, leading to noise. This is totally absent in the direct conversion X-ray detection system, especially at high spatial frequency.

In the direct system, the number electrons produced, and lateral spread are independent of depth.

Selenium detector has high quantum efficiency and dynamic range compared to others. It does not require a readout facility. It is not influenced by light scatter and detector thickness. The detector receives X-rays without much loss. Hence, it is superior to other detectors in terms of noise reduction and an image quality. The DQE of *Selenium* decreases both in terms of higher spatial resolution and higher photon energy. The decrease at high spatial frequency is due to an increased noise in an image. It scores well in terms of spatial resolution over gadolinium detector. Gadolinium scores over Selenium in terms of photon energy. However, Selenium is susceptible to humidity and temperature, compared to other detectors. Hence, it should be protected from an environmental factors.

RADIATION EXPOSURE

Both an indirect and direct digital radiography (DR) likely to reduce radiation exposure to the patients, compared to computed radiography (CR) and screen-film radiography (SFR) systems. This is possible without loss of an image quality. Reduction of number of retakes is the main cause of dose reduction in digital radiography system. In addition, it has wider dynamic range and superior quantum detection efficiency that also helps the dose reduction. Studies have been undertaken to compare an *entrance skin dose (ESD) and effective doses (ED)* of patients with standard operating conditions **(Table 7.7).** It is found that the patient doses were in higher CR, compared to screen-film radiography and direct digital radiography. In DR, the effective doses were found to be −29% and −43% lower compared to screen-film radiography, and computed radiography. The computed offers much higher dose compared to screen-film radiography.

Table 7.7: Comparison of patient effective doses in mSv in digital radiography (DDR) vs computed radiography (CR) vs screen-film radiography (SFR).

Examination	DDR	CR	SFR	DDR vs CR, Dose reduction, %	DDR vs SFR, Dose reduction, %	CR vs SFR, Dose increase, %
Abdomen (AP)	0.223	0.358	0.280	−38	−20	+28
Chest (PA, Lat)	0.023	0.041	0.029	−44	−21	+41
Lumbar spine (AP, Lat)	0.179	0.476	0.309	−62	−42	+54
Pelvis (AP)	0.168	0.326	0.295	−48	−43	+11
Skull (AP, Lat)	0.022	0.029	0.027	−24	−19	+7

(*Courtesy:* Compagnone G et al, 2006)

DIGITAL IMAGE: VIEWING AND RECORDING

Digital Image Viewing

In screen-film radiography, all images are made in the X-ray film, as hard copy. However, in DR, an image is displayed on a monitor, pre and postprocessed and then printed on a special film by a *dry/laser printer*. The detail and design of the printer is explained in the latter paragraphs. This is the final hard copy, which is viewed with the help of a viewing box. They are generally known as *medical imaging workstations*. A typical workstation consists of following:

❑ Computer
❑ Operating system software
❑ Display processing software
❑ Display controller
❑ Display device

The medical imaging image display devices are of *three types*, namely:

❑ Cathode-ray tube (CRT)
❑ Active matrix liquid crystal display (AMLCD)
❑ Flat panel display

Computer

The computer includes a central processing unit (CPU), mathematical computation modules, input/output (I/O) controllers, and network communication hardware. It also has keyboard, mouse, trackball or wheel, joystick, and barcode scanner. Storage or recording devices such as hard disk, digital video disk (DVD), compact disk (CD) and output devices such as display monitors, printers, and speakers are also incorporated. There are also supporting hardware and software components. The display controller hardware converts digital information into analog or digital signal, suitable to the display device. Software module allows programs to assess controller hardware. The user application program accesses an image data and sends it to display controller in a suitable format. The special feature of medical imaging computer is that it uses special display software, high resolution display device, and high-performance display controller device. The above is the basic difference from general computer.

Operating System Software

An operating system (OS) software is required to perform the function of hard disk, CPU, I/O devices, and printer. It is a low-level program that controls the resources of computer. It supports network communication, security, display, and file management and execution of application programs. OS also provides time sharing, so that multiple programs are processed simultaneously. It also monitors keyboard, mouse, network, and other devices. Thus, OS creates an operating environment for the user and for application programs. The software in medical devices is *UNIX, LINUX, Macintosh, and Microsoft windows systems.*

Display Processing Software

Digital image consists of array of digital grayscale values. The display device should transform the grayscale values to luminance values. The values used by different modalities like CT and DR are different. In general, images are stored initially with specific values, and converted into analog or digital voltages for presentation on a display device. In DR, the stored images are converted to *digital driving levels (DDLs)*, before obtaining analog or digital images with the help of OS. In addition, coloring the image is also done in display processing.

Display Controller

The display controller is nothing but video card or graphic card. It is a combination of hardware and software to transform DDLs to appropriate signals for display device. Most of the display devices accept only analog video signals. In that case, the controller performs digital-analog (D-A) conversion. In flat panel devices, the controller sends digital signal to display device, and the device converts this into a suitable signal to control luminance.

Display Device

The display device generates a visible image from analog video signals. In addition, it has an internal software to respond to controller commands. A single workstation can have multiple display devices, e.g., 1–2. Either CRT or flat panels are used as the display device.

Flat Panel Monitor

The purpose of the monitor is to convert an electronic signal into visual display. Earlier CRT was used and slowly replaced by flat monitor systems. They basically use liquid crystals or plasma to give better images. The flat panel systems are divided into following categories:

❏ Liquid crystal display (LCD)
❏ Plasma display panel (PDP)
❏ Light emitting diode (LED)

The LCD monitor screens consist of a back light and liquid crystal. Back light is a series of light tubes placed behind the screen. They are like fluorescent lamps, but smaller in size. LCD screen does not emit light by itself it acts only as filter to block the light on per pixel basis. The fluorescent lamps that are used are called *cold-cathode fluorescent lamps* (CCFL). The liquid crystal system acts as a filter and either block or permits light transmission.

The liquid crystals are in the form of semi liquid. It is a thin nematic crystal, like rod shaped and exists in an unorganized state. The LCD has several layers as shown in **Figure 7.17.** The liquid crystal is the main component, and it is sandwiched between polarized films/filter.

The crystal has electrodes both in front and back. The liquid crystal exists initially in an unorganized state. When an electric current is passed, the crystal

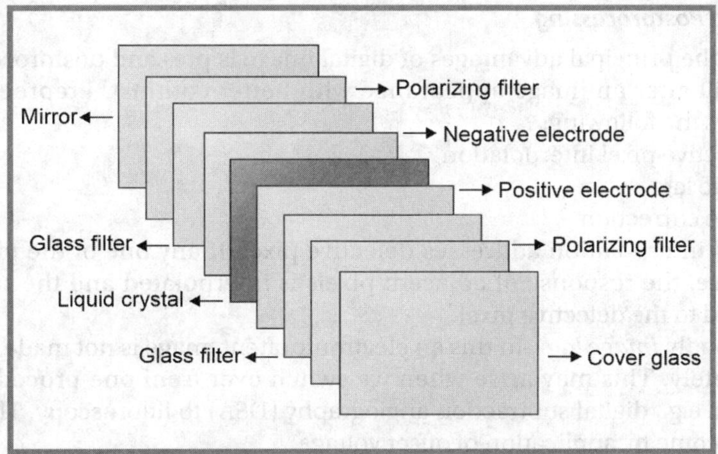

Fig. 7.17: Flat panel display system: Liquid crystal display (LCD) and its components.

undergoes a twist. In addition, it has a mirror, glass filter and cover glass. The polarizing filter is rod shaped and both filters are kept at 90°. That is, if one filter is in vertical and other one is in horizontal orientation. TFT panel is there behind the liquid crystal and each pixel has one TFT. The TFT controls the current to each pixel. When there is no electric current, the light emission is blocked by the polarizing filter. Once the TFT supplies an electric current, the crystal undergoes a twist and permits the light to transmit. Thus, switching ON and from the TFT, make an electric current either absent or present in the liquid crystal. Therefore, the crystal undergoes no twist or twist; other words either block or permit light transmission forward. The degree of twist depends on an electric current supplied by TFT. Thus, the TFT controls an electric current, crystal twist and light intensity.

In plasma display panel, thin layer of pixel is used, and each pixel is made of 3 Neon and Xenon gas filled cells. Each cell is coated with different phosphor layer, that will produce red, green, and blue light. The plasma layer is sandwiched between dielectric layers. If current is passed through dielectric layer, it passes through pixels, and ionizes the gas. As a result, electrons are liberated, which release an ultraviolet (UV) light. The UV light stimulates the phosphor to emit light. The color of light emission depends on phosphor for which it is coded. The current through pixel is modulated by the electrodes at a high rate (>1000 time/sec). Thus, an emitted light intensity is controlled. Plasma monitors can produce billions of color shades. Though the motion blur is less in the system, they suffer from an image retention. Hence, this type of monitor is no longer available in the market.

The light emitting diode monitor is like that of LCD monitor. The only difference is the back light. It uses light emitting diodes as back light, instead of CCFL. The LED is more energy efficient and smaller than CCFL. This enabled to make smaller TV monitors. There is not much improvement in picture quality between LCD and LED.

Pre- and Postprocessing

One of the principal advantages of digital image is pre- and postprocessing. This will alter an image appearance with better contrast. Preprocessing includes the following:

- ❑ Defective pixel interpolation
- ❑ Image lag
- ❑ Noise correction

Pixel interpolation addresses defective pixel. If any one of the pixels is defective, the response of adjacent pixels is interpolated and the same is assigned to the defective pixel.

Secondly *image lag*—in this an electronic latent image is not made visible completely. This may arise when we switch over from one procedure to another, e.g., digital subtraction angiography (DSA) to fluoroscopy. This can be overcome by application of offset voltage.

Thirdly *noise correction*—any voltage variation leads to line noise, resulting in an image artifacts. All the above preprocessing is done automatically in the system before the image display.

Postprocessing is done after an image display. It is performed with the help of technologists or radiologists. The purpose of postprocessing is to optimize an image appearance, to detect pathology. Various postprocessing steps are annotation, window width and window level, magnification, image flip, image inversion, subtraction, pixel shift, region of interest, edge enhancement and smoothening equalization.

Annotation is labelling an image by adding text. This contains patient information, examination, site, reference, etc. Text can be added to the image to identify regions of interest. Adjusting window width and window level, one can easily see all shades of gray up to 16,000. For example, 16-bit image may have 65,536 gray shades, which can be seen fully with window width and level adjustments. This is the most important advantage of digital image.

Magnification helps to see smallest detail of an image. This will improve visualization and spatial resolution. A small electronic magnifying lens is provided in the system, to see fine details. The image flip is the process in which an image is flipped either horizontally or vertically. This will standardize an image viewing order, so that proper orientation of an image is obtained for further interpretation. Generally, bone appears as white and soft tissue as black. In image inversion, an image can be changed from negative to positive or vice-versa. That is, bone appears as black and soft tissue as white which will help to identify pathology more visible.

The purpose of image subtraction is to improve an image contrast. One can easily see anatomy or pathology easily. Sometimes misregistration occurs in subtraction images, which can be rectified by pixel shift. Radiology needs quantitative imaging with measurements. This is possible by defining *region of interest* (ROI). That ROI may have multiple pixels. The mean value of all pixels may be assigned to that ROI. It has clinical application in bone mineral study, calcified lung nodule detection, and renal stone identification, including disease characteristics.

Edge enhancement is a software by which contrast of an edge can be increased. It must satisfy two conditions, first the part should be fully exposed, secondly its SNR must be low. Otherwise, noise can be enhanced along with an edge enhancement. Smoothening is a software function by which image noise is reduced. Noise lies in the high frequency domain of the histogram. Adjusting the high frequency, noise can be eliminated. Equalization is the technique in which an underexposed region is made darker and an overexposed region is made lighter. Though this appears with lower contrast, it is useful to identify dense and lucent structures.

Recording of Digital Image

Medical digital image can be printed directly using printers from the display monitors. The printers used in radiology may be divided into nonlaser and laser types. Nonlaser includes video monitor, thermal print heads, or an inject technology. Laser printers are further divided into wet laser and dry laser category. Wet laser basically uses chemicals like darkroom film processing. In this, the film is exposed to a laser beam that modulates an image; later film is subjected to developing, fixing, and washing. This technology is now phasing out. Dry laser employs laser-induced thermal technology. A typical laser printer consists of the following parts: (1) electronic data, (2) corona wires, (3) photoreceptor drum, (4) laser and mirror, (5) ink roller, (6) paper tray, and (7) fuser unit.

During the printing, the computer sends large number of electronic data of the order of few megabytes to the printer. The electronic circuit in the printer analyses the above data and plans how it should appear correctly on the page. This electronic circuit in the printer resembles a small computer. The electronic circuit also activates a corona wire, which is a high voltage wire. It can give static electricity to anything nearby. A photoreceptor drum is kept nearby, which gains positive charge from the corona wire. Thus, the drum gains positive charge spread uniformly across its surface.

The electronic circuit also activates a laser which can draw an image of the paper onto the drum. The laser is not moving, instead the beam falls on a mirror and the mirror scans over the drum. The laser erases the positive charge in the drum and creates area of negative charge. Gradually, an image of the page is built up on the drum. The area of positive charge appears as white, whereas areas of negative charge appear as black. An ink roller touching the drum coats it with powdered ink (*toner*). The tonner is basically positively charged. When the toner and drum is in contact, the toner gives an ink to the drum, only to the area where negative charge is present. No ink is attracted to the drum area where positive charge is present. Thus, an inked page of the drum is developed.

A sheet of paper from the hopper is fed forward to the drum. As the paper moves forward, an uniform positive charge is given to the paper by another corona wire. Therefore, the positively charged paper attracts the negatively charged toner particles. Thus, an image of the drum is transferred into the paper, but the toner particles are resting lightly on the paper. The inked paper is passed on between two hot rollers, where the heat (120–140°C) and pressure permanently fix the toner particles into the paper. This makes the latent image into a permanent image. The final printout comes from the printer, still it is warm. The following paragraph will explain step-by-step function of the laser printer **(Fig. 7.18A):**

❑ Computer data of several MB reaches the printer.
❑ Printer electronic circuit plans how to correctly print an image.
❑ Printer electronic circuit activates a corona wire to give positive charge to the photoreceptor drum.
❑ The photoreceptor drum gets an uniform positive charge across its surface.
❑ Printer electronic circuit makes laser and mirror to draw the page of the image on the drum. It makes area of negative charge on the drum.
❑ The ink roller touching the photoreceptor drum coats it with tiny particles of powdered ink, wherever area of negative charge is present.
❑ A positively charged paper is fed forward to the drum. The paper attracts tonner particles only from the area of the negative charge. Thus, an image is transferred from the drum to paper.
❑ The paper is moved between two hot rollers. The heat and pressure from the rollers fuse the toner particles in the paper permanently.
❑ The final printout comes out of the printer.

The dry laser printers are basically made up of solid-state technology and not involving any optical components. They are heat-sensitive, instead of light-sensitive. It uses multiple technologies, including radiographic, thermal, mechanical, and digital process. It offers daylight loading facility. They provide printing for MRI, CT, DSA, picture archiving and communication system (PACS), computed radiography (CR) and DR systems. They offer high-resolution images with fast throughputs of multiformat multimodality printouts. A laser printer image may contain 325 pixels per inch. One can print 45–140 films per hour, depending on film size. They are highly reliable, durable and user friendly. There is no wet process in this, and no chemicals involved. Hence, the size is small, occupies lesser space.

Advantages of hard copy are; films are instantly readable, it can be prepared at any time, film is a physical record, it makes physician job easier, films are not subjected to system failure, films cannot be corrupted like computer, and serve the purpose of medicolegal cases.

Disadvantages of hard copy are, involve high cost, it is time consuming, printer is space occupying, films can be easily destroyed or lost, and film may degrade image quality with storage.

Commercial Dry Laser Printers

The commercial dry laser printers that are used in hospital setup. They are basically DICOM-native imager, facilitates network connectivity easily.

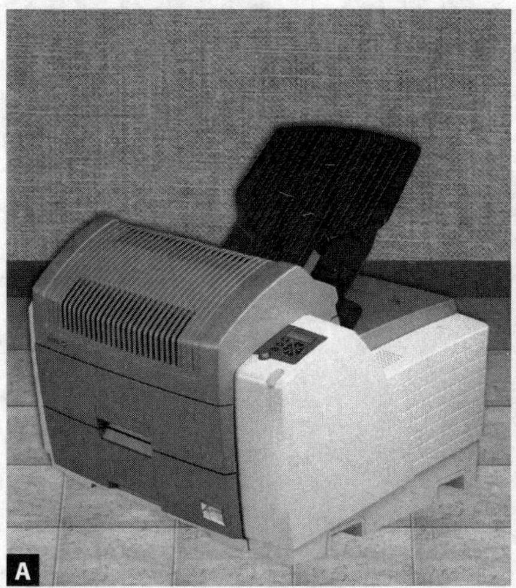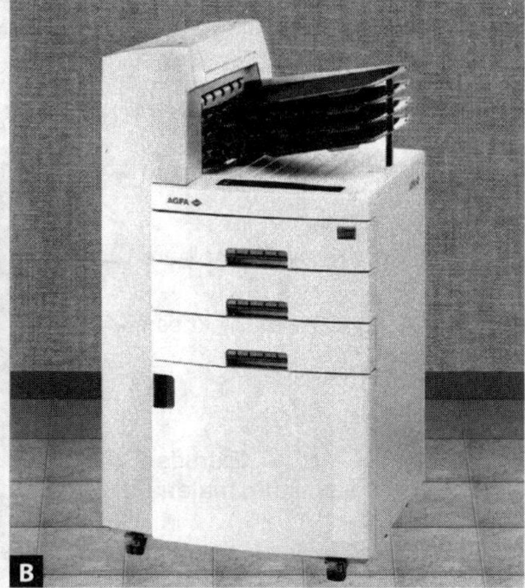

Figs. 7.18A and B: (A) Direct digital imager and (B) High-resolution digital imager. (*Courtesy:* Agfa Healthcare India Pvt Ltd)

They provide 2–5 media sizes of different image sizes. The printing time is ultrashort, e.g., 75 sheets/hr for a size of 14 × 17 inch. Thus, it can handle 11 × 14 inch (86 sheets/hr) and 8 × 10 inch (140 sheets/hr) and enhance throughput. A 10 × 12 inch-film imager may have 3070 × 3653 pixels of diagnostic area. The minimum printing resolution of 32 PPi (pixels per inch) and contrast resolution of 12 bits can be achieved.

Multiple media size direct digital imager **(Fig. 7.18B)** is also available. They have multiformat architecture, sorting function, and take printing work from different sources. Thus, an imager is capable of printing CT, MRI, DSA, digital radiography (CR and DR) and digital mammography images.

X-ray Film Viewer

X-ray films and digital image printout films are examined by using a viewing light box **(Figs. 7.19A and B).** While reading the X-ray film on an view box, magnification and an external light influences the information. Use of low-ambient light and restricting light from the surroundings of view box, will improve its performance. A typical view box consists of a light source of variable intensity. It is fitted in an Aluminum box with glass or acrylic front screen.

Initially, ordinary light bulbs/tube lights of multiple numbers are used to match the view box size. Off late light-emitting diode (LED) lamp is used, which can serve to 200,000 hours, longer than the cold cathode fluorescent (CCFL) lamp. The light intensity can be varied from 300 cd/m^2 to 4500 cd/m^2, to reduce eye's fatigue. Generally, this is achieved by ON/OFF individual switch, with feather touch dimmer. The light source should spread the light uniformly on the screen, without any dark spot. It can provide nine digital grades to adjust brightness, to view different density of X-ray films.

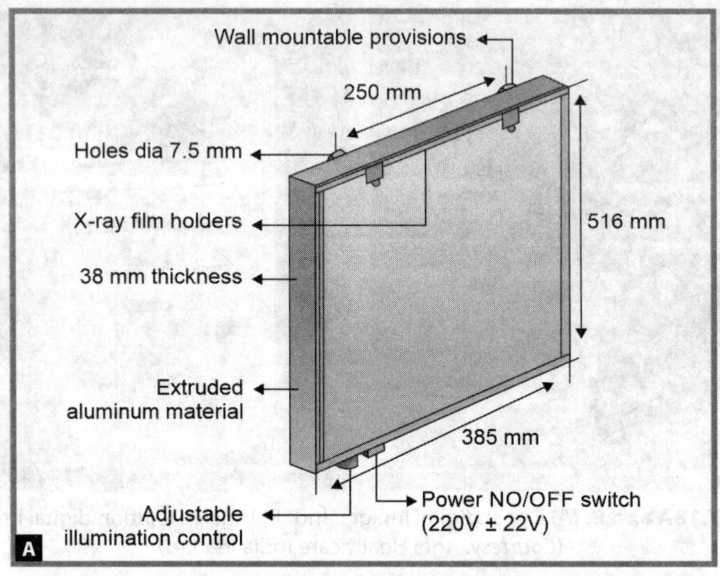

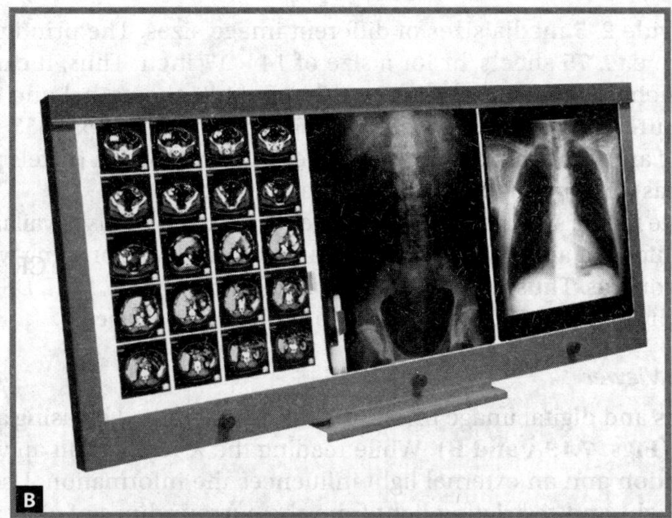

Figs. 7.19A and B: (A) View box dimensions, parts (B) X-ray film viewing.

It is fitted with an automatic film sensor. When the film is inserted, it starts working and turns off automatically, while the film is removed. In addition, it has close timer function, brightness memory function, etc. The close timer function will help to save power. When it works continuously for more than an hour, it will switch OFF automatically. The film viewer can remember the brightness; if the film is inserted again, it will show the same brightness. There is no need of brightness adjustment again. It is available in different sizes to read single or multiple or multiformat films. It has holders for X-ray films and wall mounting facility.

PICTURE ARCHIVING AND COMMUNICATION SYSTEM

Patient may undergo multiple investigations with different modalities. Multiple radiologist or physicians from different locations may need access to patient image. There is a need to maintain quality of images in such situations. Hard copy images are difficult to store and archive and its quality deteriorates over time. Hence, *picture archiving and communication system (PACS)* is used as a provision in radiology. It is a computerized way of replacing the roles of conventional films.

PACS helps transmission of images from an image acquisition location to different remote locations. It provides cost effective and easy access to images from multiple imaging tools. It is simultaneously available to different locations within the hospitals or across the globe. Basically, PACS mainly requires four components namely, (1) imaging acquisition devices, (2) communication network system, (3) display workstation, and (4) archive and server/storage. PACS integrates the following:

❑ Input from digital devices of radiological modalities, e.g., CR/DR, CT, MRI, etc.
❑ Image acquisition device
❑ Image storage device/server
❑ Transmission network
❑ Display stations/imaging workstation
❑ Camera that convers hard copy images
❑ Radiology information system or hospital information system

Radiological images and reports are transmitted digitally through PACS. It eliminates manual filing, retrieving and transport of films. DICOM (*digital imaging and communications in medicine)* is an universal format for an image storage and transfer, which is used in PACS. Imaging tools include CR/DR, cath lab, CT, ultrasound, MRI, and PET-CT, etc. The images from the modalities are sent to the quality assurance workstation, called PACS gateway **(Fig. 7.20).** It checks the patient demographics as well as attributes of the study. If the study information is correct, images are passed to the archive for storage. Then, the radiologist reviews the images through their workstations and make the final report. The workstation and an archive are a bidirectional transmission.

Storage for PACS includes online, near line and offline storage. Online storage permits an immediate access to data. It includes hard discs to store data which can be connected to resemble the function of a hard disc with large storage capacity. It is referred to as *redundant array of inexpensive discs (RAID).* Data not required for immediate access is stored in near line, namely *magnetic tapes and an optical jukebox.* Offline storage refers to *magnetic tapes and an optical disc* that are useful to long-term storage and data backup. However, an offline storage takes long time to an access data.

PACS uses web-based interfaces to use an internet or wide area network (WAN) as their way of communication, via virtual private network (VPN) or secure sockets layer (SSL). The client-side software includes *ActiveX, JavaScript, and Java Applet.* Very good backup for patient images is required,

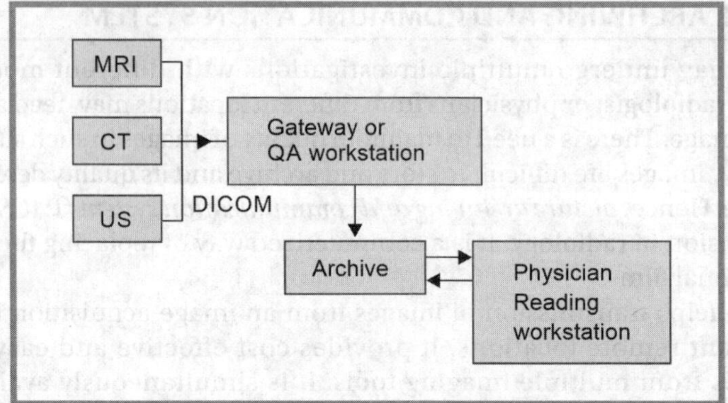

Fig. 7.20: Picture archiving and communication system, block diagram.

in case of loss of images from PACS. Hence, the images are automatically sending their copies to a separate computer for storage.

PACS finds variety of use that includes: replacing hard copy such as films, providing remote access, including distance education and teleradiology, providing electronic image integration platform with easy access to hospital information system (HIS), radiology information system (RIS), and helping radiology workflow management such as patient examinations.

PACS delivers images timely and provides an easy access to images and interpretations. It avoids traditional film-based image retrieval, distribution, and display. Benefits include an enhanced analysis and viewing, improved data management, unmatched mobility, user-friendly and streamlined workflow, etc. Limitations of PACS include high capital investment, quality of images displayed by suboptimal resolution monitors at different location, technical failure, and improper backup storage, etc. It may lead to hamper of data retravel and involves risk of massive data loss.

Teleradiology

Teleradiology (TR) is the transmission of patient images from one location to another location using PACS. The images include CR/DR, CT, ultrasound, MRI, PET-CT, etc. Main purpose is to share an image or study with other radiologists and physicians. Since, the number of radiologists is lesser than an image imaging procedure, teleradiology fill the shortage of radiologists. It helps remote diagnosis and treatment.

Teleradiology improves patient care, by allowing radiologist services, who is physically not present at that location. This is highly true in specialist such as MR radiologist or Neuroradiologist, or Periodic radiologist, etc., who are available only in urban cities. Teleradiology allows round the clock service of the specialists without interruption.

Teleradiology uses an internet, telephone, wide area network (WAN) and local area network (LAN). Specialized software is used to transmit images. Advanced technologies such as graphic processing, voice recognition, and an image compressions are also used in teleradiology.

BIBLIOGRAPHY

1. Bushberg JT, Seibert JA, Leidholdt EM Jr, Boone JM. The Essential Physics of Medical Imaging, 3rd edn, Lippincott Williams and Wilkins; 2012.
2. Compagnone G, Casadio baleni M, Pagan L, Calzolaio FL, Barozzi L, Bergamini C. Comparison of radiation doses to patients undergoing standard radiographic examinations with conventional screen–film radiography, computed radiography and direct *radiography*. The British Journal of Radiology, 79 (2006), 899–904 [accessed Oct 12, 2023].
3. Dowsett DJ, Patrick AK, Johnston RE. The Physics of Diagnostic Imaging, 2nd edn, NY; Hodder Arnold; 2006.
4. Thayalan K. Basic Radiological Physics, 2nd ed. Jaypee Brothers Medical Publishers (P) Ltd, New Delhi; 2017.
5. Thayalan K. Medical X-ray Film Processing, 2nd ed. Jaypee Brothers Medical Publishers (P) Ltd, New Delhi; 2021.
6. Xiangyu Ou, Xue Chen, Xianning Xu, Lili Xie, Xiaofeng Chen, Zhongzhu Hong, Hua Bai, Xiaowang Liu, Qiushui Chen, Lin Li and Huanghao Yang. Recent developments in X-ray imaging technology: Future and challenges. Research (Walsh DC), Science Partner Journal; 2021.

Mammography

BASIS FOR MAMMOGRAPHY

Soft tissues have similar effective atomic number and similar mass density. It is difficult to create difference in such tissue composition with conventional radiography. Hence, soft tissue radiographic techniques like mammography were attempted (1920). X-ray imaging of breast organ is called mammography which gives good subject contrast. **Solomon A** (1913), a pathologist observed microcalcifications in breast carcinoma after analyzing about 3,000 gross mastectomy specimens. **Warran S (1930)** described a stereotactic system by using double emulsion film for imaging breast with 70 kV. In 1938, **Gershen J and Cohen** published radiographic image of normal breast with age.

Robert Egan (1950) attempted to have soft tissue mammography with low kV, high mAs with direct film exposure. He used *Tungsten target, Beryllium window X-ray tube with minimum Al filtration* and metal extension cones, long source to image distance (SID) to reduce focal spot blurring and field coverage. Fine-grain industrial film was exposed to 6 seconds without grid. Its image quality was poor with little medical benefit.

Wolf and Ruzicka (1960) came with *xero mammography* techniques. It had good resolution and edge enhancement. However, it involves higher dose and poor contrast sensitivity. Single screen-film mammography succeeded xero mammography since it offered better images with lower radiation dose. Dedicated mammography units were designed by **Charles Gros and Strasbourg** in 1965. He used Molybdenum target with Molybdenum filter. *Picker, Siemens, Philips, and GE* started manufacturing such units. It becomes popular after the introduction of *Molybdenum target*, single-emulsion screen-film system (1972), and arrival of grid and automatic exposure control (1990). The mammography units undergone several modifications over a period before coming to the present status. Mammography enhances differential absorption in soft tissues. It provides high contrast between normal and cancer tissues and detects calcifications. It helps to detect breast cancer early and reduces mortality rates for women. If the disease is detected early, treatment is much more effective and curable.

Breast cancer arises in the *lining cells of the ducts and lobules in the glandular tissue.* Initially, it is in situ, then invades the surrounding breast tissue or lymph nodes or other organs of the body **(Fig. 8.1).** As on 2020, there were 2.3 million breast cancer and 685,000 death reported globally (WHO). Breast cancer is a second leading cancer in women next to lung cancer. Chances of breast cancer increases with age, one out of 7 women likely to develop breast cancer. Chances of death in women is one in 33. In early detection, the chance of 5-year survival rate is about 98%.

Role of mammography is much important to diagnose breast cancer and it is a golden standard. Radiation dose is a much concern in mammography however, it is a safe and an effective method of breast imaging today. Generally, base line mammogram is recommended for women of age >40. It is useful to compare with future mammogram images. There are two types of mammography, namely, (1) screening mammography and (2) diagnostic mammography.

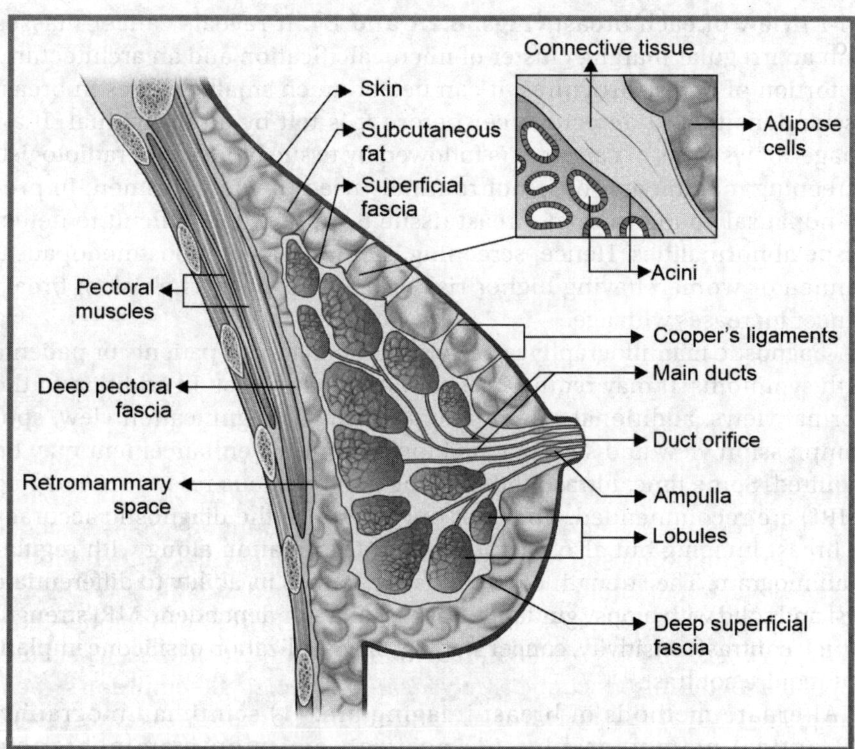

Fig. 8.1: Anatomy of human breast.

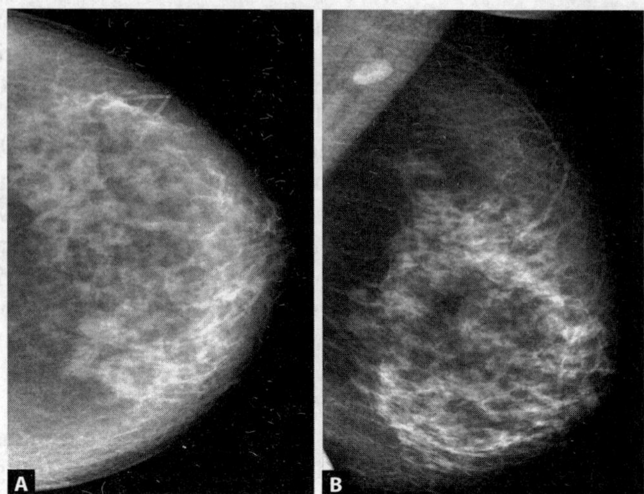

Figs. 8.2A and B: Breast mammogram: (A) Craniocaudal view; (B) Mediolateral oblique view.

Screening mammography is performed in asymptomatic patients with two views. It includes a craniocaudal (C-C) and mediolateral oblique (M-L) view of each breast **(Figs. 8.2A and B)**. It reveals cancer masses with an irregular margin, cluster of microcalcification and an architectural distortion of breast structures. It can detect much small changes in breast tissue density and detect cancer before it is felt by an individual. If an image shows signs of cancer, it is followed by tissue biopsy by a radiologist. Screening mammography is not routinely used in young women. In premenopausal young women, breast tissue is harder, it is difficult to detect tissue abnormalities. Hence, screening is emphasized in postmenopausal women or women having higher risk of breast cancer. The risk of breast cancer increases with age.

Diagnostic mammography is performed on high-risk patients or patients with symptoms. It may require 2–3 views of each breast. In addition to the normal views, additional examinations, such as magnification view, spot compression view and stereotactic biopsy, contrast enhancement may be required. Some time, ultrasound imaging and magnetic resonance imaging (MRI) are recommended. They not only enhance the diagnostic accuracy of breast imaging but also useful for an interpretation along with regular mammogram. The strength of an ultrasonogram is its ability to differentiate cyst and solid with biopsy guidance but it is operator dependent. MRI strength is high contrast sensitivity, cancer staging, an visualization of silicone implant but require contrast.

Alternate methods of breast imaging are: (1) scintimammography, (2) optical mammography, (3) positron emission mammography, (4) thermography, and (5) electrical impedance scanning.

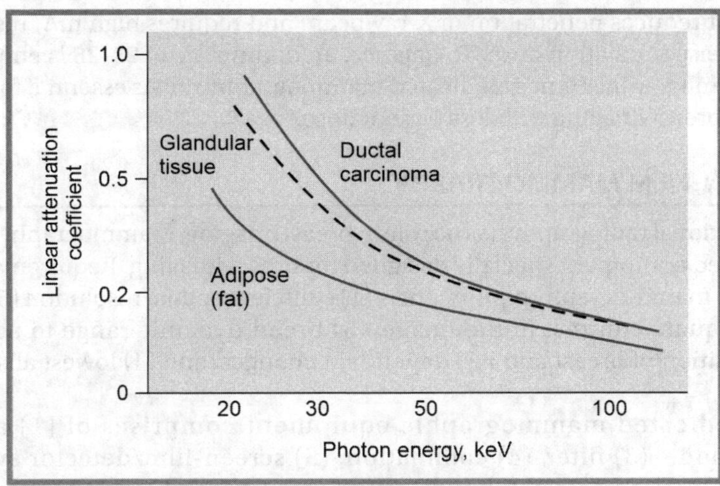

Fig. 8.3: Variation of attenuation coefficient of breast tissues at low photon energy.

Breast Anatomy

The breast consists of three tissues, namely, *fibrous tissue, glandular tissue, and an adipose (fat) tissue*. In premenopausal women, the fibrous and glandular tissues are characterized with ducts, glands and connective tissues that are surrounded by fat layer. Postmenopausal breast appears with degeneration of fibro glandular tissue and an increase of adipose tissue. In addition, young age breast is dense and hard to image due to glandular tissue, but older age breast is fattier and easier to image.

The most sensitive tissue to radiation is glandular tissue. Mammography radiation dose is enough to induce cancer in glandular tissue. Hence, mammogram is not recommended for women of <40 age. Even in older patients, the mammogram frequency and interval are restricted. Adipose tissue requires lesser radiation exposure. Normal ductal and connective tissues appear distorted in malignant breast. Majority of breast cancer is due to ductal tissue and related microcalcification, which appear as small grains of varying sizes (μm). The incidence of breast cancer is higher in an upper lateral quadrant of the breast.

The mass density and atomic number of the breast components are similar. It is necessary to image blood vessels, ducts, and microcalcifications as small as <μm. Hence, general radiography with 70–100 kV is not useful in breast imaging. *Compton interaction* dominates in soft tissue and differential absorption is much minimal **(Fig. 8.3).** Hence, low kV must be used to visualize above structures (soft tissues). Low kV radiation maximizes *photoelectric effect*, increases differential absorption, and differentiates attenuation coefficient of various breast tissues. At low X-ray energy, photoelectric absorption dominates over Compton scattering. It is known that the absorption differences in an atomic number is proportional to Z^3 for photoelectric effect. Though low kV is useful, it reduces penetration of X-ray beam and requires high mA, resulting an increased radiation dose. To balance, an optimal kV of 23–28 is employed in mammography. Hence, dedicated mammography unit is essential for good quality breast imaging with less patient dose.

SCREEN-FILM MAMMOGRAPHY

Conventional radiography has no role in breast imaging. Mammography needs dedicated equipment specially designed for breast imaging. Requirements of an ideal mammography equipment is (1) sufficient spatial resolution (50μm), (2) adequate contrast in the image, (3) broad dynamic range to address composition of breast and age dependent changes, and (4) lowest absorbed dose.

A dedicated mammographic equipment comprises of (1) anode (2) cathode, (3) filter, (4) collimation, (5) screen-film/detector system, (6) grid, (7) compression paddle, (8) X-ray generator, and (9) automatic exposure control **(Figs. 8.4A and B).** The equipment should provide range of energies to balance radiation dose and image quality. The X-ray spectrum is decided by the target, filter, and tube voltage. For screen-film mammography 18 and 23 keV energy is sufficient, whereas digital mammography demands higher energies.

Mammography employs small focal spots, low kV technique, low grid ratio, and special single side screen-film system. It is basically a 2D imaging system. The control console is provided with Lead glass protection which eliminates requirement of large room space. Newer machines are provided with an automatic selection of target/filter combination to have lowest breast dose to an individual patient, e.g., Mo/Mo or Mo/Rh or Rh/Rh or W/Rh. Isocentric and motorized swivel movements are provided which enables precise and easy positioning of breast. The differences between the conventional and mammography X-ray tubes is given in **Table 8.1**.

Anode

X-ray tube is a rotating anode type, the anode is mounted on a *Molybdenum stem*, which is attached to a *bearing* with rotor and *stator assembly*. Anode angles vary from 16° to 0° with a source to image distance of 65 cm. In addition to an anode tilt, tube tilt is also incorporated to have an adequate anterior field size. Hence, the term *effective anode angle* is used. It is defined as anode angle relative to the horizontal tube mount. It includes an anode angle + physical tube tilt. The effective anode angle is about 22°–24°, for a field coverage of 24 cm × 30 cm area. This can be achieved either by 0° anode angle and 24° tube tilt or 16° anode angle and 6° tube tilt. The anode is often grounded with zero potential whereas the cathode is given higher negative potential.

Target

Mammography X-ray tubes are designed with Tungsten (W, Z = 74) in earlier days. Tungsten target X-ray tube was operated under 30 kV with 0.5 mm

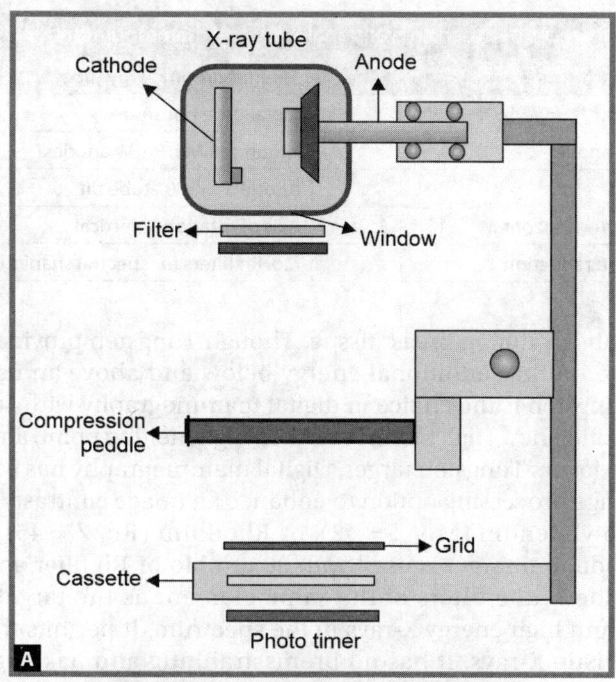

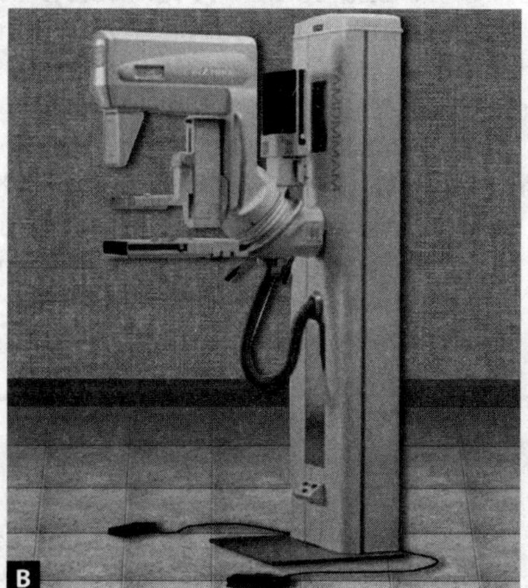

Figs. 8.4A and B: Mammography X-ray equipment: (A) Anatomy of mammography machine; (B) Commercial mammogram unit.
(*Courtesy:* M/s Siemens Healthineers)

Al filter. It gave bremsstrahlung, and 12 keV, L-shell characteristic X-rays. Bremsstrahlung X-ray is useful for mammogram and L characteristic X-ray have too low penetration for an image formation and gives only patient radiation dose. The useful energy range for mammogram is 17–24 keV, to have

Table 8.1: Differences between conventional X-ray and mammography X-ray tubes.

Conventional X-ray tube	Mammography X-ray tube
Glass envelope	Metal tube housing
Tungsten (W) anode	Grounded Mo, Rh, W anodes
Anode angle, 7°–16°	Anode angle, 0°-tube tilt 26°
Axis of rotation—horizontal	Axis of rotation—vertical
Al filter for dose reduction	Mo, Rh filters for spectral shaping

differential absorption in breast tissue. Though Tungsten provides sufficient energy range but has additional energy below and above an useful range. However, Tungsten is the choice in digital mammography with an increased production efficiency. High atomic number, high melting point, and improved heat loading favors Tungsten target. Digital mammography has wide latitude and post image processing option to enhance an image contrast.

Later, Molybdenum (Mo, Z = 42), or Rhodium (Rh, Z = 45) targets are used. Molybdenum target is used with 30 μm Mo or Rh filter and operated at 26 kV. Added tube filters of the same element as the target is used to reduce low and high energy X-rays in the spectrum. It permits transmission of characteristic X-rays. It has no bremsstrahlung and has strong K-shell characteristic X-rays of 17 and 19 keV **(Fig. 8.5A).** This energy range is more suitable for mammography. The spectral variation between Tungsten (Z = 74) and Molybdenum (Z = 42) is due to their atomic number which make the spectrum different.

Rhodium target is operated at 28 kV, filtered with Rhodium (25 μm) gives similar spectrum of Molybdenum and gives K-shell characteristic X-rays of energy 20.2 keV and 22.7 keV **(Fig. 8.5B).** Since the atomic number of Rhodium is slightly higher, its bremsstrahlung spectrum and k-edge are slightly higher than that of Molybdenum.

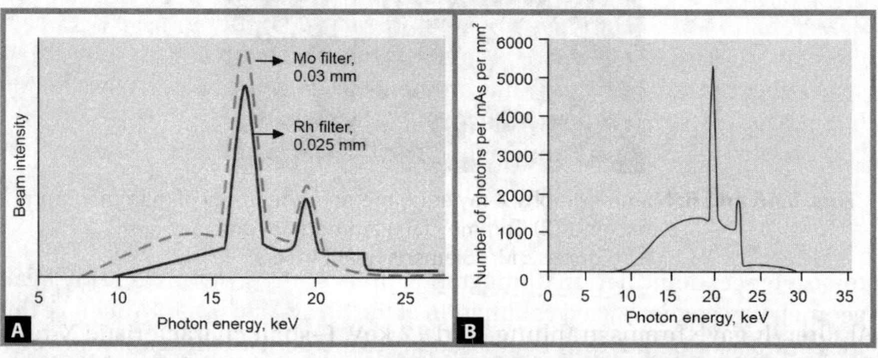

Figs. 8.5A and B: (A) X-ray spectrum of Mo target with Mo and Rh filters with applied voltage of 30 kV; (B) X-ray spectrum of Rh target with Rh filter at 30 kV. (*Courtesy:* Radiology key)

Table 8.2: Target/Filter material properties used in mammography X-ray tube.

Properties	Molybdenum (Mo)	Rhodium (Rh)	Tungsten (W)
Atomic number, Z	42	45	74
Physical density, g/cm³	10.2	12.4	19.3
K_α X-ray energy, keV	17.5	20.2	59.3
K_β X-ray energy, keV	19.6	22.7	67.2
K-edge, KeV	20	23.2	69.5
Melting point, °C	2620	1966	3410

(*Courtesy:* Radiology key)

Molybdenum and Rhodium characteristic X-rays arise from K-shell, and the energies lie in the useful range of mammography. Their bremsstrahlung spectrum is smaller than that of Tungsten. Hence, most of the X-ray tubes are designed with Mo target with Mo filter or Mo target with Rh filter or Rh target with Rh filter. Somes times Tungsten anode is used with a Silver or Rhodium filter for greater penetration. Some other systems use Molybdenum anode with Aluminum filter for an increased penetration which is needed for denser breasts. The properties of various target materials used in mammography is given in **Table 8.2.**

Focal Spot

Focal spot size is very critical in mammography, where high spatial resolution is required. Filament is positioned within a focusing cup, which offer two focal spot sizes, namely, 0.3–0.4 mm and 0.1–0.15 mm, respectively. Smaller focal spot is required to reduce blurring and have magnification mammography. Focal spot size depends on nature of use, SID, and position of the field. Focal spot size of 0.3–0.4 mm is used in contact imaging whereas 0.1–0.15 mm is used in magnification mammography. Machines with <65 cm SID uses 0.3 mm whereas > 66 cm uses 0.4 mm focal spot.

The filament types are either *double wound filament* to increase electron density or *flat ribbon filament* to give more focused uniform beam or circular filament to create *camel hump profile* (two focal spots). Focal spot size can be selected either by a negative bias on the cathode or by having two separate filaments with two focal spots. Magnification mammography uses lower focal spot size, longer exposure time with reduced tube current, e.g., Mo target uses 25 mA with a small focal spot. It also reduces geometric blurring and help an easy visualization of microcalcifications.

Full field mammography gives high exposure to chest wall area and torso. Hence, dedicated mammography units employ half-field X-ray beam geometry by having a fixed collimation at the X-ray tube level. To achieve this, the central axis of the X-ray beam is made to incident on the chest wall's edge side of the detector **(Fig. 8.6).** It is also perpendicular to the plane of an image detector. This will make the patient positioning easy and take care of the *heel effect*. However, full field is used in digital mammography units.

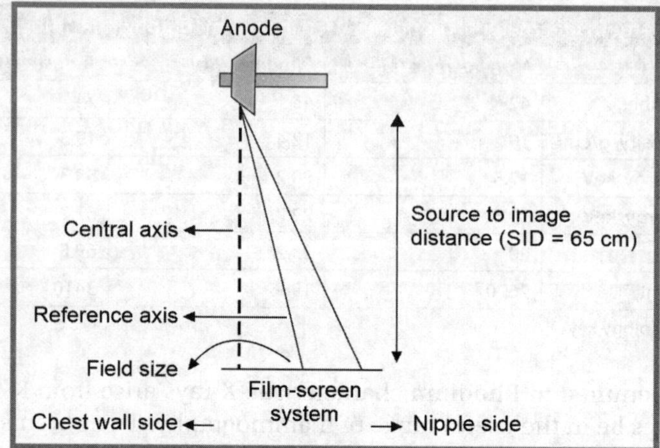

Fig. 8.6: Collimation of X-ray beam at 65 cm SID, so that central beam incident on the chest wall side.

A reference axis is one which bisects the X-ray field along an anterior chest wall–nipple direction. Nominal focal spot is measured at the reference axis. Reference angle is the sum of the target angle and tube tilt. The focal spot size is not constant, and it decreases from cathode to an anode side. It is smaller at the reference axis compared to chest wall position. Hence, sharper images are obtained at the anode side of the field, towards nipple. High resolution *par phantom* having 20 lp/mm is used to measure focal spot size.

Heel Effect

Heel effect causes the X-ray intensity higher at cathode side, and lower at an anode side. Target's self-absorption reduces the X-ray intensity relative to cathode side and requires >20° target angle for full field coverage. The shape of the breast requires higher intensity of radiation near chest wall side, to create an uniform exposure to screen-film system. However, breast compression provides an uniform thickness of breast and near an uniform exposure to screen-film system. To achieve better uniformity, the cathode is positioned towards chest wall and anode is towards the nipple side. This will permit easy positioning of patient since the anode side is bulky and is away from patient. This will also increase an intensity of radiation near the chest wall, where greater penetration is needed.

However, an effective focal spot size is higher at the chest wall side, which reduces spatial resolution. It is due to an increased focal spot blur by large focal spot size at the cathode side of the tube. Hence, mammography systems use tilted X-ray tubes with long SID of 60–80 cm, to overcome the above problem. Thus, the effective focal spot is made smaller to image the tissue near the chest wall. Since, the patient head is always closer to X-ray tube housing, it is convenient to the patients. Other issue is variation of focal spot size over the detector. It is minimized by using long SID and an optimal breast compression.

Filter

Thin *Beryllium* (Z = 4, thickness 0.5–1 mm) window or *borosilicate glass* window is used as tube port window. It acts as an inherent filter of the order of 0.1 mm Al equivalent and permits all low energy photons including the bremsstrahlung energy of < 5 keV. In addition, added filters are used to remove unwanted high energy bremsstrahlung X-rays. It improves energy distribution by selective absorption of lowest and highest energy X-rays. However, the total beam filtration should not be lesser than 0.5 mm Al equivalent. Generally, filter material is same as target material. This will allow its K-characteristic X-rays to reach the breast and suppress low and high energy bremsstrahlung X-rays. These filters remove the bremsstrahlung photons above the K-edge energy.

Mo produces useful K-characteristic X-rays of 17.5 and 19.6 keV with Mo filter. Rh target gives K characteristic X-rays of 20.2 and 22.7 keV with Rh filters. Hence, material having K-absorption of edge energies at 20 and 27 keV are suitable for filters in mammography. Since, Mo, Rh and Silver (Ag) satisfy, they are used as filters in mammography.

Molybdenum target requires 0.03 mm thick Mo filter or 0.025 mm thick Rh filter. Mo target with Mo filter is commonly used for thin fatty breast (up to 4 cm) with 24–26 kV whereas Mo target and Rh filter is used for glandular breast up to 5–7 cm with 27–31 kV. If breast thickness is >7 cm, Rh target with Rh filter is recommended. The unfiltered beam of Molybdenum has both dominant characteristic X-rays and substantial bremsstrahlung X-rays. Use of Mo filter has K absorption edge at the K-characteristic X-ray energy. It promotes the dominant characteristic X-rays with suppressed bremsstrahlung spectrum.

Rh target tube uses Rhodium filters of 0.025 mm thickness. It gives high quality X-rays with higher penetration. This combination is suitable for thicker and dense breast imaging. The half value layer of the beam is very low. Mo filter should not be used with Rh target X-ray tube. It attenuates the K characteristic X-rays since their energies are above the K edge absorption energy of Mo.

Tungsten target is used in digital mammography due to its X-ray production efficiency and high tube loading. However, its unfiltered spectrum consists of L-characteristics X-rays of 8–12 keV which is unwanted. For a Tungsten target X-ray tube, 0.05 mm thick Rh or 0.05 mm thick Ag or 0.7 mm Al can be used. It attenuates the unwanted L-characteristic X-rays. In *tomosynthesis, Al filter* is used since it involves reconstruction process.

Generally, stationary anode tube is used in mammography. Nowadays, *bi-angle and double track anode* X-ray tubes are used with rotating anode X-ray tubes. One track is meant for Mo and other is for Rh. Such tubes have both small and large filaments for each track, totaling four focal spots. In general, thick, dense breast is best imaged with Rh/Rh combination, whereas thin, fatty breast is best imaged with Mo/Mo combination.

Collimation

Metal apertures or variable shutters are used to collimate the X-ray beam. It matches the cassette sizes of 18 cm × 24 cm or 24 cm × 30 cm. Nowadays, an automatic collimation system are used to sense the cassette size. Collimator light and mirror assembly uses low attenuation mirror to reflect the light. The light field should match the radiation field within 2% of SID. The useful X-ray beam must extend to the chest wall edge of the cassette without field cutoff as shown in **Figure 8.6**. This can be achieved by placing the central axis over the chest wall at the cassette edge. The reference axis that bisects the field, specify the field size. Since, the focal spot varies along cathode-anode direction, it is smaller at the reference axis than at central axis. The nominal focal spot is specified at the reference axis.

The half value layer (HVL) of the mammographic beam is about 0.3–0.4 mm Al. It varies with machine and HVL of the breast tissue depends on its composition. This depends upon kV range and type of target, filter material and thickness used in the X-ray tube. HVL is measured with compression paddle by using pure Al sheets and it increases with an increase of kV. HVL value of the X-ray beam for various target combination under same compression peddle are as follows:

❑ Mo target, 0.03 mm Mo filter 26 kV: 0.30 mm Al
❑ Mo target, 0.025 mm Rh filter at 26 kV: 0.35 mm Al
❑ W target, 0.05 mm Rh filter, 26 kV: 0.51 mm Al

X-ray Generator

A generator modulates, regulates, and delivers an electrical energy required for mammography X-ray unit. It should support cathode-heating current, tube current, anode drive, and automatic exposure control. It has a control unit, power unit, an anode control unit, an energy storage unit and tank.

The operating voltage ranges from 25–30 kV with tube current of 80–100 mAs. The exposure times are about 1–4 sec. The tube is operated with less than 35 kV, within the space charge effect. Hence, there is no linear relation between filament current and tube current. Feedback circuit is used to adjust the filament current as a function of kV, to deliver a tube current. Three-phase or high frequency generators are used to minimize voltage fluctuation and reduce exposure time. *Photo timers and automatic exposure control (AEC) systems* are used to operate correctly at low energies.

Nowadays high frequency generator is used in mammography machines which was introduced in 1984 by **Lorad**. High frequency generator works from a single-phase supply and provides rectified smoothed DC voltage supply. For example, a 60 Hz is rectified, smoothed, chopped to a frequency of 6 kHz or higher. The ripple factor of about 1% that provides constant voltage supply to the X-ray tube. It provides superior quality of kV, close to a constant voltage. It gives an improved image quality with less patient dose. It also provides an exceptional exposure reproducibility, that is essential for consistent image quality. It is smaller in size due to higher efficiency with good reproducibility, less expensive, and capable of providing up to 600 mAs at 25–35 kV range.

Compression Peddle

Breast compression is required in all mammography examinations, to get good quality images. Compression also ensures that tissues near the chest wall are not underexposed and tissues near the nipple are not overexposed. **Leborgne R** (1949), a radiologist first used breast compression and becomes a popular technique in 1970. Breast compression improves contrast and conspicuity. Two types of compression are there, namely (1) area compression and (2) spot compression.

All mammography units are provided with an area compression device that is parallel to receptor surface **(Fig. 8.7A).** The compression paddle (*Lexan plate of polycarbonate*) is a radiotranslucent plate of 0.3 cm thick attached to a mechanical assembly. It has flat and parallel geometry to the breast support table with deflection <1 cm. It should match the cassette size of 18 cm × 24 cm or 24 cm × 30 cm. It can be operated by radiographer's foot from either side of the patient. Compression gives a force of 10–20 Newton (N) that spreads the breast tissue out. Nowadays pressure can be measured directly instead of force which can be displayed digitally.

Spot compression paddle **(Fig. 8.7B)** gives better compression over a small area (about 5 cm diameter), is also used to provide compression in a particular region of interest in the breast. It is very useful to reduce thickness locally, which needs further examination. It will eliminate super imposed anatomy by spreading the tissue further. This makes it easier to detect any pathologic conditions. The optimum degree of compression is unknown; sometimes over compression may lead to patient discomfort.

Compression peddle can slow down its speed after its initial contact with breast. Then adjust the speed according to compression resistance. It compresses only as long as the breast is soft and pliable. It stops at a point of an optimal compression for maximum image quality. Overall, breast compression provides an improved image quality that helps to detect small, low contrast lesions and high contrast microcalcifications. It also improves spatial resolution and contrast resolution and reduces patient radiation dose. Breast compression have the following advantages:

- ❑ It reduces breast thickness, lowers the radiation dose and spread the breast tissue apart.
- ❑ Reduces superimposition of tissues: Overlapping or superimposition of anatomy is spread out the tissue, e.g., separates glandular tissue.
- ❑ Produces more uniform thickness: reduce the dynamic range of exposures.
- ❑ Reduces motion and geometric unsharpness.
- ❑ Reduces scatter and beam hardening—contrast resolution is improved.
- ❑ Reduces magnification: since breast is closer to the receptor, minimizes magnification and reduces focal spot blurring with lesser radiation dose to the breast.

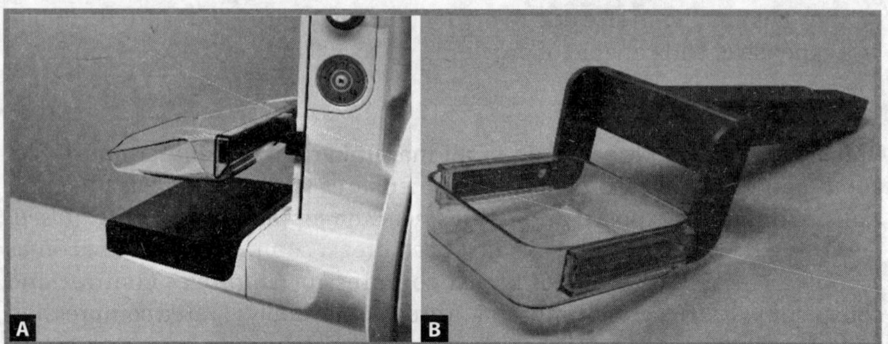

Figs. 8.7A and B: Compression peddle: (A) Whole breast compression peddle;
(B) Spot compression peddle.
(*Courtesy:* Siemens Healthineers)

Compressed breast requires only low kV thereby improving subject contrast to visualize subtle differences in tissue. It offers an uniform attenuation over an image, thereby reducing exposure range. Since, it also immobilizes the breast, minimizes motion related blur, and reduces exposure times. Overall, it offers an improved resolution or clarity of an image.

Grid

Scattered radiation is an important factor that reduces contrast in mammography. Scatter increases with breast thickness, breast area and independent of kV. Scatter can be reduced by a grid, or air gap technique with breast compression. It reduces the ratio of scattered to transmitted radiation that reaches the receptor. Hence, special grids are made for mammography, and are placed between the breast and cassette. Moving grid was first introduced by *Philips* (1978), followed by fine-line stationary grid by ***Leibel-Flarsheim*** (1984).

Generally, moving grids with grid ratio 4:1, focused to the SID is used to improve an image contrast. Grid moves during exposure to blur image of the grid septa. Its motion must be uniform and sufficient amplitude, to avoid nonuniformities in an image. Focused linear grid with ratio 5:1, of frequency >30 lines/cm can also be used. *Aluminum, wood, paper, or Carbon fiber* are used as an interface material for grid. Moving grids have line densities of about 30–60 lines per cm, whereas stationary grid have about 80 lines per cm. Currently, high transmission *cellular grid (HTC)* is employed. It is basically crossed grid with grid ratio of 3.8:1, which reduces radiation in two directions. *Copper and Air* are used as grid strips and an inter space material with 15 cells /cm density.

Use of grid decreases scatter but increases patient dose up to 2–3 times. Generally, grid controls scatter to primary ratio which depends on field diameter and breast thickness. The use of grid reduces scatter and improves contrast to about 40%. However, compared to dose, the improvement of contrast is significant. In an air gap technique, the breast is positioned away from the cassette and closer to the X-ray tube. This will also reduce scatter effectively and reduce patient radiation dose. However, the patient is closer to the focal spot and facing higher X-ray output, which contributes radiation dose to the breast.

Automatic Exposure Control

Automatic exposure control (AEC) is a radiographic density control device which terminates an exposure if a predetermined radiation quantity has been reached. It can control kV, mA, and an exposure time. Its aim is to produce high quality radiographic images consistently with minimal technical factors. It is provided with a backup timer. AEC employs photo timers to measure the X-ray intensity and quality **(Fig. 8.8).** It is like an automatic brightness control (ABC) in fluoroscopy.

Usually, AEC sensor is kept closer to the screen-film system, underneath the cassette to avoid shadow on an image. It minimizes object to image distance (OID), thereby improving spatial resolution. It sense the amount of radiation in front of the receptor and adjust dose or dose rate to the patient so that enough photons reaches the receptor. Sensor terminates an exposure when predetermined amount of radiation is received. The location of sensor is adjustable. AEC is microprocessor controlled, it has correction for reciprocity failure of the film, and address breast thickness and its composition.

The typical radiation exposure is about 5–10 mR at the detector level and vary based on sensor position. It is better to locate the sensor under densest tissue below the detector. AEC modes of operation includes (1) auto time, (2) auto kV, and (3) fully automatic. In the former, kV, target/filter is selected by the radiographer. In an auto time, kV is chosen based on breast thickness. In fully automatic, kV, and target/filter is chosen by the machine.

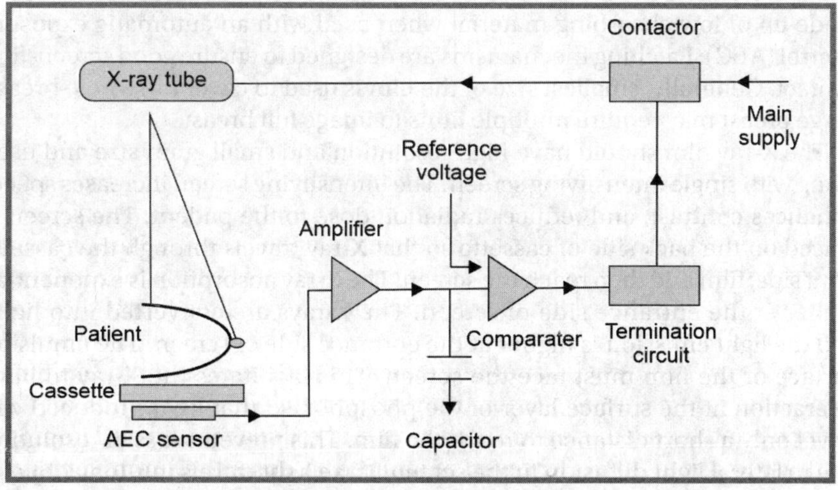

Fig. 8.8: Automatic exposure control principle in mammography.

There are two types of AEC available, namely, (1) ionization chamber type and (2) solid state diode type and the former is commonly used. Each type will have single or multiple detectors along the chest wall-nipple axis. The detectors are filtered differentially to assess the beam quality. It will also assess the level of compression and type target/filter combination that is employed. AEC must be an accurate and reproducible with lesser radiation dose. It should hold an optical density within 0.1 OD, when the voltage is varied from 23–32 kV, for a breast thickness of 2–8 cm, regardless of compression. The disadvantage of AEC is that it is prone to an operator error like misposition of an anatomy and improper detector selection. Radiographers shall be aware of sensor selection, suitable kV and mA selection, density control adjustment and patient positioning.

Screen-Film System

Initially, nonscreen industrial film is used to record breast images in 1960 with manual processing time of 5 minutes and an entrance skin dose of 3–10 R. Later, xeroradiography used blue powder with a skin entrance dose of 2–4 R. In 1972, low dose screen-film, with *Calcium tungstate* screen was used which reduced the radiation to 1–1.5 R. It is replaced by rare earth screen *(Gadolinium oxysulfide)* cassette with significant reduction of dose. The cassette, screens and films are specially made for mammography. Single sided emulsion film with single back screen is enclosed in a light-proof cassette **(Fig. 8.9).** This is to avoid light cross over. This screen-film system gives very low blurring and good visibility of microcalcifications. It is also capable of detecting small differences at a low dose. Cubic grain emulsion is used instead of tabular grain. It increases the contrast in the toe region of the characteristic curve, which is useful for mammography.

The cassette is made up *Carbon fiber*, to have low attenuation (low Z) and are available in 18 cm × 24 cm and 24 cm × 30 cm sizes. Its back side is made up of low absorbing material when used with an automatic exposure control (AEC). Latching mechanisms are designed to ensure good screen-film contact. Generally, smallest size of the film is used to cover the whole breast. Large breast may require multiple films to image full breast.

The X-ray film should have high resolution and small grain size and used along with single intensifying screen. The intensifying screen increases speed, enhances contrast, and reduces radiation dose to the patient. The screen is placed on the back side of cassette so that X-ray travels through the cassette front side, film and then reach the screen. The X-ray absorption is exponential, higher at the entrance side of screen. The X-rays are converted into light, and the light emission is higher at the entrance side of screen. The emulsion surface of the film must face the screen. This facilitates the X-ray to have interaction at the surface layer of the phosphor, so that light produced will travel only a short distance to reach the film. This prevents loss of resolution due to lateral light diffusion in the screen. If the light travels in a long oblique path, it is absorbed by the dye coated in the phosphor. It ensures sharper

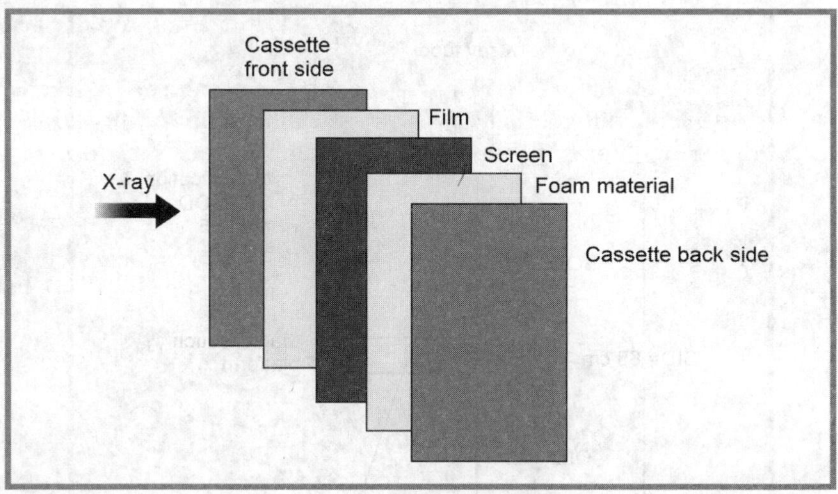

Fig. 8.9: Mammography cassette and screen-film placement: Single emulsion film with single side screen.

image. If the screen is placed between the patient and film, then an excess screen blur occurs that will reduce spatial resolution.

Gadolinium oxysulfide activated with terbium (Gd_2O_2S: Tb) is used as screen phosphor, since it emits green light to match the green sensitive film. It has main emission at 545 nm to match the film spectral sensitivity. It is dense and have good conversion efficiency. Its X-ray absorption efficiency is 40–60% with a conversion efficiency of 15%. Mammography films have low film latitude, higher resolution and higher contrast compared to conventional films. The contrast displayed may be inadequate due to limited latitude. Fixed pattern of noise due to granularity of the screen-film emulsion, can impair detectability of microcalcifications. The speed of the screen-film systems in mammography ranges from 100–150. It can give satisfactory images with a resolution about 15 lp/mm (MTF of 10%) for a given radiation dose of 15 mR.

Screen-film system requires film processing with a dark room or an automatic film processor which involves the steps; developing, fixing, washing, and drying. Temperature, time, and rate of replacement are important parameters. Normal film processing can be used but the quality of an image may not be satisfactory. Hence, dedicated film processor is required for mammography. However, it requires strict quality control to ensure an optimum processing. Film not only detects an image but also store and display an image.

Magnification Mammography

Magnification mammography is done after an initial mammogram. It can be done on magnification mode to improve visualization of mass margins and fine calcifications number and its extents. The prime aim is to magnify the breast or a specific area of breast tissue to better evaluate a previously an unclear abnormality. It produces twice the size of the normal image.

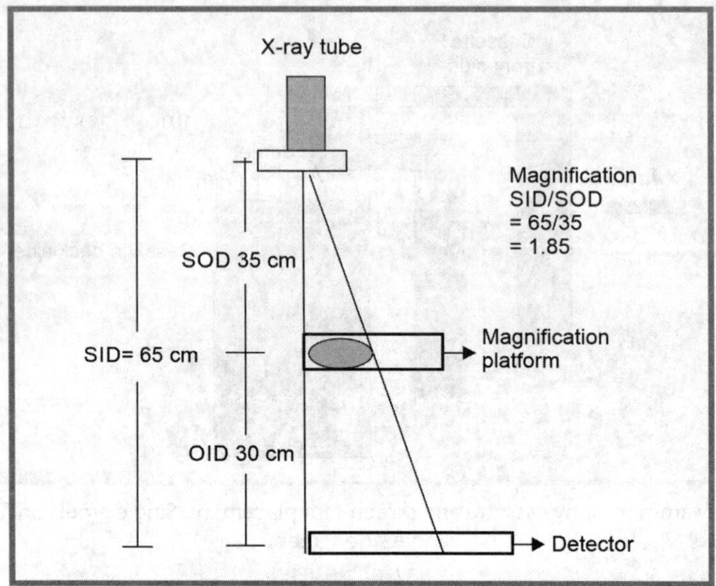

Fig. 8.10: Magnification mammography geometric setup.

The purpose of magnification mammography is to examine in depth a small, *suspicious lesions or microcalcifications* seen in the normal mammogram. In this mode, the breast support platform is raised and kept midway between the focus and cassette **(Fig. 8.10).** The spatial resolution in magnification mammography is limited by focal spot size. Examination is done with smaller focal spot (0.1 mm) with compression paddle and without the use of grid. As the breast is closer to the X-ray tube, dose to the breast is higher. Anti-scatter grid is not used since there is an air gap between an object and screen-film which reduces scatter. A magnification of about 1.5–2 can be achieved.

Magnification has lot of advantages that include, increased resolution of film, reduction of noise, reduction of scattered radiation and reduction rate of biopsy procedure. Scatter radiation is mainly reduced because of the air gap between the cassette and the magnification stand. It also has disadvantages, which include, geometric blurring, poor spatial resolution on the cathode side due to bigger focal spot size, and increased patient dose.

Therefore, small focal spot should be used to reduce geometric blurring. Use of small focal spot may limit the current to 25 mA and warrant higher exposure times. Longer exposure time causes not only motion unsharpness and an additional radiation dose to the patient. Hence, screen-film systems of higher speed are recommended in magnification mode. This procedure is used only at special circumstances.

Viewing Conditions

Mammography X-ray film, analog and digital printout films are exposed to high optical densities; hence, their viewing conditions should be an optimal.

Magnification and an external light may influence the viewing condition. Use of low-ambient light and restricting light from the surroundings of view box will improve its performance. Generally, X-ray film view boxes are made with source of variable intensity which is fitted in an Aluminum box with glass or acrylic front screen.

Nowadays light emitting diode (LED) lamps are used as source of light. Its light intensity can be varied from 300–4500 cd/m^2, to reduce eye fatigue. It can be achieved by an ON/OFF individual switch, with feather touch dimmer. Light source should spread the light uniformly on the front screen without any dark spot. It should be fitted with an automatic film sensor. It should provide 9 digital grades to adjust brightness.

Mammography view boxes should have a minimum luminance of 3000 cd per m^2. This is two times higher than the view boxes used in general radiography. Ambient light intensity should be < 20 lux. High intensity spotlight should be available. Masking is essential to preserve visibility of low contrast objects. It clears portion of a film and an area of view box which improves an image contrast. Use of magnifying glass may help to visualize fine details including microcalcifications. Hence, conventional radiography view boxes should not be used in mammography.

DIGITAL MAMMOGRAPHY

Screen-film mammography (SFM) has been used since 1950. However, up to 20–30% of malignancies were missed in SFM mammography. One of the drawbacks of screen-film mammography is its contrast resolution. Breast has tissues of contrasting density. Glandular tissue often interspersed with fat. Women with dense breast have 4–6 times higher risk for breast cancer compared to women with little or no glandular tissue. The sensitivity of SFM mammogram is generally limited, there is a reduction of 62.9% sensitivity in dense breast, compared to 87.0% in breast with fatty involution. Hence, digital mammography (DM) was introduced in breast for better imaging. Instead of screen-film systems, digital detector is used in this mammography.

Digital mammography performs image acquisition, display, and storage separately to have an individual optimization. Acquisition is done with low noise detectors with wide dynamic range. Once the image is stored digitally, it can be displayed with contrast that is independent of detector properties, and an useful image processing techniques might be applied before an image display.

Digital system uses full field of X-rays and hence often called *full field digital mammography (FFDM)*. FFDM employs W/Rh target combination and it has better signal to noise ratio than screen-film mammography. Silver and Aluminum filters can also be employed in Tungsten target **(Fig. 8.11)**. Since, it gives an instantaneous image, it saves time and cost. Generally, there are two ways of detection in digital mammography namely, (1) area detector, and (2) scanning detector. The former acquires entire image simultaneously and it is a fast acquisition. In the later, an image is obtained by scanning the

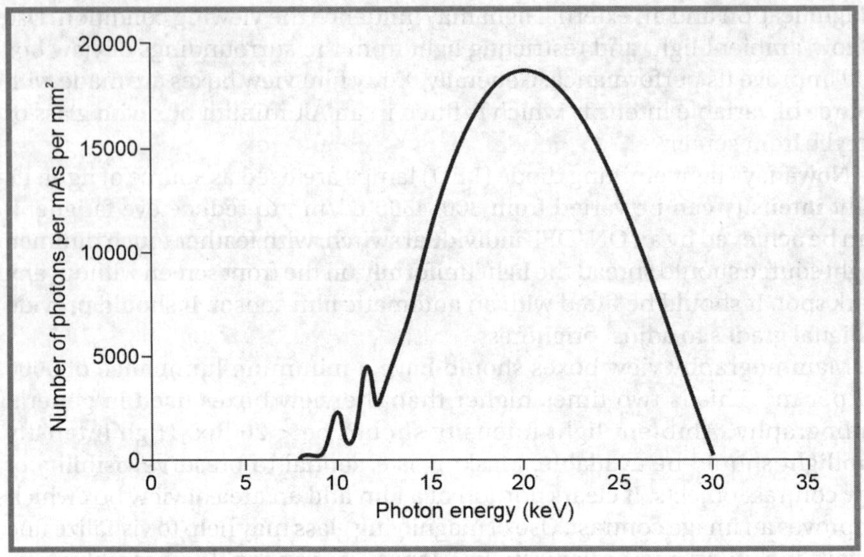

Fig. 8.11: X-ray spectrum of Tungsten target with Al filter, operated at 30 kV. (*Courtesy:* Radiology key)

X-ray beam and detector across the breast. It uses simple detectors, takes longer time with an intrinsic scatter reduction.

In area detectors, X-rays are an indirectly or directly converted into digital signal. It has large dynamic range with spatial resolution of 300 μm. It can be fed to a computer aided detection system for interpretation. The detector should have the following characteristics:

❑ Efficient absorption of an incident radiation
❑ Linear or logarithmic response over a wide range of radiation intensity
❑ Low intrinsic noise and no fixed pattern of noise, to limit quantum noise
❑ Limiting spatial resolution is 5–10 cycles/mm
❑ Field size of 18 cm × 24 cm and 24 cm × 30 cm
❑ Image immediately adjacent to chest wall

Indirect Capture

In an indirect capture, X-rays incident on a scintillator (CsI:Tl), which emits light. This light is further detected by an *Amorphous Silicon* (a-*Si*) photodiode or a charged-coupled device (CCD) which gives digitized signal. This is like that of flat panel detector used digital radiography. The CsI behaves like a fiber-optics, conducts light to the photocathode with less lateral spread and permit increase of phosphor thickness to improve quantum detection efficiency. This system uses a-Si thin film transistor (TFT). The a-Si diode arrays are constructed from a matrix of a-Si TFT deposited on a glass substrate. The CsI crystals are deposited as linear columns on the a-Si detector array. When light falls on the diode, it liberates charge. It is readout sequentially along the bottom row. The charge is transferred column wise through the bottom row which makes the final digital signal.

It consists of 1920 × 2304 detector elements on 19.2 × 23 cm area with each pixel size of 100 μm. There is close bonding between CsI and photodiode and hence light loss is lesser. Since Silicon diode gives strong signal, the detective quantum efficiency is also higher. The digital detector is linear over wide range exposures. The limitation includes smaller image receptor size and large pixel size. Of course, decreasing the pixel size may increase spatial resolution with increased noise. Hence, there is trade off between resolution and SNR.

Direct Capture

In direct capture, the X-rays incident directly on a photoconductor, which converts the X-rays into digital signal directly. No scintillator is used in this detector. Photoconductor is *Amorphous Selenium* (a-*Se*) of detector size 24 cm × 29 cm with a pixel matrix of 2400 × 2900. Absorbed X-rays liberate electron hole pairs in the Selenium. Charged particles are drawn on the opposite face of the detector by an external applied electric field. To collect the signal an array of electrode pads forms the detector elements. The electric field can be tailored to collect the charge with minimum lateral spread. Thus, use of thick detector is possible to have good detective quantum efficiency. Detail description of indirect and direct conversion digital radiography systems are given in Chapter 7.

It is a good photoconductor with high X-ray absorption capability (95%). Its quantum efficiency is higher than that of film-screens and CsI. Even with an increasing thickness, it maintains its sharpness. Its limitation is that it requires large storage space per an examination. In an indirect system, there is some degree of light spread which degrades resolution. This is eliminated in the direct capture system. In addition, spatial resolution is limited to pixel size, not to the thickness of photoconductor.

Digital mammography captures areas of contrasting densities since the contrast resolution is much higher. The spatial resolution of screen-film mammogram is about 16 lp/mm, whereas it is limited for DM. However, the ability of detection of macrocalcification is equal in both cases. This is due to high contrast resolution of DM which enhances its ability to visualize small high contrast structures like microcalcification. There is a reduction of 45% time in DM to perform breast examination, compared to SFM. The disadvantage of digital mammography includes an expensive equipment and less accurate in fatty breast patients. Advantages of digital mammography are:

❑ Higher contrast resolution
❑ Ability to manipulate to improve quality and visibility
❑ Reduced false positive and increased positive predicted value
❑ Lesser repeat examinations
❑ High patient throughput
❑ Eliminate X-ray film processing
❑ Simplify an image storage and retrieval

❏ Helps remote accessing of an image
❏ Better an image acquisition
❏ Enable stereotactic biopsy
❏ Availability of computer-aided detection (CAD)

Digital mammography can be used for magnification mammography. Its advantages are film grain size is eliminated, limiting spatial resolution of detector is lower than the screen-film receptor, and the increased anatomical size improves an effective resolution of the detector.

AEC principle is also used in digital mammography to ensure constant pixel signal-to-noise ratio throughout an image. The SNR for each image is based on the breast thickness, its composition, and beam quality. Generally digital detector can act as AEC sensor with pre-exposure concept. Digital detector captures entire low dose image and determines the overall signal-difference-to-noise ratio (SDNR) or minimum SDNR over a small region of an interest. Target, kV, and filter is selected to give desired SDNR. It can be operated at a wide range of an input dose levels.

Stereotactic Biopsy System

Mammography can also be used to perform stereotactic biopsy, to differentiate benign and malignant tissues. Biopsy is used to sample suspicious nonpalpable lesion detected in the mammogram. This avoids surgery and differentiates benign and malignant lesions. There are four parts in the system, namely (1) stereotactic unit, (2) device for patient positioning, (3) computer, and (4) biopsy device. Stereotactic biopsy can be done by using a prone table in which patient is lying in prone position and the breast hangs through an aperture inferiorly. The biopsy is performed by an operator by sitting underneath an elevated table. In this procedure, patient motion is minimal, patient cannot see the biopsy needle and has minimal vasovagal reactions. Alternatively, an upright add on system with the patient in sitting or lateral decubitus position can be used.

Stereotactic localization unit is fitted to the mammographic unit before biopsy. Craniocaudal, mediolateral, lateromedial or oblique views of breast can also be used for the procedure. Needle can be inserted either vertical or lateral directions. If the breast is compressed in craniocaudal direction, needle is inserted in the lateral direction, parallel to the compression peddle.

Alternatively, 3D X-ray technique is used to guide a core needle to the biopsy site. The patient is positioned at 0° so that the target is at the center of the biopsy window. The breast is X-rayed at two different angles, ±15° by moving the X-ray tube which give two digital stereo images in a same screen. This is displayed on the computer monitor and the suspicious area is marked on the image. The x, y and z coordinates of the lesion center is calculated from the computer. It is transformed to the upright add-on stereotactic biopsy unit.

Breast skin is cleaned and injected with local anesthesia. A small nick (2 mm) is made at the skin to insert the needle. The radiologist inserts the needle and advances it to the suspicious lesion. The biopsy system is moved towards the suspicious area with computer generated x, y and z coordinates. Again, X-ray is performed to verify the needle tip position. Thus, tissue sample is collected, kept in 10% formalin solution, and sent for pathologist opinion. Biopsy samples can be taken either with core needle biopsy or vacuum assisted device. Earlier FNAC device is used to take biopsy, off late replaced by 14 Guage CB needle which is reliable and reproducible.

DIGITAL BREAST TOMOSYNTHESIS

Breast tomosynthesis is an extension of full field digital mammography (FFDM) that gives slice wise examination but eliminates overlapping of breast tissues (2011). It is basically a 3D imaging of breast tissue, often called 3D digital mammography (3DDM) or digital breast tomosynthesis (DBT). It permits visualizing multiple images of breast instead of a single image. In this, X-ray tube is rotated around the patient isocentrically and multiple quasi 3D images are taken. These images are reconstructed to get multiple slices for noise reduction or overlap of fibro glandular tissue. Finally, an image is viewed by the radiologist for an interpretation.

The X-ray tube, target/filter, an exposure time and compression methods of FFDM can be used in 3DDM also. In addition, it has provision for X-ray tube motion, sweep angle and number of projection. The breast is positioned like normal mammogram, but with little compression. The X-ray tube moves isocentrically in an arc around the breast and it takes multiple X-ray images, say 15, from many angles **(Fig. 8.12).** Tube motion is either continuous or step and shoot techniques. Continuous X-ray emission technique is faster, has focal spot blur and limits number of projections. On the other hand, step and shoot technique reduces focal spot blur but exposure time is longer. It also involves the possibility of motion related artifacts.

Tomosynthesis gives images from a moving X-ray source. Unlike CT scan, the sweep angle is restricted with 15°–50°. The X-ray tube moves symmetrically in an arch both in clockwise and anticlockwise directions from the center of the detector. If 50° is the sweep angle, the tube moves +25° and -25° from the center of the detector. Smaller sweep angle gives better in-plane resolution and ability to visualize microcalcification. Larger sweep angle gives better out of plane resolution for large objects. Another limiting factor for sweep angle is the field of view. At a wide sweep angle, parts of breast projection can go out of the field of view. Most of the vendors use stationary detectors in tomosynthesis.

The higher the number of projections, better the image quality. It increases in-plane resolution and decreases out of plane blur for low contrast objects. However, the radiation dose is higher as number of projection increases. If the radiation dose per projection is kept constant, number of projections will increase the total radiation dose. If the dose per projection is kept lower, the image noise increases with poor contrast

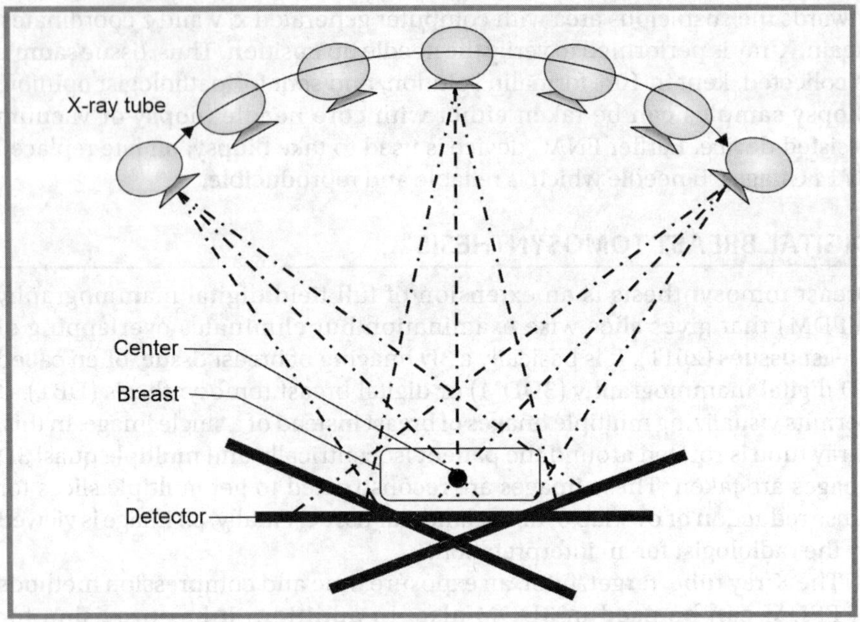

Fig. 8.12: Principle of breast tomosynthesis with multiple projections.

to noise ratio. Hence, vendor limits the number of projections based on sweep angle, radiation dose and acquisition parameters for each type of equipment.

DBT units are fitted with Tungsten target with Rh or Al filter, offering higher photon energies. Hence, use of higher photon energies gives lesser image noise. It gives less mean glandular dose than SFM. Combined dose of FFDM and DBT may increase the dose by a factor of 2.5. However, it is still less than the recommended standard of 3 mGy per view.

The computer collects the data and use CT based reconstruction algorithm to construct 3D images, throughout the breast. *Filtered back projection (FBP)* method involves application of convolution filter for each projection. *High pass filter* is used to improve sharpness and an iterative reconstruction can improve an image quality. Reconstructed thin slices of 0.1 to 0.5 mm parallel to the detector plane can be viewed. Thin slices allow visualization of *amorphous microcalcifications*. Synthesized mammography allows a global visual assessment of the whole breast.

Tomosynthesis can be used for screening, diagnostic, and stereotactic biopsy. It provides clear, accurate view of the breast. Combined use of FFDM and DBT give superior detection of malignancy in cancer screening. Hence, radiologists can effectively diagnose the size, shape, and location of an abnormalities. This will benefit young women especially with dense breast. Artifacts in DBT are *blurring ripple, and truncation with loss of skin and superficial tissue resolution.* Special training of staff and strict quality control is required. Advantages and disadvantages of DBT are given below:

Advantages

- Early detection of breast cancer
- Avoids unnecessary biopsies
- Reduce tissue superimposition
- Contrast enhancement of lesion
- High depth and contrast resolution
- Better depiction of smallest calcification
- Total radiation exposure to the patient from a two-view tomosynthesis is similar or less than the conventional mammogram
- Requires less compression than SFM mammography

Disadvantages

- Special training of technologist is required for patient positioning
- More artifacts are likely due to long exposure time
- Large calcification may cause significant artifacts
- Reconstructed images may lengthen interpretation time

CONTRAST-ENHANCED DIGITAL MAMMOGRAPHY

Screen-film mammography followed by full field digital mammography have been used over the years. FFDM provides image storage and display, improved efficiency, and elimination of film processing. It has shown an improved sensitivity in pre-and perimenopausal women. However, it has no improved diagnostic accuracy compared to that of SFM. MRI breast imaging used contrast media as an alternative. Though its sensitivity is higher, specificity is lower compared to SFM, due to false positive cases. There was a need to search for a technique with contrast media in breast imaging.

Contrast-enhanced digital mammography (CEDM) is a recent development in digital mammogram. It uses an intravenous injection of *Iodinated contrast agent* in conjunction with a mammogram procedure. It is based on the principle that rapidly growing tumors require an increased blood supply to support growth. When contrast is injected, it leaks into an interstitial space and selectively accumulates around the tumor. Since Iodine atomic number is higher it increases the chance of photoelectric absorption in such areas. Hence, the X-absorption is more in contrast enhanced tissue compared to non- enhanced tissue. It enables a method of contrast distribution in breast tissues.

It provides morphologic data with physiological information which will help to understand if a suspected lesion is growing or not. It provides better visibility of cancer in diagnostic mammography, especially in women of dense breast who have high-risk. It may be an alternative to magnetic resonance imaging (MRI) in imaging of high-risk patients. This technique can increase

mammographic lesion conspicuity. Two types of techniques are employed in CEDM:
- ❑ Temporal subtraction
- ❑ Dual energy CEDM

Temporal Subtraction

Temporal subtraction is like digital subtraction angiography. It employs a technique with an acquisition of high energy images before and after an injection of contrast agent. First noncontrast breast image obtained followed by contrast enhanced image by keeping the patient in the same position. These two images are subtracted from one another resulting only Iodine signal image. Number of such sequential images are obtained at a high energy, above the K-edge of iodine, after an intravenous nonionic Iodine contrast. It is possible to analyze the kinetic curve of enhancement of breast tissues. Patient must maintain a particular position like MLO for a prolonged period. Hence, only single view can be imaged, is the main disadvantage of this technique. Motion artifacts are more as breast is under compression while contrast arrives in the blood stream. If there is a movement between two images, it may lead to misregistration artifacts.

Dual Energy CEDM

Dual energy CEDM overcomes the limitations of temporal subtraction technique. It relies on attenuation properties and k-edge of iodine. In this, dual images are acquired, below and above the k-edge of Iodine that provides traditional low energy image and contrast enhanced image.

In practice, nonionic iodinated contrast agent is administered at a dose of 1.5 mL per kilogram of body weight at a rate of 3 mL/sec. Image is obtained as follows: (1) one high energy (high kV with strong filtration) and (2) one by using distinct low energy (standard kV and filtration). The first image is above the k-edge energy and Iodine has strong attenuation. The image contrast seen in the high energy image is due to Iodine attenuation and breast tissue attenuation. The second image is taken below the k-edge energy and an image contrast seen only due to by breast tissue attenuation but not due to contrast medium. The low energy image is then subtracted from the high energy image. The difference between the X-ray attenuation of Iodine and breast tissues of these two energy levels are used to suppress the background breast tissues. The images are acquired after 2 minutes of contrast injection. This method depicts areas in the breast associated with an increased vascularity.

Absence of compression during contrast injection ensures nonocclusion of small tumor feeders. It provides enough uptake even in small lesions. The overall procedure takes only about 10 minutes, it can be followed by a stereotactic biopsy or ultrasonography guided biopsy in the same appointment. This technique will not provide information about the kinetics of tumor enhancement but permits acquisition of multiple views of the same breast or bilateral examination. It is less sensitive to patient motion, compared

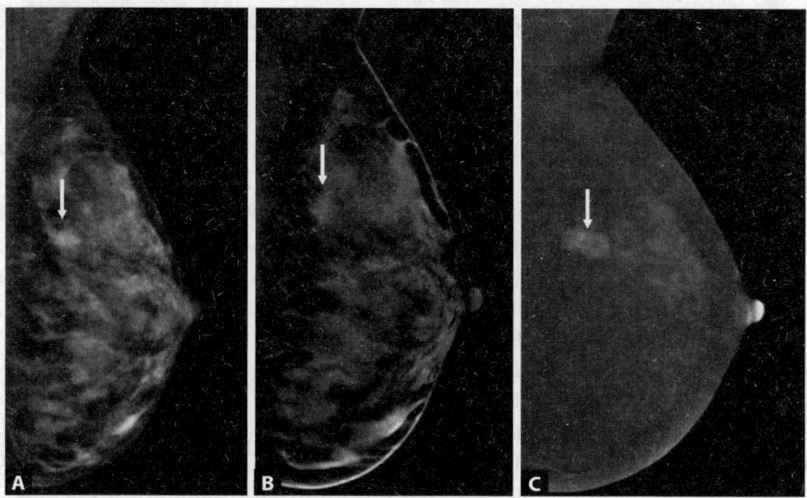

Figs. 8.13A to C: Breast lesion appearance: (A) Digital mammography; (B) Digital breast tomosynthesis; (C) Contrast-enhanced mammography.
(*Courtesy:* Nicosia L et al, 2023)

to temporal CEDM. Image is superior due to an elimination of misregistration artifacts. CEDM has low sensitivity and high specificity, especially in high dense breast patients. It can be reported alone or with standard mammogram. Difference between the digital, tomosynthesis and contrast-enhanced mammography images are shown in **Figures 8.13 A to C.**

RADIATION DOSE

Mammography involves low kV X-rays and hence photoelectric absorption mostly accounts for radiation dose. Low energy scatter also contributes to radiation dose to tissue. The radiation dose to the tissue depends on (1) speed of imaging system, (2) intended image density, (3) breast thickness, (4) breast composition, (5) kV selection, (6) filter, (7) type of grid, and (8) detector sensitivity. Mammography warrants images with high contrast sensitivity, high detail, and low visual noise. This requires high X-ray exposure compared to other radiographic examinations. Low penetrating X-rays, visualization of microcalcification, and type of receptor accounts such high X-ray exposures.

Tissue compression lowers radiation dose, by minimizing photon scatter especially the low energy scatter. If efficient screen-film system is used, then lesser photon density is enough to give an optimal image. This will reduce radiation dose to the patient. The nature of anode material and filter also influence patient dose. Choice of *Carbon fiber grid and cassette* will also reduce radiation dose. To improve film sensitivity, longer developing time and higher developer temperature are recommended. However, digital mammography can reduce such radiation doses to patients due to lesser retakes.

Radiation dose, which can induce cancer in breast, is the main risk in mammography. Glandular tissue is the site for carcinogenesis, compared to an adipose tissue, hence it is taken as reference tissue for radiation dose. Whole breast is approximated near homogeneous with mixture of glandular and an adipose tissue. Dosimetric studies were carried out with *Monte carlo* simulations. The dosimetric approximation and using a single value for the whole breast leads to *mean glandular dose (MGD)*, which is considered as dose index to evaluate risk. The glandular dose varies with depth, beam quality, breast thickness, and optical density of an image. Since, glandular tissue is lying at different depths, the dose also varies and hence measurement is difficult. Therefore, MGD is estimated as follows:

$$MGD \text{ (mrad)} = D_{gN} \times ESE \text{ (R)}$$

where, D_{gN} is the factor used to convert an entrance skin exposure to mean glandular dose in mrad or mGy. It is determined by Monte carlo simulations and measurements. It depends on kV, target, filter, breast compression and thickness. The above conversion factor is available in the ACR QC manual, 1999. The entrance skin expose (ESE) can be measured by keeping a standard breast phantom. Alternatively, the following equation can be used for quick estimation:

$$MGD \text{ (mrad)} = 0.5 \times HVL \text{ (mm)} \times ESE \text{ (mR)}$$

where, HVL of the beam and ESE can be measured locally. This gives MGD values with in 2–3% for all target and filters. Maximum allowed MGD for 4.2 cm breast thickness containing 50% adipose and 50% glandular tissue is 300 mrad or 3 mGy. A typical mammography screening involves two views of each breast which accounts 3–5 mGy to the glandular tissue. It is an accepted risk, where the benefit of breast cancer screening far exceeds the radiation risks.

In tomosynthesis, multiple exposures are given with changing geometry in the same breast which warrants different of dose estimation. *American association of Physicists in medicine Task Group-223* (APPM-223) suggested a concept of *normalized mean glandular dose* $(D_g N)$, where D_g is the glandular dose, and N is the number of projections. The mean glandular dose is normalized by a reference exposure in an imaging technique for a given pre-fixed point or area. It is dose/exposure expressed in mGy/R or mGy/mGy-air kerma. The reference exposure is nothing but entrance surface exposure (ESE) of the breast. Usually, the above radiation exposure is measured few centimeters above the entrance surface of the breast by a detector and reduced to ESE by inverse square law.

In tomosynthesis, distance between the X-ray tube and breast entrance surface, sweep angle is changing during an acquisition. To address this, *relative glandular dose (RGD)* is suggested as an index. RGD describes the change in the mean glandular dose between a zero-degree projection and nonzero degree projection during acquisition. Mean $\overline{RGD}$ (for a complete tomosynthesis is given by the relation:

$$D_g N_{TOMO} = D_g N_{MAMMO} \times \overline{RGD}$$

where, D_gN_{TOMO} is the normalized glandular dose for a complete tomosynthesis acquisition, and D_gN_{MAMMO} is the normalized glandular dose for a mammography acquisition. D_gN_{TOMO} values are given in the AAPM –223 report in mGy/mGy-airkerma for various slice thickness (2–9 cm) over wide range of kV (26–38). The $\overline{RGD}$ values vary from 0.997–0.995 (nearer to unity) for varying thickness of breast from 2 to 9 cm and it vary with vendor's model.

PHANTOM AND IMAGE QUALITY ASSURANCE

The objective of quality assurance (QA) in mammography is to obtain high quality images with lesser patient dose. *American College of Radiology (ACR)* has recommended QA programs for mammography that includes daily, weekly, monthly, quarterly, and annually. Daily QA includes cleaning of darkroom and checking the processor quality. Screens, view boxes and phantom images are to be checked on weekly basis. Repeat analysis, fixer retention in film is to be carried out quarterly. Darkroom fog, screen-film contact, and compression must be checked half early. Nowadays, CR and DR detectors are used in mammography and the dark room related QA are not much important.

Mammography phantom simulates the breast for a radiography examination. It is made up of an acrylic block, a wax insert, and an acrylic disk attached to the top of the phantom. It represents a standard breast of 4.2 cm thickness composed of 50% adipose and 50% glandular tissue. There are two types of phantoms, namely (1) small ACR mammography phantom, and (2) ACR digital mammography phantom. Both can stimulate a compressed breast of 4.2 cm thick of average density.

Small ACR phantom consists of a wax insert that contains fibers, specks, and masses. Generally, phantom is made up of 6 cylindrical nylon fibers of decreasing diameter, 5 speck groups of decreasing order (Al_2O_3 specks), and 5 solid discs of decreasing diameter **(Fig. 8.14)**. Phantom configuration is as follows: Thickness of fiber diameter are 1.56 mm, 1.12 mm, 0.89 mm, 0.75 mm, 0.54 and 0.42 mm, respectively. The diameter of speck group is 0.54 mm, 0.40 mm, 0.32 mm, 0.24 mm and 0.16 mm, respectively. The diameter of masses are 2 mm, 1 mm, 0.75 mm, 0.50 mm, and 0.25 mm, respectively.

In the case of ACR DBT mammography phantom, fiber diameter varies from 0.89 mm to 0.3 mm, specks diameter from 0.33 mm to 0.14 and mass diameter from 1.00 to 0.2 mm, respectively.

The phantom is positioned so that the chest wall side of the phantom and detector must flush to each other. Compression paddle is used to offer suitable compression. In the case of ACR digital mammography phantom, 5 daN (12 pound-force) compression force is used. AEC detector is positioned below the phantom at the center. Now, the phantom is exposed to radiation with suitable technical factors. If AEC is used, record the technical factors of phantom test. The exposure time or mAs reproducibility should be within ±15%. Identification of smallest size for each category reveals the performance of the mammography unit. Some vendors suggest placement of acrylic plate of

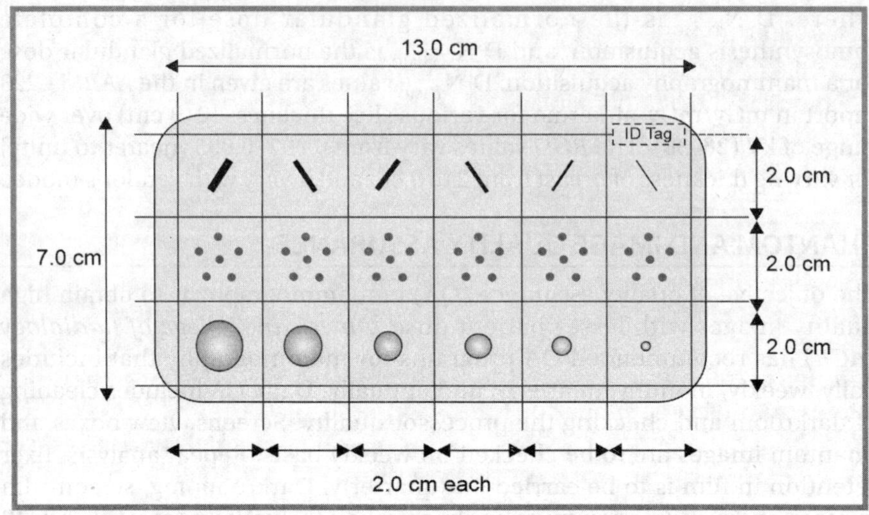

Fig. 8.14: Model of digital mammography phantom with fibers, specks, and masses of different diameter with decreasing order.
(*Courtesy:* American College of Radiology, 2023)

4 cm on an image receptor. It is useful to find the manual technique for those who use an automatic optimization parameter with AEC. The phantom image is analyzed for as per ACR test pass criteria:

❑ Small ACR mammography phantom: 4 largest fibers, 3 largest speck groups and 3 largest masses must be visualized.

❑ ACR digital mammography phantom: 2 largest fibers, 3 largest speck groups and 2 largest masses must be visualized with no clinically significant artifact. Mammography unit should be tested twice if used for both DBT and FFDM. Similarly, the CR unit is tested twice, one for screen-film and one for CR.

The images should be counted from larger to smaller size, with ACR recommended scoring. The pattern of scoring varies with type of phantom.

In the case of ACR digital phantom, full score is given for the following:

❑ If full length of fiber is visible with location and orientation. One break is allowed if it is ≤ then the fiber width.

❑ If 4–6 specks are visible with correct locations.

❑ Mass density difference is visible in correct location and border is continuous or generally circular (≥ ¾ border visible).

The following is eligible for half score:

❑ Half-length of fiber is visible (≥ 5 and <8 mm long) in correct location and orientation. One break is allowed if it is ≤ then the fiber width.

❑ If 2–3 specks are visible with correct locations.

❑ Mass density difference is visible in correct location and border is not continuous or generally circular (< ¾ border visible).

Then, using a magnifying glass an image is checked for an artifact. The artifact test is failed if:

❑ Artifacts are as prominent as (or more prominent than) the visible test objects in the phantom image, or
❑ Artifacts obscure test objects in the phantom, or
❑ Artifacts could affect clinical interpretation.

BI-RADS CLASSIFICATION

Breast imaging report and data system (BI-RADS) is the concept of *American College of Radiology (ACR)* which is largely used today for mammography reporting. It is a tool to reduce variability between radiologist while reporting mammography, ultrasonography, and MRI. BI-RADS lexicon includes (1) micro/macrocalcifications, etc., (2) architectural distortions, etc., (3) special cases: ductal ectasia, an intramammary lymph node, or focal asymmetric density, etc., and (4) associated findings: skin or nipple retraction, skin thickening, cutaneous lesions, an axillary lymph nodes, etc. According to the composition of breast four categories recommended for reporting:

❑ Type 1: fatty breast, < 10–49% of dense tissue
❑ Type 2: Fibro glandular, 10–49% of dense breast
❑ Type 3: Heterogeneously dense, 49–90% of dense tissue
❑ Type 4: Dense and homogeneous, >90% of dense tissue

The accuracy of mammogram decreases in type 3 and 4 which require an ultrasonography information for reporting. The probability of malignancy is large at type 4, hence, it is subdivided into 4a, 4b, and 4c. The classification of BI-RADS score is given in the **Table 8.3.**

Table 8.3: Classification of BI-RADS score.

Category	Definition	Likelihood of cancer
BI-RADS 0	Incomplete	N/A
BI-RADS 1	Negative	Essentially 0%
BI-RADS 2	Benign	Essentially 0%
BI-RADS 3	Probably benign	>0 % but ≤2%
BI-RADS 4	Suspicious	>2 % but <95%
BI-RADS 5	Highly suggestive of malignancy	≥ 95%
BI-RADS 6	Known biopsy proven malignancy	N/A

(*Courtesy:* American college of radiology BI-RADS Atlas: Breast imaging reporting and data system)

BIBLIOGRAPHY

1. Albus K. Phantom testing: Mammography revised, American college of radiology (Revised 8-31-2023); 2023.
2. Bushberg JT, Seibert JA, Leidholdt EM Jr, Boone JM. The Essential Physics of Medical Imaging, 3rd edn. Lippincott Williams and Wilkin; 2012.
3. De Marco P et al. Breast Digital Tomosynthesis versus Contrast-Enhanced Mammography: Comparison of Diagnostic Application and Radiation Dose in a Screening Setting. *Cancers* 2023, *15*, 2413.
4. Digital mammography quality control ACR manual, American college of radiology; 2018.
5. https://radiologykey.com/X-ray-imaging-mammography
6. Nicosia L., Bozzini AC, Pesapane F, Rotili A, Marinucci I, Signorelli G, Frassoni S, Bagnardi V, Origgi, D. Radiation dosimetry in digital breast tomosynthesis: Report of AAPM Tomosynthesis Subcommittee Task Group 223, Medical physics: Volume 41, Issue 9, September 2014
7. Thayalan K. Basic Radiological Physics, 2nd edn. Jaypee Brothers Medical Publishers (P) Ltd, New Delhi; 2017

Fluoroscopy Imaging

EVALUATION OF FLUOROSCOPY

Fluoroscopy is an imaging technique used to obtain real-time moving images of an internal structure of a patient. It was invented by **Thomas A Edison (1896)** after an input from **Enrico Salvioni**. Edison also designed the first fluoroscope equipment and *Zinc-cadmium sulfide screen* in the same year. Though he used *Barium platinocyanide* initially, he studied more than 1800 materials with X-rays including *Cadmium sulfide and Calcium tungstate*. However, he abandoned his X-ray studies after the demise of his friend, **Clarence Dally** (1904), whose both arms were amputated due to severe X-ray burns.

Fluoroscopy is a type an imaging which shows continuous X-ray image like a X-ray movie. The X-rays enter the human body, transmit and incident on a fluorescent screen to form X-ray live image. However, it requires flow of contrast materials such as *Barium or Iodine* through the body. In radiography, images are made with transmission of X-rays through the body with screen-film or CR cassette as detectors and it produces only static images. The former needs a darkroom and later needs a reader to process an image whereas fluoroscopy does not require such provisions.

Fluoroscopy is basically dynamic imaging, where the radiologist views images of moving organs or fluids continuously, while the X-ray beam is ON. Fluorescent phosphors, like *Calcium tungstate* are used as detectors which emits instant images directly or indirectly. Fluoroscopy is used to view an internal organs, insert catheters, place stents, study blood vessels, guide surgical procedures especially in orthopedics, in addition to as an imaging system and therapeutic tool. Real-time imaging requires 30 frames per second like that of television technology. This will facilitate to follow motion of an organ over a period. Hence, fluoroscopy imaging has higher temporal resolution, to follow motion. Since fluoroscopy is a dynamic process, the radiologist must adapt the moving images, even though image is dull. This requires knowledge of image illumination and visual physiology.

Generally, fluoroscopy is performed at low doses and the images are formed relatively with few X-rays. Hence, quantum mottle is higher in fluoroscopy. Fluoroscopy X-ray tubes are operated at 1–5mA current, high tube voltage with higher grid ratio of 10:1.

Generally, this equipment is made as a radiographic and fluoroscopic (R and F) imaging system. It is available as portable C-arm devices and cardiac catheterization laboratories and an interventional radiology equipment. Fluoroscopy can be discussed in three headings, namely, (1) direct vision fluoroscopy (2) image intensifier fluoroscopy, and (3) digital fluoroscopy.

Visual Physiology

Vision is one of the five senses in the body by which human eye differentiate colors. Physical properties of eye are important to understand vision. Human eyes consist of a series of lenses and spaces that focus the images like a camera. It contains *vitreous humor, aqueous humor, crystalline lens, and the cornea* and each one has its refractive index. There is a structure called *iris* between the cornea and crystalline lens, which control the light that falls on the eye. Light from an object passes through *cornea, lens,* undergo refraction and focused upon the retina. Retina has two types of photoreceptors, namely *rods and cones*. There are about 91 million rods and 4.5 million cones in the retina. The image on the retina is an inverted one, and the energy is converted into an electrical impulse by rods and cones of the retina. Then it goes to the brain through an *optic nerve* as *action potential* to process eye vision. In bright light, an iris contracts, allows less light to the eye. In low light, the iris expands and allows large light. Retina can adjust to various levels of light which is referred to as *visual physiology*.

Human vision is due to rods and cones in the retina of the eye. Basically, rods and cones are very small structures and there are about 10^5 numbers per square mm in the retina. Cones are present at the center of the retina (*fovea centralis*), whereas rods are present at the periphery. Rods are responsible for vision at low light levels whereas cones are responsible at higher light levels. Thus, cones help for day light vision (*photopic vision*) and rods are responsible for night vision (*scotopic vision*). Cones detect small objects better and differentiate brightness levels. It is sensitive to wide range of wavelength of light and capable of detecting color. Its ability to preserve fine detail is referred to as *visual acuity*. Rods unable to detect color and hence become color blind. In scotopic vision, eyes are sensitive to green light ($\lambda = 555$ nm). The transformation of scotopic vision into photopic vision is called *dark adaptation*, which finds application in direct vision fluoroscopy.

DIRECT VISION FLUOROSCOPY

Direct vision fluoroscopy device consists of an under-couch X-ray source and a fluorescent screen above the table. The X-rays incident on the human body gets attenuated differently by different tissues, and transmitted rays are passed on to a scintillation phosphor screen, *Zinc-cadmium sulfide (ZnCdS)* which gives an image as faint scintillations. The screen was backed with a Lead glass to reduce radiation dose to eyes. It converts an incident X-ray energy into visible light. Transmitted rays interact with screen atoms by photoelectric absorption and give energy to the electrons. Most of the electron energy is dissipated as heat, and only less energy appears as visible light. The radiologists used to view faint yellowish-green fluoroscopic image directly with *red goggles* in a darkroom. To record an image a spot film radiography is performed. The thick phosphor converts the X-rays into light proportionally, but the brightness is too low. In addition, it requires radiation protection devices like Lead curtain, bucky slot cover, Leaded apron and gloves and protective viewing window. This type of fluoroscopy had been in use until 1950, which is called as direct vision fluoroscopy. It was discontinued due to the following reasons.

The light output of the fluorescent screen is very poor for a given exposure rate. The light conversion efficiency of the screen is also much lower, and the spatial resolution is very poor. The radiologists can see only a small percentage of light from the screen, due to narrow viewing angle (6°) to light photons. The image quality of a fluorescent screen is also poor since visual acuity of eye is 10 times lesser at such low light levels. Fluoroscopy screens are not used now a days since it offers higher radiation dose to the operator. Contrast of fluoroscopic image is 1/10th of radiographic image, since the images are so faint, it must be viewed under dark conditions with red goggles. However, radiologist should adopt their eyes to dark before 10–20 minutes, to adopt full darkness. One can visualize fine details and differences in brightness levels of anatomical parts. In addition, the patient may receive higher dose of radiation and hence this modality is not in use today.

IMAGE INTENSIFIER FLUOROSCOPY

In the beginning, fluoroscopy was performed by viewing the live image, produced by X-rays on a thick intensifying screen. The room must be completely dark so that faint glow of the screen could be seen. The radiologists also wear red goggles for dark adaptation. The difficulties involved in dark adaptation and working in dark lead to the development of an image intensifier (II).

When X-rays pass through human body it is transmitted with varying intensity. This transmitted radiation is made to fall on an II tube. Collimator limits the size of the X-ray beam automatically to proper field of view (FOV). II tube converts an incident radiation into an electron image, in turn an optical image. As a result, visible image is formed in an exit fluorescent screen. This image can be viewed directly or indirectly by the radiologist. The image can be observed by a video camera and be presented on a television monitor **(Fig. 9.1)**.

Fluoroscopy must have maximum image detail, for which greater image brightness is required. The image intensifier fulfills the above requirement. Image brightness mostly depends on anatomy, kV, and mA. Hence, by

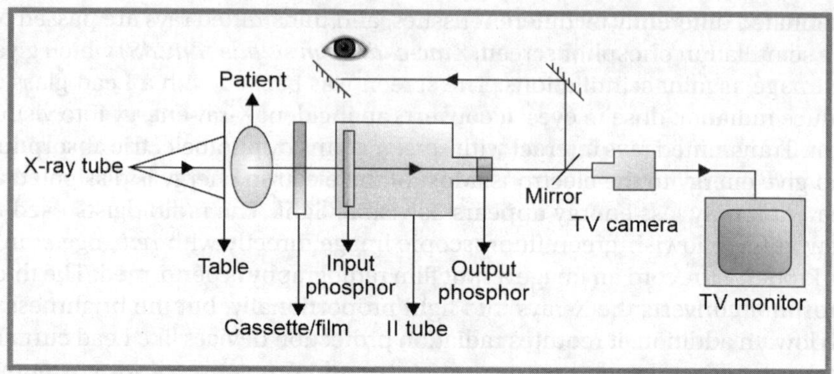

Fig. 9.1: Fluoroscopy imaging with image intensifier and TV system.

controlling the kV and mA, an image brightness can be varied in fluoroscopy. Fluoroscopy examination requires several minutes to hours, and the radiation dose to the patient is higher. To reduce patient dose, the exposure rate (200 mGy/sec) must be lower in fluoroscopy. Fluoroscopic system uses low current (1–5 mA), low output and typically produces 30 images/sec. This shows that only fewer X-ray photons are used in forming a single fluoroscopic image. Therefore, fluoroscopic images are statistically inferior to radiographic images. Hence, there is a search for high gain detector systems in fluoroscopy.

Fluoroscopy Equipment

Fluoroscopy X-ray equipment is like a general radiography unit however, X-ray tubes of higher heat capacity and dissipation is needed. This is to get sequence of higher dose radiographic images in rapid succession to visualize *opacified vessels*. Hence, specially made X-ray tubes are used in fluoroscopy. X-ray generator for fluoroscopy consists of X-ray tube, high frequency generator, image intensifier, video camera, TV monitor for real-time display, and film camera for hard copy. Dual focal spots, namely 1.2 mm and 0.3 mm are used with anode angles of 8°–12°. The focal spot size is not a limiting factor for resolution, since II tube has an upper resolution of 4 lp/mm. However, large focal spot under the magnification mode create image unsharpness which reduce resolution.

High frequency power supply of 15 kW–80 kW is recommended. This will provide a maximum power of 450 W–2000 W for continuous operation. The heat storage capacity range is 0.4 MJ–1 MJ. The advantage of a high frequency generator is less patient radiation dose due to lesser ripple factor and small size. *Automatic exposure system (AES)* is used to maintain radiation dose per frame, address the attenuation of internal structures and provide consistent quality image.

Fluoroscopy equipment uses beam *hardening filters, added filters and wedge filters.* Mostly they are made with *Al or Cu* materials as fixed filters.

Added filters are manually selectable or auto selectable to switch over from low to higher dose mode conditions. Wedge filter is movable which can attenuate the beam in a selected area.

Collimator in fluoroscopy collimates the X-ray beam, it is either circular or rectangular to match the II tube entrance window. Once FOV is selected, the collimator blades automatically adjust and set a field just larger than the visible field. If source to image distance (SID) changes, the collimator maintains the FOV and reduces spillover radiation outside the visible area.

Patient tables should have enough strength to support patient weight. It should offer lesser attenuation to avoid shadows, loss of signal and loss of contrast in an image. Tables made with *Carbon fiber* material will satisfy the above condition. In addition, *foam pads* of minimal attenuation can be used to position patients on the table.

Antiscatter grids are very important in fluoroscopy, since scatter radiation is more, especially in an abdominal procedure. Typical grid ratio used are 6:1 to 10:1, either circular or rectangular pattern.

The image receptor is either an image intensifier tube (II tube) with TV system or digital fluoroscopy system. The latter uses either *charge-coupled device* (CCD) or *flat panel detectors* of rectangular size to generate digital output. The optical image from the II tube output photocathode can be viewed or recorded by a simple optical system.

The methods of converting the II tube's visible optical image into an electronic signal are (1) thermionic camera tube, and (2) *CCD* cameras. The camera captures an image, converts it into an analog electrical signal which is fed to a television monitor for viewing. *Vidicon cameras* are commonly used which have same sensitive size as that of an output phosphor. The advantage is that it can control the brightness and contrast electronically. Several people can monitor an image at a time and provide image storage facility with postprocessing. These cameras are discussed in detail in subsequent paragraphs.

Image Intensifier Tube

The image intensifier is an evacuated glass envelope (vacuum bottle), which contains three basic elements. They are (1) input phosphor and photocathode, (2) electrostatic focusing lenses, (3) anode and output phosphor **(Fig. 9.2)**. The patient side of the vacuum bottle has an *Al window (1 mm)*, which is a curved one to withstand air pressure. The evacuated glass envelope limits the size of II and its diameter ranges from 23 to 57 cm. The field size can be reduced electronically by using an electrostatic focusing. The glass envelope is mounted inside a metal container, which will avoid damage and rough handling.

Input Phosphor and Photocathode

The input phosphor follows the *Al window* and has three layers, namely, a curved substrate layer (0.5 mm Al) to support the phosphor, *CsI input*

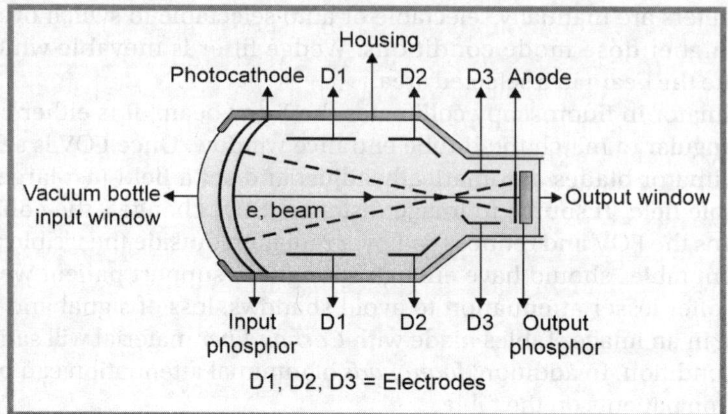

Fig. 9.2: Image intensifier and its components.

phosphor (200–400 µm) and a *photocathode* (**Fig. 9.3**). X-rays from the patient passes through an Al window and falls on an input phosphor. This phosphor absorbs X-rays and converts the X-ray energy into light photons. This is like the action of an intensifying screen in cassette. The input phosphor is thick enough to absorbs large X-rays and thin enough to preserve resolution. It should ensure that greater photons are passed to the photocathode with less lateral spread.

The *photocathode* is coated on the inner side of the phosphor. It is a thin metal layer, and the commonly used photocathode is *Antimony and Cesium* (Sb_2Cs_3) compounds. The light photons are absorbed by the photocathode which converts the light into an electron. Many light photons emit one electron. The number of electrons that is emitted is directly proportional to light intensity, in turn is proportional to an intensity of input X-rays. For example, a 60 kV X-ray photon can emit about 8000 light photons, followed by emission of 400 electrons.

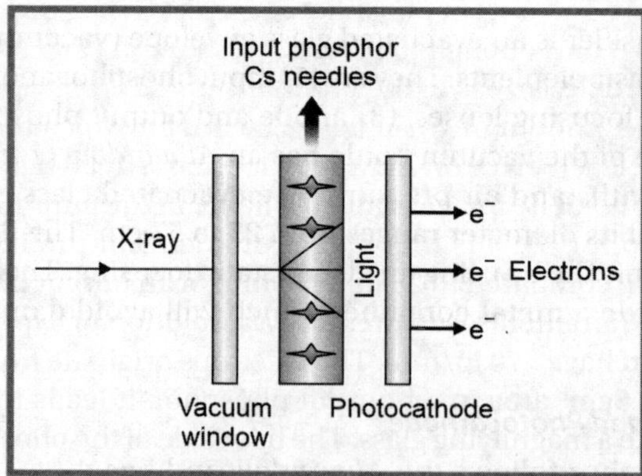

Fig. 9.3: The input screen of the image intensifier tube.

CsI phosphor is commonly used as an input phosphor, because of its special property. It is a vertically grown needle like crystal (5 µm, dia.), tightly packed, that can push the light in the forward direction. It also reduces lateral spread of light, resulting lesser unsharpness. The K-edges of Cesium (36 keV) and Iodine (33 keV) falls under the bremsstrahlung spectrum of fluoroscopy X-rays, which increases its absorption efficiency (60%). This will reduce patient dose. The input screen is maintained at a high negative potential compared to anode, to accelerate electrons. The screen size may vary from 150–400 mm in diameter, depending upon the clinical application.

Electrostatic Focusing lens

There are 3 electrodes (D1, D2, and D3) between an input phosphor and an anode. They are basically metal rings, which are given positive voltage with respect to photocathode. They accelerate electrons and focus them on the output phosphor through an anode. The image intensifier is about 50 cm long, and a potential difference of about 25,000 V-35,000 V is maintained between photocathode and the anode. Voltage difference between the cathode and the anode accelerates electrons with an increasing kinetic energy. This is referred to as an *electronic gain.* The electrons arrive at the anode with high velocity and strike the output phosphor. Visible light is emitted which contains an image of the input phosphor. Thus, the electrons gain energy and form a minified and an inverted image at the output phosphor. The electrodes focus the electrons on the output phosphor and acts as an electrostatic lens.

Anode and Output Phosphor

The anode is a circular plate with a hole in the middle to permit the flow of electrons. It is made with a thin coating of *Al* (0.2 µm) on the vacuum side of an output phosphor. It is electrically conductive, and its potential is 25 kV higher than an input screen. The anode receives accelerated electrons, so that they deposit their energy in an output phosphor.

The output phosphor most widely used is *Zinc cadmium sulfide doped with silver (ZnCdS:Ag).* The output phosphor is small, 25 mm–35 mm in diameter and thin (4 µm –8 µm) enough to preserve resolution **(Fig. 9.4).** The ZnCdS: Ag phosphor particles size is of the order of 1 µm–2 µm. It absorbs electrons and emits a large amount of green light, 530 nm for which the video camera is very sensitive. Each electron may produce about 1000 light photons from an output phosphor. The image is much smaller in the output phosphor than the input phosphor. This is due bigger diameter of the input phosphor, 150 mm–400 mm compared to 25 mm–35 mm of an output phosphor.

One of the requirements is to preserve a resolution of 5 lp/mm, an output phosphor should have >70 lp/mm. The electrons originate from 410 cm^2 area and focused on 5cm^2 area in an output phosphor. It leads to light intensity amplification like a magnifying glass. The back side of the phosphor is covered with Al (0.5 µm) to prevent backward light emission. If there is backward light emission, it leads to *veiling glare.* The image signal passes through transparent

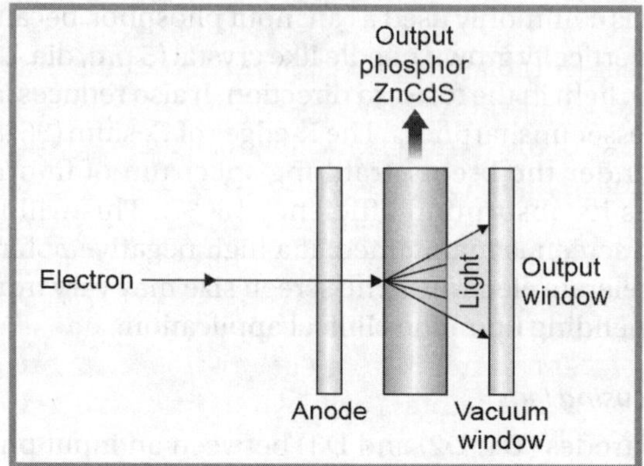

Fig. 9.4: Output screen of the image intensifier tube.

Al window which is part of a vacuum tube. The total light emission of an output phosphor is proportional to the input X-ray intensity.

Image Intensification

Intensification of II tube is due to its increased illumination of an image, which is caused by multiplication of light photons at an output phosphor and image minification. Absorption X-rays is greater if the thickness of an input phosphor is higher. However, resolution is poor due to light diffusion. Central portion of a II tube has spatial resolution of 4–5 lp/mm, whereas it is reduced at the edges. Spatial resolution varies with II tube diameter: lesser the diameter higher the resolution. The II tube performance is estimated with (1) flux gain, (2) minification gain, (3), brightness gain, (4) conversion factor, and (5) contrast ratio.

Flux Gain

Flux gain or an electronic gain is the ratio of an output phosphor light photons to an input phosphor light photons and it is of an order of 50:

$$\text{Flux gain} = \frac{\text{Number of an output light photons}}{\text{Number of an input light photons}}$$

Minification Gain

Minification gain describes an intensification caused by smaller size of an output phosphor. It is ratio of square of the diameter of an input phosphor to the square of the diameter of an output phosphor. If d_1 and d_2 are an area of an input and output phosphors, then:

$$\text{Minification gain} = \frac{d_1^2}{d_2^2}$$

If d_1 and d_2 are 300 and 30 mm respectively, then the minification gain is $\left(\frac{300}{30}\right)^2 = 100$.

Brightness Gain

The light image at an output phosphor is several thousand times brighter than an input phosphor. The ability to increase an illumination depends on the brightness gain (BG) of the II tube. It is the ratio of the brightness of an output phosphor to that of an input phosphor:

$$\text{Brightness gain} = \frac{\text{Brightness of an output phosphor}}{\text{Brightness of an input phosphor}}$$

$$\text{Overall brightness gain} = \text{Flux gain} \times \text{Minification gain.}$$

If the flex gain is 50 and minification gain is 100 then, brightness gain is equal to $50 \times 100 = 5000$. Brightness gain of the II tube is of the order of 5000–30,000 and it decreases with age. It is not a measurable quantity hence the term *conversion factor* is introduced to evaluate the performance of a II tube.

Conversion Factor

Conversion factor or gain is a modern method of accessing the performance of an II tube. It is defined as the ratio of brightness (luminance, cd/m²) of an output phosphor to X-ray exposure rate (μGy/sec) at an input phosphor:

$$\text{Conversion factor} = \frac{\text{Brightness of an output phosphor, } cd/m^2}{\text{input X-ray exposure rate, μGy/sec}}$$

Luminescence of light intensity is measured in *candela (cd)*. Typical values of conversion factor are 50–300 (cd/m²) per μGy/sec., which is equal to a brightness gain of 5000–30,000. Conversion gain varies with II tube size: higher the II tube diameter higher the conversion gain and vice versa. If the field size is reduced, an input exposure rate must be increased to maintain constant brightness level at an output phosphor. If II tube size is reduced by a factor of 2, an input exposure rate must be increased 4 times. The brightness of an II tube deteriorates over a period and requires periodic quality assurance.

Contrast Ratio

Contrast ratio is the ratio of periphery to central light intensity at an output phosphor. Typical contrast ratio is 20:1. It can be checked by imaging a *Lead disc* having one-tenth area of an input phosphor. The image appears behind an image of a Lead disc is called an *veiling glare*. It is due to an internal scatter of X-rays, that is few X-rays passes through an input phosphor, photocathode, and strike the inner part of the II tube, and are scattered back to an input phosphor which may cause loss of contrast. Light scattered and reflected within the II tube and output window can also cause loss of contrast.

Magnification Mode

When electron travels from an input phosphor to an output phosphor the beam gets focused at certain distance before an anode. This point is referred to as *cross over point*. By changing the voltage of an intermediate electrodes, the electron crossover point can be moved nearer the patient. This will reduce the FOV and irradiates only a smaller volume of tissue. The image appears magnified since it fills the entire screen on the monitor. If the input FOV is reduced to half, then the size of the patient image also viewed half. It will offer two-fold magnification of an image. It also increases spatial resolution by two-fold.

In normal fluoroscopy, the spatial resolution is 0.7 lp/mm, whereas in magnification mode it increases to 1.4 lp/mm. Magnification will minimize scatter and increase an image contrast. Thus, magnified images can be obtained on the output screen, with higher spatial and contrast resolution but with higher patient dose. However, the magnification mode will reduce minification gain, resulting in lesser brightness of an image. Halving the FOV reduces the brightness by one-fourth on the output screen. Hence, an input X-ray exposure requires four-fold increase to keep the same brightness. This is generally achieved by an automatic exposure system (AES) in modern fluoroscopy machines.

To restore the brightness, higher tube voltages are employed in magnification mode. Use of magnification mode goes with an increase of tube voltage due to two reasons: an increase of tube voltage reduces entrance skin air kerma rate (35–60 mGy/min), and the tube current must be kept below 5 mA to reduce an input power to the tube without an overheating the anode, within 190–260 watts. If magnification is performed with constant tube voltage, it will increase an entrance skin air-kerma rate.

The magnification factor is directly proportional to the diameters of the II tube. If an II tube of 25 cm diameter is operated in 12 cm mode, then an image magnification is 25 ÷ 12 = 2.1. For a magnification of 1.5, tubes are operated at 85 kV and 2.7 mA with an entrance skin exposure of 50 mGy/min. For a magnification of 2.5, the tube requires 94 kV and 2.8 mA with an entrance skin exposure of 61 mGy/min. In general, II tubes are provided with 1–4 magnified fields, which are called *multifield image intensifiers*. They provide different magnification of an image with higher flexibility.

For example, II tube of 25/17/12 cm is *tri-field tube*, which can be operated with 25 cm, 17 cm, and 12 cm FOV. When it is operated in 25 cm FOV all photoelectrons from the whole input phosphor are accelerated towards an output phosphor. If an operator switches over to 17 cm FOV, the voltage of the *electrostatic focusing lens* gets increased. It causes the focal point to move towards the patient side. Now only electron from the center of 17 cm diameter of the input phosphor is accelerated towards the output phosphor **(Fig. 9.5)**.

Overall, magnification fluoroscopy offers better spatial resolution, better contrast resolution but higher patient radiation dose.

Television System

Television (TV) system consists of a *video camera, monitor and optical coupling*. The video camera converts light image from an output phosphor into an electrical signal, which is proportional to light falling on the camera plate. This can be viewed on a TV monitor, which enlarges an image to

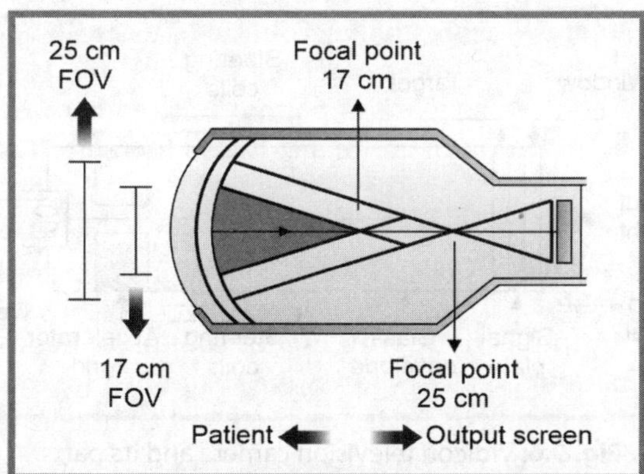

Fig. 9.5: Magnification of II tube changes the focal point towards the patient.

an original size with real-time image display. There are two methods of producing an electrical signal, namely, (1) thermionic television camera, and (2) charge-coupled device (CCD). However, the TV camera is an vacuum device that produces only analog video signal whereas CCD gives digital image.

Thermionic Television Camera

Vidicon (Sb_2S_3) or its modified version, and *Plumbicon (PbO)* are used as cameras in fluoroscopy. This camera consists of cylindrical housing of dimension 1.5 mm diameter and 25 cm length. It contains camera tube and electromagnetic coils to steer electron beams. A glass envelope maintains necessary vacuum and supports mechanically an internal parts of the tube.

Vidicon tube consists of *cathode, an electron gun, electronic grids,* and *target* which serves as an anode **(Fig. 9.6).** The electron gun is a hot filament that produces electrons by thermionic emission. Electron beam is accelerated towards an anode with the help of grids. The electrons are further accelerated and focused by additional electrostatic grids. The size of an electron beam and position is controlled by an external electromagnetic coils namely, *deflection coils, focusing coils,* and *alignment coils.*

Target assembly consists of three layers, a *thin window, signal plate, and target.* The window is outside, it is a thin part of glass envelope, and the target is inside of the target assembly. The inner side of window is coated with a thin layer of *metal or graphite* which acts as signal plate. Signal plate is thin enough to pass light and thick enough to conduct electricity. It conducts the video signals to an external video circuit. The inner side of the signal plate is coated with a photoconductive layer of *Antimony trisulfide* which act as a target. It is a photoconductor, during illumination it conducts an electron but in dark behave as an insulator.

When II tube's output light comes, it passes through window, signal plate and interacts with the target. If an electron beam is incident on a same point

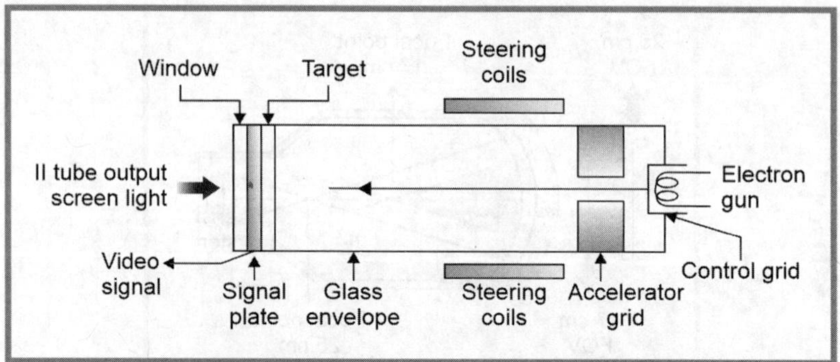

Fig. 9.6: Vidicon television camera and its parts.

of the target at same time, part of the electrons is conducted to the signal plate through the target. The signal plate transfers this video signal to an external circuit. If the point on the target is dark, no video signal is generated.

Television camera and II tubes are manufactured so that an output phosphor and the window of the television camera are of same size (2.5 cm–5 cm). Coupling between the television camera and II tube is very important. There are two ways of coupling, namely (1) *lens coupling*, and (2) *fiber optic coupling* which will be discussed later.

Thermionic Television Camara and Image Intensifier Coupling

The television camera and II tube should be coupled properly. It should ensure that there is no loss of light at the joint portion. The output phosphor diameter should be equal to the window of television camera tube. Either *lens coupling* or *fiber optic coupling* can be used to achieve this.

The lens system is a traditional method, bigger in size, suitable for cine or photo spot camera **(Fig. 9.7)**. This system consists of (1) collimating lens to shape the divergent beam into parallel beam, (2) an aperture to limit the light to video camera which can be fixed or adjustable one, and (3) a lens to focus an image on to the video camera. The objective lens receives light from an output phosphor and converts into a parallel beam. Whenever an image is recorded on the film, the mirror split the beam, and sends a part of a beam to the video camera and the remaining portion to the film camera. This will enable us to view images during recording by the radiologist. The video signal is amplified and transmitted to the TV monitor for display.

The *beam splitting mirror* is retracted from the beam when the film camera is not in use. Both television camera and film camera are coupled to the lenses. The lens focusses the parallel light on the film and camera. The lens and mirror position needs to be very precise to produce good images. The lens is a compound lens made of several individual lenses.

The fiberoptic system is efficient in light collection, which improves geometrical integrity. It is a simplest method with bundle of fiberoptics, which

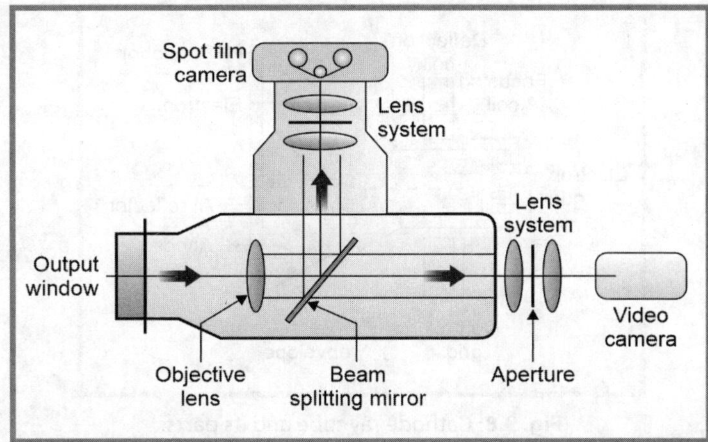

Fig. 9.7: Image intensifier and the video camera is coupled with a lens system.

is only few mm thick and contains 1000 of *glass fibers* per square mm cross section. This coupling is compact, easy to move the II tube tower. It is a rugged coupling for rough handling. The disadvantage is that it cannot accommodate additional optics like *photo spot or cine camera.*

Television Monitor

The video signal from the television camera is amplified and passed on to the monitor by means of cable for display. The main part of the monitor is the *picture tube or cathode ray tube (CRT).* It consists of an *electron gun, control grid in a glass envelope* and *external coils* to steer and focus electron beam **(Fig. 9.8).** It is different from the normal TV monitor in which the anode assembly consists of a *fluorescent screen and graphite lining.*

The video signal received by the picture tube is modulated which is proportional to the light intensity received by the camera. The electron beam intensity varies proportional to modulation of video signal. The control grid attached to an electron gun modulates an electron intensity. The electron beam is focused on a fluorescent screen by an external coils. The electron interacts with phosphor and emits visible light. The phosphor contains linear crystals which are aligned perpendicular to the glass envelope, to reduce lateral dispersion. It is backed by thin layer of Al which transmits only an electron beam but reflects light.

Understanding the television image is complex one. The optical signal from an output phosphor is converted into an electronic video signal in the television camera by a constant electron beam. This video signal modulates an electron beam in the TV picture tube and transforms an electron image into visible image. Electron beams both in camera and in picture tube are finely focused pencil beams. They are synchronously directed by an external coils of each tube. These beams are always in the same position at same time and precisely move in same fashion.

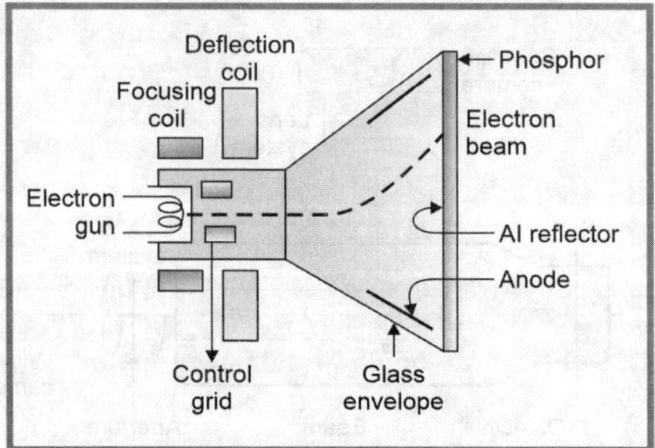

Fig. 9.8: Cathode ray tube and its parts.

Movement of an electron beam follows *raster pattern* on the screen of the picture tube. That is, an electron beam begins in an upper left corner of the screen and moves to an upper right corner, creates a varying intensity of light as it moves. This is called an *active trace*. Then, an electron beam is turned OFF and returns to the left side of the screen, known as *horizontal retrace*. A series of active traces and horizontal retraces are repeated until an electron beam is at the bottom of the screen. Thus, one television field is completed.

The electron beam is turned OFF and goes to the top of the screen referred to as an *vertical retrace*. The electron beam then performs second television field with an active trace and horizontal retraces. The only difference is that the present active trace is in between an adjacent active traces of the first television field. This movement of an electron beam is called an *interlace* and two interlaced television fields form a single *television frame*.

In practice, 525 lines of active trace per frame is available, however only 480 lines per frame is used due to an additional time for retracing. Some systems have 875 or 1024 lines per frame to have better spatial resolution. Such systems find application in digital fluoroscopy. Human eye cannot detect flickering if the frame rate is >20 frames per second. Generally, 30 frames/sec is used in video monitoring. If the power supply frequency is 50 Hz, then there are 50 television fields per second. This may give 25 television frames per second.

The vertical resolution of the monitor depends on the number of scan lines. The horizontal resolution depends on the band pass, which is expressed in Hz. It describes the number of times per second that the electron beam is modulated. For example, band pass of 1 MHz refers to the electron beam that is modulated million times in each second. Higher the band pass, the better the horizontal resolution. Usually, fluoroscopy monitors will have a band pass of 4.5 MHz against the 3.5 MHz of normal TV monitor. Up to 20 MHz band pass is possible with high resolution systems.

In general, TV monitor is the weakest link in an image intensifier fluoroscopy. The spatial resolution of the monitor is lower than that of II tube.

For example, a 525-line system, two fields of 262.5 lines are read in 1/60 sec = 17 msec and form a 525-video frame in 1/30s = 33 msec. If the TV monitor uses 625-line systems, then two fields of 312.5 lines are read to form a 625-video frame in 40 msec. The spatial resolution is 1 lp/mm, compared to 5 lp/mm for to II tube. Thus, TV monitor degrades to image quality hence, the image must be recorded on film by a photographic camera to get the benefit an II tube's higher resolution.

Television camera tubes are basically noisy. Due to involvement of filament heat and voltage difference, a small electric current always flow in any circuit. It is called *background electronic noise.* It will interfere with an electronic signal and reduce contrast. Above type of video display has two limitations: (1) an interlaced mode of reading degrades digital image, restrict the use in digital fluoroscopy and (2) camera tubes are relatively noisy, its SNR is 200:1. This means that an output signal is 200 times greater than the background signal.

The advantage of TV monitor display includes (1) the brightness level can be adjusted, (2) multiple observers can see the display at same time, and (3) image is stored in an electronic format.

Image Recording

Fluoroscopy images can be recorded by means of (1) spot film, (2) photo spot camera, and (3) cine fluoroscopy. In spot-film, the cassette loaded with film is positioned in between the patient and II tube. Normally, this device is covered by Lead, so that it cannot be exposed unintentionally during fluoroscopy mode. When an exposure is desired, a control moves the spot film cassette sideways, and position it in the path of the X-rays. The control changes the fluoroscopic mA (3 mA) exposure mode into high radiographic mA (300 mA). It takes one or two seconds to complete an exposure. The area of film can be selected by masking with Lead diaphragm so that multiple images can be recorded. If only one image is recorded it is called *one-on-one mode.* If two images are exposed, it is called *two-on-one mode.* Thus, 1–6 images can be recorded in a single film. During the cassette movement and recording, an image cannot be viewed on the monitor, thus it interrupts fluoroscopy examination. It gives 2D life size image format for easy interpretation with higher patient radiation exposure.

Photo spot is like a movie camera which exposes one frame while activated. It gets image from an output phosphor of II tube through the split mirror and involves lesser patient radiation dose. It would not interrupt fluoroscopy examination while recording. It also avoids additional heat loading on the X-ray tube. This camera uses 70 mm or 105 mm roll film sizes at the rate of 12 images per second. Larger the film size, better the image quality with an increased patient dose. However, in 105 mm film recording, the patient radiation exposure is only 50% of the spot film radiation exposure. Required exposure is about 1 µGy per frame with 50 msec exposure time.

Photo spot camera can also be used for spot filming with an adequate image quality but gives only minified image compared to life size image of the spot film. Spot film recording gives a spatial resolution of 8 lp/mm, frame rate of 1/sec and patient entrance skin dose of 2 mGy. In the case of photo spot camera, it is 5 lp/mm, 12/sec and 1 mGy, respectively.

Cine fluoroscopy records series of photo spot images in rapid sequence. Grid controlled X-ray tube with small focus is used. X-ray pulses needs to be synchronized with cine shutter. It records moving images on a 35 mm cinematographic film with images of 18 × 24 mm size. Frame rates are of 15, 30, 60 or 90 frames per second and 30 frame/sec is often used. The image intensifier circle should fit exactly within the film. After processing, the images can be viewed on cine mode. Heart examinations are performed with cine fluoroscopy. The images have good contrast with reduced geometric blurring.

Automatic Exposure Systems

In fluoroscopy imaging, if an image intensifier moves from a thinner to thicker region of the patient, higher the amount of attenuation of X-rays. This will reduce the brightness of an output screen. Automatic exposure system (AES) previously known as an automatic brightness control (ABC) is a mechanism, which can keep the brightness of the image constant at the monitor. It is basically a feedback circuit, which measure the light intensity of an output screen or video camera signal. *A photomultiplier or a photodiode* is used to monitor the light output of II tube. The corresponding changes will be feedback to the generator for an adjustment. The generator will regulate the X-ray exposure rate incident on an input phosphor of II tube, by changing the kV or mA automatically. In system with fiber optic coupling, video signal from a central area of an image is monitored. Thus, AES ensures a constant average dose rate at an input window of an image intensifier, so that an image brightness is independent of X-ray attenuation in patient.

In general, the brightness of central area of an output phosphor is considered for an adjustment. Brightness can be adjusted by both kV and mA, which has influence on contrast and patient dose, respectively. The three methods of adjustments are possible, (1) change of kV at constant mA, (2) change of mA at constant kV, and (3) change of both kV and mA. If the II tube moves from thinner to thicker part of the patient, an increase of kV may result in lower dose with lesser contrast, but an increase of mA may result in better contrast with higher dose.

Alternatively, the brightness of an image on the monitor can be adjusted by varying the gain of TV system, which is called an *automatic gain control (AGC)*. This will result in an increased image noise and an unwanted radiation dose. Generally, mA is adjusted as a first step to obtain an input dose rate of II tube. If the current limit is reached, then kV is adjusted to get an input dose rate. Even it is not sufficient then, an AGC option is used to adjust the video display brightness. Thus, an AES provides constant image brightness on the television or flat panel monitor systems, irrespective of an anatomical thickness.

Image Intensifier Image Quality and Artifacts

The fluoroscopic image quality can be described by (1) *spatial resolution,* (2) *contrast,* (3) *noise,* (4) *sharpness,* and (5) *artifacts. Various artifacts include:* (1) *lag,* (2) *veiling glare,* (3) *vignetting,* (4) *blooming,* (5) *pincushion distortion,* and (6) *S-distortion.*

Spatial resolution is the ability to detect fine detail and it is 3–5 lp/mm for II tube. However, CCD (1.7 lp/mm), an video camera and TV monitor (1.2–3 lp/mm) will degrade an image quality in conventional fluoroscopy. Lesser diameter of II tube will offer higher resolution. However, II tube with CCD in digital fluoroscopy may offer much improved resolution.

Subject contrast in fluoroscopy is low compared with radiography because low exposure levels produce images with relatively low signal-to-noise ratio (SNR). However, contrast is improved by using radiopaque markers and contrast agents like Iodine. Excellent temporal resolution of fluoroscopy is its strength and its reason for an existence.

Generally, fluoroscopy image is noisy which influences the contrast resolution. Noise can be reduced by increasing an input dose rate, increasing mA, resulting in higher dose to the patient. Alternatively, noise can be reduced by *frame averaging.* In this, successive images are added together pixel by pixel and an average value is displayed as an image. There should be no movement between the frames, otherwise blurring may occur in an image. Flat panel systems suffer from high electronic noise.

Image sharpness is influenced by several factors. Noise interacts with sharpness and obscure and blur small details in the image. Multiple signal conversions in the II tube degrades sharpness. In flat panel, sharpness is affected by display matrix and pixel size.

Artifacts

II tube's output phosphor continues to emit light even after the X-ray has stopped. This is known as referred to as *lag* in fluoroscopy. The lag time is low for CsI tubes, it is about 1 msec.

Veiling glare is due to scattering in the II tube, which reduces an image contrast. It causes an central area of an image brighter than the periphery. Scattering of light at an input phosphor and output window and electron scattering in the II tube accounts for the above effect. The larger the II tube size, the greater the veiling glare. It can be minimized by using a thick output window in II tube, but it should have *Dopants* to absorb light and sides coated with light absorbing materials. Fiber optic coupling instead of lens may be beneficial.

Vignetting is fall off brightness at the periphery of an image intensifier and it is about 25%. It is due to an optical distortion which produces darkening near the edges. It is caused by lenses, and video camera. It can be minimized by reducing an aperture size.

Blooming is caused when an input signal to the video camera exceeds its dynamic range. It creates lateral charge spread within the camera target, resulting diffuse image which is larger than an original image.

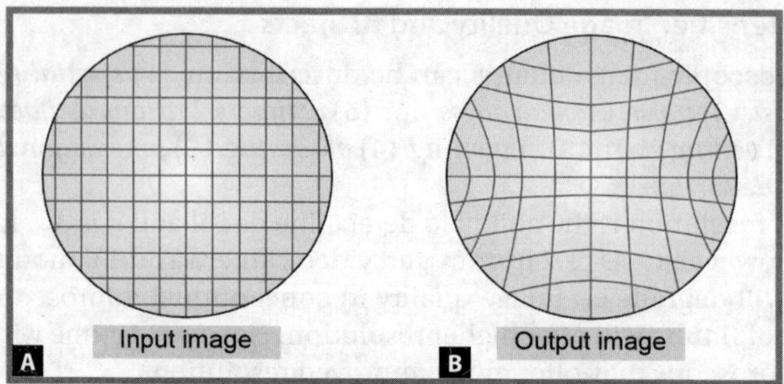

Figs. 9.9A and B: Pincushion distortion.

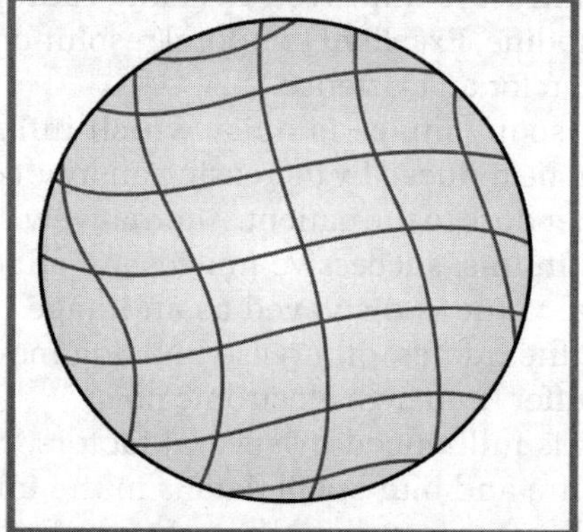

Fig. 9.10: S-type distortion.

Pincushion distortion is due to curved geometry of an input screen. Straight line appears as curved, and it is 3% for a 23 cm II tube. Though curved nature of II tube enhances an electron focusing but results in pincushion distortion. The resultant image at an output phosphor appears as distorted **(Figs. 9.9A and B).** The II tube base plate is also curved, it produces both *pincushion and vignetting*. Imperfection in an electron focusing and optical system may also influence this.

S-type distortion is caused by the effect of magnetic field on an electron paths **(Fig. 9.10).** Pincushion distortion and S-type distortion are combinedly referred to as *geometric distortion*. These distortions are not visible and less significant during fluoroscopy imaging.

Limitations of Image Intensifier Systems

❑ The device is large, and difficult to position during the procedure.
❑ If there is air leak in the II tube, the vacuum is destroyed, resulting in degraded image quality.

❏ If the voltage of an electrode is not correctly adjusted, an electron will not reach the focal point (defocusing effect). It may result in blurred image with loss of spatial resolution.
❏ Variation of magnetic and stray electromagnetic fields from power supply may give defocusing effect.
❏ The television system depends upon the raster lines and bandwidth frequency for spatial resolution. Its resolution is always lesser than II tube's output screen image.

DIGITAL FLUOROSCOPY

Digital fluoroscopy is a digital X-ray imaging that produces dynamic images. The nature of an image and the way in which it is digitized is different from conventional fluoroscopy. It was developed by the *University of Wisconsin* and *Arizona* (1970). Initially, the signal from a video camera is routed through a computer for manipulation and transmitted to the monitor for display. In this, an image acquisition is fast with postprocessing techniques which improves an image contrast. Spatial resolution is limited by the pixel size:

$$\text{Pixel size} = \frac{\text{Image intensifier size}}{\text{Matrix}}$$

Generally, 1024 × 1024 matrix size is used, referred to as 100-line system in fluoroscopy. Its advantages include: (1) image storage facility, (2) image processing such as noise reduction, and edge enhancement, (3) black and white reversal, i.e., display of – and + images, (4) geometrical inversion, i.e., left to right and top to bottom, (5) dose reduction, (6) wide dynamic range, (7) dynamic imaging, and (8) filmless imaging. The images are compatible to picture archiving and communication systems (PACS).

The digital fluoroscopy is same as conventional fluoroscopy but added with computer and multiple monitors. Operating consoles have provision for entering patient data and communication with computer. It also has an interactive video control, pad for curser and region of an interest marking. Other part of the console has provision for data acquisition and an image display. There are two monitors, one to edit patient and examination data and to the other annotate final images. The other monitor is used to display subtracted images.

During the fluoroscopy operation, the X-ray tube operates in radiography mode with few 100-mA tube current. If tube is energized continuously, it may fail due to an overheating and the patient radiation is higher. Hence, X-rays are pulsed in nature which is referred to *pulse progressive fluoroscopy*. Generally, the image acquisition rate is 1–10 per second and 33 msec is required to produce a video frame.

If the system uses flat panel image receptor instead of II tube, an exposure time varies. The X-ray generator must have rapid ON and OFF provision. The duration from the ON condition to reach the peak kV is called an *interrogation time*. The time required to switch OFF the X-ray tube is called an *extinction time* (<1 msec). *Duty cycle* is the fraction of time the X-ray tube is energized.

Usually, the tube is energized for 100 msec in every second, it is roughly 10% duty cycle.

In digital fluoroscopy, either charge-coupled device (CCD) or flat panel image receptor are used and the latter is most common.

Charge-coupled Device as Receptor

Charge-coupled device (CCD) is used to get digital signal of II tube output light. CCD replaces the thermionic television camera system in II tube **(Fig. 9.11).** It is a solid-state imaging sensor without an electron gun and deflection coils and an evacuation, etc. When light incident on the CCD, an electrical charge is generated which is processed to have a digital signal. This signal is proportional to an intensity of light from II tube's output screen.

CDD is mounted on an output phosphor of II tube and coupled with a lens system or fiber optics. In the case of lens coupling, it is possible to sense the entire CCD input light by a sensor to operate an AES system. The input screen of CCD camera is a semiconductor photosensitive surface, which is divided into thousands of an individual photodiodes and arranged in rows and columns.

Generally, an *amorphous Silicon* (thin) is used as an input screen, which is divided into number of pixels (1024 × 1024). The camera is operated under 12 V supply and a fiber optic system is used to focus the light on an input screen. The CCD camera is having 12-bit image depth, so that the dynamic range is higher.

When an output phosphor light incident on CCD, an electrical charge is generated. Each pixel acts as capacitor and charge are collected pixel by pixel. The collected charge on each pixel is readout row by row. The readout can be

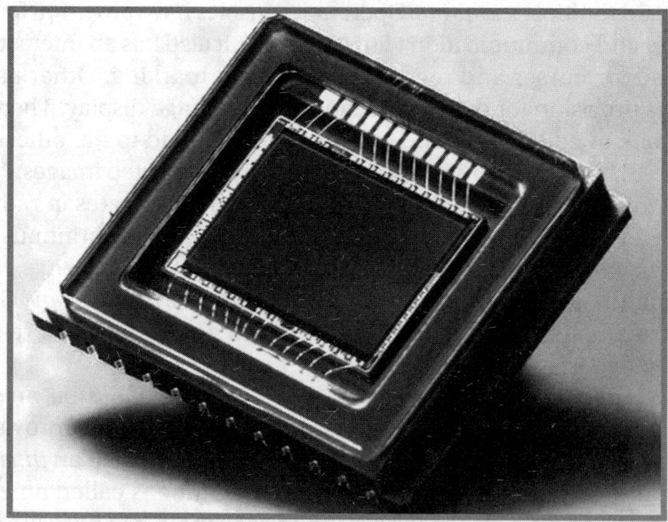

Fig. 9.11: Charge-coupled device (CCD).

done quickly at the rate of 30 frames per second. The stored information in each row is shifted electronically and readout as video waveform.

CCD is simple, small size and rugged system. Its spatial resolution depends on its physical size and pixel count. Systems with 1024×1024 matrix size can able to provide a spatial resolution of 10 lp/mm. There is no pincushion or barrel artifacts. It has greater sensitivity to light with lesser electronic noise compared to television camera. Thus, it provides higher signal to noise ratio (SNR), linear response, and better contrast. Its linear response is much useful in digital subtraction angiography (DSA). Some of the advantage of CCD digital fluoroscopy are:

❑ High spatial resolution
❑ High DQE and SNR
❑ Extended life
❑ Lower radiation dose to patient
❑ No lag and spatial distortion

Flat Panel Image Receptor

In an image intensifier receptor technology, the spatial and contrast resolution is nonuniform from the center to periphery of the circular image. Veiling glare and pincushion distortion increases with age of II tube. Hence, flat panel image receptors (FPIR) replace II tube with CCD camera in digital fluoroscopy. They directly absorbs X-rays emits light in turn an electronic signal **(Fig. 9.12)**.

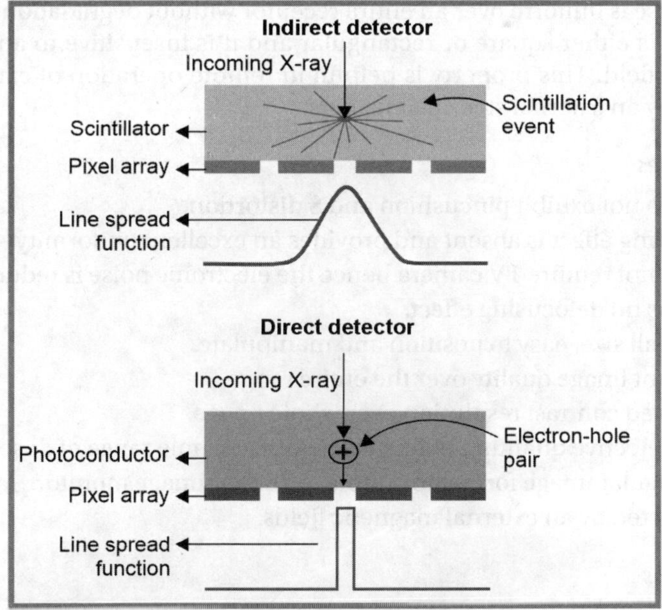

Fig. 9.12: Flat panel detector principle (top) an indirect detector, and (bottom) direct detector.

The commonly used detectors are an indirect solid-state system. It is a *Cesium iodide (CsI)* phosphor with an *amorphous Silicon (a-Si)* pixels. FPIR consists of an array of individual detector elements (DEL), of varying size of 200–140 μm. The size of array ranges from 25 × 25 to 40 × 40 cm. A typical FPIR may contain 1.5–5 million DEL's.

The transmitted X-ray from the patient incident on the CsI phosphor which emits light proportional to X-ray intensity. This light falls on an *amorphous Silicon photodiode* and electrons are released. The conduction of photodiode varies in proportion to light intensity. The electrons reach the fully charged capacitor and neutralize some of the charges. The remaining charge in the capacitor is drained out and sent to readout electronics which measure the change caused by the X-rays. This is repeated many times per second. By reading the DEL row by row, an electronic image distribution of X-rays that are incident on the FPIR can be formed. Thus, FPIR forms an image without TV camera.

CsI phosphor's detective quantum efficiency is 65% and having advantages of an increased dynamic range and improved spatial resolution. Hence, flat panel detects greater range of signal and its contrast resolution is about 3 lp/mm for a pixel size of 150 μm. Image intensifier's maximum spatial resolution is 1.2 lp/mm for a given largest FOV, which is equal to a pixel size of 400 μm. In the case of magnification, flat panel does not improve spatial resolution since the pixel size remains the same. Alternatively, an image intensifier improves the resolution with magnification.

FPIR is much smaller and light weight which can be easily manipulated. Its response is uniform over an entire receptor without degradation over age. Its image is either square or rectangular and it is insensitive to an external magnetic field. This property is helpful in remote operation of catheters in patients by an external steering magnets.

Advantages

- They do not exhibit pincushion and S distortion.
- Vignetting effect is absent and provides an excellent uniformity.
- It does not require TV camera hence the electronic noise is reduced.
- There is no defocusing effect.
- It is small size, easy to position and manipulate.
- Constant image quality over the entire range.
- Improved contrast resolution over whole image.
- High detective quantum efficiency (DQE) at whole range of dose levels.
- Rectangular image format to couple to similar image monitor.
- Unaffected by an external magnetic fields.

Limitations

- It is difficult to manufacture a flat panel detector without defective detector element.

❑ Software interpolates values for defective detector element which may create artifacts.
❑ Flat panel is sensitive to temperature and mechanical shock.
❑ Its resolution is limited by the size of detective element.

Digital Image Display

Digital fluoroscopy requires SNR of 1000:1, to preserve lower signals against noise. In high SNR, an image contrast will not be degraded. Its dynamic range is about 2^{10}, the SNR gives 5 times more information. It is much important in digital subtraction techniques.

Image can be displayed either by video or flat panel format. Video system used in the conventional fluoroscopy is not suitable. Here, TV camera tube operates in progressive mode and form an image on the monitor. When a video signal is read in a progressive mode, an electron beam of the TV camera sweeps the target continuously from top to bottom in 533 msec. There is no interlace of one field to another field here.

Flat panel image display replaces cathode ray tubes in digital fluoroscopy. It is easier to view, postprocessing and provide better images. They are light weight, easily mounted in suspended position for an angiography procedure.

DIGITAL FLUOROSCOPY EQUIPMENT

Typical digital fluoroscopy equipment used today are C-arm geometry with following configurations: (1) X-ray tube plus II tube with fiberoptic coupling with CCD, (2) cantilevered C-arm having an X-ray tube with flat panel detector system embedded with DSA, and (3) cardiovascular system having an X-ray tube with flat panel image receptor system.

The first type is used for *orthopedic intervention, foreign body localization, cholangiography, cystography, pyelography, and cardiac pacemaker implantation.* Mostly, they are mobile fluoroscopy C-arm machines often used in an operation theaters and intensive care units. These machine employes 15–23 cm detector system.

The second type finds application in vascular intervention studies, neurovascular imaging and peripheral angiography. In this, the table does not rotate but floats; the patient is allowed to move in lateral and longitudinal directions. It is a C-arm unit which can be rotated and skewed, to take posteroanterior, lateral and an oblique views. The power injectors are table or ceiling mounted. Detector size of 30–44 cm is used in peripheral angiogram whereas 23 cm–30 cm size is used in neuro angiogram.

The third type is used exclusively for cardiac angiography, as cardiology catheterization suite **(Fig. 9.13).** Such units have small flat panel detectors (23 cm), permits more cranial caudal tilt, high frame rates, with pulsed X-ray cineradiography. Nowadays biplane systems are used to reduce the amount of contrast. It has one table with two X-ray generators and two detectors set-up. It gives two orthogonal views of an area of interest simultaneously with single

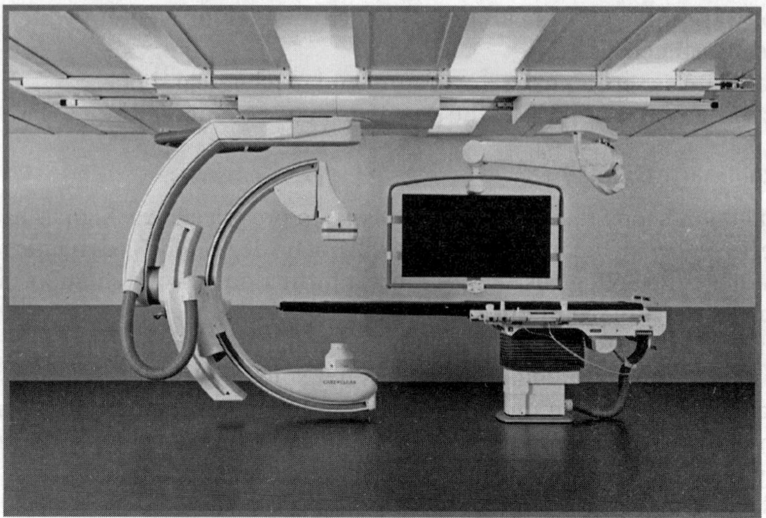

Fig. 9.13: Cardiac catheterization laboratory for interventional cardiology procedures.
(*Courtesy:* GE Healthcare)

contrast injection. It reduces the use of contrast material and its reactions and permits the evaluation of more vessels. It excludes scattered radiation of other imaging chain and permit the use of single plane studies.

Basic principle of *arterial access* interventional procedure was provided first by **Ivar Seldinger** (1953). An 18-gauze needle is inserted with stylet in the *femoral artery*. Once the *pulsating blood* returns, the *stylet* is removed. A *guide wire* (145 cm long) is then inserted through the needle into an *arterial path*. Now the needle is removed, and the *catheter* (10 cm long, 3Fr dia.) is threaded onto the guide wire. Under fluoroscopy, the catheter is advanced along the guide wire. Guide wire helps in placing the catheter within the blood vessel. After the catheter is placed the guide wire is removed. *Heparinized saline* use is used to flush catheter to prevent blood clotting. Finally, a test injection is given to check the correct position of the catheter under fluoroscopy.

DIGITAL MODES OF OPERATION

Continuous Fluoroscopy

Continuous fluoroscopy is a basic form of fluoroscopy imaging. The X-ray beam is always ON and gives continuous exposure. The video camera refreshes at the rate of 25–30 frames/sec. The frame integration time is 40 or 33 msec which may lead to blurring of moving objects.

Pulsed Fluoroscopy

Pulse fluoroscopy uses short pulses of X-rays. It is obtained with *grid-controlled or grid-switched X-ray tube* or operating a generator in pulsed mode. Many photons are produced within short time intervals of each pulse without increasing the kilovoltage. Thus, it offers a great degree of dose reduction to the patient with an improved temporal resolution. The production of pulses and the video system need to be synchronized. The pulses may be seen as a *tooth or square wave pulse* and is generated before the start of each readout cycle. The duration of pulse should be lesser than that of readout cycle.

In practice, the pulse gets distorted due to the capacitance of long high-tension cable hence, and the pulse has longer rise and decay time. This may cause production of low energy X-ray, which will increase the patient dose. It has the following advantages:

❏ Reduces radiation dose
❏ Improved image quality due to reduced integration time
❏ Freezes object motion and gives sharper images
❏ Reduce temporal resolution at low frame rates

Frame Averaging

Frame averaging is an algorithm assisted preprocessing. It is known that fluoroscopy has high temporal resolution and relatively high noise. Sometimes, the temporal resolution is intentionally lowered to reduce noise. This is possible by averaging series of images which causes an image *lag*. It refers to fraction of an image data from one frame to next frame. Commonly used algorithm is *recursive filtering* in which just acquired image is added together with last displayed image. X-ray photons of several images are combined into one image which is known as *frame averaging* which is a common future in mobile C-arm units. Frame averaging is based on specific application and objective.

Last Frame Hold

When the fluoroscopy mode is switched OFF, the monitor displays the last acquired image. It is a standard future in all modern fluoroscopy units. Fluoroscopy machine continuously digitizes image in real time and temporarily store on the video frame memory. When the mode is switched OFF, the last image is displayed on the monitor without showing patient anatomy. Last frame hold feature permits an examination of images as long as necessary without radiation. It is a necessary feature for dose reduction in fluoroscopy.

Road Mapping

Road mapping is a software and video enhanced assisted variation of the last frame hold feature. It is much useful in angiography. There are two ways of doing it: (1) positioning side by side video monitors and capture an image then shown on the monitor next to the live fluoroscopy monitor. In this, the path of a vessel is seen in one monitor and the catheter advances real time on an other monitor. (2) Capturing a contrast injected image or subtracted image and use this as overlay on the live fluoroscopy monitor image. This method gives an vascular roadmap superimposed on the live fluoroscopy image. It is useful to guide the catheter tip to negotiate into the patient.

DIGITAL SUBTRACTION ANGIOGRAPHY

Digital subtraction angiography (DSA) is a type of fluoroscopy technique used in an interventional radiology/cardiology (1970). In this, one can visualize an image of the blood vessels that are filled with contrast, in a boney or soft tissue environment. Angiography is the study of blood vessels in the body after an injection of Iodine contrast (Angio = blood vessel). Subtraction is a technique in which images of bone are subtracted to clearly visualize images of an unobscured vessels. Hence, DSA is an acquisition of fluoroscopic images along with an injection of contrast and real time subtraction of pre-and postcontrast images.

For example, it is helpful to identify narrowing of proximal internal carotid artery. It gives an enhanced visualization of vasculature because of an injection of contrast in the vessel. Blood vessels normally not seen in the X-ray because of low atomic number and low contrast. Dense fluid like Iodine of high atomic number and density increases contrast. Iodine contrast absorbs many-fold X-ray photos than blood and tissue. Generally, Compton scatter in a X-ray beam area reduces an image contrast. It is possible to improve the contrast by electronically to some extent. However, digital subtraction gives better contrast enhancement for the visualization of vessels. DSA requires injection of contrast material in blood vessel, image subtraction and postprocessing. It can be used in both diagnostic and therapeutic indications. However, caution is needed in patients with poor renal reserve, deranged coagulogram and allergic to contrast media.

DSA Equipment

Digital subtraction angiography equipment is basically a fluoroscopy X-ray machine, with X-ray tube, X-ray generator, an image intensifier with video camera or flat panel system. It is a C-arm type X-ray machine which can rotate axially and sagittally around a floating-top table. The II tube is coupled with CCD camera or replaced by a flat panel image receptor system. It has collimators and filters, pulsed fluoroscopy with an variety of frame rates for dose reduction. It also has provision to change and display collimator position without fluoroscopy, road mapping and land marking, last image hold and frame grab, an image enhancement and display of images side by side. It also has masks, different range manipulations, cine and quantification and measurement facility.

Video camera generates an analog electronic signal proportional to an input light received by its camera target. Digital image processing is a vital system which acquires images from the video camera, digitizes and store them in the computer memory. There are two memories, one for the mask image and the other for contrast image. The image content is subtracted in an arithmetic unit, processed, and converted back into an analog signal. Then,

Table 9.1: Comparison of temporal and energy subtraction techniques.

Temporal subtraction	*Energy subtraction*
Single kV$_p$ setting is used	Rapid kV$_p$ switching is needed
Normal X-ray filtration is enough	X-ray beam filter switching is preferred
Contrast resolution is 1 mm at 1%	Higher intensity is required for comparable contrast resolution
Simple arithmetic subtraction is needed	Complex image subtraction is necessary
Motion artifact is an issue	Motion artifacts are greatly reduced
Total subtraction of common structures is possible	Some residual bone may survive subtraction
Subtraction capability is limited by the number of images	Many more types of subtraction images are possible

(*Courtesy:* Stewart Carlyle Bushong et al, 2017)

the signal is displayed on a high-resolution monitor. Images can be stored on a magnetic hard disk and computer but needs large memory of the order of 512 MB–1GB. The acquisition and processing are controlled by the CPU of the computer.

DSA Procedure

The patient is laid on the table and local anesthesia or general anesthesia is given. Blood vessel is accessed for puncturing by using an ultrasound. Standard access kit consists of 18-gauge needle and 0.035″ guide wires through which an interventional catheter is threaded. Noncontrast image is taken before injecting contrast material which shows only an anatomy and other foreign bodies as regular X-rays. After contrast injection, contrast image is taken, which shows an opacified vessels super imposed on an anatomy and are stored in the computer. The first image (mask) is subtracted from the contrast image by pixel by pixel. This image shows only filled vessels which can be viewed on real time. The subtracted image looks nosier. After the procedure *hemostasis* is applied on the puncture site.

Digital Subtraction Methods

There are two methods of digital subtraction, namely (1) *temporal subtraction, and (2) energy subtraction* and former is commonly used. If both techniques are combined it is referred as *hybrid subtraction* which gives still enhanced contrast image. Comparison of above two techniques is given in **Table 9.1.**

Temporal subtraction refers to subtraction of image obtained at one time from an image obtained later. It highlights changes over time by performing subtraction process. If contrast is injected before the second image, subtracted image shows only the vessel filled with contrast. There are two methods of temporal subtraction, namely (1) *mask mode,* (2) *time-interval difference (TID) mode.*

Logarithmic Subtraction

Attenuation of X-rays is an exponential and subtraction should fulfill the following conditions: (1) the subtracted image signal must be linear to the concentration of the contrast medium, and (2) subtracted image should be independent of an overlying tissue. Hence, direct linear subtraction of images is not used, instead logarithmic subtraction is used. The mask image and the contrast image are converted into their logarithms initially and then subtracted. Logarithmic subtraction ensures a vessel of uniform diameter with an uniform contrast; even it passes through regions of varying thickness. It does not retain stationary anatomical structures, which may obscure small signals. Finally, the signal is converted into an intensity level for display, which is independent of patient size. The intensity depends on the product of vessel thickness and an attenuation coefficient of the contrast medium.

Mask Mode

Digital images are obtained before and after an injection of contrast medium, to differentiate vascular pathology from surrounding anatomy. It is a noninvasive procedure, that provides an improved image quality with lesser use of contrast medium. The following steps are carried out:

Step 1: The patient is positioned on the couch so that the region of an interest is within the field of view. Imaging system is changed from fluoroscopy to digital fluoroscopy mode. In this mode, X-tube draws about 20–100 times more current. The image of a particular anatomical region is taken by using pulsed X-rays. The image is recorded and stored in the primary memory which is displayed on the first video monitor. This is called preinjection mask image (A), which shows normal anatomy of the region. It requires 2 frames, the first is used to stabilize the system (technical factors) and the second frame is stored as preinjection mask image.

Step 2: With the help of a power injector about 30–50 mL of contrast, at the rate of 15–20 mL/s is injected through an venous. If artery is chosen, about 10–25 mL of diluted contrast is injected at the rate of 10–12 mL/s. After the injection of contrast, confirming that the contrast reaches the anatomical site, series of an additional images are taken with pulsed X-rays. These images are stored in an adjacent memory. It is called contrast image (B), which shows contrast filled vessels, superimposed on an anatomy.

Step 3: The mask image is subtracted from each contrast image (B-A), by pixel by pixel basis and stored in the primary memory as contrast-mask image (C). The subtracted images are displayed on the second monitor. This image reveals only vessels filled with contrast medium **(Figs. 9.14A to C).**

The final image is viewed in real time. There should not be any movement of patient during the above procedure and an image is obtained rapidly. Movement between frames may lead to misregistration of an image especially at the bone edge. This can be minimized by movement of mask, which is called *pixel shifting* that can be done manually of automatically.

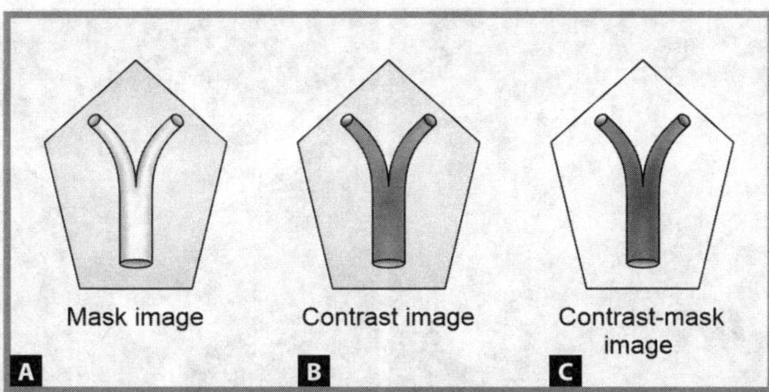

Figs. 9.14A to C: Principle of digital subtraction angiography: (A) Mask image; (B) Contrast image, (C) Contrast-mask image.

Digital subtraction is good for static objects, it provides better analysis of an opacified arteries. Patient motion or inadequate technique may give an insufficient mask image. In that case, later images are taken as mask image, known as *demasking.* Typical procedure may need about 30 images apart from the mask image. Since the duration of X-ray pulse is 33 ms, the time required for one video frame is 33 msec. Generally, video system is not only slow but also involves higher noise. Hence, several video frames are summed to create a single image. This process is called an *image integration.* Manually or preprogrammed control of an imaging sequence is possible, after taking the mask image.

To reduce scatter, special algorithm is used. Taking successive frames reduce quantum mottle and increases SNR. However, subtracted image reduces SNR and an image looks noisier. Hence, higher mA is used in DSA.

If the length of an anatomy is greater than the FOV (e.g., leg), then multiple images are taken to cover the entire anatomy. Each time, the contrast is injected to that region. However, modern machine provides software that acquires several mask images and contrast images over the full length of an anatomy. This is facilitated by table movement and its position for each image. Appropriate mask image for a given table position is subtracted from the contrast image. There is a chance of movement during the above procedure. The temporal subtraction has an advantage of changing contrast during the procedure and has no dements on the nature of high voltage generator.

Time-interval Difference Mode

In the time-interval difference (TID), region of an interest is exposed to higher kV (120–130 kV) and lower kV (70 kV) at very short interval (50 msec). Then, high kV image is subtracted from the lower kV image. The only difference is each subtracted image is made from different mask, called *progressive masks.* The mask image is obtained before contrast injection. After contrast injection, an image is acquired for 5 seconds. In 4 seconds, about 60 images are obtained

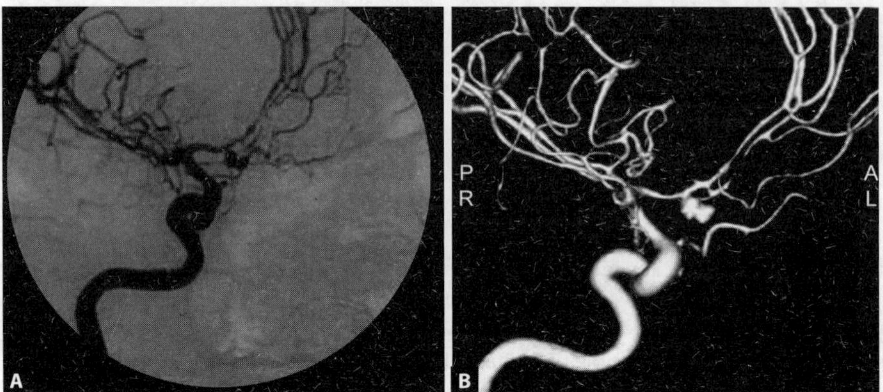

Figs. 9.15A and B: Rotational angiogram: Cerebral angiogram, endovascular coiling anterior communicating aneurysm: (A) Preprocessed image; (B) Postprocessed image.

at the rate of 15 images per second. If TID of 4 images is required, then frame 1 is subtracted from frame 5, frame 2 is subtracted from 6, 3 is subtracted from 7, and 4 is subtracted from 8, respectively.

The real time images show dynamic flow of contrast. It is free from motion artifacts but with less contrast compared to mask mode subtraction. This technique is mainly used in cardiac evaluation. If motion arises between the mask and subsequent image, misregistration artifacts may occur in the subtracted images.

Rotational Angiography

Rotational angiography is a medical imaging technique by using X-rays, which creates 3D volume like CT scan. A fixed C-arm machine rotates around the patient and generates a series of X-ray images which are reconstructed by software to get 3D image. It can be done for a patient during surgery or during catheter insertion.

For example, mask images are taken at several angles, by rotating the X-ray tube and II tube for a 90° rotation. Similarly, postcontrast images are taken from each angle and subtracted suitably. This may be used for 3D reconstruction of vessels, which can be viewed at any angle (**Figs. 9.15A and B**). This is a useful technique when there is a superposition of vessels that are lying one over the other.

Energy Subtraction Mode

Energy subtraction technique uses two different X-ray beams (energies) alternatively to create images. The subtracted image is a result of differences in photoelectric absorption. Generally, 32 and 34 keV X-ray beam are used. Since Iodine k-edge is 33 keV, there will be sudden absorption at the 33 keV for Iodine contrast. The subsequent image will have higher contrast but in bone and soft tissue, the absorption is moderate. In practice, it is done in two ways

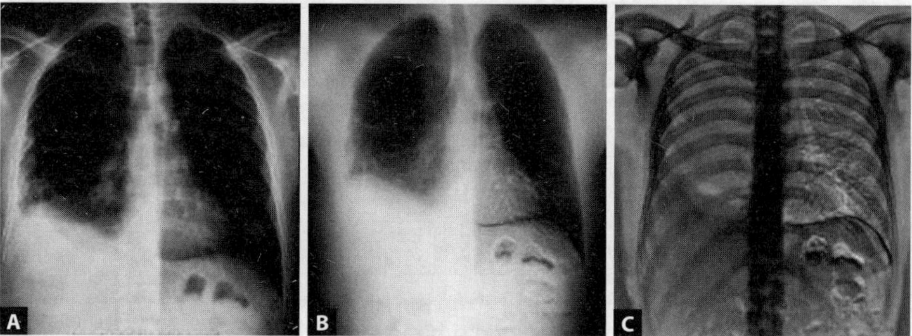

Figs. 9.16A to C: (A) Normal chest radiograph; (B) Bone subtracted; (C) Soft tissue subtracted.

(1) alternatively pulsing the X-ray beam at 70 kV and 90 kV, and (2) having dissimilar filters on fly wheel, into the X-ray beam.

The first method is called *dual energy subtraction technique* it is based on the concept that linear attenuation coefficient decreases with an increase of energy. The decrease is greater in bone than in soft tissue. In this technique, images of the same anatomical region are taken rapidly at low kV and high kV. When the low kV image is subtracted from the high kV image, soft tissue details get canceled, and gives only bone details **(Figs. 9.16A to C)**. Similarly, subtraction of high kV images from the low kV image, cancels details of bone anatomy and highlights only soft tissue. This technique is insensitive to patient motion and remove effects due to an involuntary motion of bowel gas.

Hybrid Subtraction

Hybrid subtraction is dual-energy digital fluoroscopy to provide pre- and postcontrast images with the soft tissues subtracted. These pre-and postcontrast soft-tissue-cancelled images are then subtracted by temporal subtraction.

Step 1: Mask image is taken with low kV and high kV. Then low kV- high kV subtraction is obtained. Energy subtraction gives the bone mask image. In this process, the soft tissue is eliminated.

Step 2: Idoine contrast is injected, and contrast image is obtained at low and high kV. Low kV contrast-high kV contrast subtraction is done. Energy subtraction gives bone + Iodine contrast image. In this process, the soft tissue is eliminated.

Step 3: Now temporal subtraction is performed. That is bone mask image is subtracted from the bone + Iodine contrast image. It provides only Iodine contrast image which is a hybrid one. In this process, the bone is eliminated but gives only vessel details **(Fig. 9.17)**.

It eliminates overlying bone and movement related misregistration issues. It also eliminates the artifact related to soft tissue motion. However, there is an increased noise with higher radiation exposure to the patient.

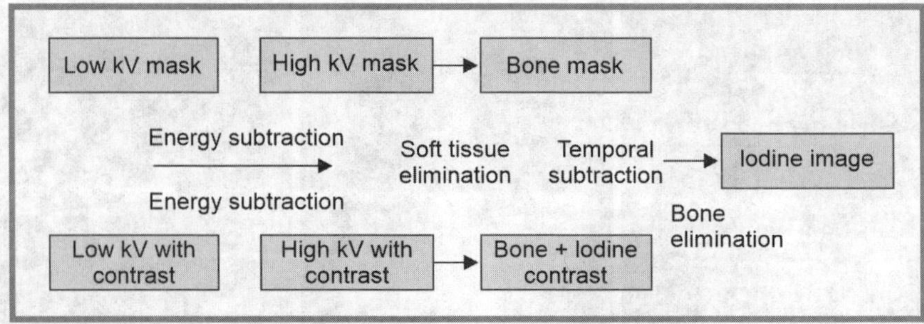

Fig. 9.17: Hybrid subtraction principle.

DIGITAL FLUOROSCOPY IMAGE QUALITY

Image quality in digital fluoroscopy is analyzed based on (1) spatial resolution, (2) contrast resolution, and (3) temporal resolution.

Spatial Resolution

Spatial resolution is 2.2 lp/mm for 23 cm FOV of II/TV system of matrix size 1024×1024 that has a pixel dimension of 230 mm/1024 = 0.22 mm, resulting a resolution of 2.2 lp/mm. However, resolution is limited by the sampling frequency, namely:

$$\text{Nyquist frequency} = 1/2\Delta$$

where, Δ is the size of the detector element. For a 30 cm FOV and 1024×1024 matrix size, $\Delta = 300$ mm/1024 = 0.29 mm. The corresponding Nyquist frequency $= 1/2\Delta = 1/(2 \times 0.29) = 1.7$ lp/mm. This is the maximum resolution possible in a digitally sampled system. Flat panels are so designed to have same or better resolution in digital fluoroscopy. In the case of a flat panel system, the sampling frequency is fixed. Hence, its resolution is independent of FOV.

Contrast Resolution

Contrast resolution is low in fluoroscopy due to low SNR. Use of high exposure rates improves contrast resolution, but patient dose also increases. Scattered radiation also contributes to low contrast resolution. Use of an antiscatter grid ratio of 6:1 to 12:1 will improve resolution. However, it increases patient dose 2–4 times hence, it is not recommended in pediatrics and an extremity in digital fluoroscopy.

Temporal Resolution

Fluoroscopy has an excellent temporal resolution by which it gives real time images. Temporal blurring is referred to as *lag*. This is intentionally done by using *recursive filtering*. It causes blurring in several temporal frame images together and increases SNR. Human eye also has lag of 0.2 sec so that six frames are averaged together which also increases SNR 2.5 times. Thus, an increase in SNR improves contrast resolution at an expense of temporal resolution. Lag is not always beneficial, and it is not desirable while recording dynamic events in DSA.

RADIATION DOSIMETRY

Benefit and Risk

Fluoroscopy has wide applications, such as photo spot imaging, spot film acquisition, digital subtraction angiography (DSA), an endoscopic examination, lithotripsy, and cineradiography. Fluoroscopy has both benefits and risks. Fluoroscopy finds clinical application in Barium enema, Barium swallow, interventional radiology, cardiology, and neuroradiology, enteroclysis, lumbar puncture, myelogram, location of foreign bodies, image guided anesthetic injections, percutaneous vertebroplasty, intravenous pyelogram, anthography, hysterosalpingogram, biopsy, and an upper gastrointestinal and small bowel series.

Cardiac catheterization is a procedure in which an intravenous catheter is inserted to see the blood flow in coronary arteries with fluoroscopy assistance. Fluoroscopy examination which visualizes a vessel is called *angiography*. It has application in neuroradiology and vascular radiology. The benefits are:

❑ To study movement and function
❑ Guide lifesaving surgical treatments

The associated risks are:

❑ High radiation exposure
❑ Longer exposure time
❑ Use of contrast material

Radiation induced cancer and skin injuries have been reported earlier. Pregnant women should notify the physician before the procedure. Patients allergic to sensitive medications, contrast or Iodine should also notify to the physician.

Radiation Dose

Fluoroscopy imaging is increasingly used in cardiology and radiology. Its imaging time is higher, and it may vary from 1–3 minutes for a simple examination to 15–60 minutes for an interventional procedure. Exposure time in fluoroscopy is longer than that of radiography. Therefore, the radiation dose is higher for both patient and the operator.

Skin is a vital tissue in fluoroscopy hence, an *entrance skin exposure (ESE)* is considered as parameter for dose estimation in fluoroscopy. Since X-ray field moves with varying size, it is difficult to access an ESE. If one field size is used in stationary mode, an ESE is directly related to an exposure time. High dose rate fluoroscopy is the choice to maintain an image quality. The maximum legal limit of an ESE is 100 mGy/min (10 R/min) for normal fluoroscopy and 200 mGy/min (20 R/min) for high dose fluoroscopy (FDA, USA). Any skin dose exceeding 15 Gy should be reported as a *sentinel event*, recommends the center for devices and radiation health (CDRH), USA .

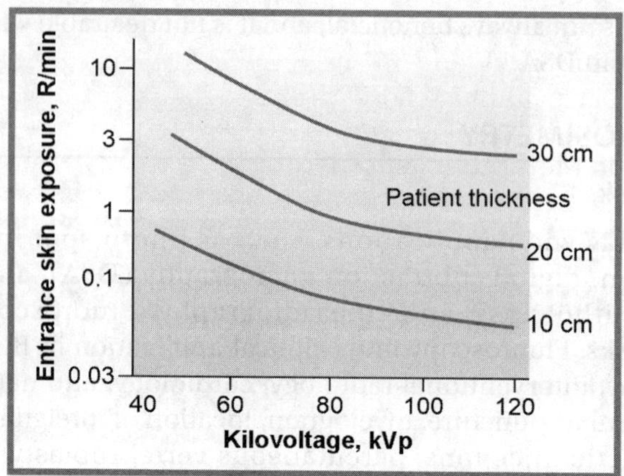

Fig. 9.18: Variation of entrance skin exposure (ESE) with kVp and patient thickness.

A typical ESE rate in fluoroscopy examination is 9–17 mGy/min (1–2 R/min) for thin body parts and 26–44 mGy/min (3–5 R/min) for an average patient (Dose in air = 0.00876 Gy/R). It will vary with kV and patient thickness. Higher the kV and lesser the patient thickness, lesser the radiation dose to patient **(Fig. 9.18).** ESE will be higher for an oblique and lateral projections. Average skin entrance dose should not exceed 40 mGy/min to the patient. A procedure with 1 minute screening, at the rate of 50 mGy/min dose rate is equal to 15 pelvis radiographs.

Digital fluoroscopy offers lesser patient dose even though high mA is used. In this, X-rays beams are pulsed and takes 33 msec for a video frame. Static images are also made with lower patient dose per frame. Both television camera and CCD have greater sensitivity than spot film. Digital fluoroscopy dose is about 50% lesser than the conventional fluoroscopy.

Generally, ESE is measured by using a phantom made up of *Lucite or Perspex* or PMMA with an ionization chamber. It is to be measured for all modes: magnification, low dose and high contrast, cine, and *data acquisition system (DAS)*. To address different patient thickness various phantom thickness like 10 cm, 20 cm, and 30 cm is used.

Nowadays, all fluoroscopy machines are attached with *dose area product (DAP)* meter. Large ion chambers are placed below the collimator whose signal is proportional to the beam area. It displays an output air-kerma in $mGy.m^2$ for each examination which is an independent of distance from the source. The ion chamber is not fully exposed here as collimator, patient position, and technical factors are changing continuously. If the area is known, an air-kerma at a point is obtained by simply dividing the DAP value by an area. It is helpful to the physician to modify the procedure or estimate skin injuries.

Cumulative air-kerma in mGy at a distance is recommended in some countries. This distance is 15 cm from an isocentre, towards the X-ray tube. This may be over estimate or underestimate due to few uncertainties.

Alternatively, cumulative air-kerma can be estimated from exposure parameters: mA, time, kV, and SID values. Effective dose is difficult to access in fluoroscopy since number of organs are irradiated of unknown time.

Dose Reduction Methods in Fluoroscopy

The X-ray beam passing through the II tube is heavily filtered by 1.5 Al window. The fluoroscopy dose rate depends upon the *quantum detection efficiency (QDE)* of II tube, which is kV dependent. For a II tube with CsI output window, the QDE is about 65% and it is maximum at 60 kV. Hence, use of higher kV > 60 is recommended. This will reduce patient dose drastically and dose reduction methods are:

❑ Employ high kV.
❑ Heavy X-ray beam filtration (0.2 mm Cu).
❑ Shorter exposure time.
❑ Keep patient's arms out of X-ray beam.
❑ Remove antiscatter grid in small patients or thin body parts.
❑ Collimate X-ray beam just sufficient to cover the region of interest.
❑ Keep X-ray tube as far from the patient's skin.
❑ Place an image receptor close to patient as possible.
❑ Minimize the use of steep angle of X-ray beam.
❑ Minimize the use of cine mode.
❑ Use of low frame rate pulsed fluoroscopy (DSA).
❑ Use of lower-dose ABC options.
❑ Use of lowest or no magnification mode.
❑ Use of last-frame-hold features.
❑ Use of frame averaging.
❑ Use the largest FOV suitable for a given clinical study.

The occupational exposure of physicians, nurses, technologists, and other personnel who routinely work in fluoroscopic suite is much high. A technologist/nurse standing at 1 m from the patient may receive 1/1000 of the patient exposure. Reducing the patient exposure will certainly help in reducing an occupational exposure too. Hence, an occupational worker should adhere the following:

❑ Wear collar level TLD above the Lead apron, body TLD below the apron and finger TLD.
❑ Wear wrap around or skirt type Lead aprons.
❑ Effective use of ceiling mounted Lead glass.
❑ Use of portable Lead glass shields for additional protection to staff members observing or participating in the procedure.
❑ Standing on the receptor side is safer but away from the direct X-beam.
❑ Keep the table height comfortable for the operator.
❑ Collimating the X-ray beam tightly as sufficient for clinical use.
❑ Follow the cardinal rules: Time, distance and shielding.
❑ Reducing total fluoroscopy time is beneficial to everyone.

WORKED EXAMPLE 9.1

A digital fluoroscopy procedure is done for 3 minutes at 100 kV and 2 mA. What is an entrance skin entrance exposure (ESE)? (Assume the exposure rate as 40 mGy/minute)

ESE = Exposure rate × Exposure time

= 40 mGy/minute × 3 minutes

= 120 mGy.

BIBLIOGRAPHY

1. Bushberg JT, Seibert JA, Leidholdt EM Jr, Boone JM. The Essential Physics of Medical Imaging, 4th edn. Lippincott Williams and Wilkins; 2012.
2. Bushong SC. Radiologic Science for Technologists, 11th edn. Elsevier; 2017.
3. Thayalan K. Basic Radiological Physics, 2nd edn. Jaypee Brothers Medical Publishers (P) Ltd, New Delhi; 2017.

Computed Tomography

TOMOGRAPHY

In radiography, all structures of the patient are exposed to X-rays. Image is formed on a detector with low contrast due to Compton scatter. Since, the beam area is larger, an intensity of scattered radiation is high. Structure within a patient is obscured by an overlying and underlying objects, resulting superimposition of an anatomy. Lastly, radiography image is a 2-Dimensional (2D) one whereas anatomical structures in the human body are 3-Dimensional (3D) in nature.

To overcome this, an image of an overlying and underlying objects may be blurred by moving the X-ray tube and film during an exposure, about an axis through the structure of an interest. The blurring of an undesired image by movement of X-ray tube and film is referred to as *tomography*. **Andre Bocage (1917),** physician first devised a X-ray tube and detector motion principle. Tomography refers to slice view or sectional imaging and is usually referred to as *body section radiography or linear tomography*. The linear tomography is an imaging technique that produces sectional view of a patient in a plane, parallel to long axis of the patient or table. One can able to produce sagittal and coronal images. It is referred to by many other names: *tomography, stratigraphy, and planigraphy*.

The essential parts of a linear tomography system are X-ray tube, X-ray film and a rigid connecting rod that rotates about a fixed fulcrum. If the tube moves in one orientation, the film moves in the opposite direction. The film is placed in a tray under the X-ray table, so that it is free to move without disturbing the patient. The fulcrum refers to the sectional plane of the patient and it is the only point in the system that remains stationary. The amplitude of the tube travel is measured in degrees and is called the *tomography angle*. The plane

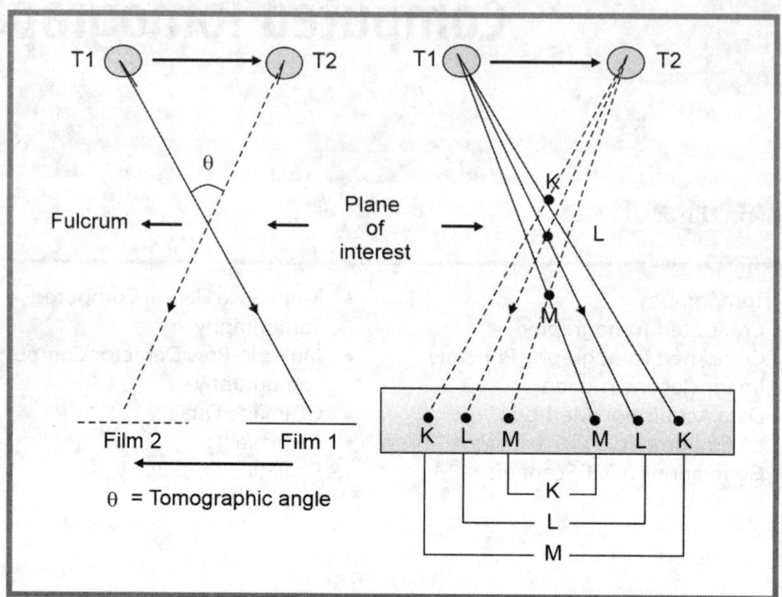

Fig. 10.1: Linear tomography principle.

of an interest within the patient is positioned at the level of the fulcrum, and it is the only plane that remains in sharp focus **(Fig. 10.1).** All the points above and below this plane get blurred.

In the figure, point K is above, and point M is below the focal plane. As the X-ray tube moves, only an image of point L, which is in the focal plane remains at sharp focus. This is because L is the only image plane that moves the same distance as the film. The image of point K moves more than the film, and an image of point M moves lesser than the film, hence both images are blurred. Object in the pivot plane for which the tube travel is equal to film travel, that is why it is in sharp focus.

The image represents the total attenuation of the X-ray beam within the patient. Structures whose tube travel is higher or smaller than the film travel gets blurred. It gives only images of longitudinal section. The thickness of the section that is in focus depends on the amplitude of tube travel. The longer an amplitude, thinner the section. The amount of blurring depends on an amplitude of tube travel, distance of an object from focal plane and film. Tube travel can be *linear, elliptical, circular, hypocycloidal, and Lissajous.* Linear tomography cannot produce trans axial images, and not in use today due to an arrival of computed tomography.

COMPUTED TOMOGRAPHY

Linear tomography overcomes the limitations of radiography to certain extent. However, an image remains dull and blurred due to use of screen-film systems. Computed tomography (CT) is a special form of tomography in which a computer is used to make cross-sectional images of an anatomy. Coronal and sagittal images can be reconstructed further from the tans axial slice data.

In CT, the X-ray source and a detector rotates synchronously around the patient. A collimated X-ray beam incident on the patient, get attenuated and transmitted. A detector captures the transmitted X-rays for further analysis by a computer. The computer reconstructs an anatomical image and displays the same on a monitor. It is a *trans axial image*, i.e., perpendicular to the axis of rotation of the X-ray tube.

CT scanner was invented by **Sir Godfrey N Hounsfield** in 1970 and was initially named *computerized axial tomography (CAT)*, now known as computed tomography. He was a physicist cum engineer, worked in the EMI, Ltd, a British company famous for recording Beatles. **Allen Cormack,** a physicist, *Tufts University (USA)* earlier developed the reconstruction mathematics of CT images (1963). It is a laboratory model for an image reconstruction. The Nobel prize was given to the discovery in 1979, for both **GN Hounsfield (UK)** *and* **Alan M Cormack (USA)** *in physiology and Medicine.* The first commercial machine was designed to study head (1973), and later it was modified to whole body scan (1975).

Its contrast resolution superior compared to screen-film radiography. The acquisition time is a few msec, which is suitable to freeze any physiologic motion. In medicine, CT is used for cancer diagnosis, trauma, and osteoporosis. In industry, it is used for nondestructive testing and soil core analysis. The special features of CT image include the following:

❑ Images are cross-sectional.
❑ Eliminate superimposition of structures.
❑ Not influenced by the properties of neighboring region.
❑ Subtle differences in X-ray attenuation are 10 times higher than radiographic image, due to scatter elimination.
❑ No use of screen-film system.
❑ 3D information of anatomical structures.

Terminology

Translation is a linear movement of X-ray tube and detector. *Rotation* is a rotary movement of X-ray tube and the detector **(Figs. 10.2A and B)**. *Ray* refers to single transmission measurement and *projection* refers to series of ray measurement that pass through the patient at the same orientation. There are two projections, namely, *parallel beam geometry* and *fan beam geometry* **(Figs. 10.3A and B)**.

The human body is imagined as a matrix and is divided into numbers of columns and rows. In general, 512×512 or 1024×1024 matrix of columns and rows are used. Each matrix element is named as *pixel (picture element)* in a 2D concept. Each pixel is assigned a number that is displayed as brightness level in a digital monitor. Numerical information in a pixel represents a CT number.

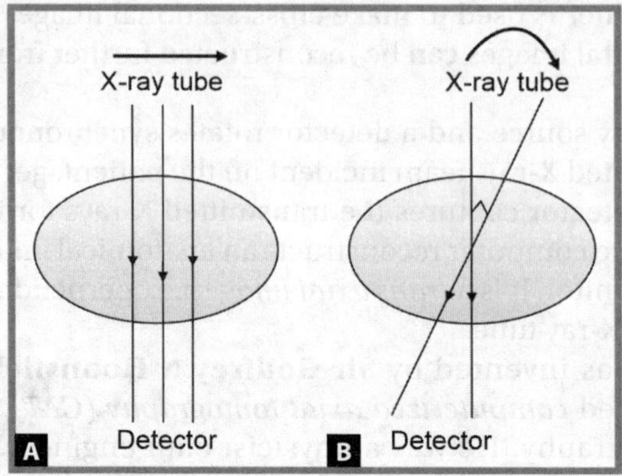

Figs. 10.2A and B: (A) Translation, and (B) Rotation in computed tomography scanning.

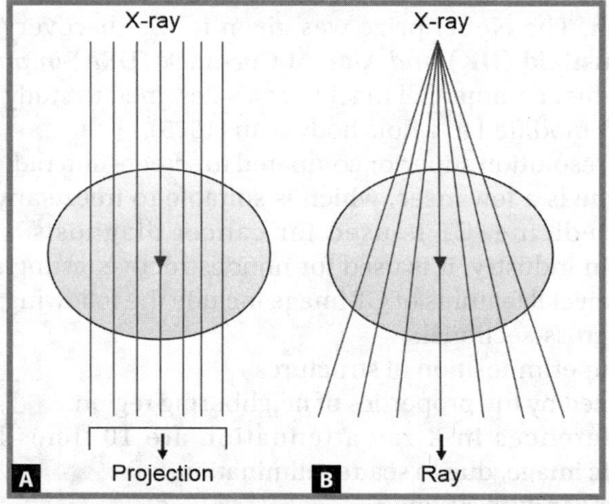

Figs. 10.3A and B: (A) Parallel beam geometry, and (B) Fan beam geometry of computed tomography.

Field of view (FOV) is the diameter of an area being seen by the X-ray beam at an isocenter. The isocenter is the center point of the CT gantry bore. A *fan beam geometry* with *top angle* 50° gives a FOV of 50 cm diameter at an isocenter. Normally, multiple FOV are provided in the CT, namely 250 mm, 350 mm, and 450 mm. The relation between the matrix size, pixel size, and FOV is given as follows:

$$\text{Pixel size} = \frac{\text{Field of view (FOV)}}{\text{Matrix size}}$$

If a CT scans a patient with a FOV of 250 mm and has a matrix element of 512, then the pixel size is calculated as:

$$\text{Pixel size} = \frac{250 \text{ mm}}{512} \approx 0.5 \text{ mm}$$

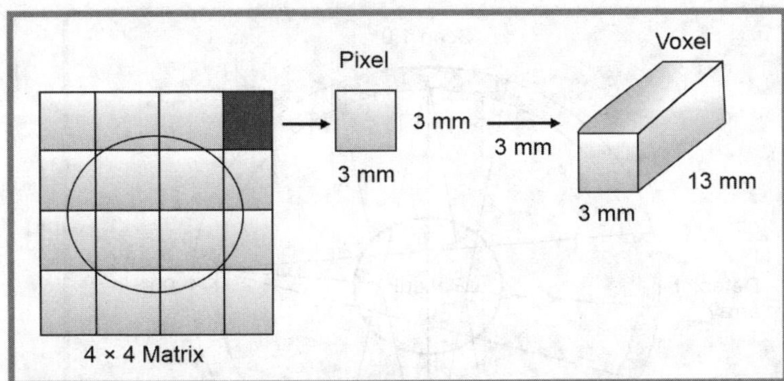

Fig. 10.4: A 4 × 4 matrix shows a pixel of 3 mm × 3 mm which represents a voxel of 3 mm × 3 mm × 13 mm.

If the FOV is increased to 350 mm, the pixel size increases to 0.7 mm, on the other hand, if the matrix size is increased to 1024, the pixel size decreases to 0.24 mm. Lower pixel size gives better resolution which is always beneficial. *Voxel (Volume element)* represents a volume of tissue within patient, it is a 3D concept which accounts slice thickness:

$$\text{Voxel size} = \text{Pixel size} \times \text{Slice thickness}$$

Each pixel displayed on the monitor represents the voxel within the patient **(Fig. 10.4)**.

COMPUTED TOMOGRAPHY PRINCIPLE

Basic principle behind CT is that an internal structure of an object can be reconstructed from multiple projections of an object. X-ray tube emitting a fan beam from a small focus is coupled to a radiation detector. Both are moved together on a carriage, so that a plane of an interest is scanned by rotation or translation around a patient **(Fig. 10.5)**. Heavily filtered, pulsed X-ray beam passes through several voxels of the body and undergo an absorption and scattering. Human body attenuates X-rays based on its mass number and an effective atomic number. Detector measures the varying intensity of transmitted X-ray beam called projections. It depends upon an attenuation pattern in the body.

After one rotation, the X-ray tube-detector assembly returns to an original position (zero) and repeat the scan resulting another projection profile. This is repeated so that large number of projections are obtained. The detector signal is always proportional to X-ray beam attenuation in each projection. Generally, detector measures sum of an absorption in an each voxel from each beam in multiple projections. It measures the linear attenuation coefficient (μ) of the structures in the voxel.

These projections are not viewed physically but stored in the computer in digital format. CT uses 1000 projections of each 800 detector measurements. A computer solves the simultaneous equation of 512 variables having μ in

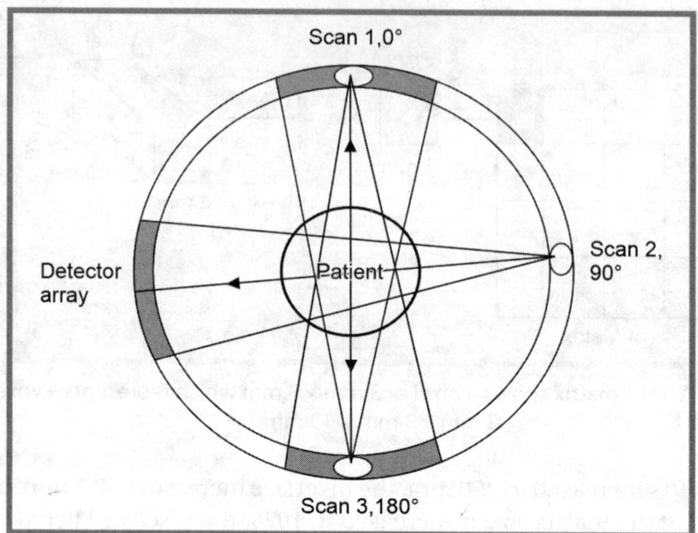

Fig. 10.5: Computed tomography scanning principle with patient at an isocenter.

each beam. It also analyzes the projection to have effective superimposition of each projection to reconstruct an image. Detector signal has a dynamic range of 12-bit with 4096 gray levels. Each increment of gray level is related to an attenuation coefficient of the total path of the beam in tissue. Computer algorithm reconstructs an image and assigns *Hounsfield unit* (HU) for each individual voxel. Each HU is allotted a gray shade for an image display on a TV monitor.

Hounsfield Units and Grayscale

Hounsfield Units

Attenuation coefficient, μ is useful for computation, not for display of images. Hence, an average linear attenuation coefficient of a tissue in an each voxel (μ_t) is normalized to that of water (μ_w), to get an integer value:

$$\text{CT number} = \frac{(\mu_t - \mu_w)}{\mu_w} \times k$$

where, K is a constant. If k =1000, then CT number is called HU number:

$$\text{HU} = \frac{(\mu_t - \mu_w)}{\mu_w} \times 1000$$

The HU is quantitative, and its range is from −1000 to +3000. CT number of a pixel represents an attenuation coefficient of the tissue in the voxel. However, an attenuation pattern in a voxel is decided by an effective X-ray energy and effective atomic number of an object. Attenuation coefficient of water (0.195) is obtained during CT calibration with phantom. HU of −1000 represents air that appear black, +3000 represents dense bone that appear

Table 10.1: CT numbers of human body organs.		
Tissue	*CT Number (HU)*	*μ , @100 kVp*
Bone	1000	0.528
Muscle	50	0.237
White matter	45	0.213
Gray matter	40	0.212
Blood	20	0.208
CSF	15	0.207
Water	0	0.206
Fat	−100	0.185
Lung	−200	0.093
Air	−1000	0.0004

(*Courtesy:* Lee W Goldman, 2007)

white, and HU of 0 refers to water. Generally, CT provides wider range HUs up to + 4000 to include foreign bodies of high Z.

Attenuation coefficient of body organs vary with kV and filtration. Conversion of attenuation coefficient into CT number makes an image independent of machine parameters (kV) but more dependent on patient anatomy **(Table 10.1).** However, CT numbers of the human body organs vary due to heterogeneity.

CT numbers drive their contrast from physical properties of the tissue that influence Compton scatter, e.g., *density, electron density, relative abundance of Hydrogen*. It is quantitative, useful for clinical diagnosis such as *pulmonary nodule, levels of calcification, bone density, fracture risk, and tumor volume or lesion diame*ter.

CT numbers also vary with photon energy. When photon of certain energy enters the body, it gets attenuated, and an average energy of the beam is higher at the beam exit (removal of low energy photons). Hence, it alters the attenuation coefficient in turn the CT number of the tissue. Same structure placed at an entry and exit of the beam appears differently in an image. This is called *beam hardening* artifacts.

Grayscale

HU is proportional to degree of X-ray attenuation in tissue and is represented by *gray shades*. There are 256 shades of gray (black- white) in the system and each HU number is allotted one shades of gray between 0 to 255. Pixel shows grayscale image relative to the density of tissue that represents the X-ray beam attenuation in tissue. Pixels assigned 0 grayscale (Dark pixel) indicates lesser attenuation of beam, e.g., soft tissue. Pixels assigned 255 grayscale (light pixel) refers to high attenuation, e.g., calcifications.

Image display

CT image is not a projected image and different from a radiography image. CT gives an electronic image from the data received that is displayed as a matrix of intensities. Such reconstructed image is displayed on a cathode ray tube (CRT) monitor, by allotting shades of gray to each CT number. In a matrix size of 512×512, each pixel represents 12-bits or 4096 gray levels, which is greater than the display range of monitor.

CT images are viewed on *stock mode* which is ideal to follow arteries. *Dynamic range* is the ratio of largest signal to smallest signal that is detected. Digital systems need wide dynamic range to accept wider attenuation of body tissue. If the dynamic range of CT number exceeds grayscale, all the numbers cannot be accommodated in the grayscale. Human eye unable to distinguish the range of gray shade levels >50. To overcome this, the map of CT numbers is adjusted with *window level* and *window width*.

Window Level and Window Width

Window level is a CT number by which the window is centered. Range of CT numbers above and below the center number is called *window width*. The former dictates an image brightness and the later determines contrast **(Fig. 10.6)**. A narrow window width provides higher contrast than wide window width. The window level and width can be set to any desired value of CT number as per the radiologist wish. Their settings affect only displayed image, not the reconstructed image data.

For example, abdomen CT is allotted a window level of 20. Then the computer is instructed to assign one shades of gray to each CT number from −108 to +148 (total 256). The range of CT numbers from −108 to +148 refers to window width. Individual pixel brightness is related to an average attenuation coefficient of each tissue voxel. In this, −108 gray shade is pure black and that of +148 appears pure white.

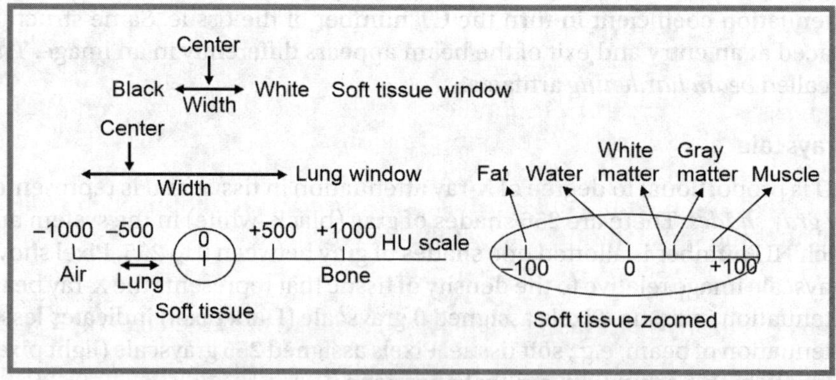

Fig. 10.6: Window level and window width in a computed tomography which influences brightness and contrast on the image display.

A narrow window width spreads large number of grayscale values over a small range of CT numbers. It provides higher contrast and detect small differences in tissue density, e.g., *liver mass*. Wider window is used to evaluate fat containing *medullary bone*. Typical window level of head, chest, lung, liver is 40, 40, –500, and 60, respectively. Their corresponding window widths are 80, 450, 1500 and 150, respectively. Final image is displayed on a monitor which can be stored permanently in the system or copied in a CD or film.

IMAGE RECONSTRUCTION

Reconstruction refers to (1) determination of linear attenuation coefficient (μ) of an individual pixel of the matrix, and (2) construction of cross-sectional image data from multiple projection raw data. It involves millions of raw data, needs to be reconstructed within a second by using *array processors*.

When source-detector makes one sweep across the patient, the internal structures of the body attenuate X-ray beam according to their *mass density and effective Z*. The intensity of radiation detected varies according to this attenuation pattern and an intensity profile or projection is obtained. The computer processes the projections that involve super position of each projection to reconstruct image of anatomic structures within that slice. Individual value of the matrix elements (μ) are obtained by solving the simultaneous equations. The matrix of values that are obtained represents the cross-sectional anatomy. Dedicated array processor is used to do calculation and instantaneous image display. Reconstruction creates X-ray attenuation map in turn map of CT number of the tissue in the plane of an interest. This is done with the help of mathematical reconstruction algorithms, namely (1) *iterative method,* (2) *back projection,* and (3) *filtered back projection.* Most modern scanners use filtered back projection image reconstruction.

Determination of μ

X-ray beam projection is transmitted through a body voxel, is given by the relation:

$$I = g\,I_O\,e^{-\mu x}$$

where, g is detector gain, I_O is number of initial X-ray photons, I, is number of transmitted photon, e is base of natural logarithm = 2.718, x is voxel thickness, and μ is voxel's linear attenuation coefficient. Values of I_O, I and x can be measured, and the only unknown is μ. *Reference detector* outside the FOV measures the signal during scan without attenuation:

$$I_r = g_r I_O$$

where, g_r is the *reference detector gain,* and *gain ratio* of the detector (β) = $\dfrac{g_r}{g}$, is found during air calibration scan. Air calibration scan is done to characteristic *bow tie filter* and to know differences in detector response. Gain ratio corrects difference in gain between detectors, difference in bow-tie filters, and difference

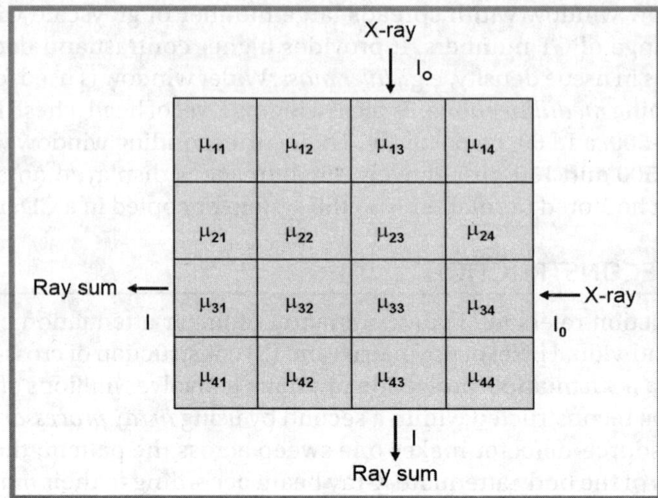

Fig. 10.7: Scanning voxels in different directions to get total attenuation coefficient along the ray path/projection.

in source to detector distances, if any. If the X-ray beam passes through few voxels as shown in the **Figure 10.7**, then:

$$I = g\,I_0\,e^{-\left(\mu_{13}\,x_{13} + \mu_{23}\,x_{23} + \mu_{33}\,x_{33} + \ldots \mu_{nn}\,x_{nn}\right)}$$

In simultaneous equation, the number of equations should be equal or greater than the variables to get a solution. To solve the above equation, additional equations are required. Hence, the voxels are scanned in different directions with additional X-ray projections, which give rise to few more equations. Thus, more than 100,000 equations are generated, by increasing the scan orientations. By solving these equations, the values of μ_{13}, μ_{23}, μ_{33}, and μ_{43}.... μ_{nn} of individual voxels are found.

Preprocessing

Before reconstruction, there are four steps of preprocessing of raw projection data. Firstly, the measured projection data is normalized by *air calibration scans* which corrects inherent inhomogeneity of the field. Secondly, *dead pixel algorithm* is applied to identify and correct dead pixels. Thirdly, *scatter correction algorithm* needs to be applied. Fourthly, *noise filtration* is done to identify low signal areas and apply smoothing. After preprocessing, the projection data undergoes logarithmic transformation and normalization. This will correct an exponential attenuation of X-rays interaction, so that μ becomes linear sum of attenuation coefficients. Projection measurement of an individual detector element (P), after preprocessing and logarithmic conversion becomes:

$$P = \ln\left(\frac{I_r}{\beta I}\right) = t \times \left(\mu_{13} + \mu_{23} + \mu_{33} \ldots.. + \mu_{nn}\right)$$

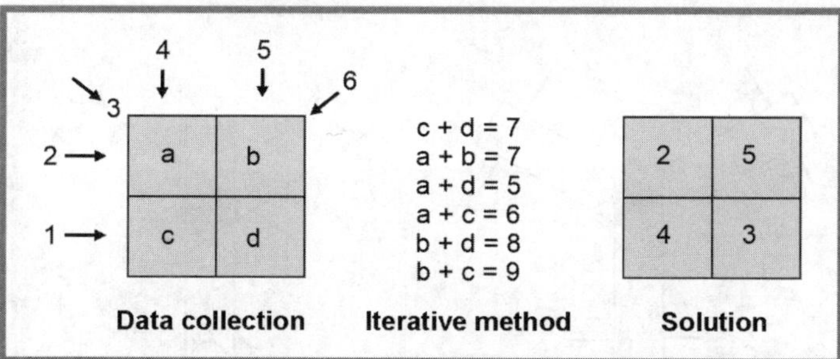

Fig. 10.8: Iterative reconstruction principle used by Hounsfield.

where, I_r is reference detector signal, and I is detector element signal and β is the gain ratio of the detector element.

Iterative Method

Iterative method was used by **G. Hounsfield,** which gives exact mathematical solution for reconstructing image from an attenuation data **(Fig. 10.8)**. One such method is an *algebraic reconstruction technique (ART)*. To obtain a solution, it starts with an assumption that all the pixels have the same value. These assumed values are compared with measured or collected data. Then, corrections are made in the assumed values so that the assumed and collected data come closer. This is repeated until all the pixel values are equal to the collected data with reasonable accuracy. It is slow, takes longer time, and gives imprecise values due to rounding of errors (e. g., 0.95 = 1). All the data must be collected before reconstruction.

Back Projection

Back projection is a mathematical process (algorithm) barrowed from trigonometry in which the collected data are back projected to produce an image. Computing projection values from the matrix elements is called *forward projection*. Alternatively, computing matrix values from projection values is known as *back projection.*

In this method, required projections of an object are obtained by multiple scans. Then, the projections are back projected to produce an image of that object. All the points in the back projected image receive density contribution from neighboring structures and creates noise. Hence, an image quality is poor and large number of projections are required to improve an image quality. Disadvantage is that it gives blurred image of the object, due to variation of image density along the radius, referred as *1/r blurring*. The image does not represent the exact structure hence, it is not used today. It is replaced by filtered back projection.

Filtered Back Projection

Process of removing blurring in the back projection data is called *filtered back projection* **(Figs. 10.9A and B).** This type of alternation of data by

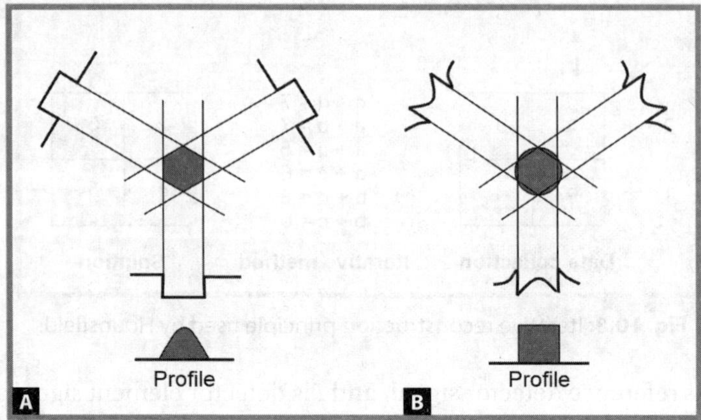

Figs. 10.9A and B: Image reconstruction: (A) Back projection; (B) Filtered back projection of a cylindrical rod object.

mathematically is referred as de*convolution kernel or filter. Convolution* is an integral calculus procedure that mathematically describes blurring process, and it is a type of mathematical multiplication. Deconvolution or filtration is the reverse of convolution and is aimed to undo the 1/r blurring. It is a one-dimensional function, compensates sudden density changes that causes image blurring. Inside margins of dense areas are enhanced, while the central region is repressed. Now the data is back projected to form a sharp image, it reveres image blurring and restores the properties of an anatomical structure.

Kernel refers to shape of the filter function in the *spatial domain*. Filtering is to be performed in the *frequency domain*, whereas the data are in spatial domain. Hence, *Fourier transform (FT)* is used to convert the data from the spatial domain into frequency domain:

$$P'(x) = \frac{1}{FT} \{FT[p(x)] *FT[k(x)]\}$$

where, $p(x)$ is the projection data in spatial domain, $k(x)$ is the kernel in spatial domain and $\frac{1}{FT}$ is used to convert the projection data back to the spatial domain. $P'(x)$ is the back projected data after filtration.

Deconvolution can also be done by Fourier transform which is faster. However, Fourier transform amplifies high frequency and creates quantum noise. Hence, various reconstruction filters, namely (1) *Lak filter,* (2) *Shepp-Logan filter and* (3) *Hamming filter* are used. *Lak filter* increases an amplitude linearly as a function of frequency and works well when there is no noise in the data. However, X-ray images involve noise which is more at high frequencies. *Shepp-Logan* filter incorporates some roll-off at higher frequencies, reducing high-frequency noise in the final CT image. *Hamming filter* has even more pronounced high-frequency roll-off, with better high-frequency noise suppression.

Bone filter has less high frequency roll off and accentuates higher frequencies in an image at the expense of an increased noise by decreasing the SNR. Bone has very high contrast so available SNR is good. Slight decrease in SNR is accepted to get sharper detail in the bone regions of the image. Thus, bone filters balance the resolution and noise and can produce fine detail (resolution) with low contrast and increased noise, e.g., bone.

Use of *soft tissue filter* gives images with reduced noise and an increased SNR. It is used in situations where high spatial resolution is less important than high contrast resolution, e.g., *metastatic liver*. It gives images with reduced noise and lower spatial resolution. Soft filters smoothen an image by decreasing an image noise and resolution, but improve image contrast, e.g., *lung*. Individual clinical work decides the nature of a filter to be used.

DATA ACQUISITION METHODS

CT has variety acquisition modes, namely (1) projection radiograph, (2) axial/sequential mode, (3) helical mode, (4) cone beam mode, (5) dual energy mode, and (6) CT fluoroscopy.

Projection Radiograph

CT radiography is obtained by advancing the patient couch through the gantry while tube and detector are stationary. It is an image of raw data acquired by CT before reconstruction. The tube is in a fixed position (0 degree) and a digital radiographic image is generated which is referred as *scout view or scanogram or topogram* which is an analogue to anterior-posterior screen-film radiograph. It is not used for clinical purpose but useful to understand tomographic principle. In regular practice, it is used to identify an upper and lower anatomical borders or scanning geometry.

Axial/Sequential Mode

In axial/sequential mode (*step-and shoot-mode*), the tube rotates at a speed of 0.5 sec through 360° and acquires data for one slice while the table and the patient are stationary. Then the couch moves to different position for another acquisition of data for second slice and so on. Thus, multiple slices are generated to cover the anatomy. Opening the collimator in a single array scanner increases slice thickness but reduces spatial resolution in the slice thickness dimension.

Table increment is equal to the beam width (W) or slice thickness. In some situations, the table increment is > slice thickness. High resolution CT is performed with table increment of 10 mm while the beam width is 1 mm. This is known as sampling of anatomy, but it may miss lesions and reduce dose. Number of tube rotations required to cover the anatomy = scan length/beam width = L/W, where *L* is the scan length and *W* is the beam width. The patient slices are perfect circle since table is stationary during scanning and the image acquisition time is long.

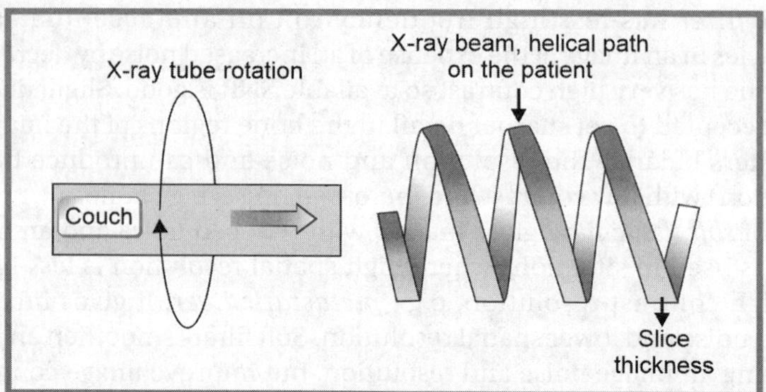

Fig. 10.10: Helical CT: Couch motion and corresponding X-ray beam path.

Helical Mode

Helical CT scanners acquire data while the couch is moving at constant speed and the gantry is rotating around the patient (1990). It has continuous acquisition of data, while couch moves and gives complete volume data in a single exposure. The X-ray beam inside the patient moves in a helical trajectory around the patient, and hence it is called as helical CT. It is worth to understand that X-ray tube is not moving in helical path **(Fig. 10.10).** Though it is called spiral CT, the name helical CT is more appropriate. In spiral, the diameter is increasing from zero from starting to end whereas helical the path diameter is same throughout.

The scanning speed increases due to an elimination of table's stop/start motion. Raw data from helical scans are interpolated to approximate acquisition of planar reconstruction data. This *interpolating projection data* is used for an image reconstruction. Methods of an interpolation includes *linear filtering and z-filtering*. Image can be reconstructed at any level at any increment above the collimation level. Helical CT uses third generation CT scan with slipring technology. It is coupled with multi-row detector array (MDA) to scan multiple slices at a time. They are often referred as either multi-slice CT (MSCT) or multi-row detector CT (MDCT).

The advantages of a helical scan are the scan speed and patient throughput, e.g., a chest scan with 10 mm slice can be done within 15–20 sec (couch motion 10 mm/sec, pitch 1.5) and avoids slice misregistration. In some instances, the entire scan can be done within a single breath-hold of a patient. It allows the use of less contrast agent and increases patient throughput. It is a good feature for pediatric patients. The couch motion can have variable speed which is defined by *pitch*. It relates the couch motion with X-ray beam width. There are two types of pitches, namely (1) collimator pitch and (2) detector pitch.

Collimator Pitch

Collimator pitch is the ratio of the table increment per rotation to slice thickness or beam width:

$$\text{Collimator Pitch (P)} = \frac{\text{Couch movement per } 360° \text{ gantry rotation}}{\text{Detector width at the isocenter or nT}}$$

where, nT is the collimated beam width, n is the number of detector arrays, and T is the detector width. It can also be stated that nT = number of slices × slice width, if n = 1, it refers to an axial/sequential CT scanner. If the table moves 10 mm in one rotation and the beam width is 5 mm, then pitch = 10/5 = 2. Pitch is expressed as ratio: 0.5:1, 1.0:1, 1.5:1, or 2:1. Pitch ratio of 0.5: 1 gives overlapping images with higher patient dose. On the other hand, pitch ratio of 2: 1 gives an extended imaging with reduced radiation dose. Pitch influences radiation dose, an image quality and scan time, its relations with radiation dose is given by the relation:

$$\text{Dose} \propto \frac{1}{\text{Pitch}}$$

Pitch = 1, refers to normal scanning which resembles axial/sequential CT scanner. Pitch = 0.75 refers to *over scanning;* table motion is slow, e. g., *cardiac imaging.* This gives an increased image quality with an increased radiation dose. If pitch = 1.5, it is said to be *under scanning;* table motion and scanning is faster with lesser patient motion, e.g., *thoracic, and pediatric patients.* Thus, higher pitch reduces scan time with lesser radiation dose to patients. It consumes smaller volume of contrast agent and good for pediatric patients. It is useful to calculate table speed (T_s) for a given slice thickness (S) and pitch value (P):

$$T_s = \frac{P \times M \times S}{\text{Rotation time}}$$

where, M is number of slices per rotation, and it may be 4 or more for modern CT scanner.

Cone Beam CT

CT scan with >64 detector elements employed in cone beam X-rays. The reconstruction algorithm that converts the raw data into CT images accounts the cone angle. Cone angles of 2° and 10° are used by the vendors and 10° cone angle is referred as *true cone beam CT.* Wider cone angle increases X-ray scatter and cone beam artifacts. However, it is beneficial to cover the whole organ without table motion, e.g., CT angiography, and perfusion study. Filtered back projection is applicable for fan beams, while cone beam uses *Feldkamp algorithm (FDK).* It takes care of beam divergence in Z direction and compute both fan beam and cone beam angles. It finds application in image guided radiation therapy.

Dual Energy CT

Dual energy CT comes as dual source CT (DSCT) or single source CT. DSCT uses two X-ray tubes on same gantry and two detector arrays to acquire data from low kV and high kV in single acquisition. Tubes are mounted with angular offset of 90° with two generators of 80 kW each. FOV of the tubes are 50 cm and 26 cm, respectively. In single source CT, it is possible to switch kV to get dual energy acquisition. However, it is difficult to switch the tube current and (mA) correspondingly. Dual energy data are logarithmically subtracted and then reconstructed for image formation.

Dual energy CT is mainly developed for cardiac studies to improve temporal resolution. Temporal resolution is quarter of the gantry rotation time (83 msec) and is independent of heart rate. *Multi-segment reconstruction* is used to improve temporal resolution. Cardiac study employs scans with ECG gating within one cardiac cycle. Its FOV is smaller and scatter from one source influences the other. Hence, *scatter correction technique* is required. Since additional filtration is possible for high kV, it increases energy separation and energy subtraction. Dual energy CT improves delineation of two different material of same attenuation.

CT Fluoroscopy

CT fluoroscopy provides an image sequence over the same region of tissue. It is a pseudo-real-time tomography images, and there is no table movement. Images are reconstructed nearly real time during continuous rotation of X-ray tube. CT images are constantly updated to include the latest projection data at the rate of 6 frames per second. Hence, 6 images are obtained in 1 sec for a 360° rotation. The time taken for 1 image = 1/6 sec = 167 msec and the angle is 60°.

After 1 sec, the CT scans 60° arc (167 msec), creates a subframe and the old is discarded. Thus, new subframe is added to the old 5 subframes accounting 17% new information and 83% old information. Most recent 6 subframes are summed to produce the CT display. CT fluoroscopy images has an excellent temporal resolution, and motion at an image level can be followed in real time. The X-ray tube is operated with a current of 20–50 mA, whereas regular CT uses 150–400 mA. This procedure is commonly used for taking needle biopsies or to drain fluids.

CT EQUIPMENT

CT scanners are available as single slice scanner (CT), multi-slice helical scanner (MSHCT), multi-row detector scanner (MDCT) and cone beam CT (CBCT) in the market. CT equipment consists of (1) X-ray tube, (2) collimator and filtration, (3) slip rings, (4) X-ray detector, (5) gantry and voltage generator, (6) couch, (7) control console, and (8) computer. Recent developments have brought slip ring technology and multidetector array in day-to-day use. The Z-axis is the gantry rotation axis, longitudinal one, and runs along foot to head of the patient. The Y-axis is perpendicular to the patient in the direction of ground to ceiling. The X-axis runs from side-to-side of the patient.

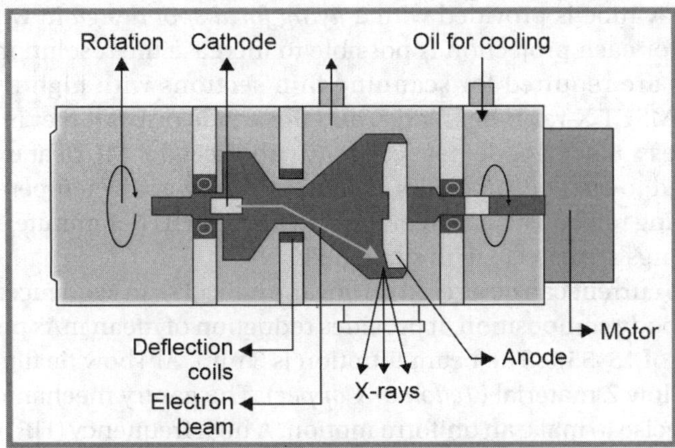

Fig. 10.11: Typical CT X-ray tube.
(*Courtesy:* M/s Siemens Healthineers)

X-ray Tube

X-ray tube is mounted with its anode-cathode axis, parallel to an axis of rotation, to reduce *heel effect* **(Fig. 10.11).** Tube potential is about 120–140 kV and mA is up to 400 and X-ray beam is pulsed at the rate of 100 pulses/sec. X-ray pluses are stable, and their intensity will not vary over an image acquisition cycle and X-ray spectrum should be narrow (does not alter μ). The current can be modulated during imaging based on patient thickness to reduce radiation dose.

Anode is flat for easy heat dissipation and its angle is smaller. High speed rotors are recommended for heat dissipation to avoid tube failure. This property is much important for sequential imaging frequency. Generally, it has large anode diameter and thicker, resulting higher mass. The anode heat capacity is > 8 MHU and the anode cooling is about 1 MHU. It can be energized up to 60 sec continuously and needs high instantaneous power capacity.

Cathode is angled, and the focal spot position can be switched magnetically. Focal spot determines the amount of information distributed over the detector array. As focal spot increases the information spread over large number of detectors and limit the resolution. Vendors offers cooling algorithms to access focal spot thermal state so that mA is adjusted suitably. There are two focal spots within 0.6-1.6 mm range and small focal spot mut be robust to use in high-resolution CT (HRCT). Life of X-ray tube is about 50,000 exposures to a minimum.

Multi-slice X-ray Tube

Multi-slice CT (MSCT) requires higher X-ray power, due to continuous large volume data acquisition. The thermal capacity of the X-ray tube is different, they are energized up to 60 sec continuously and the instantaneous power capacity must be higher. The focal spot design and heat dissipation are vital factors. X-ray tube is provided with a *flying focal spot design* in which rapid deflection for each projection is possible to increase the resolution. Smaller focal spots are required for scanning thin sections with high resolution. Generally, MSCT X-ray tube is large, and the anode disc is larger in diameter and thickness. Since anode heat capacity can exceed 8 MJ, heat exchangers are provided to cool oil, air, and to maintain gantry at low temperatures. An anode cooling rate must be high in the order of 1 MHU per minute and liquid metal bearings are used to with stand heat.

The tube current can be altered during the helical scan sequence, to suit an individual body composition. It provides reduction of mean mAs per rotation of an order of 15–55%. The beam filtration is 3 mm, Al +bow tie filter, usually made with low Z material (*Teflon or Copper*). The gantry mechanical design must be precise to make an uniform motion. A high frequency (HF) generator is employed since it is small and is mounted in the gantry itself. The HF generator and the X-ray tube should be matched properly to have maximum capacity, 50 kW.

Collimator and Filtration

Optimal collimation minimizes the volume of tissue and improves an image contrast. CT scanner uses two collimators of 100 μm thick, made up of *Tantalum* of low Z, to limits scatter radiation. X-ray beam is collimated both at the X-ray tube and at the detector level. It defines the slice thickness in a single slice scanner and beam width in a MDCT. Additionally, an *anti-scatter collimation* is also available.

Single slice scanner uses 2 collimators as pre-and post-patient collimation. One collimator is placed after the X-ray tube housing which limits an area of anatomy. It is referred as pre-patient collimator which provides parallel X-ray beams. It decides the beam profile and radiation dose. The other collimator is placed above the detector, known as pre-detector collimator. This collimator restricts the X-rays viewed by the detector and reduces scattered radiation. If properly coupled with pre-patient collimator one can select slice thickness, referred to as sensitivity profile. Since it reduces scatter radiation, an image contrast is improved.

X-ray beam is heavily filtered, and detectors are individually collimated. The X-ray beam is not mono energetic hence, filters are used to remove low energy photons. *Aluminum (2.5 mm) + Copper (0.4 mm)* are used as filters and modern CT units uses 6 mm Al with an algorithm's help. Since patient cross section is an elliptical, X-ray beam passes through lesser tissue at periphery than at the center of the body. Hence, the noise levels may vary, and it is highest at the center than at periphery. As a result, the dose is higher at periphery than at center. To overcome this issue *bowtie filters* of different sizes for head and body scanning are used **(Fig. 10.12A).** It reduces the dynamic range of exposures at the detector and reduces scatter and patient dose.

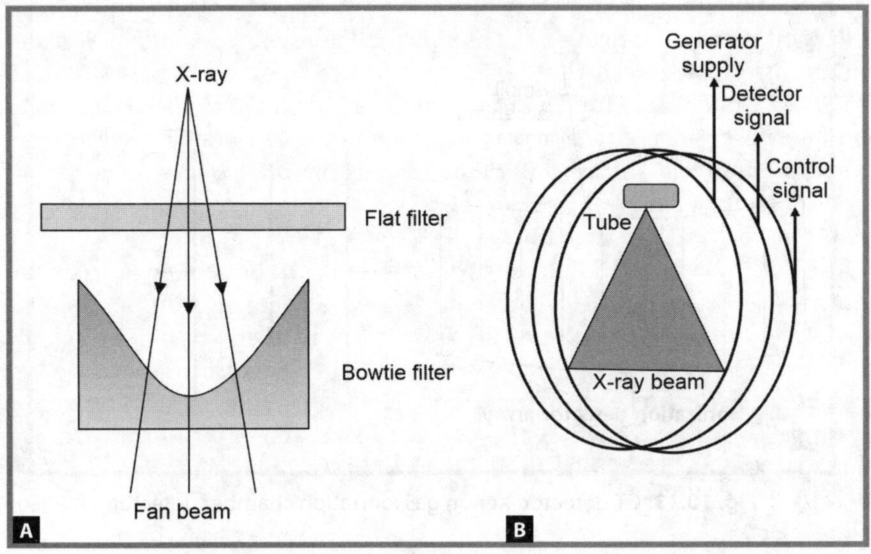

Figs. 10.12A and B: (A) Bowtie filter; (B) Slip rings in helical CT.

Slip Rings

Generally, CT scan cannot be rotated continuously beyond 360° due to an inertial limitation. After an end of each slice, gantry needs to come to zero to begin an another slice. It increases scanning time and decreases through put hence, *slip ring technology* was introduced (1980).

Slip rings are an electromechanical device which conducts electricity. It conducts an electrical signal from a rotating surface to a fixed surface. One surface of the ring is smooth, and other rings have sliding contactors by means of *Carbon brushes or small metal* **(Fig. 10.12B)**. The later ring sweeps the former continuously without an interruption. The power is transmitted through stationary rings. The *brushes (Silver graphite alloy)* transmit power to the gantry, glide in contact grooves on the stationary slip ring.

Slip ring is a three-layer parallel conductive rings concentric to gantry axis. Each ring provides connectivity to X-ray tube, detector, and control circuits, that supply electric power. This permits rotation of X-ray tube and detectors while maintaining an electrical contact with stationary slip ring system. It is used to energize tubes and collect data continuously without interscan delay.

Slip ring eliminates an inertial limitations at the end of each slice and has greater rotational velocities, with shorter scan time. If slip rings arrangement is in place, the X-ray tube can rotate faster (5 sec per rotation) and move more than 360°. It is used in multi-slice helical CT that allows the gantry to rotate continuously. It eliminates the need of an electrical cable, which restrict continuous rotation. It overcomes the limitations of an earlier versions and has greater rotational velocities of 1sec rotation time.

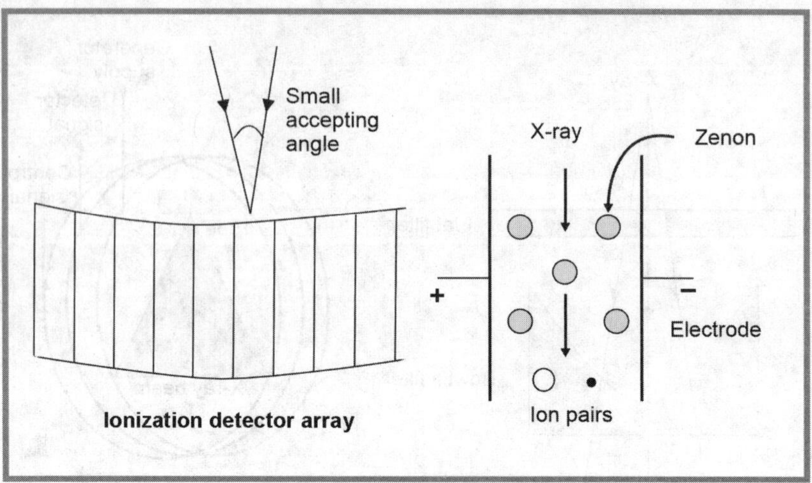

Fig. 10.13: CT detector: Xenon gas ionization chamber detector.

X-ray Detectors

Detector requirements of CT scan are (1) small size with good resolution (600–900 numbers for single slice, width <1.5 mm), (2) high detection efficiency, (3) fast response and negligible after glow, (4) wide dynamic range and (5) stable noise free response. There are two types of detectors, namely (1) *single detector array,* and (2) *multidetector array.* Single detector array is made either with *Xenon gas ionization chamber or solid-state detector* and multidetector array is made only with *solid state devices.*

Xenon Gas Ionization Chamber

Xenon gas filled ionization chamber detector is made with high atomic number (54) and its K-shell binding energy is 35 keV. High atomic number facilitates photoelectric absorption as main interaction in the detector. Xenon gas is kept under high pressure of about 2 MPa and its detection efficiency is about 60%. When X-ray incident on the detector, ionization takes place and electric charges are produced **(Fig. 10.13)**. These charges constitute an electric signal that is amplified and digitized. The digitized electronic signal is proportional to incident X-ray intensity.

Xenon detector is small and is elongated in the beam direction. It is aligned with the focal spot, uniform, less dependent on stable high voltage, and has in-built collimation. The number of chambers is up to 1000 and the detector aperture is 1–2 mm with 100 mm length. It has low detection efficiency due to thin septa and its sensitivity is about 50% relative to scintillation detector. It is highly directional, and it should be positioned in a fixed orientation.

Solid-state Detector

Solid-state detectors are basically scintillation detectors coupled with *photomultiplier tube (PMT) or photodiode.* The size of the detector is about

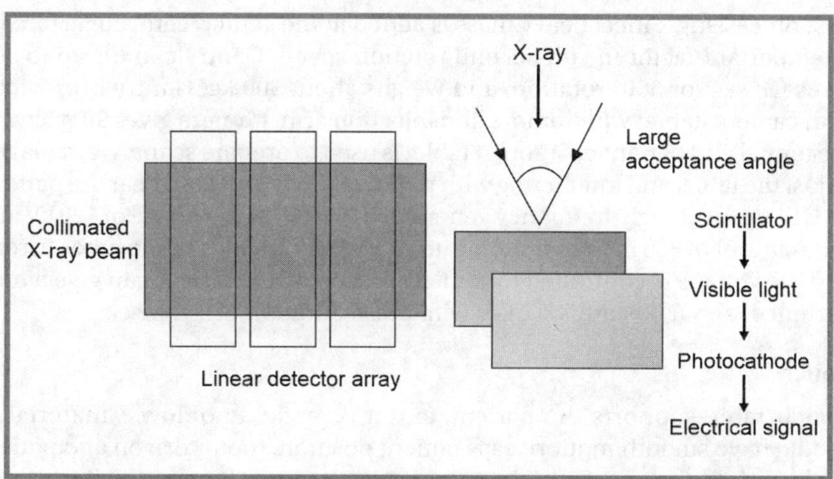

Fig. 10.14: CT detector: Solid-state detector working principle.

1.0 × 15 mm and 1.0 × 1.5 mm in the case of multidetector array. When X-ray incident on the detector, light is produced which is detected by the photodiode **(Fig. 10.14).** The photodiode gives an electric signal which is digitized. The digitized electronic signal is proportional to incident X-tray intensity. The detectors are wider (12 mm) than the collimated X-ray beam thickness.

Scintillators are used with photomultiplier tubes and converts absorbed X-ray energy into light energy, referred as *conversion efficiency.* Solid-state detectors have better X-ray absorption efficiency (90%) and large acceptance angle. Since, they are closely packed, the detection efficiency is high (90%). The geometric efficiency is less due to gap between detectors to avoid cross talk. However, now it is possible to design detectors with zero space.

It reduces patient dose, provides faster imaging rate, and improves image quality by increasing *signal-to-noise ratio (SNR).* It has negligible afterglow, and the stability of an output signal depends on high voltage supply. A detector array may contain 800 individual detectors in the axial plane. Most common is solid-state scintillators; *Bismuth germinate ($Bi_4Ge_3O_{12}$), Cesium iodide + Sodium iodide (UV light), Cadmium tungstate ($CdWO_4$), and Yttrium and Gadolinium ceramics.* Density of the detector system influence spatial resolution of the CT.

Usually, solid-state scintillation or Xenon gas ion chambers are used as detectors. Currently, ceramic scintillation phosphors are in use, which gives an absorption efficiency of about 99%. Few commonly used ceramic scintillation phosphors are: (1) *Lutetium orthosilicate (Lu_2O: Ce),* (2) *Gadolinium orthosilicate (Gd_2O: Ce),* and (3) *Yttrium aluminum perovskite ($YALO_3$: Ce).*

Gantry and Voltage Generator

Gantry consists of X-ray tube, detector array, high frequency generator, transformer, and control electronics. Subsystems receive commands from the control console and upload data to the computer for image production and post processing. Since, heavy mass is added in the gantry, centrifugal force is an important factor in sub-second rotation speed. Gantry can tilt up to 30°, takes 0.3 sec for 360° rotation, and weighs about 500 kg. Gantry is provided with camera, tablet with remote and injection arm. Camera gives 90° views of the tunnel and patient position. A tablet is used to prepare scans, view images, adjust the table, and interacting with radiologists by standing near the patient.

CT scan uses high-frequency generator of 64 kW, tube voltage of 120 kV and tube current of 830 mA corresponds to 100 kW. It provides stable tube current, and the voltage is controlled by a microprocessor. Generator can give a tube current of about 800 mA @125kV with pulse duration of 2–4 msec.

Couch

Couch/table supports the patient, and it is made up of low Z material. It should have smooth motion, easy patient position, motor driven and patient load bearing capacity of weight up to 250 kg. It moves longitudinally through gantry aperture, indexed automatically and the tabletop can be removable. It is designed for accessories like paper roll holder, infusion stand and storage box. Generally, tabletop is curved, whereas flat top preferably *Carbon fiber* is required for radiotherapy simulation. In such case, room lasers; two fixed side lasers and one moving laser in ceiling are used for patient positioning. Auto indexing of the couch must be provided so that the operator need not enter the room during imaging. In helical CT, the couch is moving while gantry is rotating, with variable speeds which can be defined by the *pitch factor*.

Control Console

There are two or three consoles in CT, one for the technologist to operate an imaging system, second for the technologist to post process the images to annotate patient data on an image. Operating console is provided with meters, controls for selection of technique factors, control for motion of gantry and couch, and computer commands for an access to an image reconstruction and transfer. Generally, each console is provided with one monitor. There are 2 monitors, one to annotate patient data (hospital, medical record number, patient name, age, gender), and an identification of image (medical record number, technique, couch position, etc.) and other for operator to view an image. Slice thickness can be selected from 0.5 to 5 mm which is achieved by an adjustment of detector rows in the collimator. The couch can be indexed so that its Z axis position, anatomy to be imaged and helical pitch etc., can be prefixed.

Third one monitor for radiologists to view images, vary the contrast, size, including visual appearance. In addition, several remote-control imaging stations are provided. This control accepts reconstructed images from an operator's control console. Physician control console is used to call up and manipulate image, optimize diagnostic information, contrast and brightness adjustments, magnification techniques, region of interest (ROI) viewing, use of online software packages, etc. Generally, physician console is kept away from the CT room with *picture archiving and communication systems (PACS) network*. All modality images are pooled here for further examination and an interpretation.

Computer

Computer is a large capacity one used to solve more than 2,50,000 equations with the help of microprocessor or an array processor and has primary memory. Microprocessor decides the reconstruction time and an efficiency of an examination. Reconstruction time is the time between an end of patient imaging and appearance of an image at the monitor. Some CT vendor uses an array processor which are faster than the microprocessor since it performs simultaneous calculations.

Computer software includes plot of CT numbers, mean and standard deviation of CT values of ROI, subtraction techniques, planner and volumetric quantitative analysis and reconstruction of images in coronal, sagittal and oblique planes.

GENERATION OF CT SCANNERS

A variety of CT geometries have been developed to acquire the X-ray transmission data for image reconstruction. These geometries are commonly called generations. The main objective of different generation is (1) scanning time reduction and (2) simplification of mechanical motion.

First Generation

First generation CT scanner is a *rotate and translate system* with finely collimated pencil beam system. It had two X-ray detectors and used parallel ray geometry with NaI: Tl as detector **(Fig. 10.15A)**. It is translated linearly to acquire 160 rays across a 24 cm FOV and rotated between translations to acquire 180 projections at 1° interval. It took about 5 minutes per scan with 1.5 minutes to reconstruct a slice with a linear measurement of 28,800 rays (160 ×180). Two contiguous slices could be imaged in each scan. It is basically a laboratory model CT scan.

There is a large change in signal due to an increased X-ray flux outside of head and hence patient's head is pressed into a flexible membrane surrounded by a water bath. The NaI: Tl detector signal decay slowly, and affects measurements. The advantage of the system is an efficient scatter reduction, and best of all scanner generations. The disadvantages include water bath acted as a bolus, long scanning time, and afterglow of NaI: Tl.

Second Generation

Second generation CT scanner is also *rotate and translate system* **(Fig. 10.15B)** with narrow fan beam geometry (10°). Linear array of 5–30 detectors were used to acquire more data, to improve an image quality (600 rays × 540 projections = 324000). These scanners provided larger rotational increments (5°) and faster scans. Advantage is its speed, shortest scan time was 18 seconds per slice. Narrow fan beam allows detection of more scattered radiation. Disadvantage of a fan shaped beam is that it gives an increased intensity at the edges of the body. Hence, requires bowtie filter

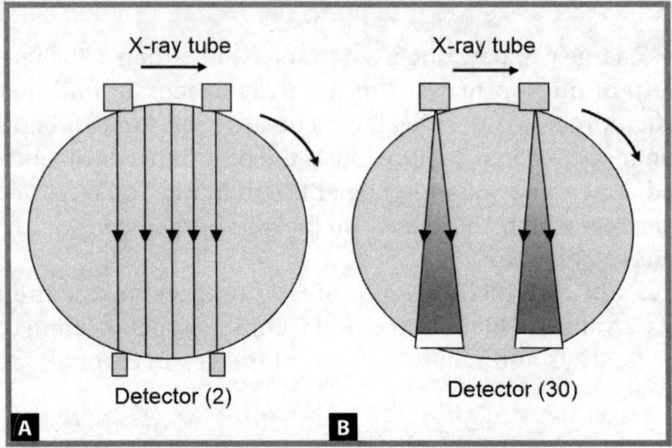

Figs. 10.15A and B: (A) First generation CT scan with pencil beam geometry; (B) Second generation CT scan with narrow fan beam geometry.

to compensate X-ray intensity at the edges of body. It involves complex mechanical motion involving rotation and translation with heavy mass of gantry system. Most of the units were designed to image for >20 minutes.

Third Generation

Third generation scanner is a *rotate and rotate system* with wide fan beam geometry **(Fig. 10.16A)**. Former term rotate refers to X-ray tube rotation and the later refers to detector rotation. There is no translation in this system. The X-ray tube and detector array are mechanically joined and rotated together. Its detector is curvilinear and has an increased number of detectors, > 800 detectors. Curvilinear geometry provides a constant source to detector path during the scan which helps reconstruction later. It also gives better X-ray beam collimation thereby reducing the effect of scatter radiation. The angle of

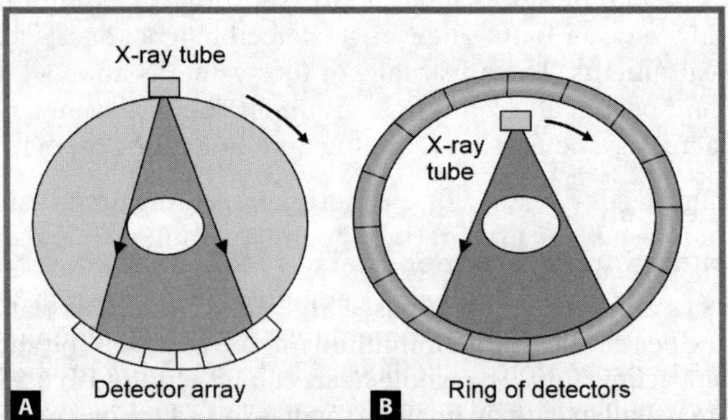

Figs. 10.16A and B: (A) Third generation is a source fan and X-ray tube is in the apex; (B) Fourth generation is a detector fan and detectors are in the apex.

fan beam is increased to cover the entire patient and common angle is 30–60°. Third generation CT scanners are sub-second system, have scan times of <100 msec.

In this generation, detector is responsible for data corresponding to a ring in an image. Any drift in the signal levels of the detectors over time affects the μt values that are back projected to produce the CT image, causing *ring artifacts*. Software is available to remove ring artefacts during the image reconstruction.

Fourth Generation

Fourth generation scanners are designed to overcome the problem of ring artifacts. It is a *rotate and stationary fan beam system*. It incorporated faster imaging, new detector design and use of large computers. It has a stationary ring of detector array of about 4,800 detectors. X-ray tube is kept inside the detector ring and complete rotation in sub-second. Since, it is rotated continuously, very fast scan time is possible. Geometrical misalignment between detector ring radius and X-ray beam origin may be possible. It has inter-scan delay times since the X-ray tube had to return to its starting position (home).

Third generation fan beam geometry has X-ray tube as *apex* of the fan. In the 4th generation, an individual detector is the apex **(Fig. 10.16B)**. Though the X-ray tube forms the fan beam, data are processed for fan beam reconstruction with each detector as *vertex* of a fan. The rays acquired by each detector are fanned out to different positions of the X-ray source. In the 3rd generation, signal data are measured at the center and at an edge of the detector array. One reference detector is employed outside the FOV as common to all individual detectors. Hence, the gain of the reference detector and the individual detector may not be equal. In the 4th generation, each detector has its own reference detector, and hence the gain of the reference and the individual detector is same. Today all helical and multi-slice CT scans are either third or fourth generation CT scanners.

Fifth Generation

Fifth generation scanner is a *stationary and stationary system*, developed specifically for cardiac tomography imaging. No conventional X-ray tube is used, instead large arc of *Tungsten* (210°) encircles patient and lies directly opposite to the detector ring. It uses an electron gun that deflects and focuses a fast-moving electron beam along Tungsten target ring in the gantry. Since, the detector is also in the form of ring, it permits simultaneous acquisition of multiple image sections.

The images are obtained in 50 msec and can produce fast frame rate CT movies of the beating heart with minimum motion artifacts. The advantage its speed of data acquisition. The whole heart can be acquired in 0.2 sec. These scanners are useful in cardiac imaging, pediatric and trauma patients. It can also be used as conventional CT by averaging multiple images with repeat scans. It becomes obsolete not in clinical use today.

Sixth Generation

To overcome the limitations of third, fourth and fifth generation CT, sixth generation was introduced:

Sixth generation = Third or fourth generation CT + Slip ring technology + Helical motion.

Before the arrival of slip ring technology, the gantry complete one rotation and have a pause before second rotation. Gantry has high voltage and data cables, and continuous rotation may harm the cables. During the pause, the couch is moved to a slice thickness increment and the gantry commons its next rotation. Hence, it consumes longer scan time, for which slip ring technology came into existence.

In helical mode, the couch moves, and the gantry is rotating during the scan. Advantages of helical CT scan are high speed, improved detection, and better contrast. It performs imaging in space and time simultaneously which is useful in 3-D examination of tissue. Total scan time required to image patient is much shorter, excluding time required to translate the patient table. In some instances, the entire scan can be done within a single breath-hold of a patient, at the rate of 1sec per slice, e.g., abdomen CT within 30 sec. It avoids misregistration of slices and handle high patient throughput.

Seventh Generation

Seventh generation uses *multi-row detector array (MDA)* and such a CT is called MDCT **(Figs. 10.17A and B).** It is a matrix of rows and columns of detectors of each element having a size of 1.25 mm. Once it is exposed, the detector collects all the X-rays and perform image processing. Detector can be binned to multiple of 1.25 mm and creates multiple slice thickness of 1.25 mm, 2.5 mm, 3.75 mm, and 5 mm, respectively. Thus, this machine uses maximum X-ray output by reducing heat loading of the machine, resulting in better efficiency.

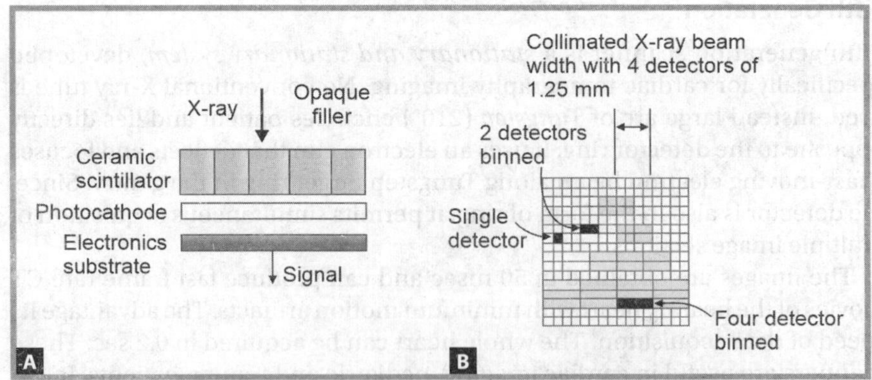

Figs. 10.17A and B: Multi-row detector array: (A) Principle of MDA; (B) 16 row multidetector array of seventh generation CT having element of 1.25 mm each.

In this, collimator spacing is wider and more X-rays are used to produce an image data. Opening the collimator in a single array scanner increases the slice thickness but reduces spatial resolution in the slice thickness dimension. Hence, slice thickness is controlled by detector size, not by the collimator here. Though it offers flexibility of CT acquisition protocol, the number of parameters has increased. It covers more volume of tissue, has better efficiency for patient imaging. There is a need to define detector pitch instead of collimator pitch.

MULTI-SLICE HELICAL COMPUTED TOMOGRAPHY

Multi-slice CT (MSCT) came to clinical use in 1992 with 2 parallel banks of detectors, that gives 2 slices. In 1998, solid state multi-row detector was introduced to make 4 slices in each rotation. Multi-slice CT generally uses third generation CT with helical scanning and low voltage slip rings. In helical scanning, the X-ray tube rotates continuously, and the couch moves the patient through a plane of rotating X-ray beam. Using a slip ring technology, the tube is energized, and data are collected continuously. Image can be reconstructed at any desired Z-axis position along the patient.

The special features of MSHCT are faster rotation sub-second times (0.5–0.8 sec), that reduces the examination time. The image quality is like that of single slice scanners, but it is different in dose, pitch, image artifacts, and method of image reconstruction. To scan longer anatomic area, more than 4 slices are required and hence gantry speed must be increased. Compared to 1 sec single slice scanner, MSCT performs 0.5 sec rotation with simultaneous acquisition of 4 slices. Thus, it gives 8 times higher performance than single slice CT, for same scanning time. For example, 4 contiguous 5 mm detector array gives 20 mm collimator spacing. The number of X-rays detected is 4 times higher than that of single array of 5 mm. If properly combined, further 10 mm, 15 mm, 20 mm slices may be obtained from the same acquisition.

Usually, MSHCT with multidetector array employs third generation CT with 16 detectors. If 750 detector elements are there in each array, then $16 \times 750 = 12,000$ detector elements are required for a 60° fan beam geometry. The 4th generation CT requires much more detector elements to cover an entire detector ring of 360°. In a single slice scanner, the detectors are wide (15 mm) and collimator determines (adjustment) slice thickness of 1–13 mm. In a MSHCT, the individual detector elements along the Z-axis are summed to get several slice thicknesses. Thus, the slice width is determined by the detector not by the collimator. The detector dimensions are always referred at an isocenter.

MSHCT can be used for conventional axial scanning and helical scanning. The width of two central detector arrays dictates the slice thickness. To keep the sensitivity profile of each detector similar, collimator is adjusted to keep the penumbra outside the detector. The radiation dose is higher with reduced artifacts. *Slice acquisition rate (SAR)* is a measure of efficiency of the MSCT system. Volume of tissue being imaged is referred as Z-axis coverage:

$$SAR = \frac{\text{Slices acquired per rotation}}{\text{Time of rotation}}$$

$$\text{Z-axis coverage} = SAR \times W \times T \times B$$

where, W is the slice width, T is the imaging time, and B is the pitch. The clinical advantages of MSHCT includes:

❏ Increased speed
❏ Shorter acquisition time with improved temporal resolution (lesser motion artifacts)
❏ High axial resolution with thinner slices in the longitudinal (Z) axis
❏ Retrospective creation of thinner or thicker sections from raw data
❏ Accurate anatomical 3D reconstruction especially in angiography and virtual endoscopy with lesser helical artifacts.
❏ Increased volume coverage per unit time.
❏ Reduced partial volume artifacts and noise.
❏ Detailed multi-planar reconstruction images.
❏ Use of lesser contrast materials and delivery of contrast material at faster rate, thus increasing contrast enhancement in images.

Detector Pitch

In MSHCT, the detector pitch influences radiation dose, image quality and scan time:

$$\text{Detector pitch} = \frac{\text{Table movement per } 360° \text{ rotation of gantry}}{\text{Detector width at an isocenter}}$$

The collimator pitch and the detector pitch of a given CT is related as follows:

$$\text{Collimator pitch} = \frac{\text{Detector pitch}}{N}$$

where, N is the number of detector arrays of multi-slice CT. MSHCT scanners with 4 detector arrays use 3–6 as detector pitch values. If a MSHCT of 4 detector arrays is scanning with a pitch of 6, then collimator pitch = 6/4 = 1.5. Hence, a pitch of 6 in MSHCT corresponds to pitch of 1.5 for conventional scanner.

Pitch helps to increase volume of tissue to be imaged for a given time. It is one of the advantages of MSHCT so that it images larger volume in a single breath hold. This finds application in angiography, radiotherapy treatment planning and noncooperative patient. The relation between the pitch and the volume of tissue is given by:

$$\text{Volume of tissue imaged} = \text{Beam width} \times \text{Pitch} \times \text{Imaging time}$$

Now it is possible to have whole body CT scan with single breath hold. In MSHCT, whole width of the detector array or central rows of the detector array receives the X-ray beam. For example, if the couch moves to 10 mm for a beam width of 10 mm in a 16 slice CT having detector width of 0.5 mm, then the pitch is 1. Pitch is nothing but the ratio of couch motion and beam width (10 mm/10 mm = 1). Alternatively, if the central rows of the detector encounter

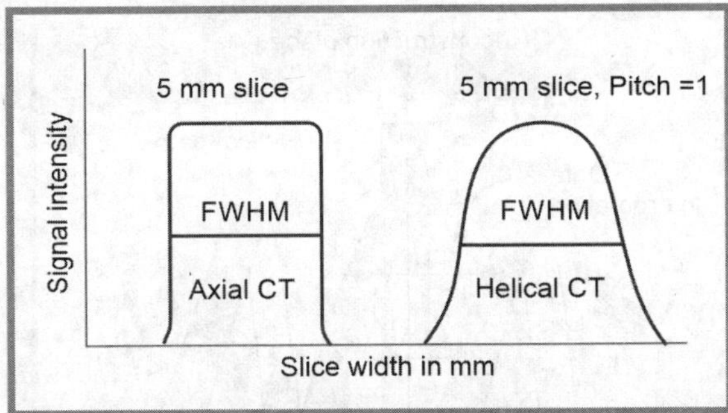

Fig. 10.18: Slice sensitivity profile for axial CT and helical CT. Axial CT profile appears as flat, and FWHM is slightly greater than the nominal slice thickness. The helical CT profile appears as an inverted bell shaped, it is wider and it increases with increasing pitch.

the X-ray beam for which the detector width is 5 mm, then the pitch is 2 (10 mm/5 mm = 2).

Generally, MSHCT have a pitch of 1 since it scans multiple slices, and the Z-axis location and reconstruction width are selected later. If the pitch is >1.0:1, the sensitivity profile gets widened, resulting reduction of Z-axis resolution. In the case of CT angiography, the pitch is < 1. This is due to multiple slice capability and need of more slices per unit time. It leads to larger imaging volume of tissue.

Slice Sensitivity Profile

The X-ray beam profile measured along Z-axis with varying signal intensity is called *slice sensitivity profile (SSP)*. It is drawn as a graph between slice width vs signal intensity. The *full width half maximum (FWHM)* of the beam profile is obtained from the graph. It is nearly rectangular for an axial CT whereas it is an inverted bell shaped for a helical CT. It is slightly greater than the set slice thickness for axial CT **(Fig. 10.18)**. Slice sensitivity profile is wider for helical CT scans, compared to axial CT and it increases with increasing pitch. Higher pitch not only increases slice sensitivity profile but also slice width.

Interpolation

CT reconstruction algorithm assumes that the X-ray source path is circular, not helical around the patient. In a helical scan, the X-ray beam path is helical in nature and gives only helical data set. Hence, before the actual CT reconstruction, the helical data set must be interpolated into a series of planar image sets. This means that raw data from helical scans are interpolated to approximate acquisition of planar reconstruction data, by an *interpolation algorithm.* Then, with the interpolated data set, CT images can be reconstructed at any position with any thickness, but equal to collimator opening **(Fig. 10.19).** This will give enough data for an image reconstruction at any position in Z-axis. Image can be reconstructed to any level image reformatting is possible to display coronal, sagittal or an oblique views.

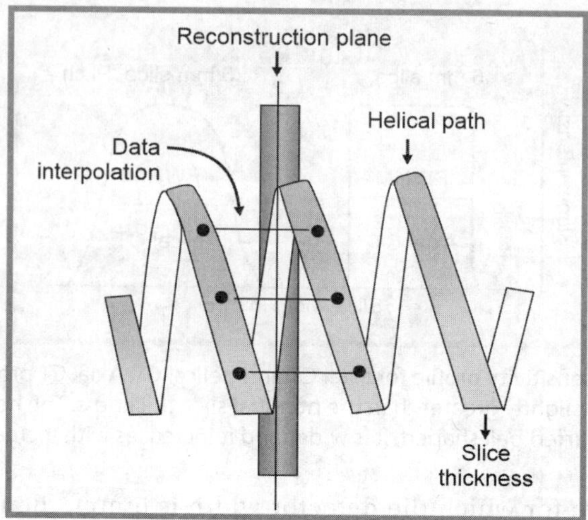

Fig. 10.19: Helical data set and interpolation for reconstruction in a multi-slice CT.

Interpolation is a weighted average of the data from either side of the reconstruction plane. It estimates values between known values. It is opposite of an *extrapolation* which estimates values beyond the range of known values. Slightly different weighing factors are used for each projection angle. Initial algorithm used 360° linear interpolation which resulted in blurring in sagittal and coronal planes. Nowadays the interpolation is done for 180°, that is for half revolution to minimize above blurring. It increases Z-axis resolution.

Interleaved reconstruction allows the placement of an additional images along the patient, so that the clinical examination is almost uniformly sensitive to subtle abnormalities **(Fig. 10.20)**. This involves no additional dose to the patient, but an additional time is required to reconstruct the images. However, slice thickness still decides the spatial resolution along the long axis of the patient.

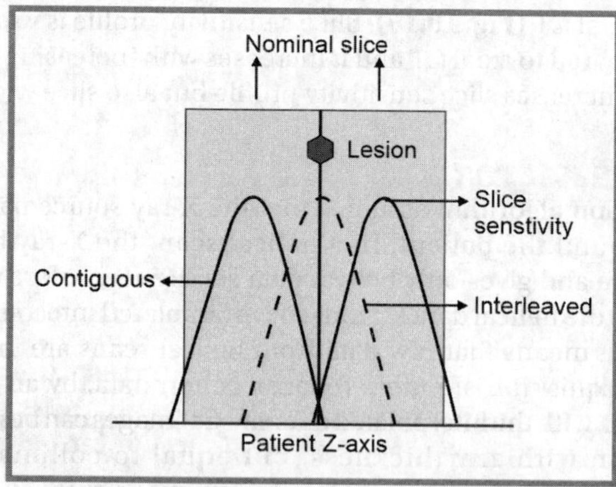

Fig. 10.20: Interleaved reconstruction predicts lesion in between the scanned slice in a multi-slice CT.

Multiplanar Reconstruction

Image can be stored permanently in the system or copied in a CD or film. Earlier, multi-format cameras (wet/dry) were used to record images on a film, now become obsolete. *Multiplanar reformatting (MPR)* is a method of converting the data acquired in one plane to an another plane. It is commonly used with thin-slices data from volumetric CT in an axil plane. Software is used to create images in different planes (coronal, sagittal, oblique). Since it uses data from an adjacent slice pixels for interpolation, and image may involve artifacts. To overcome this, the image data is segmented initially, and volume rendering is performed.

Another manipulation of data with software is *curved planar reconstruction (CPR)*. It generates a planar image that transects an organ along its short axis, e.g., blood vessel, and ureter or intestine. Other methods are (1) maximum intensity projection (MIP), (2) shaded surface display (SSD), and (3) shaded volume display (SVD).

MIP reconstructs an image by selecting the highest value of the pixels along any arbitrary line through a data set and exhibits only those pixels. It is the simplest form of 3-D imaging and widely used in CT angiogram due to quick reconstruction. It uses only 10% data but give high contrast 3D image of a contrast filled vessel. It differentiates vasculature from surrounding tissue but lacks vessel depth since superimposed vessels are not displayed. Small vessels passing obliquely through a voxel may not be imaged due to partial volume averaging.

SSD gives a real three-dimensional view of the surface of structure within the acquired volume data set. It identifies the narrow range of values of an image and displays that image. The selected range appears as an organ surface. It is borrowed from computer aided design and manufacturing applications. Initially, it is used in bone imaging and later in virtual colonoscopy.

In SVD, surface boundaries are made distinctive and provides an image that appears nearly 3D image. This concept is called *volume rendering*. It is very sensitive to the pixel range, selected by an operator and causes difficulty in the imaging of actual anatomy.

MULTI-ROW DETECTOR COMPUTED TOMOGRAPHY

Multidetector Array

Multidetector array (MDA) is a combination of several parallel detector arrays. To energize detector array quickly it requires large capacity computer. In this, the X-ray tube is directed at multiple rows of detectors along the longitudinal, Z-axis. Generally, MDA is designed in rows and columns, e.g., $16 \times 16 = 64$ pixels **(Figs. 10.21A and B)**. MDA has thousands of individual detectors of each width 0.5 to 0.625 mm:

$$\text{Beam width} = \text{Number of slices} \times \text{Detector width}$$

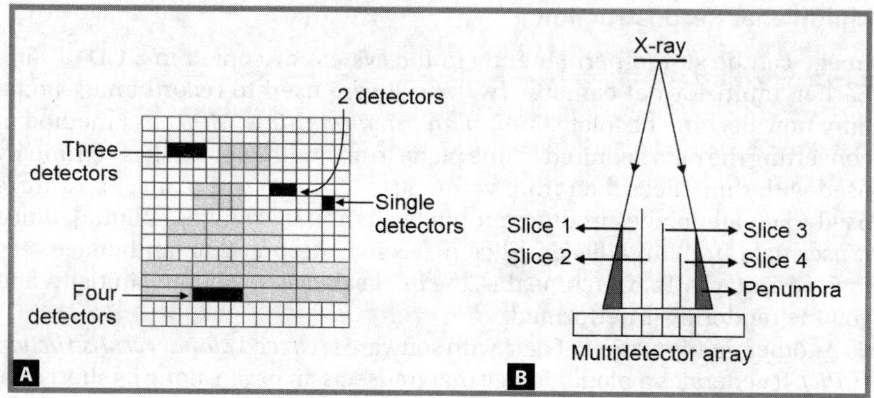

Figs. 10.21A and B: Multidetector array: (A) Detector physical view, (B) Slice selection.

It has separate data acquisition channels for each detector element and can generate multiple channels (4, 8, 16, 64) of spatial data.

MDA is available in 2 commercial designs, namely, (1) *adaptive array detector* and (2) *linear or matrix detector* **(Figs. 10.22A and B)**. In an adaptive array design, the detector width is unequal or nonuniform, e.g., it may have detector width as 1.0 mm, 1.5 mm, 2.5 mm, and 5 mm, respectively from the center to an edge. In the linear array, the width is equal or uniform, e.g., it may have 1.25 mm throughout the dimension with 16 detector modules. Hybrid design has both uniform and nonuniform element design. Generally, 8, 16, and 64 slices CT systems have the following provision with 32 mm detector in the Z-axis:

8 slice CT, Z = 32 mm   : 8 × 0.5 mm, 8 × 1 mm, 8 × 2 mm, 8 × 4 mm
16 slice CT, Z = 32 mm : 16 × 0.5 mm, 16 × 1.0 mm, 16 × 2 mm
64 slice CT, Z = 32 mm : 64 × 0.5 mm, 32 × 1 mm

A 64 slice MDA CT has 64 matrix elements of width 0.625 mm in the Z direction, so that it can cover 40 mm (64 × 0.625). Slow rotation time is used in

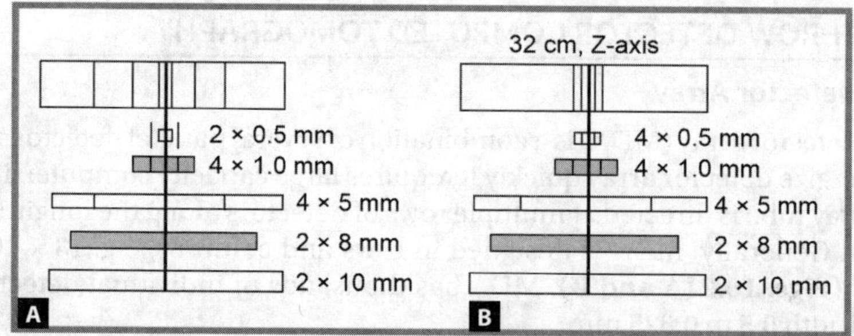

Figs. 10.22A and B: Multidetector array: (A) Adaptive array: 4 slice, unequal width, and center slice 2 × 0.5 mm, (B) Linear array: 4 slice, equal width, and center slice 4 × 0.5 mm.

head scan, whereas fast rotation times are employed in an abdomen to avoid motion artifacts. MDA detectors have high physical density and highlight output with higher detection efficiency. The quantum detection efficiency is >90% and the geometric efficiency is 80–90%. It has high homogeneity, small after glow and provides uniform response in all detector elements.

MDA is made with an indirect solid-state scintillator: *Gd_2O_2S rare earth material*. The phosphor is heated for long-period of time and converted into high-density ceramic referred to as *sintering*. Number of detector elements are created with the help of a laser or saw. Spaces between the detector elements are cut and filled with an *opaque filler (optical)* to reduce the optical *cross talk*. Then it is coupled to a *photodiode* followed by an *electronic substrate*. Electronics substrate gives power to detector array, receive signals from each photodiode, also has an analog-to-digital convertor (ADC).

Advantages of MDA is that its wider collimator spacing is suitable for large volume tissue with an increased contrast resolution. Slice thickness is controlled by detector size, not by the collimator hence, *detector pitch* is defin^e^d. It has faster rotation, shorter exposure time with improved temporal resolution, high axial resolution with thinner slices. Retrospective creation of thinner or thicker slices, 3D anatomical reconstruction, lesser volume of contrast, and increased volume coverage per unit time is possible. Its clinical application includes *angiography, virtual endoscopy,* creation of 3-D images using specialized algorithms.

MDCT

The concept of multiple-row detector CT (MDCT) was introduced in 1998, which improved the volume coverage longitudinal spatial resolution **(Figs. 10.23A and B).** Later introduction of 16 section scanner with short scan time offered thinner slices and improved Z-axial spatial resolution. They find

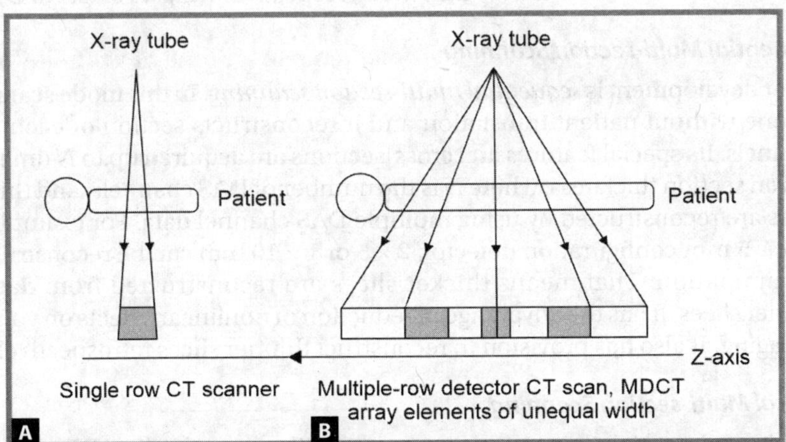

Figs. 10.23A and B: Difference between row detectors: (A) Single-row detector; (B) Multiple-row detector elements of unequal width used in MDCT.

newer application, including cardiac imaging. Detector array design includes (1) uniform, (2) nonuniform, and (3) hybrid for four section MDCT scanners. GE design has 16 × 0.625 mm, Siemens/Philips has 16 × 0.75 mm and Toshiba has 16 × 0.5 mm designs.

Advantages of MDCT are:
- Ability to get large number of thin slices, thereby increasing spatial resolution both in axial and longitudinal axis.
- Do fast scanning of large volume of tissue with variable slice thickness.
- Fast rotation of X-ray tube offer superior image with minimal artifacts.

Collimation

Multidetector array CT (MDCT) uses single collimator, known as pre-patient collimation. It limits the area of a patient, determines patient dose (dose profile). Detector serves as second collimator referred as *post-patient collimator which* restricts the X-ray beam seen by the detector array, reduces scatter and improves contrast, and defines slice thickness (sensitivity profile). Collimator width is about 50 cm at isocenter, to cover full patient and thickness in Z-axis is about 1–10 mm.

Detector Acquisition System

MDCT has multiple detector channels in both trans axial and longitudinal direction. Number of *detector acquisition system (DAS)* channels are available to sample the detector. The DAS number is independent of number of detector elements. If the number of DAS channels is less than number of detector elements, the output of the elements is summed before DAS sampling. For example, consider a MDCT employing a four DAS sample channel with 16 equal detector elements. Sampling of inner four elements results in an acquisition of four inner 1.25 mm slices per rotation. It may be summed in four groups, namely, 4 × 2.5 mm, 4 × 3.75 mm or 4 × 5 mm slices, respectively **(Figs. 10.24A to D)**.

Sequential Multi-section Scanning

Other development is *sequential multi-section scanning*. In this mode scanning is done without patient translation and it reconstructs section of each DAS channels. Its special features are: cross-sections are acquired up to N times for a given section thickness, where N is the number of DAS channels, and thicker slices are reconstructed by using multiple DAS channel data. For example, in a 4 × 2.5 mm configuration detector, 2 × 5 or 1 × 10 mm can be reconstructed by summation. That means thicker slices are reconstructed from data of thinner slices. It has the advantage of reduction of nonlinear effects on volume averaging. It also has provision to reconstruct thinner slices retrospectively.

Helical Multi-section Scanning

In this mode, patient is scanned in translation like normal helical CT scanning. The projections of a single section are interpolated from the data of single DAS channel. Data of all DAS channel is contributed to each reconstruct a slice in

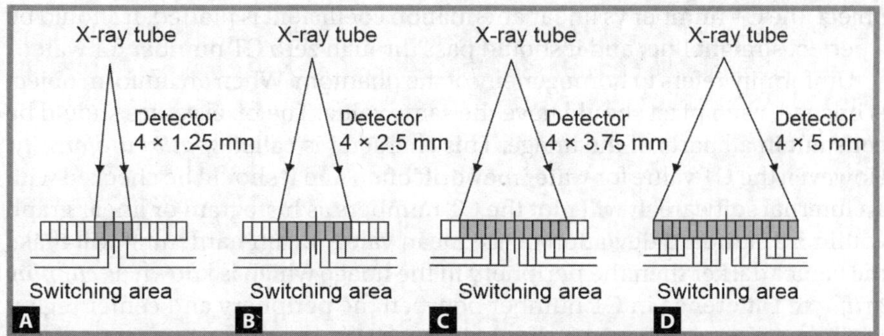

Figs. 10.24A to D: Four DAS channel scanner having 16 equal detector elements, acquisition of four 1.25 mm slices per rotation. Summing of the elements in group of 2, 3 and 4 prior to sampling gives: (A) 4 × 1.25 mm, (B) 4 × 2.5 mm, (C) 4 × 3.75 mm, and (D) 4 × 5 mm slices, respectively.

MDCT. The algorithm balances the longitudinal resolution to against noise and artifacts. It permits retrospective tailoring of section profile and select different nominal slice width. This is known as *z-filtering*. Cone beam artifacts may be significant if conventional algorithms are used. Hence, cone beam reconstruction algorithms are developed.

Helical Pitch

Generally, pitch of a computed tomography having a beam width of W is given by:

$$\text{Beam pitch} = \frac{\text{Table increment per gantry rotation, mm}}{W}$$

where, W is the beam width. There is a need to differentiate beam pitch and detector pitch to suit the MDCT. The detector pitch of MDCT having single data acquisition channel width T in mm is given by:

$$\text{Detector pitch} = \frac{\text{Table increment per gantry rotation, mm}}{T}$$

If there are N number of DAS channels in MDCT, then:

$$\text{Beam pitch} = \frac{\text{Detector pitch}}{N \times T}$$

CT IMAGE QUALITY

CT image quality is mainly controlled by: (1) linearity and uniformity, (2) slice thickness, (3) spatial resolution, (4) contrast resolution, (5) noise, and (6) artifacts.

Linearity and Uniformity

CT must be calibrated frequently to ensure that the CT number of water is zero. This is done on daily bases with suitable test object. After imaging the test object, the CT number vs linear attenuation coefficient is plotted. It should be a perfect straight line, and it should pass through zero CT number for water.

Uniformity refers to homogeneity of the phantom. When an uniform object is imaged, each pixel should have the same value. The pixel values should be constant in all parts of the image. This character is called *spatial uniformity*. However, the CT value for water may drift often and it should be checked with an internal software. It will plot the CT numbers as histogram or linear graph within ± 2 standard deviation of the mean value. Beam hardening will make the center darker than the periphery in the image which is known as *cupping artifacts*. Difference in CT number between the periphery and center region of a homogeneous phantom should be ≤ 8 HU.

Slice Thickness

Slice thickness affects quality of an image due to variation of noise with slice thickness. Thin slices have better resolution but are noisier with loss of soft tissue contrast since it collects more X-ray data. A 5 mm thick slice is 40% less noisy than 2.5 mm slice thickness. However, bone contrast is not affected by thin slice thickness due to an existence of greater image contrast. Slice thickness affects resolution in Z-axis which is important for sagittal and coronal reconstructions. Slice thickness depends on slice sensitivity profile which in turn is affected by the pitch ratio.

Spatial Resolution

Spatial resolution of a CT is the ability to differentiate small objects placed adjacent to each other and is a function of pixel size. It is a measure of degree of blurring in a CT image. It is expressed as spatial frequency in line pair per centimeter, lp/cm. Resolution is affected by pixel size, slice thickness, sampling frequency, detector width, field of view (FOV), focal spot size, and choice of an image reconstruction filter.

The range of spatial resolution in CT is 5–15 lp/cm. Limiting resolution of head and body scans are 10 lp/cm and 7 lp/cm, respectively. This is due to sampling frequency of 2 and 1.4 pixels per mm in head and body region, respectively. Though spatial resolution of CT is low compared to screen-film radiography, an acquisition time is few 100 msec, which is suitable to freeze any physiologic motion. MDCT has an isotropic resolution of 8 lp/cm.

Smaller the pixel size, higher the spatial resolution. If an anatomy does not occupy totally within the slice thickness, leads to *partial volume averaging*. Hence, the voxel size also affects spatial resolution. Collimator design, both pre-patient and pre-detector influence resolution since it has control over scatter radiation. The ability of a CT system to reproduce a high contrast edge is mathematically expressed as an *edge response function (ERF)*. The measured ERF is related to the modulation transfer function (MTF) which is used to express spatial resolution of CT.

Digital CT scan employs 512 × 512 matrix size. In head scan imaging, it covers 250 mm of an anatomical length, and the sampling frequency is about 10 lp/cm. In abdomen scan, it covers over 350 mm of anatomy, and the sampling frequency is 14 lp/cm. The achievable resolution is about 7 lp/cm. CT resolution is much lower than digital radiography (2.9 lp/mm) and screen-film radiography (5–10 lp/mm).

To improve the resolution in CT scan, large matrix size or small focal spot are used. Large matrix size does not alter resolution much, due to inbuilt focal spot and detector blur. Axial resolution can be improved by operating in high resolution mode with smaller FOV and larger matrix size. Employing small focus or smaller detector size will also improve CT resolution. To improve resolution, bone filters/detail reconstruction filters are used. The detector width may also affect resolution in the Z-axis.

Contrast Resolution

Ability of CT to differentiate one soft tissue from another is called contrast resolution. It is the difference between HU values of tissues. In a good contrast image, darker parts are much darker, and lighter parts are much lighter. Good quality image can detect even smallest size object with low contrast detectability.

Basically, CT offers superior contrast resolution compared to screen-film radiography due to well beam collimation. The reason is that an attenuation of X-ray beam is caused by difference in atomic number and mass density of the structures, e.g., fat-muscle-bone interface. Though these differences are measurable, not addressed well in radiography due to larger field area. On the other hand, CT amplifies the differences and increases their subject contrast. Ability to scan low contrast objects is limited by the size and uniformity of the object and noise of the system.

Contrast increases as tube voltage decreases, not affected by tube current or scan times. It increases with addition of *contrast medium (Iodine)* and reduces as the photon energy increases. Higher photon energy reduces contrast much more in high Z, than soft tissue lesions. Displayed image contrast on the monitor are controlled by *window level and window width*. Narrow window width offers higher contrast. Lesion that differs by 5 HU (0.5% μ) from its surroundings can be detected in CT scan, whereas the minimum difference is 3 to 5% for screen-film radiography. Thus, CT gives better contrast than screen-film radiography.

Noise

Noise defines an image content that limits ability to visualize lesion or pathology. It is fluctuation of CT number above or below the mean value. It appears as graininess on the image, low noise image appears smooth but high noise image appears spotty. CT number is a measurement of attenuation coefficient of the voxel in the tissue. Voxel value should be constant for a homogeneous object, but it fluctuates around the true value of an object, resulting in noise. It is analogy to a margin of error in a series of physical measurements. Noise depends on kV, filtration, pixel size, slice thickness, detector efficiency, and patient dose. Noise in CT is about ±3 HU and it is a fundamental limit to the quality of CT image. It reduces contrast resolution of small objects and worsens the spatial resolution of low contrast objects. There are three sources of noise, namely (1) *quantum noise,* (2) *electronic noise, and* (3) *structural noise.*

The quantum noise is the major contributor, and it is caused by random variations in the number of photons detected. Increase of mA or scan time reduces noise but also reduces spatial resolution and increases partial volume effect. Number of X-ray photons (quanta) is directly proportional to mA and gantry rotation time. Noise is inversely proportional to $mAs^{0.5}$, if mAs is reduced by 4, noise will be reduced to half.

Increase of kV reduces noise and ensures higher number of photons and penetration. Though it reduces noise, it also reduces contrast. Smaller FOV has fever number of photons per pixel, which increases noise, and it can be reduced by increasing FOV or slice thickness. Increase of voxel size will reduce noise. Noise does not change with pitch in a helical CT scan. In a multi-slice scanner, an increase of pitch increases noise, because of the cone beam effect, complex reconstruction, and data are used from all detector rows for each projection angle. Noise is apparent with lower window width but reveals low contrast detail. Noise in the reconstructed image is affected by back projection filter.

Increasing slice thickness increases X-ray photons and reduce noise. Acquisition of image with 1.25 mm slice thickness and displaying it in 5 mm slices will reduce noise by 50%. Higher kV, use of soft tissue filter reduces noise, but also reduces spatial resolution. Use of good resolution filters will increase noise, e.g., detail, lung, bone, edge filter, etc.

CT ARTIFACTS

Artifacts are errors in the representation of CT image information. It is discrepancy between CT reconstructed image and the true attenuation coefficient of an anatomy. Artifact patterns appear as lines, shades, bands, rings, dark spots, and ghost images. It degrades image quality and leads to wrong diagnosis. Knowledge of artifacts is important since they mimic pathology. Sources of artifacts are (1) *physics-based artifacts,* (2) *patient-based artifacts,* (3) *scanner-based artifacts,* and (4) *helical and multi-section technique artifacts.* Artifacts can be minimized by CT design, software, patient positioning and selection of scan parameters.

Physics-based Artifacts

Physics based artifacts arises from physical process during image acquisition. They are (1) *beam hardening artifact,* (2) *partial volume artifact,* and (3) *under sampling artifact.*

Beam hardening artifact is caused by polychromatic nature of X-ray beam (25–120 keV). As the beam passes through the patient, low energy is absorbed, and the mean energy of the beam increases **(Fig. 10.25A)**. The spectrum shifts to higher effective energy. As a result, the beam become hardened, that causes underestimation of μ and *HU*. The advantage of beam hardening is that it removes low energy X-rays which are less penetrating and offer only skin dose. On the other hand, it hardens the beam that have high penetration. This causes two effects, namely (1) *cupping artifact,* and (2) *streaks and dark bands artifact.*

X-ray beam passing through a midportion of a uniform phantom are hardened more than that passing through the edges. CT number at the center of the phantom is lower than at periphery. CT number profile has more intensity at the edges than at center. Since, the profile appears as cup, it is called cupping artifacts. This can be minimized by filtration, calibration correction and beam hardening correction software.

Streak and dark bands artifact appears at heterogeneous cross-sections between two dense objects in the image **(Fig. 10.25B)**. Part of a beam passing through one of the objects at certain tube position is hardened less, relative to when it passes through both objects at other tube position. It occurs at bony regions of the body when contrast is used.

Partial volume artifact is an averaging the CT number in an voxel which is heterogeneous in composition, e.g., presence of bone and soft tissue. This artifact increases with an increasing pixel size and slice thickness. It is pronounced for softly rounded structures that are parallel to the CT slice. For example, when cranium shares few numbers of voxel with brain tissue, there is loss of details of *brain parenchyma*. Use of thinner slices, lower FOV and helical scan with an interleaved reconstruction will reduce partial volume artifacts, e.g., 5 mm slices at an interval of every 2.5 mm. It decreases with decreasing voxel size.

Under sampling or projection/view aliasing artifact arises from the use of too few projections or large interval between projections in an image reconstruction process. It causes aliasing of high frequency objects. It appears as regular streaks projecting from hard, high contrast edges within an image. It can be minimized by high resolution techniques like flying focal spot or by software.

Patient-based Artifacts

Patient-based artifacts are caused by patient during scanning. They are (1) *motion artifact,* (2) *metal artifact* and (3) *incomplete projection artifact.*

Motion artifact is due to voluntary and involuntary patient motion, e.g., cardiac, sneezing, etc. It is random and unpredictable appears as *shading* or *streak* in the reconstructed image **(Fig. 10.25C)**. It depends on the density of an object in motion and densities much different from the surroundings produces more intense motion artifacts. High density structures or metal implants motion leads to *star artifact.* Structures move from one voxel to another and introduce errors in reconstruction. It appears as double images or an image ghosting that may leads to rescanning. Different views of the structures do not add up correctly during projection.

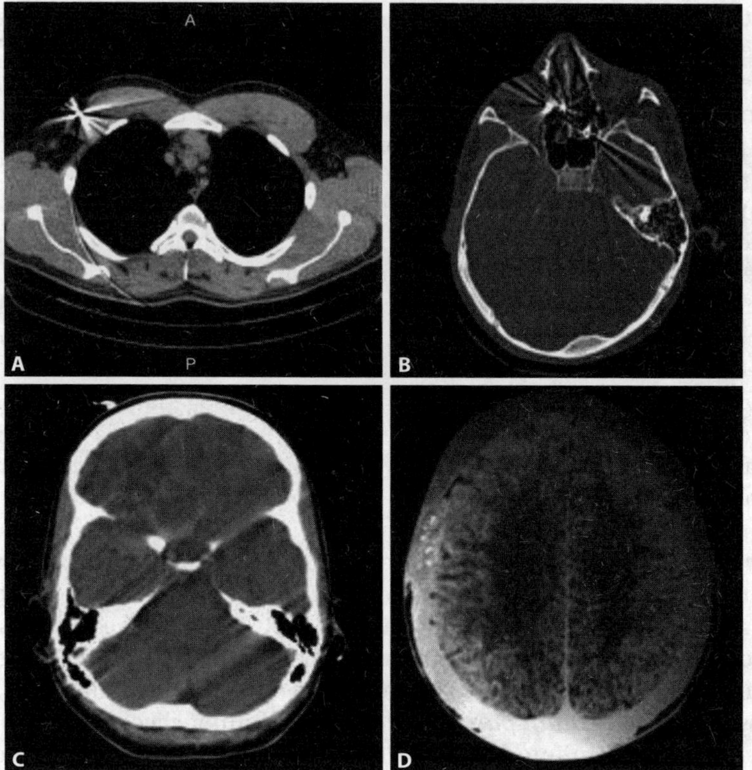

Figs. 10.25A to D: CT Artifacts: (A) Beam hardening artifact; (B) Streak artifact; (C) Motion artifacts; (D) Ring artifact.

Motion artifact can be minimized using patient immobilization, sedation, shorter scan time, patient counseling, software correction and breath hold technique. It can also be reduced by over scanning, that is adding 10° to the normal 360° rotation. Under scanning also reduce artifacts at the cost of resolution.

Metal artifact is caused by presence of metal in patient resulting *streak artifact*. Metals are high Z material gives an incomplete attenuation profile, e.g., *metal implants, dental amalgam,* and *shotgun pellet, etc.* Hence, an absence of transmitted X-rays to the detector that appears a dark and light lines. Streak artifacts projecting from the metal increase with motion and may saturate scanner. Patient is instructed to remove all metal objects before the scan. Use of gantry angle to avoid metal area, use of high kV, software, and thin slices also reduce such artifacts.

Incomplete projection artifact arises when a portion of the patient lies outside the FOV, or object not scanned lies close to the patient, resulting *streaking or shading*, e.g., thorax scanning with arms down instead. It can be avoided by proper patient position or avoiding reference data channels for inconsistency.

Scanner-based Artifacts

Scanner based artifacts arises from imperfections in scanner function. They are (1) *ring artifact,* (2) *cone beam artifact,* and (3) *under sampling artifact.*

Ring artifact is the result of mis-calibration or failure of one detector in rotate-rotate system of 3rd generation CT scanner **(Fig. 10.25D)**. Due to the failure of a particular detector, incorrect data in every projection will appear as a ring in an image. Radius of the ring is determined by the position of the detector in an array and virtually disappeared in contemporary CT units. It can be avoided by detector calibration and selecting correct FOV and using calibration data suitable to an anatomy.

Cone beam artifact arises while large number of sections are acquired with wider collimation. The X-ray beam becomes cone shaped instead of fan shaped. Divergency of the cone beam also increases when using large number of rows in the detector, it results an under sampling of object that are far from the central axis of the scanner. This means that it collects data at wide angle interval during rotation. Cone beam artifact appears as an irregular deformation of the object. It can be reduced by decreasing the pitch or increasing the sampling.

Helical and Multi-section Technique Artifacts

Helical and multi-section technique artifact arise from helical interpolation and an image reconstruction process. In helical CT, while the gantry is rotating, the couch moves in Z-axis. Since, rows of detector also moves in a helical path, the structures are changing their shape or position in the Z-axis. Image reconstruction use these structures that at different positions for different projections. It can cause an artefactual representation of structures that are changing in shape and position in the Z-axis. It is more apparent for large beam top angle, and large pitch, e.g., helical scans of top of the brain. It is seen as two crescent shaped bands of increased density along the skull-brain interface, which mimics a *subdural hematoma*. Helical interpolation causes severe distortion and appear *wind mill* like appearance in multi-slice scanners. Above artifacts can be minimized by reducing the variation in Z-axis, low pitch, 180 interpolation, thin slices or avoiding helical scans.

RADIATION DOSIMETRY

The radiation dose in CT is unique in three ways: (1) the volume of tissue irradiated by the primary X-ray is small, (2) the volume of tissue is irradiated at almost all angles (even distribution of dose), and (3) radiation dose to the slice volume is higher due to techniques used (kV, mAs). For example, a thoracic CT is performed with 120 kV, and 200 mAs, whereas a PA chest radiograph is done with 120 kV, and 5 mAs.

In CT, the scattered radiation (Compton interaction) increases the dose then the primary beam and tissues beyond the section are exposed to radiation. The dose is uniform on surface and decreases towards the center.

Since, the dose profile is not uniform along the patient axis, doses at the patient surface may be higher than dose that at center. The surface–center dose ratio may be 1:1 in head scan and 2:1 in a body scan. CT section dose profile is not perfectly square but has tails that extend beyond the section edges due to scatter. The dose increases as the number of slice increases. The *multi-slice average dose (MSAD)* is defined as the average dose, at a particular depth from the surface, resulting from a large series of CT slices (FDA, USA). MSAD is estimated by measuring (1) CT dose Index, and (2) dose-length product. Effective dose (E) in CT scan is calculated from the CT dose index (CTDI) as described below.

CT Dose Index

CT dose index (CTDI) is a radiation dose measure of an output (mGy) of a CT scanner. It is useful to compare an output of different CT scanners. Initially, $CIDI_{100}$ and $CTDI_w$ were used for effective measurements. Currently, $CIDI_{vol}$ is used for helical scanners. $CIDI_{100}$ is a linear measure of dose distribution over a pencil ionization chamber, in mGy. It is not used clinically since it is addressing the human body variations. $CTDI_w$ is closer to the human body dose profile whereas $CIDI_{vol}$ is obtained by dividing the pitch factor.

CTDI is measured both at the center or peripheral point on a head or body phantom **(Figs. 10.26A and B)**. Phantoms are made with PMMA material of diameter 16 cm, 32 cm for head and body, respectively. Phantom has multiple chambers inserts to make measurements both in center ($CIDI_{cent}$), and periphery ($CIDI_{peri}$). A 100 mm long pencil shape ion chamber covers 14 slices and measure dose while gantry is rotating. For a single scan, there are 7 CT slices in both directions. CTDI are always stated for 100 mAs value. Measurements are made at the peripheral ($CTDI_{peri}$) and at the center ($CTDI_{cent}$). $CTDI_w$ refers to CT dose index weighted which is given by:

$$CTDI_w(mGy) = \frac{2}{3(CTDI_{peri})} + \frac{1}{3(CTDI_{cent})}$$

$CTDI_w$ is always stated in air kerma in mGy and the value increases with increase of tube kilo voltage. $CTDI_w$ of body scans are lower than head scans, due to greater attenuation in the body.

Dose Length Product

$CTDI_w$ does not quantify the patient risk, since slice thickness, number of slices, and an organ sensitivity are not accounted. Hence, a term dose length product (DLP) is defined as an integrated total dose over a scan length. It refers to total energy imported to the patient and accounts the biological risk. In an axial/sequential CT, the DLP is calculated from the relation:

$$DLP\ (mGy.\ cm) = \Sigma CTDI_w \times N \times T \times C$$

where, N is the number of slices, T is the slice thickness (cm), and C is the exposure in mAs. CTDI tells the rate at which the energy is put on the patient

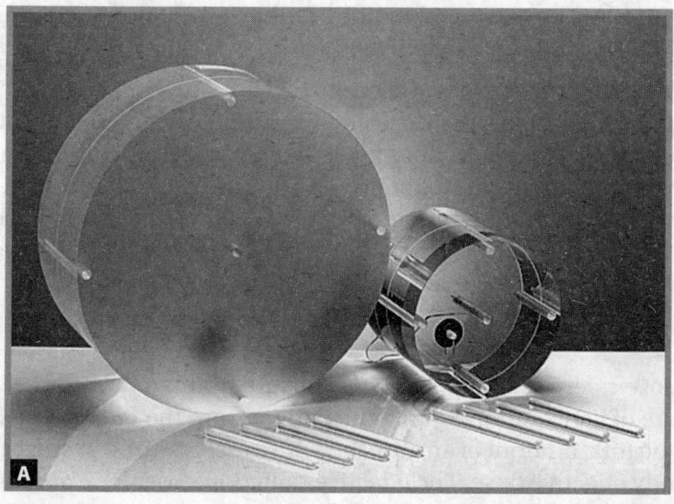

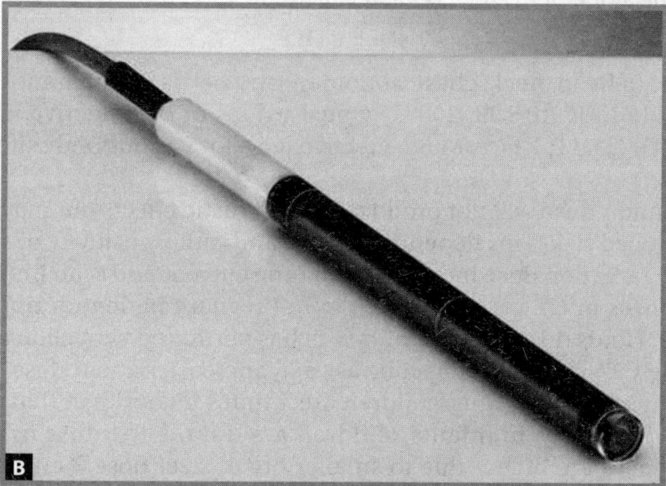

Figs. 10.26A and B: CTDI measurement: (A) Phantom for body and head for CTDI measurement, (B) Pencil 100 cm ion chamber.

whereas DLP tells the total energy imparted to the patient. Hence, DLP is an indicator of relative risk in CT.

CTDI$_{vol}$

In helical CT or MDCT, the concept of CTDI$_{vol}$ is used which is independent of total scan length, and it is related to CTDIw as given below:

$$CTDI_{vol}\ (mGy) = \frac{CTDI_w}{Pitch}$$

Typical CTDI$_{vol}$ is 80 mGy and 50 mGy for adult head and torso examinations. Brain perfusion and cardiac gating studies may increase CTDI$_{vol}$ in multiple times. It is directly proportional to mAs, and inversely proportional to pitch. Product of $CTDI_{vol}$ and scan length (L) is given by a relation:

$$DLP(mGy.cm) = CTDI_{vol} \times L$$

It is useful to compare the doses delivered by various scan protocols or to achieve specific image quality for a given patient. It cannot be used as parameter for patient dose. Generally, $CTDI_{vol}$ and DLP are displayed before the scans as *radiation dose structure report (RDSR)*. Notification/alert value can be set in the scanner which is higher than the *diagnostic reference level (DRL)*. FDA recommends an alert value 1 Gy for $CTDI_{vol}$.

Effective Dose

Effective dose refers to relative risk of exposure from an ionizing radiation. It is a measure of cancer induction in the patient from the radiation received. It accounts the total amount of an absorbed dose received and averages it to give a whole body effective dose. The effective radiation dose (E) is proportional to DLP and the slope of E/DLP is called k factor or E_{DLP} (mSv/mGy.cm):

$$E = k \times DLP$$

The *k* value of head, neck, chest, abdomen, and pelvis for different kV setting are available in ICRP 103, 2007. Typical values of kV, effective mAs, scan length, $CTDI_{vol}$, DLP, k factor and effective dose for various body site given in **Table 10.2**.

CT radiation dose will not produce deterministic effects but may increase cancer induced risk. This depends on dose and radiosensitivity of an organ/tissue. The radiation dose increases with tube current and scan time. Typical effective doses in CT vary from 2–20 mSv. Pregnant patient during CT may contribute a fetus dose of 10–15 mSv which is permitted with clinical intent.

Multiple CT scan involving contrast may increase patient dose. Effective doses for head CT in infants/children are 4 times higher than that of adults. Body CT scan doses in infants/children are double the dose of an adult. Children doses are higher due to smaller organ size (dose = energy/mass). CT accounts only 8% of all examinations but contributes 48% of total patient dose from X-rays.

Table 10.2: Typical values of kV, effective mAs, scan length, $CTDI_{vol}$, DLP, K factor and effective dose for various body site.

Tissue site	kV	Effective mAS	Scan length, cm	$CTDI_{vol}$ (mGy)	DLP (mGy-cm)	K factor	Effective dose, (mSv)
Head	120	390	17	60	1000	0.002	2
Chest	120	110	30	7.4	220	0.018	4.5
Abdomen	120	210	25	14	350	0.016	5.7
Pelvis	120	210	30	14	420	0.014	6

(*Courtesy:* Anjan Dangal)

Patient effective dose is proportional to total energy deposited and the dose is proportional to tube current and scan time. Increasing kV from 80 to 140 increases the dose by a factor of 5. Effective dose is also proportional to the product of the slice thickness and number of slices. In helical CT, the dose is inversely proportional to pitch. A pitch of 1.5, will reduce the dose to 67% compared to that of pitch 1. Similarly, a pitch of 2, reduce the dose by 50%. Pre-and postcontrast CT scans of the abdomen doubles the patient dose. Skin doses are very high in CT fluoroscopy.

MDCT radiation dose is same as that of an axial CT scans. Generally, CT scan dose is higher than radiographic X-rays. A thoracic CT scan (chest) is equal to about 100 conventional chest X-rays in terms of radiation dose.

BIBLIOGRAPHY

1. Bushberg JT, Seibert JA, Leidholdt EM Jr., Boone JM. The Essential Physics of Medical Imaging, 3rd edn. Lippincott Williams and Wilkins; 2012.
2. Bushong SC. Radiologic Science for Technologists, 11th edn. Elsevie; 2017.
3. Dowsett DJ, Kenny PA, Johnston RE. The Physics of Diagnostic Imaging, 2nd edn. Hodder Arnold; 2006.
4. Goldman LW. Journal of Nuclear Medicine Technology; 2007;35(3):115-128
5. https://www.aapm.org
6. https://www.radiologycafé.com/frcr-physics-notes/ct-imaging/ct-artefacts/
7. https://www.slideshare,net/AnjanDangal/computed-tomography-dose-index
8. Thayalan K. Basic Radiological Physics, 2nd edn. Jaypee Brothers Medical Publishers (P) Ltd, New Delhi; 2017.

Nuclear Medicine

INTRODUCTION

Nuclear medicine is a branch of medicine in which non-sealed radionuclides are used for diagnosis and therapeutic application. All the radionuclides used in the field are either liquid or colloidal form. It mostly deals with imaging of internal organs and the evaluation of various physiological functions. After injecting a radioactively labeled compound to the patient, an image of an isotope distribution is obtained. To a lesser degree radioisotopes are also used to treat specific diseases. There are about 2500 radionuclides, mostly artificially produced. They are produced by either nuclear reactors or cyclotron or radioisotope generators. This chapter explains the various imaging equipment used in nuclear medicine, namely, Gamma camera, Positron emission tomography, and hybrid imaging systems.

GAMMA CAMERA

Gamma camera was designed by **Hal O Anger** of Donner Laboratory, in Berkely, California (1950). It uses Tc-99m gamma rays (140 keV) and characteristic X-rays to form images. Tc-99m is injected intravenously to the patient which concentrates in an organ of interest and emits gamma rays. The gamma rays are detected by a gamma camera. It is a planar imaging, that produces 2D images of radionuclide distribution in the patient. The equipment consists of (1) scintillation crystal, (2) photomultiplier tune, (3) collimator, (4) digital position and logic circuits, (5) pulse height analyzer, and (6) computer and display system **(Fig. 11.1)**.

Scintillation Crystal

Scintillation crystal is a single crystal of large area: 60 cm × 40 cm of diameter of 6–12.5 mm thick and has high atomic number (Z = 53) and high density, e.g., NaI (Tl). It absorbs 90% Tc-99m gamma rays by photoelectric process,

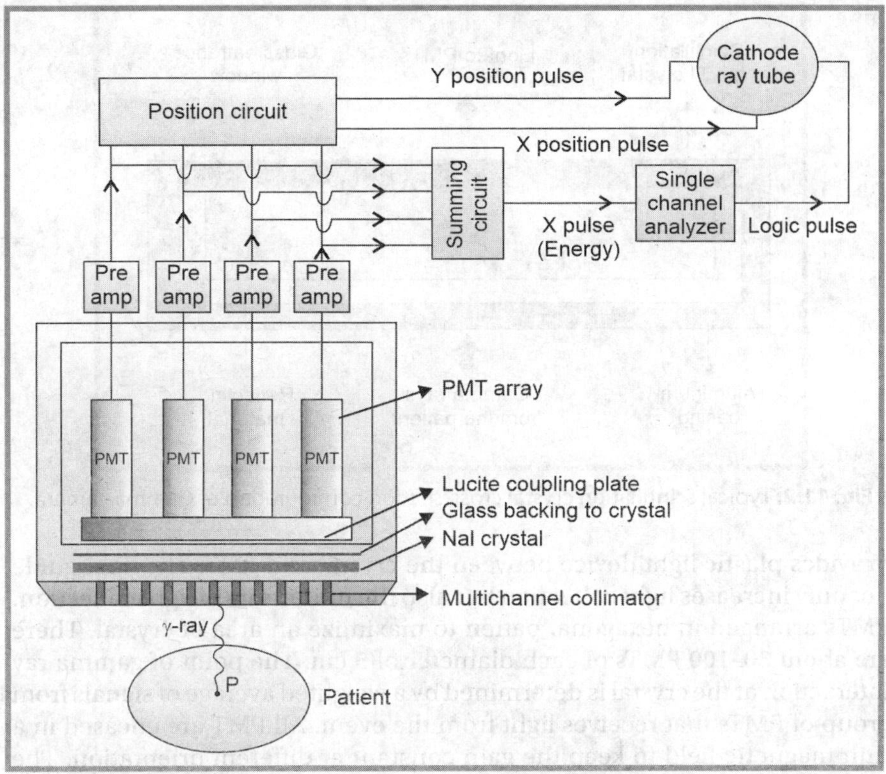

Fig. 11.1: Gamma camera with scintillation crystal and multi-hole collimator.

and 30% for I-131. The crystal is surrounded by a reflecting material like TiO_2 to maximize an output **(Fig. 11.2)**. It is hermetically sealed inside a thin Al window casing to prevent moisture deposition. One face of Al cylinder is transparent for the entry of gamma rays. It is a fragile phosphor, hygroscopic, and influenced by temperature.

Gamma ray entering the crystal does interaction at a point and gives flash of light and an ultraviolet (1:5000). These light photons undergo multiple reflections in < µs and reaches the photomultiplier tube (PMT) via transparent face of the crystal. About 4000 light photons may reach the PMT out of 5000. Distribution of light leaving the crystal depends on the collimator hole. Collimator controls the gamma ryas and forms a projected image of gamma distribution on the surface of crystal. To avoid loss of light a flat *Lucite light coupling* is provided between crystal and PMT.

Photomultiplier Tube

The crystal is coupled to several PMTs, and each PMT is an evacuated glass envelope, having a photocathode (refer **Fig. 5.7**, Chapter 5). It is coupled with crystal with *silicone based adhesive* to avoid light leak. Some vendor

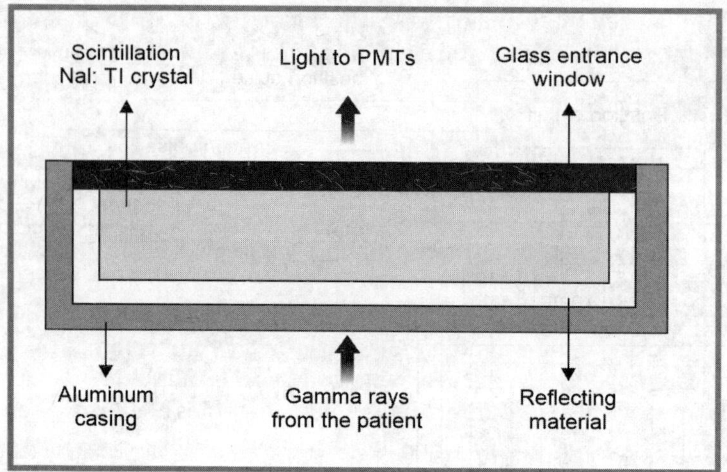

Fig. 11.2: Typical scintillation crystal cross-section configuration of Gamma camera.

provides plastic light device between the crystal and PMT. The light guide not only increases light collection but also the uniformity of light collection. PMTs arranged in hexagonal patten to maximize an area of crystal. There are about 30–100 PMTs of each diameter of 5 cm. The point of gamma ray interaction at the crystal is determined by a weighted average of signals from group of PMTs that receives light from the event. All PMT are encased in a thin magnetic field to keep the gain constant at different orientation. The crystal and PMT array are enclosed in a light-tight, Lead lined protective housing.

Gamma camera is susceptible to stary magnetic fields like magnetic resonance imaging (MRI). It absorbs light and emits photoelectrons (1 electron per 5–10 photons). The electrons pass through series of dynodes and produce additional electrons. All the electrons (10^6) are accelerated towards the anode to create a charge pulse.

Each PMT is provided with a preamplifier, by which the signals are further amplified. Most of the electronics are mounted on individual PMT base to minimize signal distortion. The light emitted by each PMT is inversely related to lateral distance between an interaction site and center of PMT. An amplitude of the pulse produced by each PMT is proportional to amount of light it receives, following a gamma interaction in the crystal. General expectation is that the light and the signal amplitude with respect to center of PMT must be linear.

The pattern of light emission in the crystal forms a 2D projection of 3D activity distribution in the patient. The PMT which is nearer to the photon interaction receive more light and produce larger voltage pulse, than those at far distance. Hence, the relative amplitude of pulses from the PMTs contains sufficient information to determine the location of each interaction in a plane of the crystal. Present gamma camera is a digital one, hence, output of the PMT is directly digitized by an analog-to-digital converter (ADC). In digital cameras, PMT output is digitized, and the event position is located by the software.

Collimator

Collimators direct the photons arising from certain directions to the crystal. It is based on the principle *absorptive collimation* which is not an efficient method. Collimator localizes the origin of gamma rays along a specific line through the patient. It is made up of high atomic number and high-density material such as *Lead*. Each hole accepts primary gamma rays, originating from perpendicular direction to the crystal. The photons originating from non-perpendicular direction, mostly scattered radiation, is absorbed by the collimator *septa*. The septa is an interspace material between two adjacent collimator holes. However, scattered rays can also pass through the collimator holes but have lesser energy, may be rejected by the pulse height analyzer at a later stage.

Digital Position Logic Circuits

The pulses from preamplifier is fed to the *digital position logic circuits*. The position logic circuit receives pulses from an individual preamplifier, after each photon interaction in the crystal and produces an X position pulse and Y position pulse respectively. The X, Y pulses together specify the location of each interaction in the plane of the crystal.

The summing circuit adds the pulses from an individual preamplifier to produce a Z pulse that refers to energy of each pulse. The amplitude (height) of Z pulse is proportional to total energy (keV) deposited in the crystal, and the pulse height is stated in keV. The Z pulse is fed to a pulse height analyzer (PHA), for an energy analysis.

Pulse Height Spectrum

Generally, to improve position accuracy, only PMT signals above certain threshold is included. It has two advantages: (1) it includes only significant pulse amplitude from PMT, and week signals of PMT involving noise is excluded, and (2) only small number of PMTs surround an interaction site is used for position calculation. This helps the camera to detect multiple events at a time and avoids overlapping. The only pulse that falls inside the PHA window (photopeak) is selected to form an image.

The plot drawn between pulse height and time is called *pulse height spectrum* **(Fig. 11.3)**. The spread of the spectrum is due to statistical fluctuations of gamma rays and electrons. The spectrum consists of *photopeak* and *tail*. The *photopeak (A)* is formed by pulses, that is produced by photoelectric absorption in the crystal. It is caused when an incident gamma rays of energy, 140 keV is completely absorbed in the crystal by photoelectric process. The peak width is measured by *full width half maximum (FWHM)* which is used to express an energy resolution of gamma camera:

$$\text{Energy resolution} = \frac{\text{FWHM}}{\text{Peak energy}} \times 100$$

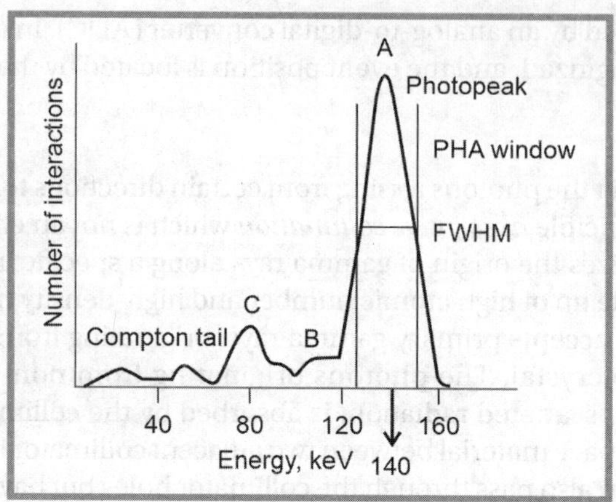

Fig. 11.3: Pulse height spectrum of NaI (Tl) detector with Tc-99m.

The *escape peak (B)* is due to Iodine K-shell characteristic X-rays (28 keV), and the measured gamma energy is only 112 keV (140–28 keV). The *X-ray peak (C)* is due to primary gamma rays that interacts with Lead shield or collimator and emits characteristic X-rays (70–90 keV).

The *tail* represents low energy gamma rays suffered by Compton interactions in the patient or crystal. Tail or Compton tail is due to Compton scatter recoil electron which is absorbed in the crystal and a peak (0–50 keV) is produced. In the spectrum, only the photopeak is used to locate the position of radioactivity within the patient, and the Compton tail is rejected.

Pulse Height Analyzer

Energy selection is much vital in gamma camera. It must delete all scattered rays within the body so that they lose their positional information. Hence, a narrow pulse height analyzer window must be selected. It must accept only gamma rays that undergo no scatter or have only small angle scatter. There are two methods of photopeak selection: (1) simple energy discrimination of Z-signal, but wider window width is necessary to account photopeak fluctuations due to non-uniformities of the crystal light collection efficiency and PMT gain, and (2) photopeak positions and discriminator level setting are computed and stored for variety of locations across the detector face. This is much suitable for digital cameras.

Modern cameras have energy resolution of 9–10% at 140 keV energy of Tc-99m. Hence, 14% *energy window* of 20 keV centered around 140 keV is sufficient. The software adjusts the discriminator levels for other isotopes. In practice, a photopeak ± 10% is set as window in the pulse height analyzer (PHA). The window for Tc-99m is 126–154 keV, that is centered at 140 keV gamma energy **(Fig. 11.4)**. The PHA gives logic pulse only if the pulse is within a preset range of energies and the selected pulse is referred as count. The pulses that are lower or higher than the preset values are rejected. More

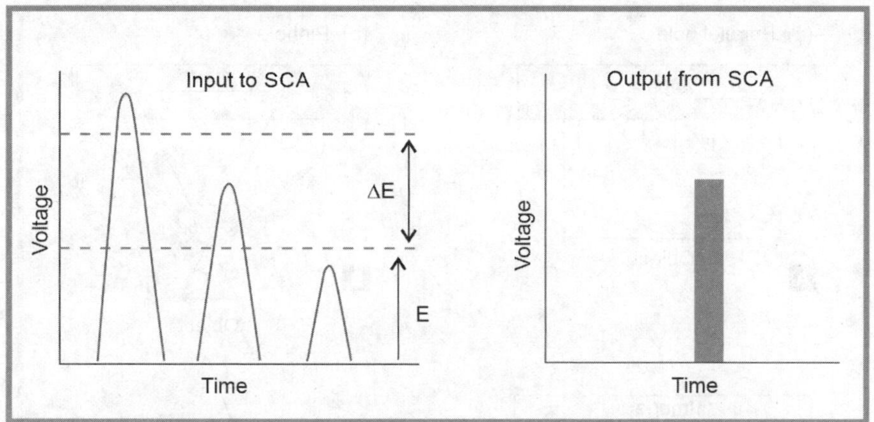

Fig. 11.4: A single channel pulse height analyzer with window width and output pulse.

number of PHA is required to detect multiple energies. Modern cameras use 2 to 4 PHAs for Ga-67 and In-111, which emits more than one energy.

Computer and Display

The pulses are digitized by an *analog-to-digital converter*. The X, Y pulses and the logic pulse of Z are then fed to a computer, which records the Z pulse as a count in memory location, corresponds to X, Y position coordinates. The X and Y values are combined into 2D array of image elements, called *pixel*. As more pulses arise, the count builds up in each memory location, and stored as digital image in 128 × 128, pixel matrix. An image is formed from the histogram of the number of events at each X and Y location. The image is displayed on a computer monitor in which the brightness and contrast can be varied.

The brightness of each pixel is proportional to number of counts, in turn to gamma rays originated from the patient and the activity at that location. Thus, images are built up by using 50,000 to 1 million counts per an image frame. If the counts are too long or short, the monitor screen would appear as uniformly bright or grainy.

Types of Collimator

There are four types of collimators, namely, (1) parallel hole, (2) pinhole, (3) converging, and (4) diverging collimators **(Figs. 11.5A to D)**. Parallel hole and pinhole collimators are commonly used in gamma camera.

Parallel Hole Collimator

Parallel hole collimator is the main collimator used today. Parallel holes are drilled or cast in Lead or made from Lead foils. Overall dimension of the collimator is 25 mm thick and 400 mm diameter. Thousands of parallel holes of round or square or triangular or hexagonal are used. Usually, 20,000 circular

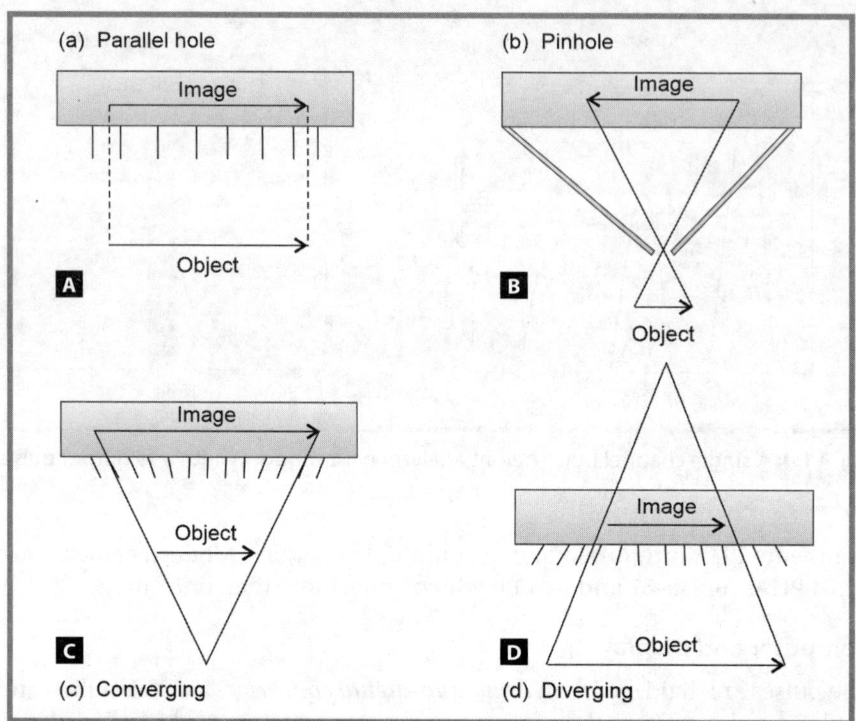

Figs. 11.5A to D: Types of collimators: (A) Parallel hole collimator; (B) Pinhole collimator; (C) Converging collimator; (D) Diverging collimator.

or hexagonal holes of diameter of 2.5 mm with septa of 0.3 mm is made. Lead walls between the holes are called septa. It must be sufficiently thick to absorb photons incident upon them. Hence, thick septa collimators are used with radiopharmaceuticals that emit high energy photons. This is suitable for Tc-99, whose *half value layer (HVL)* = 0.3 mm. This collimator projects the image so that gamma ray image size is same as the source distribution on the detector. Modification of this collimator is *slant-hole collimator* in which all holes are parallel but 25° angled from the perpendicular.

A variety of parallel hole collimators are available that includes, low energy high sensitivity (LEHS), low energy general purpose (LEGP), low energy, high sensitivity (LEHS), medium energy, high sensitivity (MEHS). Collimator to object distance (COD) will not affect the image size but degrade the spatial resolution with an increasing COD. The FOV and in air sensitivity are same at all distances from the collimator face. No collimator will give an expected spatial resolution and efficiency and there is always a compromise between them.

Pin Hole Collimator

Pin hole collimator is a cone of Lead with single hole/aperture of few mm diameter. *Tungsten and Platinum* can also be used to make the collimator. The aperture is at 20–25 cm from the detector. Pin hole size can be varied by using removable inserts. It gives magnified but an inverted image of source distribution, e.g., thyroid. The image size (I) and an object size (O) are related as follows:

$$\frac{I}{O} = \frac{f}{b}$$

where, f is collimator cone length, b is distance between the source and pin hole. The area of the detector (D) and area of projected image (D′) are different:

$$D' = \frac{D}{I/O}$$

where, D is the detector diameter. Sensitivity is a measure of gamma ray detection, and it is < 1% for this collimator. Wider and shorter the hole, the greater the sensitivity, and require only lesser radionuclide with lesser patient dose. This will reduce spatial resolution, which is the limitation of gamma camera. It is mainly used in magnification imaging and for small animal imaging, e.g., thyroid, heart. It is also available as multi-pinhole collimator which has array of multiple pin holes of hexagonal pattern.

Convergent Collimator

Convergent has holes that converge to a point at a distance of 40–50 cm after the collimator. It projects magnified, noninverted image of the source distribution in the patient. The degree of convergence follows the relation:

$$\frac{I}{O} = (f + t)(f - b)$$

where, f is distance between the front collimator and convergence point, b is source to collimator face distance, and t is collimator thickness. It reduces FOV, useful in children, or small organs. Spatial resolution deteriorates at edges of collimator and suffer from geometrical distortion. The FOV and in air sensitivity vary with distance in this type of collimator.

Divergent Collimator

Divergent hole collimator has holes that diverge from the detector. They diverge from a point at a distance 40–50 cm behind the collimator, giving a mini field, noninverted image of the source distribution on the detector. The degree of divergence follows the relation:

$$\frac{I}{O} = (f - t)(f + b)$$

where, f is distance between the front collimator and convergence point, b is source to collimator face distance, and t is collimator thickness. It is used with small diameter camera, to get larger FOV, to image large organs, e.g., lung. It suffers from geometrical distortion.

Static and Dynamic Imaging

Gamma camera is used for *static imaging* in which image of an unchanging radionuclide distribution is obtained over a time. Entire length of the patient can be studied to give a *whole-body scan*. The couch or the camera is moved across the length of the patient to perform whole-body scan. It has application in bone scan of skeleton and an identification of tumor and metastases in the body.

It can also be also used in *dynamic imaging* where the changes in the radionuclide distribution is observed rapidly (several images/sec). It gives physiological information like rate of *tracer uptake or clearance* from the organ. The function of an organ can be studied by acquiring series of separate image frames rapidly, e.g., kidney, lung, heart, etc. It can be displayed on a screen as a cine loop or recorded in a multiformat film. There is a curser to define *region of interest (ROI)*, and the total count in the ROI is measured and can be displayed over time, e.g., renogram. In multi-gated cardiac study (MUGA), each image of 49 sec duration is acquired at 20–30 points in a cardiac cycle. At each point, several hundred successive images are added by pixel by pixel to improve statistics and reduce noise. Images can be synchronized to electrocardiogram signals, to have different phases of the cardiac cycle. This gated image will give cardiac function information.

Types of Gamma Camera

Gamma camera is available in the market as single head or double or triple head with different specifications. Generally, multiple head system increases sensitivity. Requirement of number of heads depends on an imaging site and specific clinical application.

In a single-headed system, the detector is mounted on a gantry so that the head is extended to different regions of the body. It basically gives planar images and can be used for dynamic studies also. Alternatively, the camera is mounted on a rotating gantry, so that multiple views are taken around a patient. This feature is helpful in taking tomographic images. In this, the camera takes 2D projection images at equal angles around the patient. This is used to reconstruct cross-sectional images.

In a dual-headed system, two gamma cameras are mounted on a gantry. In a circular gantry two heads can be positioned on variety of positions. It simultaneously takes two different views of patient. For example, in a whole-body scanning, if two heads are positioned at 180° apart, it gives both an anterior and posterior views at a time **(Fig. 11.6)**. It acquires 2 angular projections at a time, an acquisition time is reduced by a factor of 2. Dual head system provides planar images, multiple planar images over time that can give dynamic images also. It is used to create tomographic images in *single photon emission computed tomography (SPECT)* systems.

Triple headed system is used mainly for tomographic studies. It acquires three angular projections at a time. Since each projection is recorded three times, it gives 3-fold increase in total number of counts. The acquisition time is reduced by a factor of 3. This property is much useful in dynamic studies using the SPECT systems.

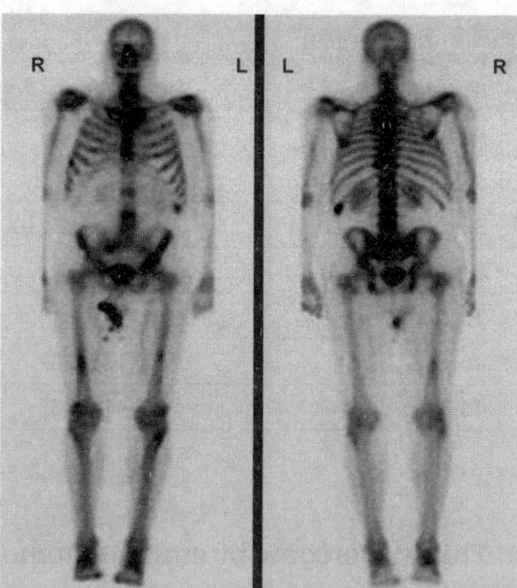

Fig. 11.6: Whole body scan of dual head gamma camera after injecting ⁹⁹ᵐTc-MDP of 25 mCi. It shows both anterior and posterior views after translating the couch through the camera, suggesting multiple metastatic lesions (ribs, sternum, spine, pelvis, femur, and left tibia) in the patient.

Cameras are made with different field of view (FOV) to suit the application. A FOV of 250 mm, as mobile camera with good resolution for *Thallium-201(Tl-201)* is used for *cardiac study*. A FOV of 400 mm, general purpose equipment is suitable for *Technitium-99m (Tc-99m) studies*. A 500 mm FOV covers whole patient width and is suitable for bone and *Gallium study*.

Performance of Gamma Camera

Gamma camera performance refers to sharpness and detail of the produced image. It includes detecting efficiency, energy measurement, and counting rates without dead time loss. Imperfections may arise due to detector, electronic circuit and collimator, and artifacts. The factors that influence the camera performance are intrinsic spatial resolution, detection efficiency, energy resolution, and high count rate performance.

There is a need of standard procedure to measure camera performance. It should give consistent results, reproducible and with simple gadgets. They are (1) intrinsic resolution, (2) system resolution, (3) spatial linearity, (4) uniformity, (5) counting rate, (6) energy resolution, and (7) system sensitivity. These measurements are done during commissioning the camera and after at regular intervals. Hence, rigorous quality assurance of the gamma camera is needed. This can be done by following an international protocol or national regulatory (AERB) recommendations for quality assurance (QA).

SINGLE PHOTON EMISSION COMPUTED TOMOGRAPHY (SPECT)

Planar imaging is a 2D projection of a 3D distribution of a radiopharmaceutical in the body. It involves superimposition of images, loss of depth information

Table 11.1: Commonly used radionuclides in gamma camera and SPECT.

Radionuclide	Half-life	Primary gamma energy, keV
Technitium-199m	6.02 h	140
Thallium-201	3.04 d	167, X-rays 68–80 keV
Gallium-67	3.26 d	93, 185, 300
Iodine-131*	8.04 d	364
Iodine-123	13.2 h	159
Indium-111	46.7 h	172, 247
Samarium-153*	46.7 h	41, 103

*Used in radionuclide therapy
(*Courtesy:* Simon R Cherry et al, 2012)

and reduction of contrast. This is overcome by emission *tomography imaging* **(Edwards and Kuhl).**

In SPECT, radionuclide is injected intravenously into the body which concentrates in an organ of interest and emits gamma rays **(Table 11.1)**. A gamma camera rotates around the patient capture gamma rays and takes many angular views called *projections.* It can rotate either 360° or 180° and 180° rotation is more common. Though 180° data acquisition is sufficient, that of 360° have advantages in terms of resolution uniformity and attenuation correction.

Imaging can be done either *continuous mode or step and shoot mode.* After getting the planar image scans, computer algorithm removes overlying structures before reconstruction. It is known as *blurring effect* which nullifies the 1/r blurring as seen in computed tomography reconstruction. Conventional SPECT systems used *filtered back projection* algorithm which is based on *radon variable formula.* It assumes linear, shift-variant, and an angular symmetry projections. SPECT imaging is not a shift-variant, angular symmetry but depth dependent. It has not addressed source depth and scatter, variable attenuation, and depth-dependent resolution.

Modern systems use an *iterative image reconstruction,* it is based on *poison statistics,* has some advantages. It accounts system resolution, patient attenuation, scattering, septal transmission, and energy resolution. Various methods of iterative reconstructions are *algebraic reconstruction technique (ART), multiplicative ART (MART), weighted least-squares conjugate gradient (WLS-CG),* and *expectation maximization (EM).* EM is further divided into *maximum likely good (ML), maximum posteriori (MP), and ordered subset (OS).*

Iterative reconstruction applies pre-filtering in projection images and post-filtering in reconstructed images to remove noise in an image. Image reconstruction creates transverse image of 3D distribution of radionuclides in that plane. Fourier transform and mathematical filtering is done to filter inherent noise in an image. Thus, SPECT creates 2D projection of 3D volume reconstruction as contiguous 2-D slices without noise.

Such a reconstruction of images from multiple projections of the detected emissions from radionuclide in the body is known as an *emission computed tomography*. Since single gamma rays gives an emission tomography image, it is referred as *single photon emission computed tomography (SPECT)*. This image excludes an activity from an overlying or adjacent planes of an object, resulting high SNR and contrast.

All SPECT system employes basically gamma camera and its detector set up. However, system needs high quality computer and software for image reconstruction, attenuation and scatter correction, image display and analysis of 3D image volume. Images are reconstructed on a matrix of 64 × 64 or 128 × 128 pixels. Cross-sectional images can be obtained in all axial locations covered by the FOV. Generally, *parallel hole collimator* is used, and the number of projections can be calculated. About 64–128 projections are needed for a FOV of 20–60 cm diameter.

For example, camera with parallel hole collimator rotates around the patient in 6° interval. In each interval, it halts to 20–30 msec, and acquires patient data, resulting 60 projections. Thus, 3 million counts are acquired in 30 minutes. After reconstruction, about 20–30 transverse parallel sections can be obtained. In addition, sagittal, coronal, and oblique sections can also be obtained. 3D display and image rotation like that of multi-slice CT is also possible.

Rotation of the gantry may be circular or an elliptical or follows body contours. Elliptical and body contour types of rotation are an efficient and improve resolution since it keeps shorter distance with the body. Body contour is obtained by initial scout scan.

The sensitivity can be improved by dual-headed or triple headed camera. They offer 2-3-fold increase in the total number of counts acquired. Converging collimator is used instead of parallel hole collimator which improve sensitivity.

SPECT Corrections

In practice, gamma rays undergo an attenuation and scattering in tissue which requires suitable corrections. It also has partial volume effects which underestimates an activity concentration for small objects which also require corrections.

Reduction of number photons passing through a thickness of tissue is called an attenuation. It is due to *photoelectric absorption* and *Compton scattering*. Photons arising from different depths in patient have different attenuation. Spatial resolution of detectors is only 10–14 mm which degrades over depth. Hence, an attenuation correction is required for quantitative accuracy.

Compton scattering reduces contrast, and it depends on photon energy, system resolution, window width, object shape and radioisotope distribution. Photons scattering before reaching the detector gives misplaced spatial information. It results in blurred images of low resolution. Though scattering correction is required, the effects of scattering are lesser in magnitude.

Attenuation and scattering causes high image noise, poor resolution, low contrast and reconstruction artifacts and distortions. Hence, an attenuation correction is applied to compensate attenuation, but still some scatter remains in the beam.

Linear attenuation coefficient of tissue for 140 keV gamma rays is 0.155 per cm. The attenuation is more severe at bone due to higher atomic number. The method of eliminating the effects of attenuation and beam divergency is called *conjugate counting*. It acquires data in 180° and combined the single data as *line of response (LOR)*. It should be done over 360° around an object. Conjugate counting is combined with either an *arithmetic mean or geometric mean* count methods. The arithmetic mean is simple, average of two counts whereas geometric mean is the root of product of two counts.

These methods of counting reduce the variation of width and amplitude of counting rate profile. One method of attenuation correction is to correct projection profiles obtained with either arithmetic or geometric mean before reconstruction. Linear attenuation coefficient (μ) and tissue thickness (D) is needed to get an *attenuation correction factor (ACF)*.

Alternative method is to have *transmission scan* with an external source for the same detector. This transmission profile, often known as an *attenuation map,* is used to reconstruct cross-sectional images based on real linear attenuation coefficient of the tissue. However, the image contrast is very poor due to high energy of gamma rays. Collimated flood source, line source, moving line source can serve as external sources for transmission scan. ^{153}Gd (half-life = 242 days, gamma energy 97 and 103 keV) and ^{123m}Tc (half-life =120 days, 159 keV) are used as an external sources. Generally, two scans are taken, one with an object and another without the object on the couch. The first one is called *reference scan* and the later, is called *transmission scan*. Attenuation map is used to compute ACF more accurately.

In partial volume effect, small objects near the resolution limit of the device appear to contain low concentration of radioactivity then the true activity. Ratio of apparent concentration to true concentration of an activity is called *recovery coefficient (RC)*. Cylinder of different diameter containing same activity is scanned in SPECT and a plot is made between cylinder diameter and recovery coefficient. Once the object size is known, the correction factor is obtained from the above plot. This can be applied partial volume correction. This correction is vital for qualitative and quantitative analysis of SPECT images.

Clinical SPECT Systems

SPECT system can be used brain imaging, cardiac imaging, and small animal studies. These systems are specially designed for each application. For brain imaging, camera with 11 detectors of each detector containing 44 thin bars of *NaI:Tl crystal* is used. Crystal dimensions of 15 mm long × 13 mm wide × 3 mm thick is coupled to a PMT of 38 mm diameter and kept in hexagonal array. The collimator has a Lead aperture ring of 12 equally spaced 2.4 mm wide axial

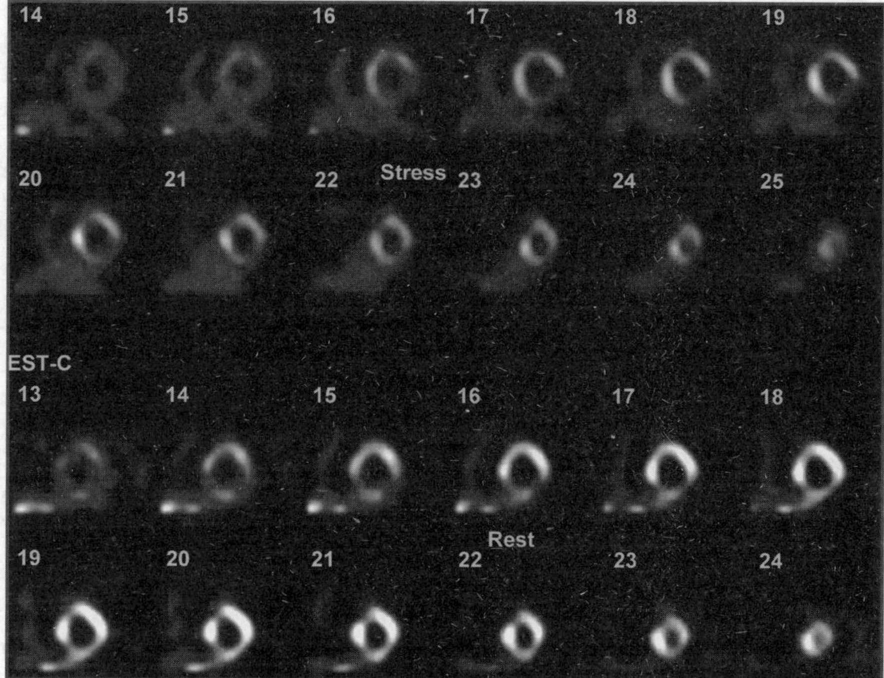

Fig. 11.7: Cardiac SPECT images showing limited perfusion suggesting single vessel coronary artery disease under stress and rest level-horseshoe shape instead donut shape (*Courtesy:* Tom Walsh et al, 2014)

slits in front side of a stationary detector array. As the collimator ring rotates at a slit interval of 30°, the camera acquires data for each projection.

Another model is designed with single *NaI:Tl crystal* of 31 cm diameter × 8 mm thick × 13 cm wide. It is coupled to 63.5 cm PMT by glass light guides. Parallel hole collimator with 6 segments rotates in front of the detector giving six angular views. Each collimator segment provides different FOV. These systems can give a resolution of 5–8 mm at the brain. They able to provide 2-3-fold higher sensitivity compared to single headed camera.

The primary application of SPECT is *myocardial perfusion* to access coronary heart disease and heart muscle damage after an infarction **(11.7).** It is done in rest condition followed by stress condition by injecting a drug that causes vasodilation. It can also be gated to an electrocardiogram in heart signal. It gives data from specific portion of the cardiac cycle.

Cardiac imaging requires a compact system with higher sensitivity. A triple headed camera with *CsI:TL crystals* of pixel size of 6 mm with *avalanche photodiodes* are used. There are about 768 pixels in each detector head providing a FOV of 16 cm × 20 cm. The detectors are stationary, and the patient sits in a chair which rotates in front of the detectors to create tomographic image data. LEHR collimator is used to give a spatial resolution of 11 mm with higher sensitivity.

Another camera for cardiac study employs a semiconductor *Cadmium zinc telluride (CZT)* arranged in an arc instead of *NaI:Tl crystal*. It has 10 small detector heads, and each head has a parallel hole collimator. Each head rotates independently to create various angular projections. Spatial resolution of 8–14 can be achieved with this system.

Thallium study of *myocardial infarctions and ischemia*, with quantitative *cerebral blood flow* are the main uses of SPECT. Detection of *tumors and bone irregularities* are possible with combination of SPECT and CT. Gated acquisition is also possible with SPECT as a planar imaging device, e.g., MUGA study. Cardiac gated myocardial SPECT can be used to obtain quantitative information of *myocardial perfusion, myocardium thickness, left ventricular ejection fraction, stroke volume and cardiac output.*

SPECT can be used in cerebral perfusion studies, including cerebrovascular, dementia, seizure diseases, and psychiatric diseases. It has role in radiation oncology with ^{67}Ga, ^{201}Tl and ^{99m}Tc radionuclides. It can reveal malignancy, metastases, especially in thorax, abdomen, and brain. It can also be used in an infection and inflammation studies and measurement of liver and kidney functions.

Advantages and Limitations of SPECT System

Advantages of SPECT system includes an improved contrast and reduced noise, precise localization of defects, background free images, noninvasive imaging technique and lower cost. It limitations are radiation exposure, limited spatial and temporal resolution, and lower spatial resolution and sensitivity.

SPECT/CT

SPECT/CT is a hybrid imaging system in which SPECT is integrated with a CT scan, the CT is at the back and the SPECT is in the front. It acquires both SPECT and CT images sequentially or simultaneously by providing functional and anatomical information. Arrival of SPECT/CT is due to two reasons, namely (1) attenuation correction in SPECT is not well addressed, and (2) image fusion requires registered dual modality data, to improve localization. Features of SPECT/CT includes attenuation correction, tumor localization and improved diagnostic accuracy. CT gives density and structure whereas SPECT gives physiology information. Additional anatomical information is added to SPECT and additional physiological information is added to CT.

SPECT/CT software employs an image registration method that include manual, semi-automated and automated. It employs registered CT image-based SPECT μ map and use an iterative reconstruction method. Original SPECT/CT was designed for cardiac study with ^{153}Gd resulted in poor resolution, noisy images, dead time and an emission contamination issues.

Present day system has dual head SPECT camera and a multi-slice CT scan (4/16 slice) in a single gantry **(Fig. 11.8)**. A single computer controls the data acquisition during scan. The scans are done sequentially by moving the patient couch. The FOV of SPECT and CT are different in the axial direction

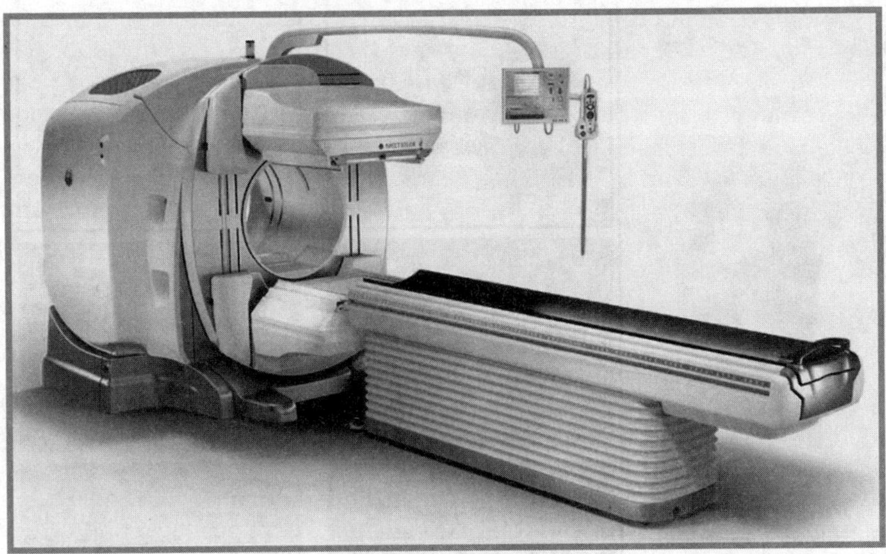

Fig. 11.8: SPECT /CT design
(*Courtesy:* GE Healthcare)

and their axial separation is 136 cm. *Low energy high resolution sensitivity (LEHRS)* collimator can be used to have step and shoot or continuous scan.

There are two detectors of 59 cm × 44 cm and 9.5 cm thick *NaI:Tl crystal.* They are basically ceramic scintillator detectors having 16 rows of 1472 detectors per row. The detectors can be rotated with 90° and 180° or different orientations. The PMT is arranged in hexagonal orientation. The source to collimator distance is 10 cm. X-ray tube focal spot size is 0.8 mm × 0.7 mm and operated with a kV of 80,110 and 130 with a tube current of 345 mA. An energy resolution is 9.5% at 140 keV. It can have one rotation in 0.5 sec and collects data with slice thickness of 0.6 mm or 1.2 mm.

In another model, dual head SPECT is combined with CT in co-planar orientation. Two heads can be put at various orientations, relative to each other. It has 54 cm and 40 cm active area in transaxial and axial direction, respectively. A flat panel detector is used with *CsI:Tl crystal* coupled with a-*Si photodiode* detector of pixel size 0.2 mm × 0.2 mm. X-ray tube has a focal spot of 0.4 mm and operated with a tube voltage of 120 kV and current of 5–80 mA. It can be rotated through 360° in 12 sec so that it makes slices of 0.3–2 mm thickness and acquires 60 frames/sec. It has high sensitivity and specificity. It can also be used to take whole body scan from head to midthigh. It involves 3 bed acquisition over axial FOV of each bed of 36.4 cm.

Modern CT systems have flexibility to reduce dose and metal artifacts. It can be switched to 2D planar mode which not only increases sensitivity but also reduces scanning time. One can review images directly or remotely from mobile services and map *standard uptake value (SUV)* data set. The console can send images to PACS or DICOM connectivity for further analysis.

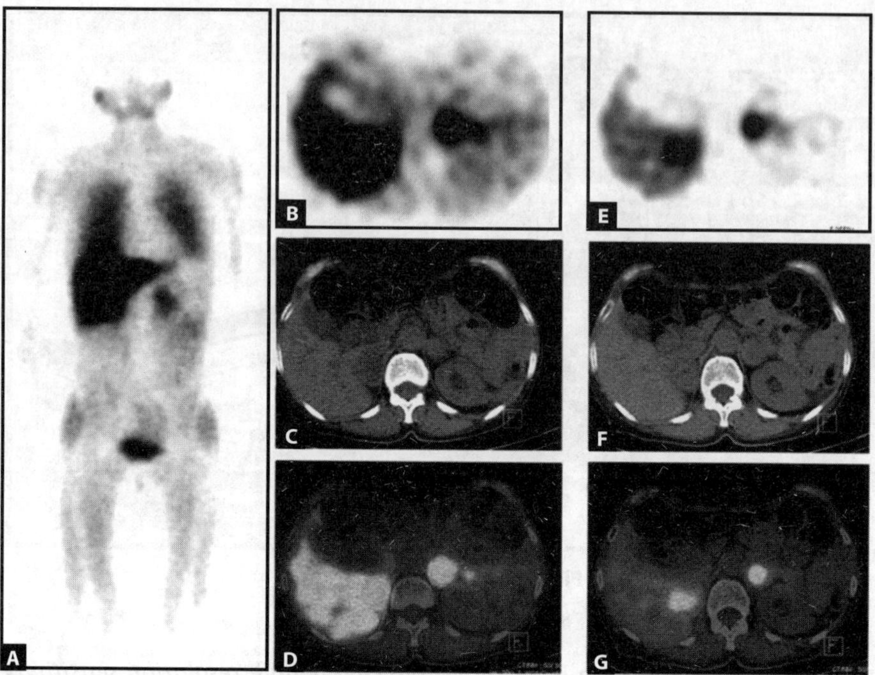

Figs. 11.9A to G: SPECT/CT image: with Tc-99m, Pheochromocytoma. (A) Planar image; (B) SPECT image of the section; (C) CT image; (D) SPECT/CT fused image, focal uptake extending to enlarged left adrenal gland, indicating pheochromocytoma; (E-G) shows transverse sections of right adrenal gland showing additional hot spot and enlargement of gland, indicating second pheochromocytoma, whereas planar image and SPECT image miss the diagnosis.
(*Courtesy:* Andreas K Buck, 2008)

The SPECT/CT has wide application in oncology, especially in thyroid, skeletal cancer, and neuroendocrine cancer **(Figs. 11.9A to G)**. It is used in cardiology by myocardial perfusion with rest and stress studies. It has roles in bone diseases, inflation, prostate cancer, thyroid cancer, hemangioma, infection, liver/spleen, brain perfusion, tumor perfusion. Up course, it requires specific radionuclides for each examination. It is also used in radionuclide therapy for radiation dosimetry, e.g., thyroid. It can be used in radiotherapy treatment planning and small animal imaging.

POSITRON EMISSION TOMOGRAPHY (PET)

Positron emission tomography (PET) is an imaging technique which uses small amount of radiopharmaceutical to get diagnosis. The radiolabeled tracer is biologically active compound which is sent to the body either by injection or inhalation of a gas. PET is used to create an image that shows the distribution of tracer in the body. It is equivalent to a CT scanner in diagnostic radiology which detects transmitted radiation from the patient. However,

PET scanner gives 3D cross-sectional view of the radionuclide distribution in an axial plane of the patient. SPECT can also be used in principle, but their detectors and collimators are inefficient at high energies, and not suitable for annihilation coincidence.

The features of PET scanner are: (1) PET image gives functional and physiological information, (2) it is a noninvasive, and an investigative procedure, and (3) it provides an absolute quantitative information on perfusion and metabolism with low noise. Usually, images are fused with CT (PET/CT) and MRI (PET/MRI). Dedicated PET/CT and PET/MRI equipment are available in the same gantry with a common couch.

Principle of PET Imaging

Radiopharmaceutical of a positron emitting radionuclide is injected into the patient intravenously. The radiotracer decays by emission of positron (+), with short half-life, e.g., *fluorodeoxyglucose (FDG)*. This is due to decay of proton into a neutron, positron, and neutrino. Positron is an anti-electron equal in mass but with positive charge. After traveling a short distance, 3–5 mm, positron joins with an electron (-) from the surrounding. The two particles combine and annihilates to each other, referred to as *positron annihilation*. It results in emission of two gamma rays of energy 511 keV each emitted in opposite directions (180°) from the body site. Their rest mass is converted into gamma energy.

Annihilation happens within a few mm from the location of position emission that depends upon an energy and effective range of positrons. The detector detects the isotope's location and concentration and emits light. PMT picks the light from the detector and converts into an electrical signal instantly. Reconstruction software takes the measured coincidence events at all angular and linear positions to reconstruct an image. Finally, visual display of the slice of interest is obtained.

Whole-body PET Equipment

PET equipment consists of a gantry, table, and computer. Gantry consists of rings of scintillation detector surrounding the patient, septa, and coincidence circuit **(Fig. 11.10)**. Ring geometry can be (1) full ring modular block detectors, (2) partial ring of modular black detectors, (3) hexagonal array of quadrant-sharing panel detectors, (4) dual-headed gamma camera with coincidence circuitry, (5) hexagonal array of gamma camera detectors, and (6) continuous detectors using curved plates of Nai:Tl. Some systems have stationary ring or polygonal array mode, can simultaneously acquire data for all projection angles. Few systems have rotating gantry for full acquisition and the former is most common.

Ring diameter of 80–90 cm is commonly used, effective bore size is 55–60 cm and the FOV in the axial direction is 15–40 cm. Inner bore of the scanner is 59 cm, and the gantry can be tilted by ± 20° from the vertical. This will help to select a scan plane with an optimal viewing angle for an organ of interest.

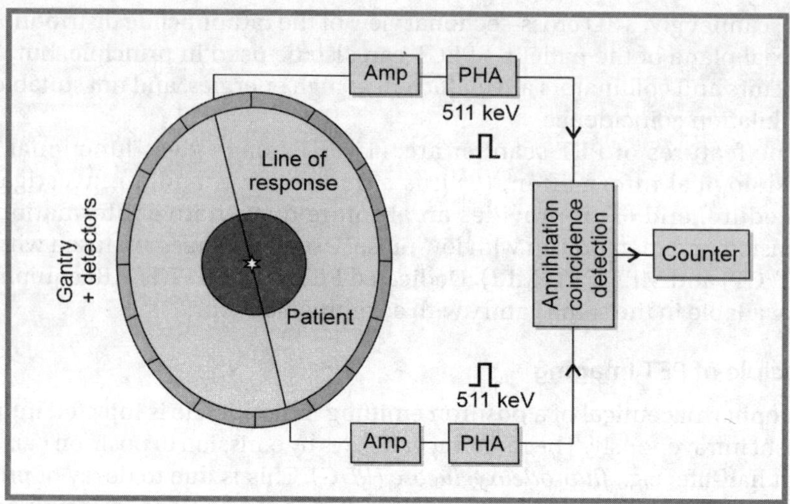

Fig. 11.10: Typical PET scanner and detector ring geometry with annihilation coincidence detection (ACD).

Detection of pairs of gamma photons in the opposite direction is known as an *annihilation coincidence detection (ACD)*. It establishes the trajectories of photons to locate the annihilation events in the body. The origin of positron annihilation event is localized along a line between two detectors without any collimator. This method of detection without collimator is called an *electronic collimation*. Hence, the sensitivity, that is the number detected events/unit activity is much higher than SPECT.

The couch moves in and out of the scanner to measure the radiopharmaceutical distribution within the body and it should have easy access to patient. A computer is used to analyze the gamma rays and uses this information to create image of a tissue of interest. PET also has a *Ge-68 source* (Half-lie = 273 days) to have transmission scans for an attenuation correction. It is permanently mounted in the system and can be retracted back into a Lead shield when not in use.

Positron

PET scanner makes use of short-lived positron emitters **(Table 11.2)**. Positron has finite range in tissue before an annihilation event. It is like a range of an electron of equal energy that travel in tissue. Since positron has a tail at the end of its path in a medium, the term *extrapolated range* is used. However, it travels in a *tortuous path* with multiple deflections, an average distance traveled is less than an extrapolated range. Hence, the term *effective positron range* is used which is an average distance drawn perpendicular to the line of an annihilation from the radionuclide emission point to an actual positron range **(Fig. 11.11)**.

Positron emitters has higher energy than SPECT radionuclides. The maximum energy and the extrapolated range of positron used in nuclear medicine is 0.5 to 5 MeV and 0.1 to 2 cm, respectively. FWHM concept of

Table 11.2: Positron emitting radionuclides used in PET and their physical characteristics.

Nuclide	Half-life, minutes	Positron energy, keV	Positron max range, mm	Tracer	Application
O–15	2	1732	8.4	Water	Cerebral blood flow
C–11	20.4	960	4.2	Methionine	Tumor protein synthesis
N–13	10	1198	5.4	Ammonia	Myocardial blood flow
F–18	110	634	2.4	FDG	Glucose metabolism
Ga–68	68.3	1900		DOTANOC	Neuroendocrine imaging
Rb–82	1.3	3356	17	Rb-82	Myocardial perfusion

(*Courtesy:* Jerrold T Bushberg et al, 2012 and Simon R Cherry et al, 2012)

spatial resolution is useful here since positron range has a tail. Hence, *Root mean square (RMS) effective range* is often used instead of FWHM value. Typical RMS effective range of positron is 0.5 to 3 mm. Since, it is inversely proportional to density, lung has higher value relative to bone. Additionally, the gamma photon emission is not exactly 180°, due to small residual momentum of positron at its path end. This is known as *noncollinearity* which leads to positioning errors. Production of short-lived radionuclides require in house medical *cyclotron* (refer **Fig. 2.15**, Chapter 2). It produces radioisotopes which are used to synthesize radiopharmaceuticals.

Detectors

Organic scintillation crystals are used as detectors which emits light photons after radiation exposure. Various scintillation detectors are *Bismuth germanate (BGO), Lutetium oxyorthosilicate (LSO), and Gadolinium oxyorthosilicate (GSO)*. A typical whole body PET scan employs 336 BGO block detectors in

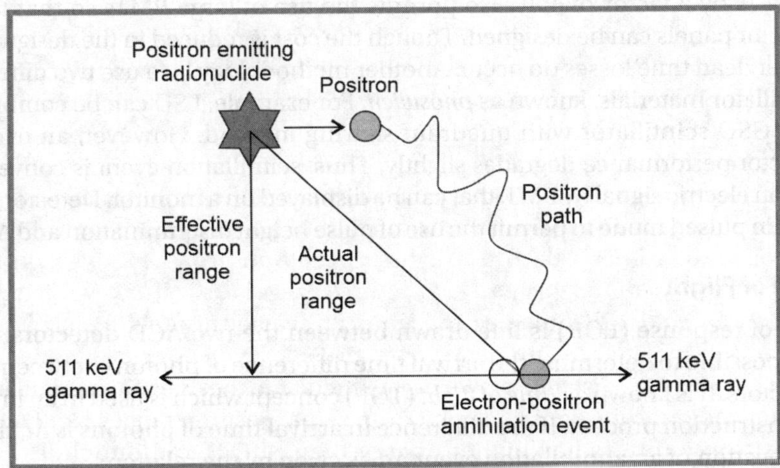

Fig. 11.11: Positron path, actual range, and effective range, causing blurring effects during an annihilation event.

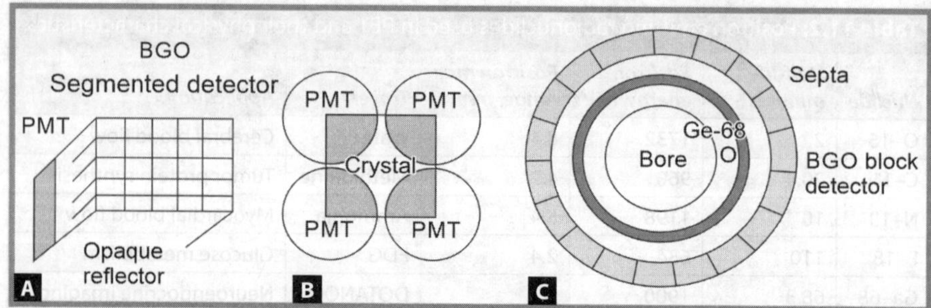

Figs. 11.12A to C: PET detector design: (A) Block detector; (B) Quadrant sharing, crystal shares four corners of the PMTs; (C) Transaxial cross-section of whole body PET scanner.

three rings of 112 blocks per ring. Each block is cut into 8 × 8 arrays of elements with each element size of 4 mm (transaxial) × 8.1 mm (axil) × 30 mm (Thick). Since, the detectors are either square or rectangular, detection also gives the volume from which they are emitted.

A large scintillation crystal is segmented into an array of many elements by making partial cuts in the crystal **(Figs. 11.12A to C)**. The cut portion is filled with a reflective material that limits an optical cross talks between detector elements. The array of crystal elements is coupled to four PMTs. The advantage of this system is that many detector elements can be decoded by using only four PMTs. Four PMTs is arranged in circular pattern around the patient. Tungsten septa of 1 mm thick × 12 mm length is kept in between the rings. The septa are pulled in and out to have different levels of scatter rejection. It not only limits the scatter radiation from an object but also serves as shield to protect organs outside the scanning volume.

In the modified version, each PMT monitor is placed at the corners of four different blocks. This is known as *quadrant sharing* which reduces the number of PMTs by a factor of 4. It also permits the use of large PMTs so that large detector panels can be designed. Though the cost is reduced in the design, but higher dead time losses do occur. Another methodology is to use two different scintillator materials, known as *phoswich*. For example, LSO can be combined with GSO scintillator with quadrant sharing method. However, an overall detector performance degrades slightly. Thus, scintillation event is converted into an electric signal by PMT, that can be displayed on a monitor. Detectors are used in pulsed mode to permit the use of pulse height discrimination and ACD.

Time of Flight

Line of response (LOR) is line drawn between the two ACD detectors. It is also possible to determine the arrival time difference of photons between two detectors. It is known as *time of flight* (TOF) concept which is used in an image reconstruction process. If the difference in arrival time of photons is Δt, then, the location of an annihilation event Δd, is given by the relation:

$$\Delta d = \frac{\Delta t \times c}{2}$$

where, c is the velocity of light which is 3×10^8 m/s. For a depth of 1 cm, a timing resolution of 0.001 ns is required. Though an electronic circuit can detect such nano seconds, scintillators find it difficult to match this timing resolution. The PET using the above concept is called *time of flight PET*. TOF PET improves image quality in terms of higher spatial resolution and contrast.

Annihilation Coincidence Detection

A coincidence circuit detects simultaneously two gamma rays emitted from an annihilation process. It is a strong signature that differentiates it from other photons. The line joins a pair of detectors that does annihilation coincidence gives *line of response (LOR)*. Image acquisition is based on coincidence detection of gamma rays. Valid coincidence takes place within 12 billion of a second. In accepted coincidences, the LOR connecting the coincidence detectors are drawn through an object and used for image reconstruction. The pair of detectors measure sum of the activity present along the LOR. Other detector pairs follow the same procedure and create hundreds of such LORs. Any pulse that does not coincide within the time window are ignored by the electronics. Annihilated photons but an unpaired is rejected, referred as *singles event*.

There are four types of coincidence, namely true, random, scatter, and multiple coincidences **(Figs. 11.13A to D)**. A *true coincidence* is a simultaneous detection of photons from a single event in the same plane. *Random coincidence* refers to detection of photons due to two independent events, not in the same plane. *Scattered coincidence* refers to detection of photons from a single event, but in different plane due to scatter. To avoid random and scatter coincidences from adjacent rings, a Lead or Tungsten septa is used between each ring detectors in the PET. Multiple coincidence is due to two lines of response, due to two separate annihilation event.

Annihilation coincidence is helpful to define a volume from which the photons are emitted. Mostly, the volume is a box of rectangular or square cross-sections. PMT reads detector response and gives signal, which is pre-amplified, amplified and energy discriminated by a *pulse height analyzer*. It accepts only photon energy of 511 keV arising from an annihilation event occurring along the LOR. Typical energy window is 300–650 keV, other photon energies are not accepted and discriminated. The size of the signal is proportional to photon energy reaching the crystal.

Coincidence circuit examines the true coincidence of the detector pair signal in terms of an amplitude. *Timing discriminator* has *timing window* by which it records the time of signal generation. Typical timing window is 12.5 ns with an energy window of 300–650 keV. A coincidence event might have occurred only if the pair of events are detected within 6–12 ns. This timing window is essential to account differences in transit time through cables and circuits, photon travel from the origin, detector finite timing resolution and other uncertainties. Timing resolution of PET is 0.5 to 5 ns based on the crystal and PMT combination. Since, the detectors are arranged in a ring geometry, all projection angles are acquired simultaneously.

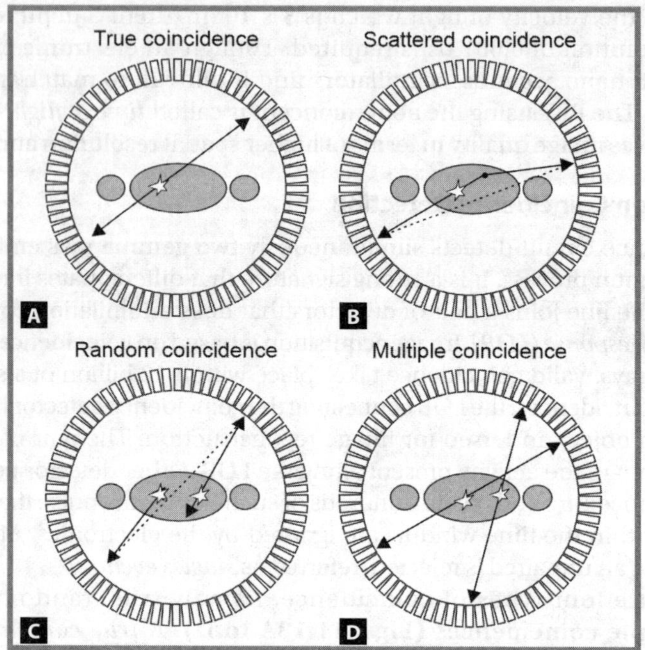

Figs. 11.13A to D: Coincidence detections: (A) True coincidence; (B) Scattered coincidence; (C) Random coincidence; (D) Multiple coincidence.

PET resolution is 4.5 mm near the center of the FOV and 6.2 mm at the periphery of the bore. It acquires 35 slices with a gap of 4.25 mm between center to center in 2D projection mode. The number of slices and slice thickness can be selected in 3D acquisition mode.

Data Acquisition

2D data is collected by using septa which permits only photons that is emitted parallel to the plane of detector. It efficiently rejects scattered annihilation photons. It also lowers single channel counting rate, resulting lesser random coincidence. It also acquires data from adjacent planes, referred to as *cross planes*. It increases two-fold sensitivity than direct plane data. Count rate is reduced and involves random and scatter coincidences resulting in loss of axial resolution. 2D data can be reconstructed into an independent parallel slices by *filtered back projection or iterative method*. Thus, it can gives series of contiguous 2D transaxial images which can be stacked together to get the volume information.

In 3D acquisition mode, the septa is removed, and data is collected from all possible lines of response. This leads to four to eight-fold increase in sensitivity. Number of scattered photons and single channel counting rate is also increased. Hence, scanning body part should be placed closer to center of the axial FOV and multi ring PET have higher sensitivity.

PET can be operated for dynamic studies with frame rate concepts. Once required frame rate is selected, the system sent acquired data to the computer at the end of each frame. Some scanner employs *list-mode acquisition*. In this, each coincidences event is sequentially written on a computer disk with time stamp. It can be integrated over any time interval so that the number and duration of frames are chosen. The frames are individually reconstructed as transverse images.

Whole-body scanning is done by moving the couch and data acquisition in multiple axial locations. The bed positions are overlapped by 1/4 or 1/3 of the axial FOV to improve uniformity in sensitivity along the axial direction. Later, data are stitched together and a single whole-body image is formed.

Image Reconstruction

Images are created from raw data collected corresponding to each annihilation event. The detector collects a series of lines of responses as LORs. Total count of each LOR is plotted as a function of its angle vs shortest distance from the central axis, referred to as *half sine wave*. Detector pair that receives coincidence from a same location in the patient will contribute to a point on the same half sin wave. The amplitude and phase of the sine wave is unique to source location for a given plane. Intensity of sine wave indicates the source strength in an organ slice. Collection of such composite intensity plot is called *sinogram* which is a 2D plot.

Thus, sinogram consists of multiple sin waves from all other data points for all the sources of an activity in an image slice. Each row in the sinogram is sequentially made relative to an individual projection profile and all LORs that are parallel to each other at same angle of orientation. It is converted into transverse slice corresponding to that angle. Each profile maps the location of the source in the direction parallel to the scan profile. Sine wave is a blurred one with different amplitude and phases. Each transverse slice has its own sinogram, which has all the data for that slice across all projection angles.

Sinogram or set of projection profiles of a slice is used to create 2D cross-sectional image activity it that slice. Simple way of reconstructing an image from the projection profile is *back projection*. Source distribution is obtained by projecting the data from each scan profile back across entire image grid. Back projection of scan profile at different angles are then added together, to get an approximation of an original radioactivity distribution. This is referred to as *linear superposition of back projection*. The image is blurred which can be improved by increasing the number of projection angle and number of samples along the profile. This is called *1/r blurring* which is suitable only for isolated object with high density.

To overcome this, *Fourier transform and filtered back projection (FBP)* reconstruction is employed. FBP employs *projection slice theorem* in combination with back projection. It involves multiple steps as follows:
❑ Acquisition of number of projection profiles
❑ Computation of 1-D FT for each profile

❑ Application of ramp filter to each k-space profile
❑ Computation of inverse FT for each filtered FT
❑ Perform conventional back projection by using filtered profiles

The end-result of PET acquisition and reconstruction is a 3D image. Each voxel represents regional tissue and radioactivity concentration. Images are displayed in an axial, coronal, and sagittal sections **(Figs. 11.14A to C)**.

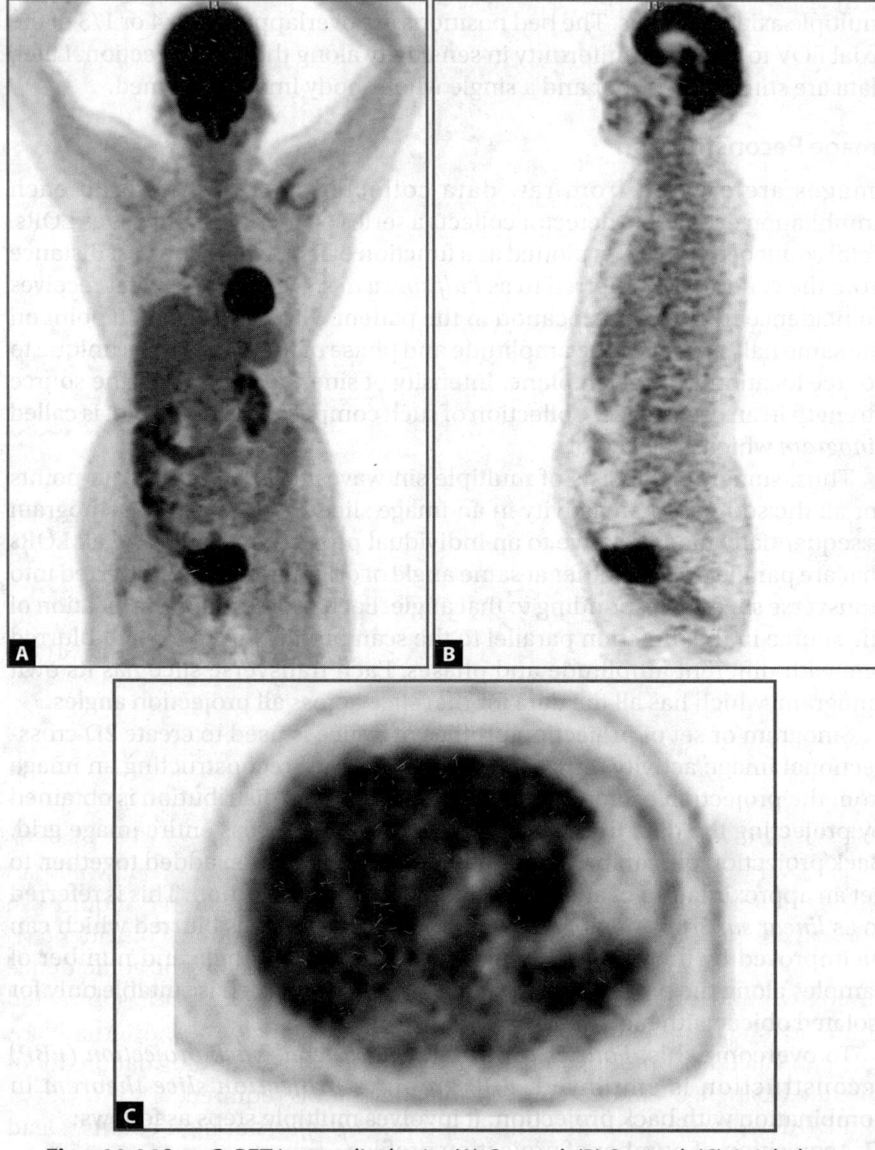

Figs. 11.14A to C: PET image display in: (A) Coronal; (B) Sagittal; (C) Axial plane.
(*Courtesy:* Dr Kamakshi Memorial Hospital, Chennai)

One can visualize the images in grayscale, and each level represents activity concentration.

Data Correction

Data correction in PET includes *(1) attenuation correction, (2) normalization, (3) scatter radiation correction, (4) random coincidence correction, and (5) dead time correction.*

Tissue attenuation correction is required, and it depends on patient dimension and tissue structure. This is done with a transmission scan before PET scan by using a long-lived *isotope (Ge-68, or Cs-137),* located in the PET gantry. It requires two scan measurements, namely blank scan, and postinjection scan. *Blank sca*n is done without an object or patient once in the morning which can be used for all patients. Source rotates around the center and measurements for all detector pair are obtained. *Postinjection transmission scan* is done immediately after PET emission scan for each patient. It avoids patient motion and misalignment between an emission and transmission scans. The ratio of the blank scan data to transmission data of a detector pair gives an attenuation correction.

PET scanners require corrections for nonlinearity and nonuniformity, otherwise artifacts may occur in images. There may be differences in an effective crystal thickness of the crystal seen by the photons while photons traveling at various angles and planes. *Normalization* correction accounts above such variation.

Scatter radiation correction overcomes hazy background in the reconstructed image, especially at the center. It also addresses decrease in image contrast and error in quantitative analysis between an image intensity and activity. Dual energy windows are incorporated to differentiate scatter events at the body and detector. Estimated scattered radiation is then subtracted from the projection profile. This scattered-corrected data is further used for reconstruction. Second correction is analysis of projection profiles outside an object. In this, scatter distribution is extrapolated from the tails of the projection profiles. It is fast but approximate of true scatter distribution.

Random coincidence contributes to an uniform background across the image, suppressing contrast. It may also distort the relation between an image intensity and actual activity in an image. The correction is required to address above issues. There are two methods by which random coincidence is estimated: delayed window and singles window. By delaying the coincidence timing window one can estimate random coincidence rate. It is subtracted from the total number of coincidence events for a detector pair. Alternatively, one can calculate random coincidences theoretically but information about the rate of single event detection by each detector is required.

PET detectors exhibit dead time and *pile-up effects* at high counts. Dead time effect underestimate concentration of an activity at high counting rates and pile-up effects cause misposition of events. Dead time losses dominate in single channel analyzer hence, corrections are required. Global or individual correction factors are employed by different vendors. Correction may be large at first-pass cardiac and bladder imaging.

Clinical Application

PET has clinical application in oncology, brain, and heart studies. In oncology it is useful to study a lesion and its characteristics, staging and assessment of therapeutic response. In brain, it is useful to study blood flow and metabolic activity. It also helps to detect nerve system issues like *Alzheimer's disease, Parkinsons disease, etc.* PET can be used to detect damaged heart tissues after heart attack and helpful to decides the best possible treatment to an individual. Specialized PET scans for brain imaging and small animal scanning are also available.

Advantages of PET include showing the chemical function of organs and tissues, detect functional changes, study metabolic functions, differentiate malignant and benign tumors, determine spread of cancer disease and heart function, detect early stages of neurological illness, e.g., epilepsy, and Alzheimer's disease. Limitations of PET include an ionizing radiation, requires short-lived radioactive compound, and local production of radioisotopes.

PET/CT

PET/CT is a medical imaging device which combines both positron emission tomography (PET) and computed tomography (CT) in a single gantry (**Fig. 11.15**). It is a *hybrid Imaging* device which has a *helical CT scanner (16-64 slice)* to produce high quality images of an anatomy and PET scanner to produce high quality images of function. In addition, CT provides attenuation correction that is required for PET images. PET/CT combines functional

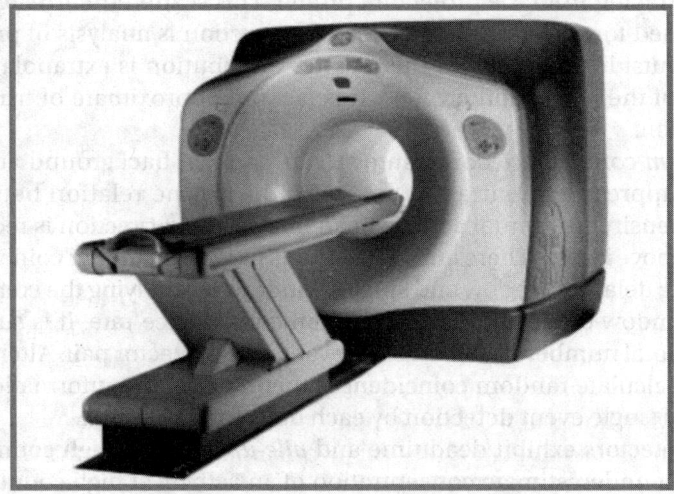

Fig. 11.15: Typical PET/CT equipment.
(*Courtesy:* GE Healthcare)

information with anatomical detail. It has accurate anatomical registration with higher diagnostic accuracy.

PET can determine the metabolic activity of the tissue but requires high resolution anatomical information. CT is the highest resolution tomographic modality and easily integrated with PET. Combination of both modality gives the best in terms of diagnostic accuracy and tumor localization.

Principle of PET/CT

A radiolabeled tracer is injected into the patient intravenously, e.g., Fluorine-18-deoxyglucose (FDG), the glucose analogue. It is absorbed by various tissues and taken up widely by most tumors. Emitted positrons undergo an annihilation with production of two gamma rays of each energy 511 keV. Images acquired from both devices by sequentially, in the same session without patient motion between the studies. First helical CT images are obtained for the patient which provides an accurate diagnostic information about the distribution of structures within the body. Then PET scan is done to detect two gamma photons as coincidence detection which gives physiological function.

Computer software is used to reconstruct and fuse both CT and PET images into a single superimposed (co-registered) image for display. Functional imaging is obtained by PET, which depicts the spatial distribution of metabolic or biochemical activity in the body that can be more precisely aligned or correlated with an anatomic imaging obtained by CT scanning. Two- and three-dimensional image reconstruction may be rendered as a function of common software and control system. It displays anatomy, function, fused images in a series of an axial, coronal, and sagittal plane, and quantitative parameters.

PET/CT Equipment

First PET/CT scanner was developed by **David Townsend, Ron Nutt et al. (1990)**. It had a partial PET scanner and a single slice CT scanner. All the components are mounted on a rotating gantry. Modern scanners follow back-to-back (Tandem) arrangement in which the FOV of the PET and CT are separated by a distance 60–120 cm in the axial direction. It has separate PET and CT components, along with a common table /bed. It is integrated in terms of mechanical and software which controls the moving bed, sequential acquisition of PET and CT data, image reconstruction, attenuation correction and display and analysis of images. Important criteria are that the bed should withstand bed deflections while it is moved in between two imaging systems.

PET system configuration is same as stated in the earlier paragraphs. System used here will have multiple rings of scintillation detectors arranged around the patient. It able to provide complete set of projection angles without any rotation of detectors. Typical PET/CT system employs 28,336 LYSO scintillator elements with dimensions of 4×4 cross-section and 22 mm thickness. They are arranged in 28 flat panel modules each containing 23×44 arrays of elements followed by 15 PMTs. PET-CT gantry bore is about 70 cm with an axial FOV of 18 cm and transverse FOV of 58 cm. It also provides TOF information.

CT has slip ring and helical technology configuration. The CT scanner has 16–64 slice detector, in a 64-slice detector there are 690 detectors in each row with an individual detector width of 0.625 mm in an axial direction. It can rotate the X-ray tube and detectors rapidly and acquires angular projections for large number of slices in few seconds to minutes. X-ray tube is operated with 140 kV with tube current of 430 mA. Tube current controls number of X-ray photons and dose, whereas kV determines energy and penetration.

Patient Preparation

Patient should have 6–12 h overnight fasting and 24 h prior to study, can have low calorie meal and avoids exercise. Blood sugar cut off level should be about 150–200 mg/mL. Patient is injected about 370 MBq (10 mCi) of radiopharmaceutical (FDG) intravenously. During postinjection, patient should relax and do not talk, and move to avoid accumulation of an activity in tissue. Patient is informed about iodine contrast related allergy if contrast necessary. He is asked to drink about 1,500 mL of oral contrast during the study. After a wait of 60–90 minutes post FDG injection the patient is kept on the table and scanning starts with CT scout image. The bladder should be emptied before the study begins. During the study patient should lie down and breathe regularly.

FDG-Glucose Metabolism

^{18}F is labeled as fluorodeoxyglucose and is commonly used to study glucose metabolism in the human body. It is produced in a medical cyclotron facility. It is like glucose molecule in the human body and undergoes metabolism as *glucose-6-phosphate* (**Fig. 11.16**). Normal glucose travels in the body and spend its energy until it become zero. Radioactive glucose follows the same path, but it gets trapped wherever a tumor or lesion is present. Trapped radionuclides emits positron which get accumulated in the site. Positron travels only 2 mm, its effective range, joins with an electron and undergoes annihilation there by resulting two gamma photons of each energy 511 keV. These gamma photons are detected by the annihilation coincidence detection (ACD).

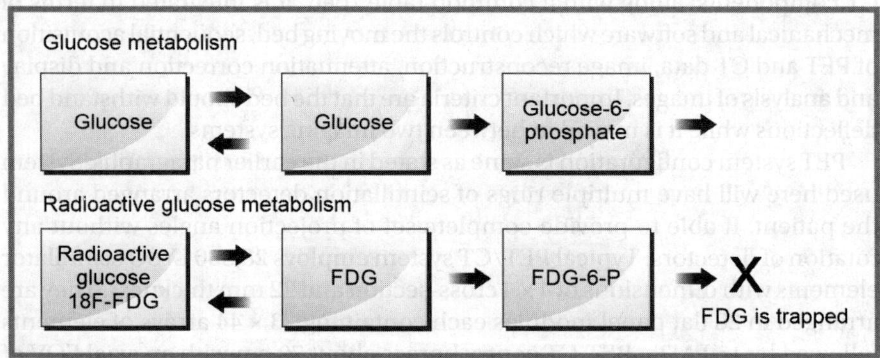

Fig. 11.16: Mechanism of FDG in human body.

Data Acquisition

Data acquisition starts with a scout image or topo gram **(Fig. 11.17)**. It is obtained by using low dose CT scans (40–80 mAs), whereas high dose CT scans (maximum 140 kV with 430 mA) is used for diagnostic images. It is used to map part of the body to be scanned and those coordinates are entered in the system. The system automatically realigns its table accordingly. Image acquisition is done sequentially, first with CT scan which generates hundreds of transaxial images of the patient. body of transmission images. Next, the table indexed back to the PET scan and the PET detects the gamma photons emitted by the patient. CT does transmission scan whereas PET perform emission scans.

The patient is stepped through the scanner and each bed step requires 2–5 minutes. Images are created over 14–15 cm body length generating about 30–45 contiguous transaxial images. It takes about 30 minutes to complete a scan and it may increase for whole-body scans. To scan whole-body about 11 detector positions are required, each detector position takes about 2–3 min. PET image depicts spatial distribution of metabolic or biochemical activity in the body that can be more precisely aligned or correlated with an anatomic images of CT scan.

The volume of data generated is much high. Transaxial CT and PET images are reconstructed. Then they are reformatted into coronal and sagittal images for an easy interpretation. For each type, sets of PET, CT and fusion images are generated. Total of 4000–8000 images are generated. After attenuation correction the PET and CT images fused together.

Other acquisition parameters are rotation speed, table motion, collimation, and scan length. Rotation speed (0.33–1 sec) affects temporal resolution, scan time, and dose, whereas table motion (10–100 mm/rotation) is proportional to scan time. Collimation affects an axial resolution and scan tine.

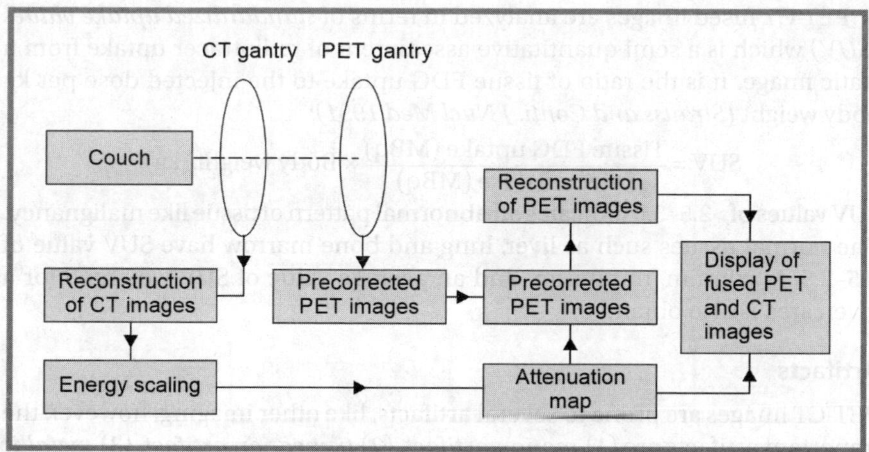

Fig. 11.17: PET-CT functional diagram.

Attenuation Correction

Photon traveling through the body gets attenuated and it is more at deeper structures and less in superficial structures. This results in depth dependent differential attenuation so that an image will show high activity near the surface and low activity near the center. Photon attenuation results in loss of counts at the detector, which is to be compensated to get the true counts, referred to as an *attenuation correction.*

High energy radioactive sources like *Germanium -68 (^{68}Ge)* or *CT transmission scan* data is used to do an attenuation correction. CT transmission data generate transaxial attenuation map of the patient which define various densities of internal structures. Usually, low dose CT scan (40–80 mAs) is performed for an attenuation correction. Since, X-ray energy of CT is 100-140 kV and gamma photon energy are 511 keV, there is a need of an *energy correction or scaling.* In CT image, pixel intensity should be converted into μ of emission photon energy. To do this, an *image segmentation* approach is used which separate tissues into air, soft tissue and bone based on their pixel values in the CT scan. Attenuation coefficient of above tissues at the emission energy is substituted for the CT number, which gives an *attenuation map.* This map is later used in an *iterative reconstruction algorithm* to compute an attenuation correction factor.

Image Display and Analysis

Image analysis parameters include fusion, color scale and SUV measurement. Fussed images are displayed as sagittal, coronal, and axial images revealing anatomy, and functional information **(Figs. 11.18A to D)**. Higher frequency filter is used to get sharp images whereas low-frequency filter is used for smoother images. Color scale of the fused image can be changed to an individual taste. Range of values representing the color scale can be adjusted by using windowing tool.

PET-CT fused images are analyzed in terms of *standardized uptake values (SUV)* which is a semi quantitative assessment of radiotracer uptake from a static image. It is the ratio of tissue FDG uptake to the injected dose per kg body weight *(Strauss and Conti. J Nucl Med 1991):*

$$SUV = \frac{\text{Tissue FDG uptake (MBq)}}{\text{Injected dose (MBq)}} \times \text{Body weight (kg)}$$

SUV values of >2.5–3.0 indicates an abnormal pattern of tissue like malignancy. The normal tissues such as liver, lung and bone marrow have SUV value of 0.5–2.5. Maximum, minimum, and an average value of SUV weighted for a given area is also obtained.

Artifacts

PET-CT images are prone to several artifacts, like other imaging, however, the important artifacts are (1) *motion artifact,* (2) *truncation artifact,* (3) *metallic artifact,* and (4) *oral contrast artifact.*

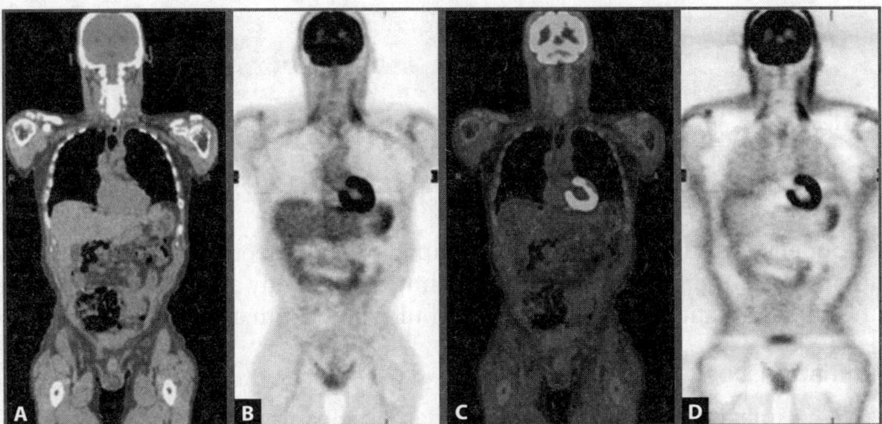

Figs. 11.18A to D: Whole-body PET-CT image: (A) CT transmission image; (B) PET emission image, with attenuation correction; (C) PET-CT fusion image; (D) PET emission scan without attenuation correction.

Motion artifact arises from change of patient position that leads to misregistration on the fusion images. It commonly occurs in head and limbs, where movement is likely to occur. This may lead to false interpretation of uptake in normal structures. Similarly, misalignment of PET and CT images can occur at the diaphragm due to respiratory motion and movement of an internal organ above and below the diaphragm. This misalignment can cause attenuation correction artifact. The liver dome and spleen may be seen 'floating' above the diaphragm.

Truncation artifact appears as dark lines extending craniocaudally along the patient. Because PET emission images are acquired over many minutes (25–40 minutes), patients are often unable to keep their arms above their head for the duration of the scan. The CT scanner has a relatively narrow axial field of view of only 50 cm and often the arms, shoulders, and hips lie outside the visualized area. Artifacts are produced at these sites because the CT attenuation correction reconstruction algorithm does not account for any attenuation of the CT X-rays by the tissues outside the field of view.

Pacemakers are one of the most common *attenuation artifact* produced by metallic implants in the body. A focus of increased activity can be seen at the site of the pacemaker on attenuation corrected PET images. In this case, a focus can be seen along the metallic pacer lead wires. This occurs because of the significantly higher radiodensity of an implant on the CT compared to normal body tissues and subsequent over correction of the PET images at this site. The nonattenuation image, however, does not show any *hot-spots* at that site and confirms it to be an artifact.

Normally, a lower-density Barium oral contrast is used in PET-CT. At normal concentrations, the diluted oral contrast is not radiodense enough to produce attenuation overcorrection artifacts. However, with time, the contrast can become compacted in the bowel with a significant increase in the

Table 11.3: Comparison of occupational radiation exposure at 0.1 m and 1 m for Tc-99m and F-18 FDG radiopharmaceutical.

Radiopharmaceutical	Dose rate at 0.1 m, µSv/h	Dose rate at 1 m, µSv/h
Tc-99m MDP (600 MBq)	114	5
F-18 FDG (350 MBq)	550	70

radiodensity and foci of an increased uptake can be seen. A radiodensity less than 400–500 Hounsfield units should not produce any artifact. Inspection of the nonattenuation corrected images would show normal uptake at the region.

Radiation Dose

PET-CT imaging is different from standard nuclear medicine imaging. In the case of PET radionuclides, 511 keV photons are used and their HVL and TVL values are 4 mm and 13.2 mm, respectively for a narrow beam geometry. It is ten times higher than that of ^{99m}Tc 140 keV photons used in gamma camera imaging. **Table 11.3** compares the radiation levels at 0.1 m and 1 m from the patient for Tc-99m and F-18 FDG. The radiation dose rate is 5–10 times higher in PET-CT scanner compared to gamma camera, which is a matter of concern.

Hospital workers radiation dose is about 3–14 μSv per study, and 50% dose arise from an administration of dose to patients. Patient radiation dose is 2–5 times higher in PET/CT and PET alone contributes about 5–11 mSv. CT contribution of dose is about 1–3 mSv for head, 5–20 mSv for abdomen, respectively. Radiation dose at 1m from the patient is 3 μSv/h/37 MBq. Patient dose is higher due to multi-slice CT which scans larger volume of patient. However, it is not a matter of concern since benefit overweighs the risk.

Clinical Application of PET-CT

PET-CT provides physicians with superior information for determining tissue characterizations and classifications, staging of cancers, restaging of cancers, patient prognosis, and monitoring effectiveness of cancer therapies. Its advantages include superior lesion localization from near-perfect anatomical and functional registration with fewer motion artifacts, better distinction between physiological uptake and pathological uptake, consolidation of patient's imaging studies, shorter scan time (30 min vs 60 min PET scan) by using CT for attenuation correction. This aids in patient comfort and minimizes claustrophobia problems. Thus, PET-CT has greater role in oncology, cardiology, and neurology patient imaging.

Advantages

- ❑ Better identification of inflammatory disease
- ❑ Confirmation of unusual or abnormal sites
- ❑ Improved localization of biopsy or radiotherapy
- ❑ Define tumor stages exactly

Limitations

❑ Claustrophobia due gantry tunnel
❑ Technical difficulties due to hybrid modality
❑ Radiation dose is relatively higher
❑ High cost

PET/MRI

PET/MRI is a medical device which combines images from positron emission tomography (PET) and magnetic resonance imaging (MRI) **(Fig. 11.19)**. They are hybrid technology which utilizes an anatomic and quantitative strengths of MRI, and physiological information of PET, to study the human body. It is useful to diagnose medical conditions and plan further treatment.

There are few limitations in PET/CT that includes, lack of soft tissue contrast, only sequential imaging is possible, an involvement of ionizing radiation, and helical CT is not flexible as that of MRI. PET imaging is done in several minutes whereas CT is done in seconds, their acquisition time is not comparable. The radiation exposure to the patient is 2–5 times higher in PET/CT. To over the above limitations PET/MRI came into existence.

Some of the features of MRI are an excellent soft tissue contrast especially in heart, lung, and liver, evaluation of function and structure, noninvasive angiography, early detection of tumors, no ionizing radiation, comparable acquisition times, motion correction and resolution recovery, and more flexible than CT, since it has multiple sequences.

PET/MRI Principle

Principle of part of PET is the same as that of PET/CT, only MRI is used instead of CT scan. Patient is injected with a radiolabeled tracer like FDG. MRI and

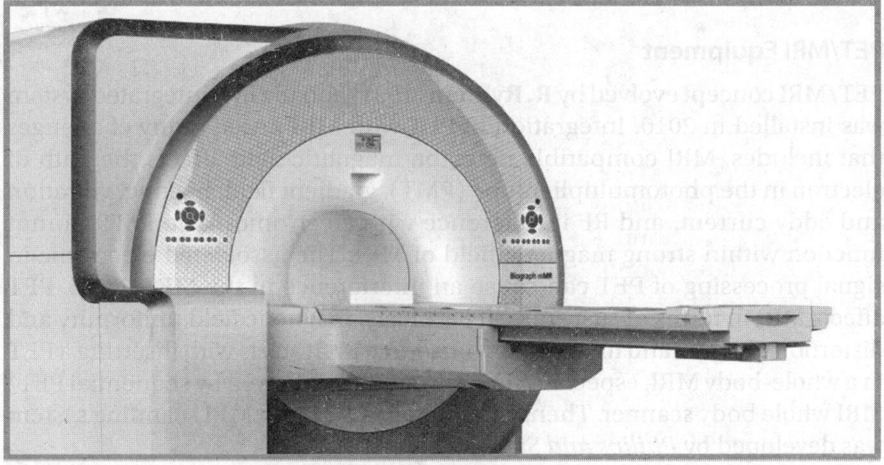

Fig. 11.19: PET/MRI commercial equipment.
(*Courtesy:* Siemens Healthineers)

PET scan are conducted sequentially or simultaneously. PET scan shows radioactive distribution in a cross section which predicts an abnormalities of tissue.

MRI is based on the principle that proton nuclei of the tissue, when placed in a strong magnetic field, selectively absorbs radio wave energy and later release energy, unique to those nuclei and their environment. It is suitable with atoms of odd atomic number like Hydrogen. Hydrogen has is more abundance with high physiological concentration of 100% in human body. MRI can be performed in *spin echo pulse sequence (SE), inversion recovery (IR)* and *gradient recalled echo (GE)*. Spin echo sequence involves application of 90° RF pulse, time gap, 180° RF pulse, and echo, referred as one cycle. Time interval between two cycle is called time of repetition (TR). Time between the 90° pulse and echo formation is called time of echo (TE).

Spin echo pulse sequence is used to offer T_1 weighted, T_2 weighted and proton density weighted images. T_1 relaxation refers to an energy exchange between spins and lattice and it is the time required to recover 63% of longitudinal magnetization. T_2 relaxation time refers to an exchange of energy between spin and spin, due to loss of phase coherence, it is the time taken to reduce the transverse magnetization to 37%. Generally, T_1 time is longer than T_2 time for body tissues. Molecular size, motion, and interaction influence T_1 and T_2 relaxation times. TE and TR are machine parameters whereas T_1 and T_2 are tissue parameters.

MRI scans use strong magnetic field (0.5–3 Tesla) and radio waves to produce cross-sectional images of an internal organ. Since, it has an inherent soft tissue contrast it shows more details of the structures. It can also give functioning information of structures also. MRI and PET images are fused together to give the final image **(Figs. 11.20A to C)**. This combines the soft tissue morphological imaging of MRI with functional imaging of PET. Usually, it takes about 45 minute or longer to complete the scans.

PET/MRI Equipment

PET/MRI concept evolved by **R. Rylman** (1991) and the first integrated system was installed in 2010. Integration of PET with MRI posed many challenges that includes, MRI compatible detector, magnetic field affects the path of electron in the photomultiplier tube (PMT), gradient field, heating, vibration and eddy current, and RF interference with electronics. The PMT cannot function within strong magnetic field of MRI. The associated electronic in signal processing of PET can cause an interference in the MRI signal. PET affects MRI in terms of susceptibility artifacts, magnetic field uniformity and distortion of signal and image by an outsource RF. It starts with inserting a PET in a whole-body MRI, especially for brain studies, followed by sequential PET/MRI whole body scanner. Then, simultaneous PET and MRI scanning system was developed by *Philips and Siemens.*

There are three possibilities of PET/MRI integration: (1) positioning the PMT outside the magnetic field with fiber optic, (2) using *solid-state*

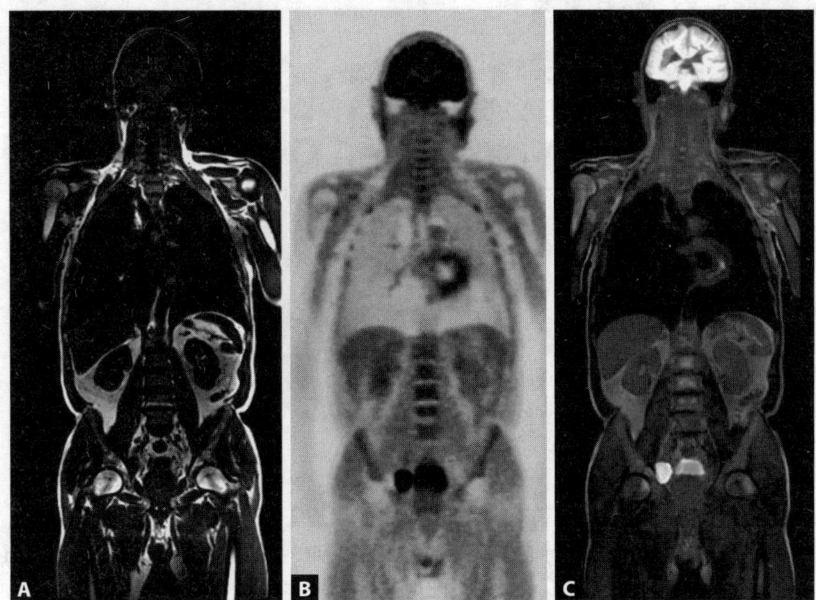

Figs. 11.20A to C: (A) MRI T_1 weighted image with higher soft tissue contrast; (B) F-18 (FDG) PET image; (C) PET/MRI fused image (Jin ho Jung et al, 2016).

photodetectors, and (3) using *avalanche photodiode (APD),* e.g., *Silicon photomultiplier (SiPM).* Initially, separate MRI and PET systems are made linked by a single patient table on rails. Secondly, the detectors are kept within the magnetic field and be coupled by optical fibers. It needs spilt-magnet design so that the fiber is shorter, and the magnet bore is wider. Attempt was made to couple the scintillation crystal directly or by an optical fiber to APD in radiofrequency shielding. Alternatively, SiPM detectors can be coupled to the scintillation detector. Thirdly, modification of detector from and to the magnetic field.

There are four commercial systems available today: The signa PET/MRI **(GE healthcare)** is a 3-Tesla equipment using SiPM detectors directly coupled to Lutetium-based crystals. It is a wide bore MRI in which SiPM PET is inserted. The biograph mMR PET/MRI **(Simens)** is a 3-Tesla equipment that uses APD detectors and *Lutetium oxyorthosilicate* crystals. The uPMR 790 PET/MRI **(United imaging)** is also a 3-Tesla equipment that uses SiPM detector directly coupled with *Lutetium-yttrium oxyorthosilicate (LYSO)* crystals. The ingenuity PET/MRI **(Philips)** is also equipped with 3-Tesla MRI coupled with LYSO crystals and PMT based PET system.

Detector

Generally, *BGO crystals* are used with PMT in traditional PET machine. Later, *Lutetium-based scintillators* like *Lutetium oxyorthosilicate (LSO)* and *Lutetium-yttrium oxyorthosilicate (LYSO) are used.* These are inorganic

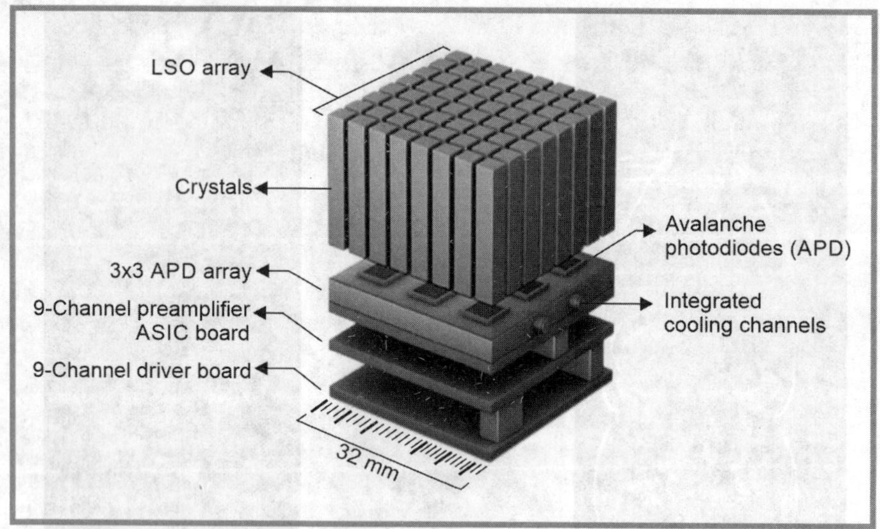

Fig. 11.21: Detector model, LSO crystal coupled with APD and integrated cooling system for PET/MRI.
(*Courtesy:* Simens Healthineers)

scintillation crystals, that have stable physical and chemical properties with detection efficiency. They have faster scintillation decay suitable for high count rates, additional LOR for 3D scanning, and longer axial FOV. They are coupled to PMTs which offer signal amplification but susceptible to magnetic fields and are bulky.

Avalanche photodetectors (APDs) are *Silicon semiconductor* can be operated within the magnetic field but also compact **(Fig. 11.21).** It is thermally sensitive, requires thermal stabilization. The signal gain is much low compared to regular PMT hence, requires additional electronic signal amplification. This property has been tested successfully in PET/CT scans.

Other alternative detector is *SiPM* which is a silicon semiconductor detector operates in Geiger mode. The detector matrix consists of 1000 of pixels that operate as photon counter in Geiger mode. These pixels are known as *single-photon avalanche diodes* which can be counted independently and simultaneously with other single-photon avalanche diodes. It is very successful, gives high resolution, high sensitivity, high signal gain, low noise, fast time response, low operating voltage, compact structure, less magnetic susceptibility, and time of flight (TOF) capability. SiPM array can be coupled with LSO/LYSO crystals to have good performance. Generally, SiPM is used with multiple crystals to reduce the readout channels. Recently, TOF PET detector is developed based on the above concept.

Patient Preparation

Patients must stop eating 4–6 hours before the scan and water can be taken as intake. Black tea and coffee are allowed since they do not contain sugar, milk, or any cream. They should stop strenuous exercises 24 hours before the scan. Patients should reveal any metals in the body, including pacemakers, surgical clips, pins or plates, cochlear implants, etc., to the doctor. It may be affected by strong magnetic field of MRI scanner. Women patients should inform the doctor about pregnancy or think she might be pregnant. It is advisable that patients should accompany an attender during the hospital visit. Some patients may feel claustrophobic during the scan.

Attenuation Correction

Attenuation correction is essential for accurate quantitation of PET data, otherwise standardized uptake value (SUV) may be underestimated. In PET/CT, transmission scans are done before or after the PET image acquisition which is used for attenuation correction. Of late, ^{68}Ge/^{68}Ga sources is used to take transmission scans before the patient is administered positron radionuclide dose. PET/MRI cannot use the above option since there is no correlation between attenuation coefficient and MRI signal intensity.

One of the advantages of PET/MRI attenuation correction are free of radiation exposure and offer more accuracy. Simultaneous acquisition may overcome mismatches compared to sequential PET/CT imaging. However, an attenuation correction is very challenging in PET/MRI since additional attenuation caused by MRI hardware and coils in the FOV. Several approaches are made to find an attenuation correction that includes: (1) simple segmentation and classification of different tissue types using T_1 signal. It suffers from lack of bone signal and associated attenuation correction. (2) Estimation methods and an attenuation formula. This is suitable for tissues with uniform attenuation, e.g., brain. (3) Use of rotating rod source of ^{68}Ge/^{68}Ga for transmission scan. Its attenuation map is noisy inferior to CT based attenuation map.

Current attenuation correction uses 3D *Dixon approach* that provides in-phase and out-of-phase data sets for water and fat. It permits segmentation of air, fat, muscle, and lung tissue for an attenuation coefficient except bone. Bone is classified as soft tissue here, which will underestimate an attenuation, may result in errors in quantitation of bone and adjacent soft tissue. This can be overcome with an atlas-based method but have limitations.

Other way of doing an attenuation correction is incorporation of *ultrashort-echo signals* to delineate bone and added to T_1 tissue segmentation. It can be combined with a Dixon sequence to produce classes of very short T_2 tissues for segmentation. This method is much useful in lung imaging.

Another way of an attenuation correction is attempting is pseudo-CT attenuation maps but there is limitation in generating such attenuation maps from MRI to PET/MRI. Deep convolutional neural network (CNNs) can produce an attenuation map which closely models CT-based approach. Secondly, integrated Dixon method with a CNN is used to generate pseudo-CT approach for pelvic PET/MRI. There is only 2% variation from the CT map. Thirdly, deep CNN combined with zero-echo time Dixon pseudo-CT. The

CNN approach can produce pseudo-CT attenuation maps from PET sinogram which is found valuable. This gives more attenuation maps.

Artifacts

PET and MRI are prone to artifacts which undermine the image quality and quantitative accuracy. Common artifact is crosstalk between PET and MRI which can be overcome by newer detectors. Misalignment may cause co-registration inaccuracies. Imperfect attenuation correction may produce artifacts and it is exaggerated with presence of contrast which will interfere with segmentation. MRI is susceptible to signal voids associated with an implant. It may produce an attenuation artifact in PET scan. MRI component's attenuation on PET can produce truncation of FOV.

Clinical Application

PET/MRI finds application in oncology, especially in head and region and pelvic malignancies due to its soft tissue contrast. Integrated PET/MRI holds great potential in the imaging of pediatric patients and young adults with potentially curable diseases. It is also used in cardiology and central nervous system studies. Another important use is MRI based motion correction however it suffers from an inaccurate attenuation correction. There is a need for development of an imaging protocol and standardization.

Advantages of PET/MRI

- More accurate diagnosis and treatment options
- Diffusion weighted images
- Dynamic contrast-enhanced imaging
- MRI and MR spectroscopy and other sequences
- Improved safety with reduced radiation exposure
- Simultaneous imaging of both PET and MRI scans
- Increased soft tissue contrast

Limitations

- It requires high initial capital cost.
- There is lack of protocol and standardization due to huge variations in MR protocols.
- No combined reporting of PET and MR components.
- Limited flexibility of combined PET/MR systems.
- High acquisition times of up to 60 min.

BIBLIOGRAPHY

1. Buck AK, Nekolla S, Ziegler S, Beer A, Krause BJ, Herrmann K, et al. Journal of Nuclear Medicine, August 2008; 49(8): 1305-1319.
2. Bushberg JT, Seibert JA, Leidholdt EM Jr, Boone JM. The Essential Physics of Medical Imaging, 3rd edn. Wolters Kluwer/Lippincott-Willimas and Wilkins, 2012.
3. Cherry SR, Sorenson JA, Phelps ME. Physics of in Nuclear Medicine, 4th edn. Elsevier, 2012.
4. Currie GM, Kamvosoulis P, Bushong S. PET/MRI, Part 2: Technologic Principles. Journal of Nuclear Medicine Technology, September 2021; 49(3) 217-225.
5. Jin Ho Jung, Yong Choi, and Ki Chun Im. PET/MRI: Technical challenges and recent advances. Nucl Med Mol Imaging. Mar 2016; 50(1): 3-12.
6. Tom Walsh, Dylan Schoo, Sean Wilson and Annie Moranski. Single Photon Emission Computed Tomography (SPECT). Slide share, 2014.

Ultrasound Imaging

PHYSICS OF ULTRASOUND

Ultrasound describes sound waves of frequencies exceeding the range of human hearing (>20 kHz). Audible sound frequency range is 15–20 kHz and the sound frequency <15 Hz is called *infrasound*. Elephants can generate and detect sound with frequencies less than 20 Hz for long-distance communication whereas *bats and dolphins* produce sounds in the range of 20 to 100 kHz for precise navigation.

Pierre and Jacques Curie discovered *piezoelectric effect* in 1880 which is the basis for ultrasound production. Ultrasound was used in the Navy to detect submarines (1915), known as *sound navigation, and ranging (SONAR)*. **Dussik brothers** got the idea of using it as diagnostic tool in 1942. However, the use of real-time B-scanner in obstetrics started only in 1965.

In medicine, ultrasound energy, and the acoustic properties of the body, produce images from stationary and moving bodies. The principle behind ultrasound imaging is *piezoelectric effect*. Diagnostic ultrasound uses 1–20 MHz frequency, and velocity depends on the nature of medium through which it travels and independent of frequency. It is not an electromagnetic radiation involving ionizing radiation but undergoes reflection, refraction, scattering and absorption at tissue interfaces. The reflection of sound from tissue is called an *echo*, which forms the basis for final image. Ultrasound is used as diagnostic tool in medicine, either continuous ultrasound or pulsed ultrasound. Knowledge of ultrasound wave emission, an interaction with body fluids, tissue, different densities, an echo signal and an instrumentation are very important.

Ultrasound contrast in soft tissue is equal to that of X-rays. Special features of ultrasound are high resolution, real-time imaging, harmonic imaging, 3-D data acquisition and Doppler ultrasound. Contrast agents can be used for better delineation of anatomy. Measurement of tissue perfusion, precise drug delivery mechanisms, and determination of elastic properties of the tissues are also possible.

Ultrasound is used in obstetrics and Gynecology for measuring the size of fetus, to determine sex of a baby, and monitor the baby for various procedures. In Cardiology, it is used to see inside of heart to identify abnormal function and measuring blood flow through heart and major block of vessels. In Urology, it is helpful to measure blood flow through kidney, locating kidney stones and detecting prostate cancer at early stage.

Ultrasound is used to guide biopsies in suspected solid mass or tissue abnormality. A fine needle or core needle gives good reflection and scattering of ultrasound which gives good visibility of needle track. It finds application in breast, prostate, thyroid, abdominal and pelvic site.

Propagation of Sound

Ultrasound (US) is produced by a transducer by *piezoelectric effect* and US pulse is passed in straight line, mostly as pulses. Sound is a mechanical energy that propagates through an elastic medium in the form of waves with *compression and rarefaction* (**Fig. 12.1**). One compression and rarefaction are referred to one *cycle*. It is a longitudinal wave (sinusoidal) in which the medium vibrates parallel to the direction of propagation. US waves have *wavelength, frequency, period, speed, amplitude, power, and intensity*.

Wavelength, Frequency and Velocity

Wavelength (λ) is the distance between successive wave crests or two maxima. Frequency (f) is the number of cycles per second, called *hertz* and one hertz

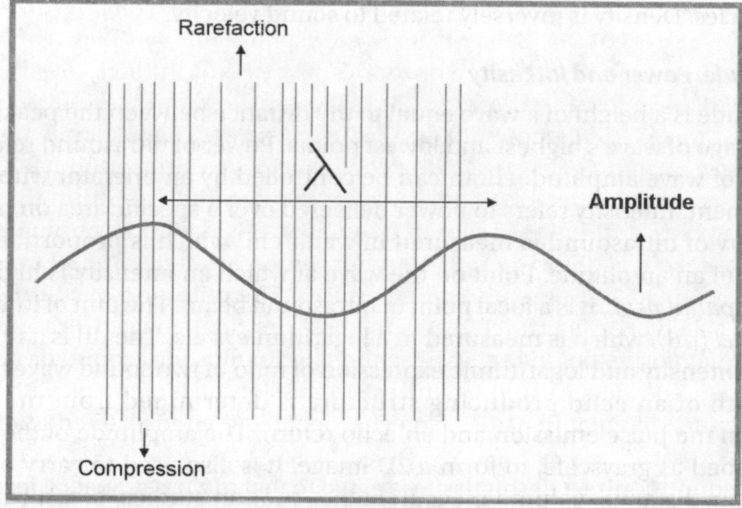

Fig. 12.1: Propagation of ultrasound as longitudinal wave with compression and rarefaction.

(Hz) = 1 cycle/sec. In practice, kHz (1000 Hz) and MHz (10^6 Hz) units are used. It depends on the emission of source and is independent of an interacting tissue. Frequencies of clinical ultrasound are from 1 MHz to 20 MHz, based on the probe type and nature application.

Period (T) is the time taken for one complete cycle and it is inversely proportional to frequency (1/f). Wavelength refers to distance whereas the period refers to time. Velocity of ultrasound (c) is the rate at which ultrasound passes through a medium. It depends on the characteristics of the medium and independent of frequency. It is related to wavelength and frequency as follows:

$$c = \lambda\, f\ m/s$$

Sound waves travel faster in solids and slower in gases. Average velocity of sound in soft tissue is 1540 m/s, and it takes 7 µs to travel 1 cm. It is higher in bone and metal, lower in lung and air (compressible). Difference in velocity (change of λ) at tissue boundaries is the basis for image contrast in ultrasound image. As tissue density increases, the propagation velocity decreases. In contrast, the velocity is higher in a stiffer tissue. Velocity depends on compressibility and density of the medium:

$$c = \sqrt{B/\rho}$$

where, B is *bulk modulus* (measure of stiffness of the medium), and ρ is *density*. Velocity is inversely $\propto$ to *compressibility* and it depends on temperature of the medium. Lesser the compressibility more the velocity of sound in a medium. Sound waves move slowly in a gas since its molecules are apart and easily compressed. Compressibility of solid >liquid >gases. Denser material has larger molecule with large inertia, it is difficult to move or stop once in motion. Propagation of sound needs rhythmic starting and stopping of particles. Density is inversely related to sound velocity.

Amplitude, Power and Intensity

Amplitude is a height of a wave equal to the distance between the peaks and an average of wave's highest and lowest points. Power of ultrasound refers to square of wave amplitude. Both can be controlled by an operator with gain adjustment. Intensity refers to power delivered over a specific area on tissue. Intensity of ultrasound is measured in watts/cm² which is proportional to square of an amplitude. Point on the wave at which an intensity is higher is called *spatial peak*, it is a focal point of ultrasound beam. The unit of intensity is *decibel (dB)*, which is measured in a logarithmic scale. The dB is a relative sound intensity and logarithmic expression of ratio of two sound waves.

Depth of an echo producing structure is determined from the time between the pulse emission and an echo return. The amplitude of the echo is encoded as grayscale, to form a 2D image. It is also used to carry out an anatomic distance, volume measurements, motion studies, blood velocity measurements and 3D-imaging.

INTERACTION OF ULTRASOUND WITH MATTER

Ultrasound undergoes reflection, refraction, scattering and absorption in a medium that depends upon the acoustic properties of medium. Reflection may be a *boundary reflection or tissue reflection* and tissue reflection mostly gives scattering. Refraction refers to change in direction of transmitted ultrasound energy. Scattering occurs by both reflection and refraction (small particles). Absorption refers to conversion of acoustic energy into thermal energy in the medium.

Acoustic Impedance

Acoustic impedance is the product of density (ρ) and velocity (c) of sound:

$$Z = \rho \times c, \, kg/m^2/s \, (Rayl)$$

It depends on density and elasticity of an interface and independent of frequency. The acoustic impedance can also be related to modulus of elasticity (E) as follows:

$$Z = \sqrt{E \times \rho}, \, Rayl$$

The acoustic impedance of various body tissues with density and sound velocity is given in **Table 12.1**.

Reflection

Reflection occurs at tissue boundary, where there is a difference in an *acoustic impedance (Z)* and it is reflected back to the probe. Reflections of sound that returns to the probe is called *echoes*. If two materials have same impedance no echo is produced. Images obtained based on the echoes give raise to structures and their varying densities, referred to as an *echogenicity*. More the difference in density stronger an echogenicity. Structures of high

Table 12.1: Acoustic properties: Density, velocity and acoustic impedance of various body tissues.

Material	Density, kg/cm³	Velocity (ms⁻¹)	Acoustic impedance × 10⁶ Rayl
Air	1.2	330	0.0004
Lung	300	600	0.18
Fat	924	1450	1.34
Water	1000	1480	1.48
Kidney	1041	1565	1.63
Blood	1058	1560	1.65
Liver	1061	1555	1.65
Muscle	1068	1600	1.71
Skull bone	1912	4080	7.8

(*Courtesy:* Jerrold T Bushberg et al, 2012)

density reflects more sound are called more *echogenic* and appear white. Thus, bone and foreign bodies gives intense echo and appear bright on the display. Fluids, water, urine has low densities, gives lower echoes, called *anechoic* and appears as black. Weaker echoes appear in *grey*. Bone and air cannot propagate sound, the echo from these structures causes *shadow* behind the interface.

The angle by which the ultrasound wave engage with a structure is called *angle of incidence*. Ideally, zero angle of incidence gives maximum echoes to the probe whereas oblique incidence gives fewer echoes which reduce brightness and resolution. In oblique incidence, the angle of reflection is equal to the angle of incidence. As angle of incidence increases the angle of reflection also increases.

As sound wave travels from medium of low Z to high Z, the reflected wave experiences a phase shift of 180° (negative sign), independent of frequency, and has directional dependence **(Fig. 12.2)**. The difference between Z, determines the amount of reflected energy at the interface. The angle of incidence (θ_i) = angle of reflection (θ_r), and it obeys **Snell's law:**

$$\frac{\text{Sin}_{\theta_i}}{\text{Sin}_{\theta_r}} = \frac{c_1}{c_2}$$

where, c_1 and c_2 are the velocity of sound in medium 1 and medium 2, respectively. The % of reflected intensity depends on the angle of incidence. The reflection coefficient (R) is given by:

$$R = \left[\frac{(Z_2 - Z_1)}{(Z_2 + Z_1)}\right]^2$$

When the beam is perpendicular to the tissue boundary, entire sound is returned as an echo. As angle of incidence increases, less likely the reflection and no reflection are detected when the angle of incidence is >3°. When $Z_1 = Z_2$, the transmission is 100% and the two mediums are said to be *acoustically matching*. This is called an acoustic window; tissue acts as conduit and allows US transmission, e.g., lung.

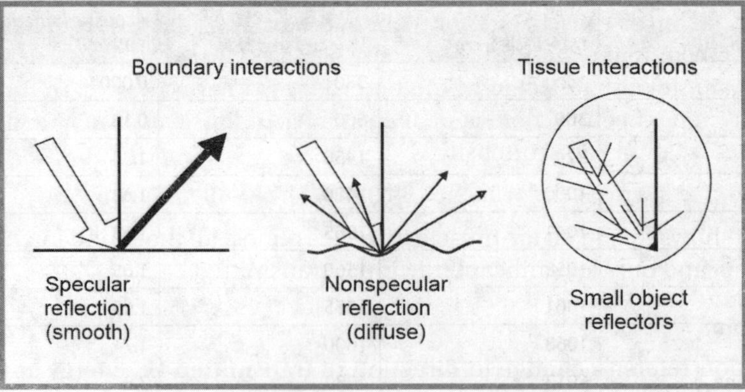

Fig. 12.2: Boundary and tissue reflections.

Table 12.2: Typical reflection factors of ultrasound at tissue interfaces.

Interface	Percentage
Gas-Tissue	99.9
Soft tissue-PZT	80
Bone-Muscle	30
Plastic-Soft tissue	10
Fat-Muscle	1
Blood-Muscle	0.1
Liver-Muscle	0.01

(*Courtesy:* Penelop Allisy-Roberts et al, 1996)

Tissue interfaces reflect ultrasound wave differently **(Table 12.2)**. Smooth interfaces are referred to as *specular reflector* which reflects large amount of sound to the probe due to large difference in an acoustic impedance. Medium reflections occur at dense tissues like muscle. *Irregular reflectors* or diffuse reflectors, reflect sound away from the probe resulting poor image quality, e.g., liver. If the object size is smaller than wavelength, **Rayleigh scattering** occurs, e.g., red blood cells.

In interface such as air or gas, nearly 100% US is reflected, and there is no transmission. They cast shadow and the underlying organs cannot be imaged hence, US imaging impossible in such cases, e.g., lung. In bone-tissue interface, there is 30% reflection and 70% transmission hence, bone imaging is difficult, an image appears as areas of void and shadowing.

Worked Example 12.1

Calculate the % of reflection and transmission coefficient in an air-muscle interface, $Z_1 = 0.0004 \times 10^6$ Rayl and $Z_2 = 1.71 \times 10^6$ Rayl.
The reflection coefficient:

$$R = \left[\frac{(1.71 - 0.0004)}{(1.71 + 0.0004)} \right]^2 = 0.998 \text{ or } 99.8\%$$

The transmission coefficient, $T = 1 - 99.8\% = 0.2\%$.

Thus, in an air-muscle interface, about 99% of sound is reflected and only <1% is transmitted.

Actual intensity reflected at the boundary is the product of an incident intensity and reflection coefficient. If an incident intensity is 40 mW/cm^2, then the reflected ultrasound intensity is:

$$40 \text{ mW/cm}^2 \times 0.998 = 39.9 \text{ mW/cm}^2 \approx 40 \text{ mW/cm}^2$$

This shows that in an air-muscle interface almost all the sound intensity is reflected, and only insignificant fraction is transmitted.

Refraction

Refraction refers to change in direction of transmitted US energy at tissue boundary when the beam is nonperpendicular. It is a deflection of US from straight line when wave velocities differ between two media. The angle by which the refracted ray deviates from the perpendicular is called an *angle of refraction*. Angle of refraction is decided by an angle of incidence and difference in wave velocity in two media. Frequency does not change but change of velocity may occur due to change of λ. Refracted beams have longer wavelength, in denser medium and it obeys **Snell's law**:

$$\frac{\mathrm{Sin}_{\theta_t}}{\mathrm{Sin}_{\theta_i}} = \frac{c_2}{c_1}$$

where, θ_t is the angle of transmission. If the angles are very small, the above equation can be written as:

$$\frac{\theta_t}{\theta_i} = \frac{c_2}{c_1}$$

When $\theta_i > \theta_c$, the critical angle, the refracted wave travels through the boundary $(\theta_t = 90°)$, then:

$$\frac{1}{\mathrm{Sin}_{\theta_i}} = \frac{c_2}{c_1}$$

Ultrasound machines assume that US beam travels in straight line propagation. Refraction is not useful for imaging, mostly gives raise to artifacts.

Scattering

Scattering occurs when the size the reflector is $<\lambda$ (10 µm), e.g., blood corpuscle, tissue parenchyma. Scattered US appear in the form of cone, and only small fraction appears as an echo. Echoes are small (1–10%), and it is frequency related, hence blood flow imaging requires high frequency. Scatter depends on λ and magnitude of roughness. It is useful in imaging of curved surfaces and boundaries, which are not right angle to an incident beam. Part of the scatter returns to the transducer and gives images called *backscatter*. Though its energy is low, it contributes to the texture of an image.

Echoes reveal tissue characteristic and organ signature. Interference of scattered echoes from different sites is called *speckle*. Speckle pattern is not related to anatomical detail, but change of pattern reveal pathology, e.g., liver. *Hyperechoic refers* to higher scatter amplitude and *hypoechoic* refers to lower scatter amplitude. Hyperechoic is due to large size and high number of scatters with large z difference.

In abdomen imaging, strong echoes arise from gas bubbles. *Kidney, pancreas, spleen, and liver* constitute complex tissues containing scattering sites that give rise to *speckled texture.* Bladder, blood vessels and cysts (fluids) have no internal structure, hence no echoes and appear as black. Vascular and perfusion imaging use contrast agents, which are encapsulated with microbubbles (3–6 µm) containing Air, Nitrogen, or insoluble gases *(per fluorocarbons)*. They permit perfusion of tissues and echoes are generated by large difference in Z, between the gas and surrounding fluids or tissues.

Attenuation

Attenuation is loss of an acoustic energy with distance, and it is exponential in nature. It refers to both absorption and scattering of ultrasound. In an absorption, energy is converted into heat due to frictional and viscous forces. When ultrasound wave interacts with a tissue and get reflected, the energy of the remaining beam decreases with an increasing depth. The strength of penetrating wave is reduced by refraction, scattering, and absorption. When waves are scattered and energy is absorbed, it results in vibration energy and heat. Multiple interfaces offer scattering and partial reflection. All the above process results in an energy reduction, called attenuation.

Attenuation is decrease in intensity over a distance and it is measured in *decibel (dB)*. It depends on viscosity, relaxation time, and US frequency. In soft tissue, an attenuation is proportional to transducer frequency. Higher the frequency, greater the attenuation **(Fig. 12.3)**. Attenuation coefficient (μ) is given by:

$$I_x = I_0 \exp(-x), \text{ dB cm}^{-1}$$

where, I_0, and I_x are initial and final ultrasound intensity in tissue, and x is the depth in cm. The thickness of tissue that reduces the sound intensity to half of its original value is called *half value layer (HVL)*. One HVL is 3 cm in soft tissue for a 1 MHz frequency probe. The depth at which 50% of the intensity is attenuated is equal to 3 dB in tissue. The attenuation coefficient for any frequency is obtained by the relation:

$$\text{Attenuation} = f \times 0.5 \text{ dB/cm}$$

where, f is an frequency. Attenuation is little in water and greater in bone **(Table 12.3)**. US is attenuated more rapidly than an audible sound. Alternatively, the attenuation rate per cm is roughly equal to frequency of the transducer. For example, a 5 MHz probe has the attenuation of 5 dB in the first cm and another 5 dB in the second cm of tissue. Higher frequency waves and

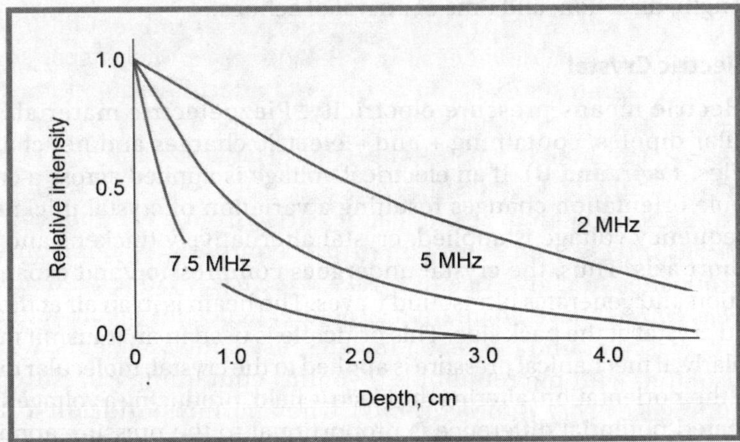

Fig. 12.3: Attenuation of US in tissue depth, higher the frequency greater the attenuation.

Table 12.3: Attenuation coefficient of various body tissues.

Tissue composition	Attenuation coefficient, dB/cm @ 1MHz
Water	0.0002
Blood	0.18
Soft tissue	0.3–0.8
Brain	0.3–0.5
Liver	0.4–0.7
Fat	0.5–1.8
Smooth muscle	0.2–0.6
Bone	13–26
Lung	40

(*Courtesy:* Jerrold T Bushberg et al, 2012)

waves used in deep seated structures are heavily attenuated, compared to low frequency waves or waves used for shallow imaging.

ULTRASOUND TRANSDUCER

Transducer is a device which converts an energy from one form to another. US transducer converts an electrical energy into sound energy and vice versa. Ultrasonic transducer contain piezoelectric crystal that works on the principle of *piezoelectric effect* (**Pierre and Jacques Curie,** *1880)*. When a crystal (quartz) is subjected to mechanical pressure, an electrical voltage is created. When an electrical pulse is applied, it produces ultrasonic waves (mechanical pressure) of predetermined frequency.

Propagation frequency is determined by the velocity divided by double the thickness of crystal. Typical crystal thickness is 0.2 mm and 2 mm. Transducer can send and receive ultrasound waves due to its pulsatile nature. It can detect the strength, direction, and time of arrival of echoes.

Piezoelectric Crystal

Piezoelectric means pressure electricity. Piezoelectric materials have molecular dipoles, containing + and – electric charges and net charge is zero (**Figs. 12.4A and B**). If an electrical voltage is applied across a crystal, the dipole orientation changes resulting a variation of crystal thickness. If high frequency voltage is applied, crystal alternatively thickens and thins in its short axis. Thus, the crystal undergoes compression and expansion/rarefaction and generates ultrasound waves. The beam is in an air at the front side and crystal at the back side. This principle is used in an transmit mode.

Similarly, if mechanical pressure is applied to the crystal, molecular dipoles change their orientation, altering the electric field, producing a voltage signal. The created potential difference is proportional to the pressure applied to the crystal. Echoes returning to the transducer produce minute voltages in

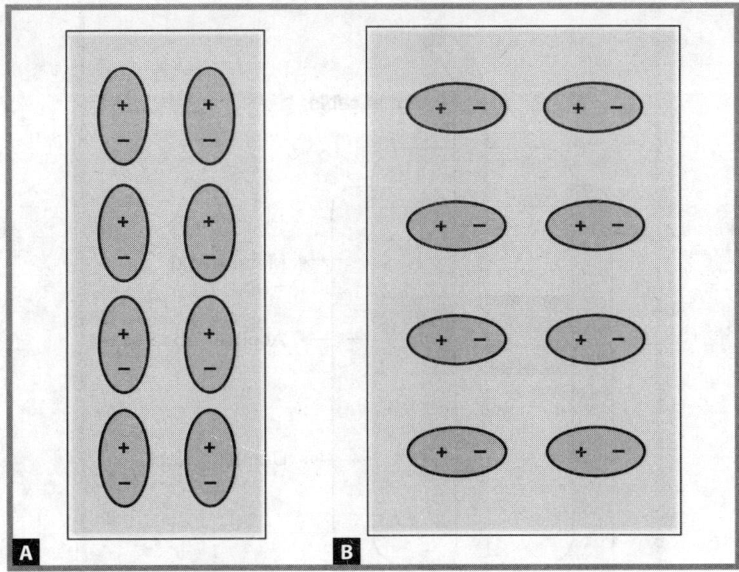

Figs. 12.4A and B: Piezoelectric effect: (A) Compression; (B) Expansion.

the crystal which is amplified to create an image. This principle is used in the receiver mode.

Natural piezoelectric material is quartz crystal and synthetic ceramic material is mostly used as crystal, e.g., *Lead zirconate titanate (PZT, PbZrTiO₄)*. PZT in its natural state has no piezoelectric properties. It is heated over its *curie temperature* (328–365°C) and an external voltage is applied, that causes the diploes to align in the ceramic. The voltage is maintained, until the ceramic is cooled below its *curie temperature*. Once it is cooled, the diploes retain their alignment.

Piezoelectric polyvinylidene fluoride (PVDF) is useful in high frequency, where high bandwidth transducer needs focusing to a certain region. It has low acoustic impedance like water, thus it is useful in making ultrasound pulses with good temporal resolution.

Transducer Design

Ultrasonic transducers consist of (1) matching layer, (2) piezoelectric crystal, (3) damping or backing block, (4) housing, and (5) signal cable. The housing generally refers to an *acoustic absorber, metal shield and a plastic case.* There are two types of transducers, namely, resonance and nonresonance transducers **(Fig. 12.5)**.

Resonant Transducer

Resonant type transducers follow the relation $\lambda = 2T$, where T is the thickness of the crystal. A potential of 150 V is applied to the crystal in 1 μs, the ceramic

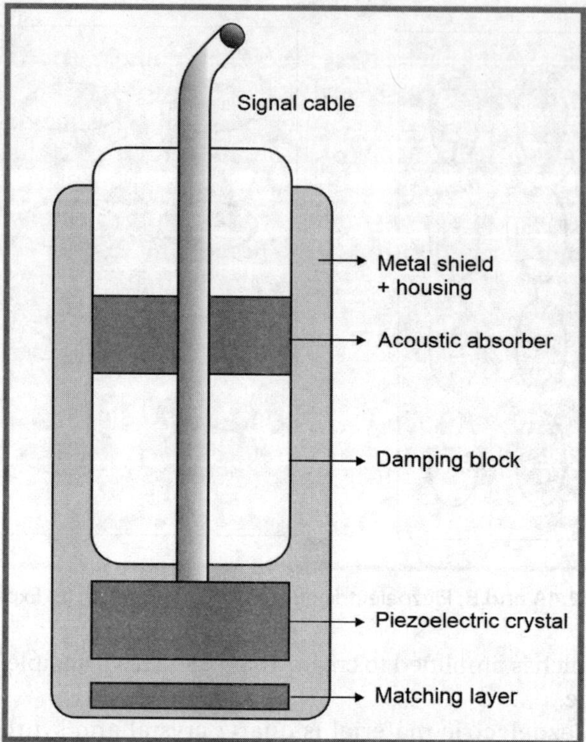

Fig. 12.5: Ultrasound transducer design.

initially contracts, later vibrates with natural frequency. It is used in pulse echo ultrasound imaging. High frequency transducer requires thinner crystals and low frequency requires thicker crystals.

Matching Layer

Matching layer consists of multiple layers of material that have an acoustic impedance between soft tissue and transducer element. It minimizes acoustic impedance difference between transducer and patient. The thickness is equal to one-fourth the wavelength for each layer, which is known as *quarter wave matching*. The matching layer impedance is obtained as follows:

$$Z_M = \sqrt{Z_T \times Z_L}$$

where, Z_T is crystal impedance and Z_L is tissue impedance, respectively. The matching layer is made up of *Perspex or plexiglass* ($Z_M = 3.2 \times 10^6$ kg/m^2/s), loaded with Aluminum powder. It acts as intermediate layer between patient and the transducer. In addition, acoustic coupling gel is used, between transducer and skin. It allows about 100% transmission of US into the tissue by reducing reflections on the skin.

Damping Block

Damping block is on the back side of the crystal behind the positive electrode, made up of Tungsten particles suspended in *epoxy resin* ($Z = 3 \times 10^7$ kg/m^2/s). It absorbs US energy directed backward and attenuates stray US signals from the housing. It dampens resonant frequency of the crystal and creates a shorter spatial pulse (SPL). Transducer and the damping block are separated from casing with an insulator (*rubber cork*). Damping lessens the purity of resonance frequency and introduces a broadband frequency spectrum. It should stop the vibration within microsecond so that the transducer is ready to receive reflected echo. The Q factor describes the bandwidth:

$$Q = \frac{f_0}{\text{Bandwidth}}$$

where, f_0 is the center frequency. High Q transducer has narrow bandwidth, little damping, and long SPL, used in velocity measurements and Doppler study. Low Q has wide bandwidth, and short SPL to receive echo signals, provides high spatial resolution in an axial direction.

Housing

Housing is made up of plastic case, metal case and acoustic insulator. It provides an electrical insulation and protects the crystal elements. Ultrasound transducers typically consist of 128–512 piezoelectric elements and each element are individually insulated. In mechanical transducer, a rotating wheel is used. In the case of electronic transducer either linear or curvilinear array is used.

Worked Example 12.2

Calculate the thickness of the matching layer of a probe with following specification: f = 7.5 MHz, c = 1540 msec^{-1}, and λ = 0.2 mm.

Answer:

As per the quarter wave matching, the thickness is equal to ¼ of wavelength:

$$\text{Thickness} = \frac{1}{4} \times 0.2 = 0.05 \text{ mm}$$

Nonresonant Transducers

Nonresonant transducers produce multiple frequency, in which the center frequency can be adjusted during transmit mode. Piezoelectric element is machined into many small rods and then filled with an *epoxy resin*, to create a smooth surface. The acoustic properties are closer to tissue than a pure PZT material. This design facilitates reduction of matching layer, with an increased transmission efficiency. The bandwidth of this transducer is about 80% of the center frequency. A short square wave burst of 150 V is used to excite the transducer. They receive echoes of wide range of frequencies and useful in *harmonic imaging*, where low frequency is transmitted, and high frequency echo is received.

Ultrasound Gel

Ultrasound cannot travel through air hence probe requires a coupling medium between an air and the skin to have propagation. Air impedes sound waves and > 99% of the beam is reflected in tissue -air interface and no beam are available for an imaging. Hence, coupling is offered through ultrasound gel or water bath which acts as a special aqueous conductive medium for sound and eliminate air pockets. Gel also prevents bubble formation between transducer and patient's skin and acts as lubricant. However, only 20% of US is transmitted and to improve transmission, matching layer design is used in the transducer.

Gel should have the following properties: nonallergenic, odorless, nonstaining, harmless, neutral pH and easily removable with tissue or towel. It is made with *water (500 mL), carbomer (10 g), EDTA (0.25 g), Propylene glycol (75 g), glycerin and trolamine (12.5 g) and colorant. Carbomer* is a synthetic high molecular weight polymer of acrylic acid, cross linked with *allyl sucrose*. It contains 50–68% of *carboxylic acid* groups. It is neutralized with an *alkali hydroxide* to make it water soluble. The propylene *glycol* is an *organic oil compound* that does not irritate the skin and helps to retain moisture. To absorbs the moisture from air *glycerin* and *trolamine* is used. The colorant is blue color which is occasionally used.

ULTRASOUND BEAM CHARACTERISTICS

Ultrasound from a point source appear as spherical. If the source is a two-dimensional (2-D) extended source, it appears as planar wavefront. If the compression zone of one wave intersects with that of an another wave, it is called *constructive interference*. As a result, wavelets of two waves reinforce on each other. If a rarefaction wave front intersects with that of an another rarefaction wave, cancellation occurs, referred to as *destructive interference*. Reinforcement and cancellation are noticeable near the source region. It is progressively lesser with distance from source. The path of the beam from the source is divided into *Fresnel and Fraunhofer zones* (**Fig. 12.6**). Fresnel zone is an initial cylindrical segment near the transducer. Fraunhofer zone is a diverging conical part away from the transducer. The length of each zone depends on frequency and crystal diameter.

Fresnel Zone

Fresnel zone or *near field* is an adjacent to the transducer face, has a converging beam profile, due to multiple constructive and destructive interference.

$$\text{Near field length} = \frac{d^2}{\lambda} = \frac{(d^2 \times f)}{4 \times c}$$

where *d,* is the diameter of the transducer. Higher frequency and larger diameter always provide longer near field length. It is lesser divergent and depth resolution increases with higher frequency. Lateral resolution depends on beam diameter, and it is best at the end of near field (single element).

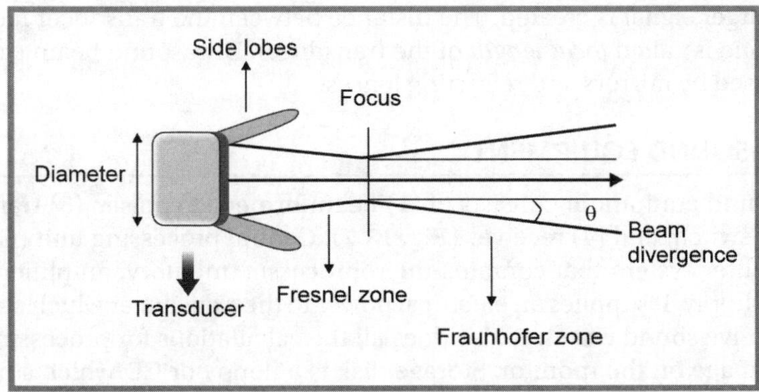

Fig. 12.6: US beam: Fresnel zone, Fraunhofer zone, and side lobes.

Though increasing the crystal diameter offers lengthy near field, it worsens the lateral resolution and depth resolution. Pressure amplitude characteristics are complex (minimum-maximum) in the near field. Peak US pressure occurs at the end of the near field, where beam diameter is minimum.

Fraunhofer Zone

Fraunhofer zone or *far field* is one in which the beam diverges and obey $\text{Sin } \theta = \dfrac{1.22\,\lambda}{d}$, where, θ is the beam divergence, d is transducer effective diameter. Less beam divergence occurs with high frequency and with large diameter. The US intensity decreases with distance.

Side Lobes

Side lobes are unwanted emissions of US energy, directed away from the main pulse. It is caused by radial expansion and contraction of crystal element. In receive mode, side lobes can create artifacts in an image. Smaller individual element width ($< \lambda$), and array transducer reduce side lobes. *Apodization* eliminates side lobes and improves an image quality. It is a method in which the transmit pulse is changed from *square to Gaussian* function.

In continuous mode, the side lobe is significant in narrow bandwidth transducers (high Q). In pulsed mode, the side lobe reduces in broad bandwidth transducers (low Q). In multi-element array, the side lobe is in forward direction. *Grating lobes* results when US energy is emitted far off-axis by multi-element arrays. It is due to noncontinuous transducer surface of the discrete elements. It creates an image of highly reflective off-axis objects in the main beam.

Focused Transducer

Ultrasound beam is narrower for a distance from the transducer face whose dimension is less than the transducer. The region where the beam narrows is called *focal zone* at which the ultrasound intensity is 100 times more, compared to that of an outside beam. If any reflector is placed at the focal zone, larger signal is created. The distance between the transducer face and focal zone is called *focal length* of the transducer. Ultrasound beam can also be focused by mirrors and refracting lenses.

ULTRASOUND EQUIPMENT

Ultrasound equipment consists of (1) beamformer, (2) pulser, (3) transmit/receive switch, and (4) receiver **(Fig. 12.7)**. Central processing unit (CPU) is a computer system that contains microprocessor, memory, amplifiers, and power supply. It supplies an electrical power to the transducer which can sent and receive sound waves. It also does all the calculations for processing and forms image on the monitor. Storage disk is a floppy or CD which store the acquired images. Transducer select is used to choose the transducer probes attached to the transducer port. CPU process the signal and display on a monitor with hard copy printout.

Beamformer

Beamformer generates an electronic delays for transducer in an array to get focusing and beam steering in phased array. Modern machines employ digital beam former for both transmit and receive modes. It has application specific integrated circuits (IC) which provide transmit/receive switches, digital-analogue, analogue-digital, preamplification and time gain compensation circuits for each element in the array.

Pulser

Pulser or transmitter gives power supply to the transducer. It controls the output transmit power by adjustment of the applied voltage to the crystal

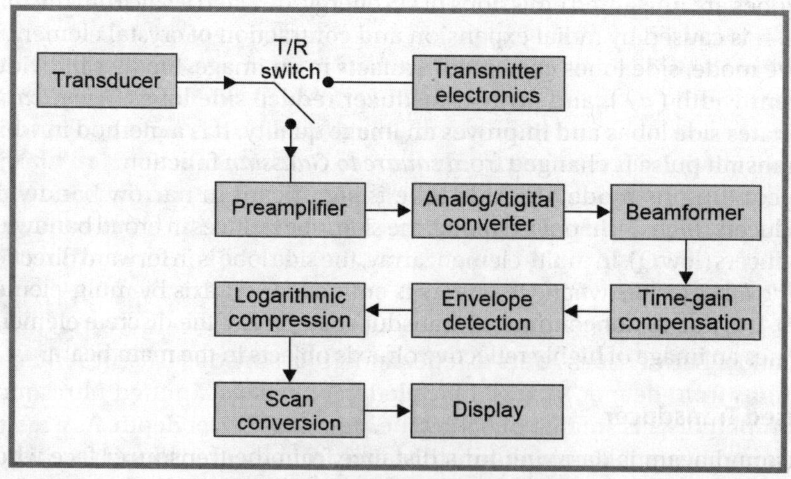

Fig. 12.7: Ultrasound block diagram.
(*Courtesy:* JC Lacefield, Diagnostic radiology physics, A Handbook for Teachers and Students, IAEA, 2014)

during pulse emission. It provides an electrical voltage for exciting the transducer elements. An increase in power creates higher intensity during transmission and reception of signals. It improves an echo detection from weaker reflectors. It provides higher signal-to-noise ratio (SNR) but the power deposition to the patient is higher. Pulser has user controls knobs such as *output, power, dB, transmit,* etc.

Hence, minimum power required for a given study is only used. It is achieved by using a low frequency transducer which offers higher imaging depth with minimal deposition of power to the patient. It helps low power setting for an obstetric imaging and has power indicators like *thermal index (TI) and mechanical index (MI).*

Transmit/Receive Switch

Generally, high voltage applied to the transducer is about 150 V whereas the induced voltages of the returning echoes is 1 V–2 µV. Transmit/receive switch isolates the high voltage during amplification stage at the receive mode. After the ring down time, the vibration of the transducer stops, it listens only the echo for about 1ms.

Receiver

Receiver consists of an amplifier, time gain compensation (TGC), compression, and rectification, demodulation and rejection and display. It also performs noise rejection, and signal processing.

Amplifier

Amplification is a preprocessing work performed parallelly. Each PZT has its own preamplifier and analog-to-digital converter (ADC). Once echo is produced, each element does preamplification, which increases the voltage to useful level. It is done by combining an amplifier and swept gain. Initial preamplification increases the detected voltages to 100 dB and swept gain compensates for an exponential attenuation of signal with distance. In doing so, large variations in echo amplitude are reduced from 1,000,000:1 to 1,000:1. Each array element also has ADC that has larger bit depth, to digitize the signals directly from the preamplification stage **(Fig. 12.8).**

Time Gain Compensation

Time gain compensation (TGC) is a method to overcome ultrasound attenuation. Early echoes refers to reflections from superficial tissues whereas reflections from deeper tissues are called later echoes. Emitted ultrasound wave amplitude gets smaller due to tissue attenuation over depth. As a result, late echoes have smaller amplitude than early echoes, even though the tissue has same echogenicity. If image is formed with these echoes, an early echo image appears lighter whereas late echo image appears darker. Hence, TGC is used to overcome this effect.

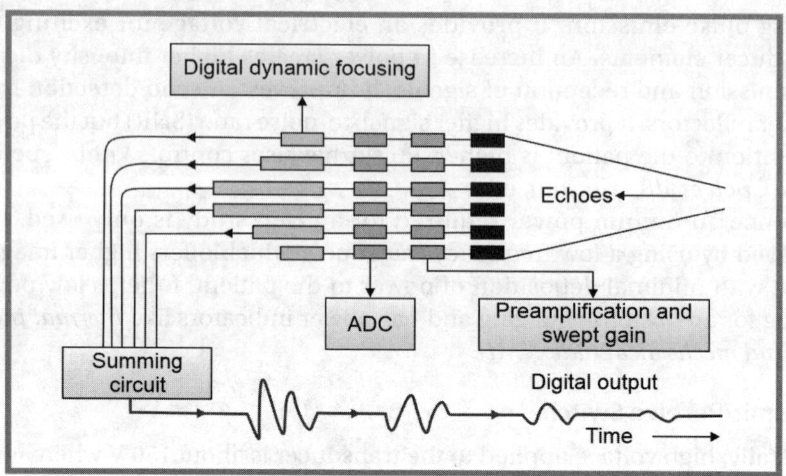

Fig. 12.8: Phased array echo processing.

TGC has gain adjustments and dynamic frequency tuning. Gain adjustment is a user-adjustable amplification of returning echo. It increases the signal gain as time passes from the emitted wave pulse. It compensates an attenuation of ultrasound energy through increased intensity of received signal that is proportional to depth. That means it normalizes the ultrasound signal amplitude with time, compensating for depth. In other words, it amplifies the signal proportional to the time delay between transmission and detection of US pulses. Amplification may be linear or nonlinear and bring the signal in the range of 40–50 dB. In linear TGC, the decibel gain is a linear function of control voltage.

Generally, TGC has multiple *slider potentiometer* and each slider meant for certain depth. It has three knobs, namely *initial gain, slope* and *far gain* of echo signals. In multiple elements, TGC is applied simultaneously for each signal from each element. TGC compensates for tissue attenuation and makes all equally reflective boundaries equal in signal amplitude, irrespective of depth **(Fig. 12.9A).** If image is formed with TGC, similar tissue will have same brightness irrespective of their depth.

Dynamic frequency focusing is a feature belongs to broad band receivers. It changes tuner sensitivity with time so that echoes of shallow depth are tuned to high frequency and that of deeper are tuned to lower frequency. This is to avoid an increased attenuation of high frequencies from deeper depth especially in a broadband pulse. Thus, a beam smoothening is done so that receiver can efficiently handle echo frequency incident at the transducer.

Compression

Ultrasound uses logarithmic compression by which week scatter signals are brought to same scale as that of strong specular reflections. It increases the smallest echo amplitudes and decreases the largest amplitudes **(Fig. 12.9B).**

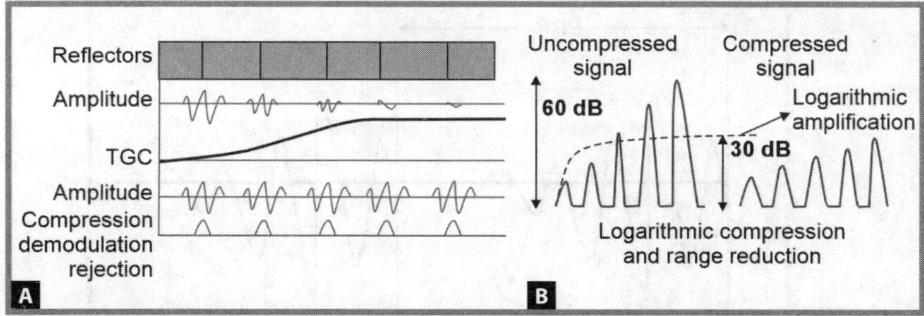

Figs. 12.9A and B: (A) Schematic description of TGC, equal reflective boundaries will have equal amplitude; (B) Logarithmic compression.

It reduces the signal range so that it fits the dynamic range of video monitor, an analog-to-digital converter (ADC), and film (20–30 dB). Dynamic range is the ratio of the highest and lowest amplitudes in decibels which is displayed on the monitor. Thus, compression changes the statistical nature of the detected signal. The output signal is proportional to the logarithm of an input signal. Analog signal processor is used to perform logarithmic compression.

Rectification, Demodulation, Rejection and Display

Compressed signal is rectified, it inverts the negative amplitude echoes to positive. Demodulation converts the rectified amplitudes into a smoothed single pulse. Rejection circuit removes a significant amount of an undesirable low-level noise and scattered sound (electronics). Processed image is optimized for grayscale and viewed within the dynamic range of the monitor. The final image is displayed on a 512 × 512 matrix with a depth of 8 bits per pixel. In color display, depth of 24 bits (3 bytes) is employed.

Pulsed Ultrasound

Ultrasound from the probe is propagated in pulses of milli second duration containing several thousand pulses per second. It is known as *pulsed ultrasound* which is essential for depth and resolution of clinical demands.

Pulse Characteristics

Ultrasound pulse raises and falls rapidly **(Fig. 12.10)**. It is characterized by the term *spatial pulse length (SPL)* which is the product of wavelength and number of cycles (n) in the pulse ($\lambda \times n$). Range of SPL of diagnostic ultrasound is 0.3–1.0 mm and it depends on the frequency. SPL gets altered during transmission through the tissue. Higher frequencies are more attenuated than low frequencies, resulting in an increased SPL which degrades an image resolution.

Pulse duration (PD) is the time taken for one spatial pulse length and its range is 0.4–1.5 ms. *Pulse repetition frequency (PRF)* is the number of pulses produced in one second and the common PRF used is 2 or 4 kHz. *Pulse repetition period (PRP)* is the time between the start of two pulses, and it is

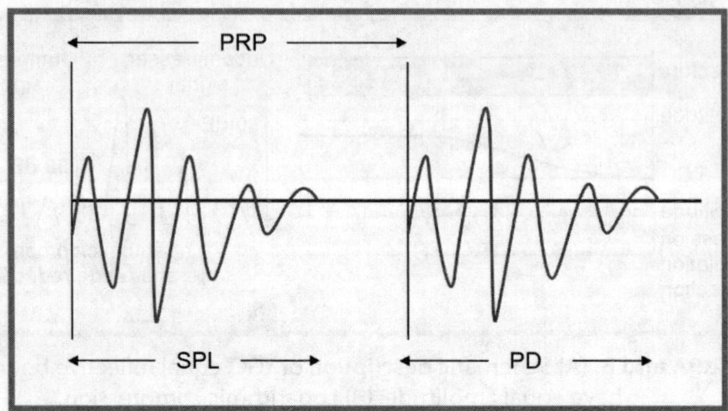

Fig. 12.10: Ultrasound characteristics, spatial pulse length (SPL), pulse repetition period (PRP) and pulse depth (PD): Increase of frequency decreases the pulse length.

inversely proportional to PRF. Higher PRF will have greater image resolution but shorter depths whereas lower PRF permits greater depths and increased listening time (0.1–0.5 ms).

Pulse-echo Operation

In pulse-echo method, each pulse is transmitted directionally into the patient, and it experiences partial reflections from tissue interfaces that create echoes, which returns to the transducer.

US is intermittently transmitted, and major time is spent for listening an echoe. The pulse is created with a short voltage waveform with 2–3 cycles long. Time delay between the transmission pulse and echo is related to depth of the interface:

$$\text{Time} = \frac{2D}{c} = \frac{2D \text{ (cm)}}{0.154 \text{ cm/μs}} = 13 \text{ μs} \times D \text{ (cm)}.$$

$$\text{Distance (cm)} = \frac{(C \times \text{Time})}{2} = \frac{\left(0.154 \left(\frac{cm}{μs}\right) \times \text{Time}\right)}{2} = 0.077 \times \text{Time (μs)}.$$

An increase in PRF results in a decrease in echo listening time. Maximum PRF is determined by the time required for echoes from most distant objects to reach transducer. High PRF limits penetration and low PRF limits line density and frame rate (ability to follow motion). The term *duty cycle* refers to fraction of beam ON time:

$$\text{Beam ON time} = \frac{\text{Pulse duration}}{\text{PRP}}$$

In real-time imaging, it is 0.2–0.4%, hence > 99.5% of the scan time is spent in listening the echoes. The PRF, PRP and duty cycle of various US modes are given in **Table 12.4**.

Table 12.4: Typical PRF, PRP, duty cycle, intensity levels and power of different ultrasound modes.

Mode	PRF (kHz)	PRP (µs)	Duty cycle (%)	Amplitude, MPa	I_{SPTA}, mW/cm²	Power, mW
M-Mode	0.5	2000	0.05	1.68	73	4
Real-time B mode	2–4	500–250	0.2–0.4	1.68	19	18
Pulsed Doppler	4–12	250–83	0.4–1.2	2.48	1440	31
Color flow Doppler	–	–	–	2.59	234	81

(*Courtesy:* Jerrold T Bushberg et al, 2012)

CLINICAL TRANSDUCERS

Clinical transducer array is made with many elements that includes (1) linear array, (2) curvilinear array, (3) phased array, (4) intracavitary probes, and (5) annular transducers. The crystal face and structural arrangement decides the area and shape of the image produced.

High frequency probes of 7–14 MHz sector transducer, more suitable for children and linear probes for superficial structure like thyroid, scrotum, etc. Medium frequency includes 3–5 MHz curvilinear or sector transducers, mostly used for adult abdominal scans. Keyboard is used to give an input data and takes measurements from the display. Low frequency transducers have 2 MHz frequency used for deeper structure imaging.

Linear Array

In linear array, many elements are arranged in groups with flat face which produces *rectangular or parallelogram image*. It produces sound waves in a straight line, parallel to each other and designed for superficial imaging. The width of an image and the number of scan lines are the same at tissue levels. Linear array uses higher frequency (5-13 MHz) giving better near field resolution with less penetration.

Individual element of the linear array gives poor beam, with short near field and widely diverging far field. Hence, they are operated in groups, say 1–6, 2–7, that gives well defined US beam (wave front). The elements are rectangular in shape and each one is individually pulsed. Only one group is excited during the scan. A single element is added to the group while the last element is removed. Thus, aperture advances along the transducer length and gives images line by line defined by an individual element (**Figs. 12.11A and B**).

Elements groups are energized from an outer to inner, pulses reinforce at same point (focus) at same time. The timing of an applied pulse can be varied to get a desired focal depth. Thus, it scans a rectangular area with large number of scan lines. Each element produces a scan line, whose length gives an image depth. It electronically sweeps the US beam across the volume of interest (VOI), enable dynamic imaging.

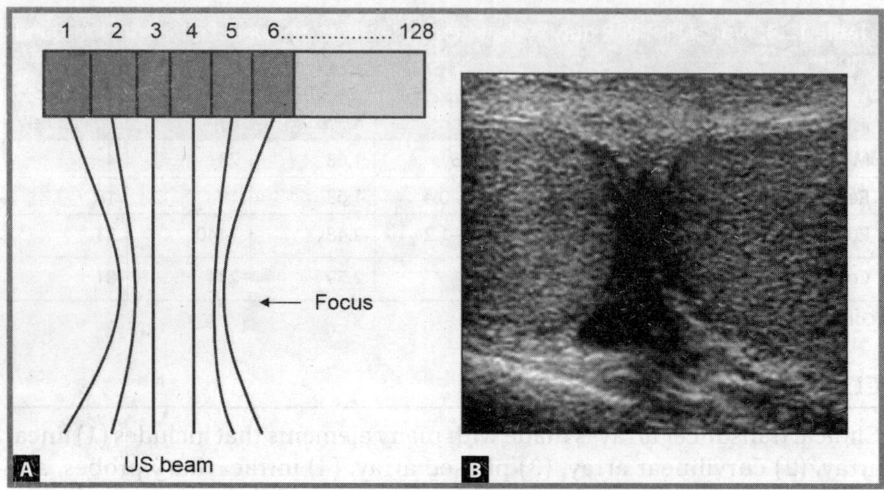

Figs. 12.11A and B: (A) Electronic scanning with linear array: In a group, outer most pair is energized, followed by inner most pair. US beam reinforces at the focus; (B) Rectangular image display.

It provides wider beam with an improved resolution and operated both in unfocused and focused mode. Focused mode is made by delaying or phasing an excitation pulse (ns) to obtain short or long focal length. If the linear array works in the above manner, it is said to be *phased linear array*. It facilitates dynamic aperture to have focus at various depths. Frame rates obey the relation with PRF and number of scan lines:

$$\text{Frame rate} = \frac{\text{PRF}}{\text{N}}$$

where, N is the number of scan lines. Application of linear array includes abdomen (large body area), gynecology, thyroid, breast, superficial vessel imaging and US guided biopsy. Advantages are good definition both in near and distant anatomy and good image quality across image depth and field of view (FOV). It can be used to view surface texture of the liver. Disadvantage is large footprint and limited FOV. It produces artifacts while scanning curved parts of the body due to air gap between skin and transducer.

Curvilinear Array

Linear array can be designed with convex transducer surface used for sector scanning, referred to as *curvilinear array (Figs. 12.12A and B).* It is smaller in size of linear array, provides sequential element switching and smaller footprint (surface contact area).

Curvilinear arrays have multiple configurations and frequencies based on application. It has curved surfaces of various radii which can be used across multiple bandwidths. For example, low frequency curvilinear probe is used for abdominal examinations due to deep penetration and wider FOV.

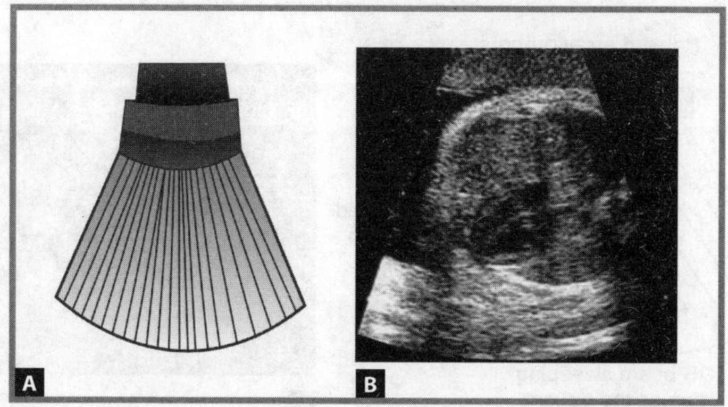

Figs. 12.12A and B: (A) Ultrasound curved array; (B) Curved array-sector image.

On the other hand, high frequency endocavitary curvilinear transducer is used for female pelvic examinations due to their higher resolution and small footprint.

The beam is wider at depth covers larger anatomy, hence used for depth examinations. It is more suitable for abdominal scanning due its curvature of abdominal wall. The scan lines decrease with increasing depth from the transducer and the image appear on the screen as curvilinear image *(convex)*.

Convex transducer's food print, frequency and application depends on either 2D or 3D imaging. In 2D imaging, convex transducer provides wide food print with central frequency of 2.5 MHz–7.5 MHz which can be used for abdominal examinations, transvaginal and transrectal examinations or organ diagnosis. Convex transducers in 3D imaging provides wide FOV with central frequency of 3.5 MHz–6.5 MHz which can be used for an abdominal examination. It is difficult to image curved regions of the body like spleen.

Phased Array

Phased array uses shorter transducer with fewer elements. A smaller number of elements (48–128) and smaller footprint with low frequency are used **(Fig. 12.13A)**. Each element has separate transmit and receive circuits. It produces both directional and focused beams. Its central frequency is 2 MHz–7.5 MHz. Beam point is narrow, but it expands based on the applied frequency.

If energized simultaneously, it acts as a single transducer and the beam travels forward. If energized separately in rapid sequence, the pulses reinforce only in one direction, called *steering*. For example, energizing 1,2,3, the reinforcement is in right, whereas energizing 3,2,1, will steer the beam to the left. Thus, scan lines sweep across the patient giving a sector field.

A *pie shaped/sector image* is formed by polar coordinates **(Fig. 12.13B)**. Image is narrower near the transducer and increase in width with depth.

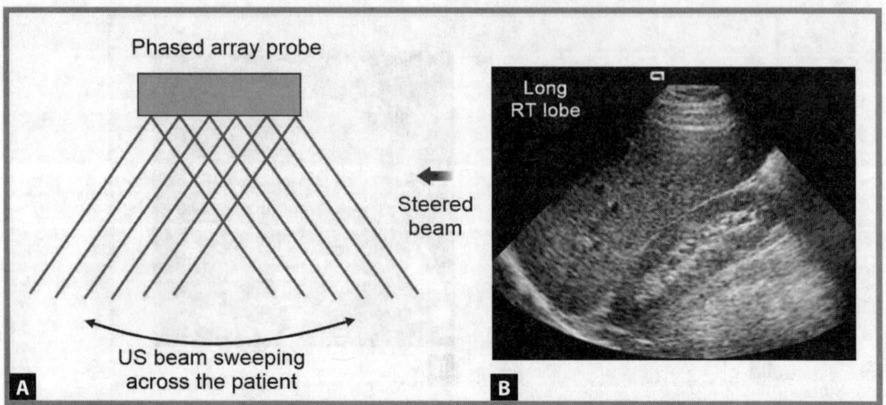

Figs. 12.13A and B: (A) Phased array with multiple elements; (B) Sector image display.

Beam shape is almost triangular and near field resolution is poor. Pulse rate determines the number of scan lines. In dynamic focusing, change of delay time during receive mode vary the focal plane but increase of focal plane decreases frame rate. It provides dynamic apertures with varying element numbers. Advantages of phased array includes large FOV and fast frame rate. The disadvantage is poor nearfield resolution. It is good while scanning the ribs as it fits in the intercostals space.

Phased array configuration and power sequences which steer US beams from a single point led to a *sector image*. Each element is excited via a delay which gives a *swiveled (angled, ±45°)* wave front. This requires narrow elements of about $\lambda/2$ dimension. The same delay is used in receive mode also and the transducer is sensitive to echo.

Focal Depth

Focal length can be altered electronically by the operator. The greater the time delay in energizing successive pair of elements, shorter the focal length. Beam is focused on an azimuthal plane (plane parallel to the length of the transducer). Focusing on an elevation plane (thickness) is done with an *acoustic lens*. Electronic focusing is also possible with *1.5-D transducer*. Focusing make the image good in the focal region and get worsened beyond the focus.

This can be overcome by multiple zones focusing facility. Multiple pulses (3–4) sent in each scan line with phase delays are altered to have different focus, both at transmission and reception mode. Each time, the transducer is gated to receive only from one focal zone. Echoes arriving from near or far distant points are blocked.

Its application includes; small array probe is used in cardiac examinations including transesophageal examinations, large array is used in abdomen and brain that gives larger FOV and phased array probe is also used for an internal examination such as rectum, vagina, and esophagus.

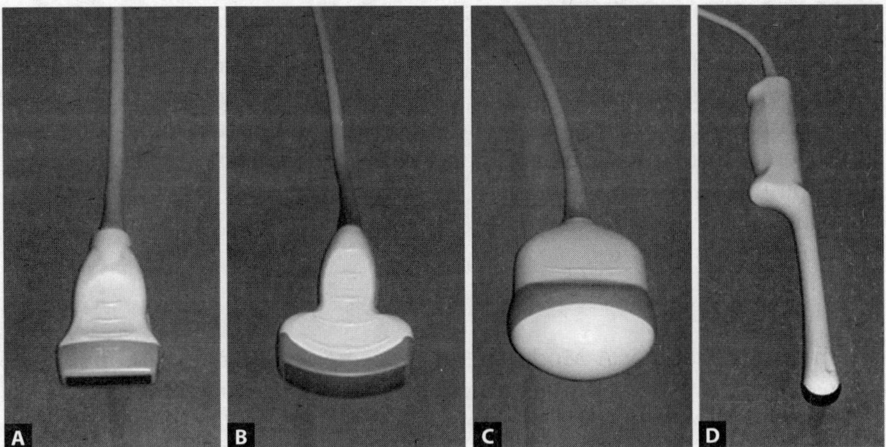

Figs. 12.14A to D: Clinical probes: (A) Rectilinear; (B) Curvilinear; (C) Real time 4D Doppler; (D) Transvaginal.

Intracavitary Probes

Pencil transducer or CW Doppler probes are used for an intraluminal study to measure blood flow and speed of sound in blood. It allows imaging both in transverse and longitudinal planes. It has small footprint with low frequency of 2 MHz–8 MHz.

Endocavitary transducer is used for internal examination of a patient which is designed to fit body orifices **(Figs. 12.14A to D)**. It includes endovaginal, endorectal, and endocavity. They have small footprint with frequency of 3.5 MHz–11.5 MHz.

Transesophageal transducer (TEE) with small footprint is used for an internal examination. It is employed in Cardiology to get image of the heart through esophagus's by using frequency of 3 MHz–10 MHz.

Annular Transducer

Annular transducer contains a series of concentric transducers that provides an *elliptical and spherical beam*. Transducer elements are shaped like rings and arranged in a concentric ring pattern around a central disk-shaped element. Each element has equal area but has different acoustic property. The signals are delayed to each ring, to create a focused beam. That is, a set of 5–10 ring elements are pulsed sequentially to move the beam from the innermost ring outwards. It produces a *symmetrical beam* which is not possible with a linear array probe.

It provides an excellent image quality with superior slice thickness uniformity. It is used in dynamic focusing, but not suitable for Doppler study. It can be either (1) annular phased transducer or (2) segmented annular phased array transducer.

Advantage is that it permits increased depth of field along a line focus with relatively limited number of elements. Disadvantage is that it must be mechanically scanned to generate a 2D image.

ULTRASOUND IMAGE DISPLAY

Ultrasound image is an electronic representation of data generated from returning echoes and displayed on a TV monitor. The image is assembled, one bit at a time like television image. Echo generates one bit of data, and many bits together form the electronic image. This image may be displayed as:
❑ Amplitude (A)-Mode
❑ Motion (M or TM)- Mode
❑ Brightness (B)-Mode

Amplitude Mode

In amplitude mode or A-Mode, the probe is held stationary, and pulses of nanosecond duration is sent into the patient and an echo is generated. Each interface gives one echo pulse. Echoes are displayed as spikes projecting from baseline, which identifies the central axis of the beam. It displays the depth on X-axis and echo intensity on Y-axis in an oscilloscope **(Fig. 12.15A)**. It is a simple US technique, shows only the position of interfaces.

Application of A-mode includes ophthalmology-distance measurements, echoencephalography, echocardiography, detecting cysts in breast and studying midline displacement in brain. It reveals the location of the echo producing structures only in the direction of the US beam.

Motion Mode

Motion mode also known as M-Mode or TM-Mode displays moving structures along a single line in an ultrasound beam. A-mode spikes are converted into dots and brightness represents amplitude in this mode. When an interface moves, the dots also move back and forth. For example, heart value can be shown as wave like structure. A single beam ultrasound scan is used to produce M-mode. Sequential US pulses are displayed adjacent to each other,

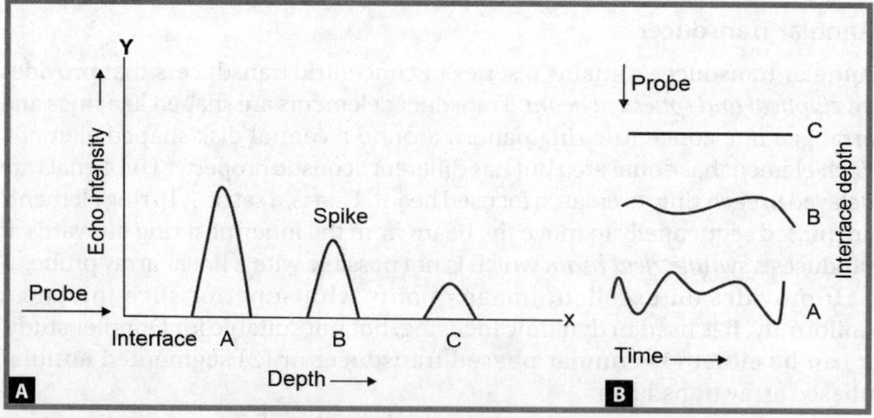

Figs. 12.15A and B: (A) A-mode display; (B) Ultrasound M-mode display: Change of position of interface over time, amplitude is replaced by brightness.

allowing the change in position of interfaces. It is recorded over a period. It provides an excellent temporal resolution of motion patterns and displays the time on X-axis and depth on Y-axis **(Fig. 12.15B)**.

Its application includes evaluation of cardiac value motion, fetal cardiac imaging, and other cardiac anatomy. Since, it has high sampling frequency of 100 pulses per second, it is useful in assessing rates and motion. Real-time 2D echocardiography, Doppler and color flow imaging reduces the importance of M-mode today.

Brightness Mode

In brightness mode or B-Mode, a slice of an anatomy of the patient is imaged. It is a 2D imaging that gives either static or real-time grayscale image. To generate a 2D image, multiple US pulses are sent as series of successive scan lines, to build a 2D representation of echoes arising from an area of an interest. To achieve this, the transducer is moved back and forth, so that beam scans a 2D section of the patient.

In static imaging, the image is compiled as the sound beam is scanning across the patient. The image presents snapshot averaged over time required to sweep the sound beam. In real-time imaging, an image is bult up as sound beam scans across the patient, while the scanning is performed quickly and automatically. One follows another image in quick succession, e.g.,30–60 complete images per second. It is useful to display moving structures like heart values.

Echoes are displayed as dots, and brightness is proportional to echo intensity **(Fig. 12.16)**. When image is displayed on a black background, signals of high intensity appear as white, absence of signal as black and an intermediate signals as shades of gray. Thus, thousands of echo signal strengths of varying brightness of points gives grayscale image. The image displays a section of an anatomy. The image depth depends on transducer

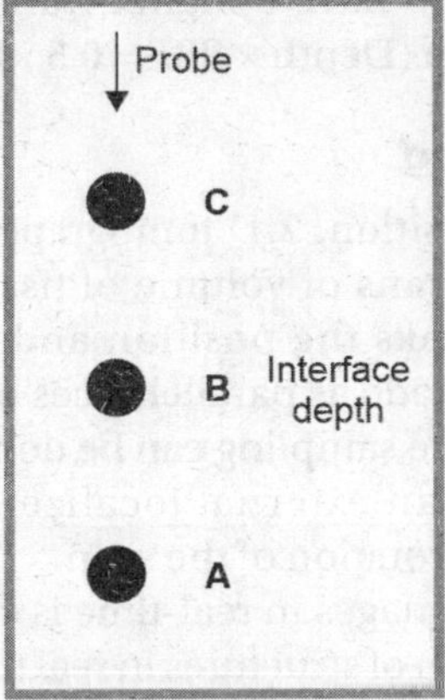

Fig. 12.16: B-mode display: The amplitude is replaced by brightness, interfaces at different depth gives varying brightness proportional to their echo intensity.

frequency, focus, etc. The B-mode scanning is usually done with an electronic scanning either with linear array or phased array.

Real-time Scanning

Real-time scanning is one in which an image is constructed instantaneously and renewed 30 times per second. It updates the position of the structures that is displayed as it happens, including an anatomical motion. Both linear array and sector probes can be used for real-time scanning. The real-time scanning image quality depends on: (1) field of view (FOV), (2) number of A lines per image (N): high resolution requires large number of lines (100) per frame, (3) line density (LN), (4) depth (D), and (5) frame rate: to follow motion large number of frames/second is required.

2D image is obtained from number of A-lines, typically 100 lines per frame, acquired across a FOV. Acquisition time for each line to collect echo from depth D is given by:

$$T_{line} = 13\ \mu s \times D\ (cm)$$

Time required per frame is: $T_{frame} = N \times T_{line} = N \times 13\ \mu s \times D\ (cm)$

Maximum possible frame rate per second with N and D is:

$$\text{Frame rate} = \frac{1}{T_{frame}} = \frac{1}{N \times 13\ \mu s \times D\ (cm)}$$

$$= \frac{0.077\ \mu s}{N \times D\ (cm)} = \frac{77000\ s}{N \times D\ (cm)}$$

The frame rate increases as *N* or *D* increases. Both high frame rate and large depth is not possible. In a real-time scanning, the following relationship is true:

$$\text{Depth} \times \text{Frame rate} \times \text{Lines per frame} = \text{Constant}$$

Higher frame rate can be obtained by decreasing *D*, *N* and or *FOV*. Frame repetition frequency depends on *N* and *PRF*, whereas PRF in turn depends on frame rate and lines per frame (PRF = Frame rate × Lines per frame). Hence, higher PRF must be used to have a higher frame rate. However, this will decrease the depth selection (Depth × PRF = 0.5 × Sound velocity).

Three-dimensional Imaging

To have a 3-D image acquisition, 2-D tomographic image data is acquired from a series of B-mode scans of volume of tissue. Electronic or manual movement of the probe links the position and an orientation with data collection. Images can be made as parallel slices or wedge-shaped slices but 3D imaging is slower. Volume sampling can be done by (1) linear translation, (2) freedom motion with an external localizer to a reference position, (3) rocking motion, and (4) rotation of the scan.

Acquisition and display images in real-time is called 4-D imaging. It gives better visualization of motion of structures in real time. It is possible to display surface by *maximal intensity projection (MPR)* processing or volume surface rendering. This finds application in an obstetric imaging.

DOPPLER ULTRASOUND

Doppler ultrasound is based on the principle of *Doppler effect* in light. Whenever there is relative motion between a light source and an object, there will be a *frequency shift*. Object moving away from the source appears to have a lower frequency and longer wavelength. Object moving towards the source appears to have high frequency and shorter wavelength. The shift in frequency is known as *Doppler shift*.

Same concept is applied in ultrasound, if there is a relative motion between a sound source and an object, there will be a frequency shift of ultrasound wave. Shift in frequency of ultrasound wave is caused by a moving reflector, e.g., blood cells. It is like a siren on a fire truck; the sound is high pitched as the truck approaches the listener (λ is compressed) and shifted to a lower pitch as it moves away from the listener (λ is expanded).

Frequency shift is useful to identify blood flow in vessels. Comparison of incident US frequency with reflected US frequency from the blood cells, gives velocity of blood. It also helps in measurement of blood flow (indirect), create color blood flow maps of the vasculature, etc. Change of frequency is proportional to velocity of an interface. Higher the transducer frequency or faster an interface moves, greater the change in frequency.

Doppler systems used in medicine may be divided as (1) continuous Doppler, (2) pulsed Doppler, (3) duplex scanning, (4) color flow imaging, and (5) power Doppler.

Doppler Shift

Doppler shift (f_d) is the difference between the incident frequency and reflected frequency. If a reflector is moving away from a source of ultrasound, then Doppler shift:

$$f_d = f_i - f_r = \frac{\text{Reflector speed} \times 2 \times f_i}{\text{Reflector speed} + \text{Speed of sound}}$$

where, f_i is frequency of an incident sound, and f_r is the frequency of reflected sound. Thus, blood moves away from the transducer expands the sound waves and produces lower frequency. Similarly, blood moving towards the transducer compresses the sound waves and produces higher frequency echoes. When the US beam and blood are not in parallel, the Doppler shift is less, and the equation needs modification **(Fig. 12.17)**. If θ is the angle between the US beam and direction of moving blood, then:

$$\text{Cos}\,\theta = \frac{\text{Adjacent side}}{\text{Hypotenuse}}$$

In the Doppler shift equation, the reflector speed is much smaller (200 cm/s) compared to ultrasound speed (154,000 cm/s) then the equation is rewritten as:

$$f_d = \frac{\text{Reflector speed (v)} \times 2 \times f_i \times \text{Cos}\,\theta}{\text{Speed of sound (c)}}$$

$$f_d = \frac{v \times 2 \times f_i \times \text{Cos}\,\theta}{c}$$

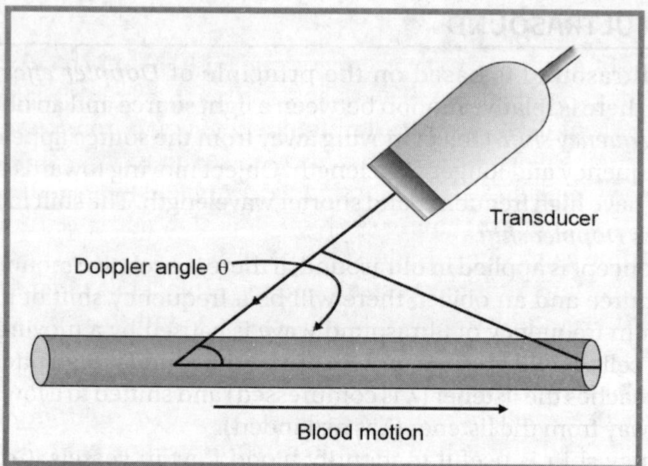

Fig. 12.17: The ultrasound and blood flow directions are not parallel; it makes an angle θ with blood flow direction.

Thus, the Doppler frequency shift, $f_d = 2\,f_i\,v \times Cos\,\theta/c$, where, v is speed of moving blood, c is speed of sound, f_i is incident sound frequency and θ is Doppler angle. Then velocity of moving blood:

$$v = \frac{f_d\,c}{2\,f_i\,Cos\,\theta}$$

If $\theta = 0, 30, 45, 60$ and 90, then $Cos\,\theta = 1, 0.87, 0.707, 0.5$ and 0, respectively. The maximum shift is found at 0 angle, that is if $\theta = 0$, $Cos\,\theta = 1$. At large angle (>60), the shift is small, minor errors in angle accuracy can result in large errors in speed estimation. Doppler frequency shift of a moving blood occurs is in an audible range, which can be converted into an audible signal through a loudspeaker. It can be heard by an operator to help in probe positioning and diagnosis.

Worked Example 12.3

In a Doppler examination $f_i = 5$ MHz, v = 25 cm/s, $\theta = 45°$, calculate the Doppler shift.

Doppler shift:

$$f_d = 2\,f_i\,v \times \frac{Cos\,\theta}{c}$$

$$= \frac{2 \times 5 \times 10^6 \times 25\,\frac{cm}{s} \times 0.707}{1540,00\,\frac{cm}{s}}, \text{ since } Cos\,45° = 0.707$$

$$= 1.14 \times 10^3$$

$$= 1.14 \text{ kHz,}$$

Thus, Doppler shift frequency lies in audible frequency range, though ultrasound is not audible.

Continuous Doppler

Continuous Doppler has two transducers, one for transmission and other for receiving echoes. Frequencies of two signals are subtracted to get the Doppler shift. A *wall filter* is used to remove low frequency signals from vessel wall and moving specular reflectors. *Low pass filter* is used to remove superimposed high frequency oscillations. Doppler signal is amplified by an audio amplifier. It is recorded as function of time to study pulsatile flow and spectrum changes. There is no time gain compensation (TGC) here.

Continuous Doppler is low cost, no aliasing artifact but suffer from depth resolution. It is suitable for measuring fast flow and studying deep lying vessels. High accuracy of Doppler shift measurement is possible since narrow bandwidth is used. It is difficult to get direction of blood flow relative to transducer hence, special signal processing method of *quadrature detection* is used. Multiple overlying vessels result in superimposition hence it is difficult to distinguish them. Spectral broadening of frequencies occurs with a large sample area across the vessel profile resulting in high velocity at the center and lower velocity at the edges of the vessel.

Pulsed Doppler

Pulsed Doppler combines continuous wave Doppler and pulse echo imaging. The former gives velocity information and the latter gives depth information. Depth selection is obtained by an electronic gate, which will reject all signals except those falling within the gate window. Alternatively, multiple gates are used to get velocity profile across a vessel.

In pulse echo format, longer SPL is used, to improve sensitivity and accuracy of frequency shift but result in loss of an axial resolution. Phase of returning echoes from a stationary object, relative to phase of the transmitted sound, does not change with time. However, the phase of returning echoes from moving objects does vary with time. Hence, sample of shifted frequencies are measured as phase change. To overcome the aliasing artifact, the PRF must be twice the highest frequency shift or Doppler signal. That is a 1 kHz Doppler shift requires at least PRF of 2 kHz otherwise it causes error in velocity estimation. As per sampling statistics theory, PRF must be at least twice the Doppler frequency shift:

$$\text{PRF} = 2f_{d(max)} = \frac{2 \times 2\, f_0\, v_{max}\, \text{Cos}\, \theta}{c}$$

$$\text{or } v_{max} = \frac{c \times \text{PRF}}{4\, f_0\, \text{Cos}\, \theta}$$

Thus, the maximum velocity, v_{max} depends on PRF, f_0 and Cos θ (for larger angles, Cos θ value is minimum). If 2 kHz is the maximum Doppler shift frequency, then the minimum PRF should be equal to 2 × 2 kHz = 4 kHz. Pulsed Doppler does not give visual display.

Duplex Scanning

Duplex scanning consists of both B-mode real-time US and a pulsed Doppler acquisition. Doppler information is obtained for a specific area called gate. Initially, it operates in 2D, B-mode to create a real-time image, to select a Doppler gate window position and then switched over to pulsed Doppler mode. Electronic array transducers are used in a group with B mode, then one or more probe is used for Doppler information. Velocity and Doppler angles are obtained from Doppler frequency shift and B-mode scan, respectively. The information of flow is obtained by the relation:

$$\text{Flow}\left(\frac{cm^3}{s}\right) = \text{Vessel cross-sectional area (cm}^2) \times \text{Velocity (cm/s)}$$

Laminar flow occurs at the center of a large smooth vessel, whereas *turbulent flow* exists in vessel containing plaque and stenoses. There may be error in flow volume due to: vessels axis might not lie totally within the scanned plane, curved vessel, and an altered flow. This gets exaggerated, if Doppler angle > 60°, misposition of Doppler gate overestimates velocity and noncircular cross-section of vessel cause errors in an area estimation.

However, Duplex scan has the following features: velocity profile can be obtained with multiple gates, mapping of velocity in color and flow in grayscale, and direction of flow by real-time color flow, etc. Doppler signal can be represented as frequency spectrum from a range of velocities in a volume.

Color Flow Imaging

Color flow imaging gives 2D visual display of Doppler data on a B-mode real-time grayscale, image. Data acquisition is interleaved with that of flow information displayed over large area superimposed on a grayscale image **(Fig. 12.18A)**. It able to gives velocity and position information simultaneously. Color coding is assigned based on blood motion in vessels. It maps the direction and velocity in each pixel using an arbitrary color scale. Blood moving towards the transducer is coded with *red (veins)*, and blood moving away (artery) from the transducer is coded with *blue*. Turbulent flow is displayed in *green or yellow*. Color intensity varies with flow velocity including an absence of flow with grayscale. There are two methods of color flow imaging, namely, (1) *phase shift autocorrelation* and (2) *time domain correlation*.

In phase shift autocorrelation, the similarity of one scan line to another, when maximum overlap exists is measured. In time domain correlation, the reflector motion over a period, λT between consecutive pulse echo amplitude is measured. The degree of similarity between the two is mathematically correlated.

Color Doppler can detect flow from small vessels. The limitation includes that clutter from slow moving solid structures and noise can suppress smaller echoes from moving blood. The spatial resolution is much lower compared to grayscale image. Velocity measurement accuracy is limited in time domain correlation.

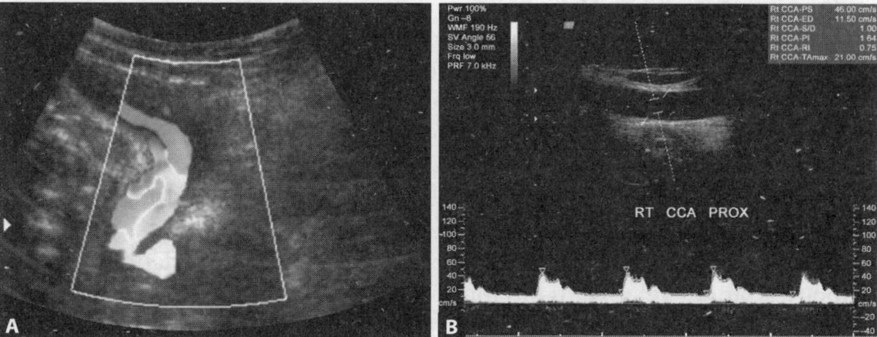

Figs. 12.18A and B: (A) Color Doppler of umbilical cord; (B) Doppler spectral display.
(For color version, see Plate 1)

Doppler Spectrum Analysis

Duplex scanning or color flow imaging is used for spectral analysis. Since blood is pulsatile, spectral characteristics also vary with time. *Laminar flow* is large flow at the center of a smooth vessel, and slower near vessel walls due to fractional forces. Presence of plaque and stenoses in a vessel, characterizes blunt or *turbulent flow*. A large Doppler gate is positioned to cover the whole lumen that contain wide range of blood velocities. Spectral characters vary with time since blood flow is pulsatile.

Duplex scan operates with multiple gates and there are several parallel channels over the vessel to get *Doppler signals*. *Fourier transform* mathematically analyzes the signal and gives an amplitude vs frequency distribution, known as *Doppler spectrum* **(Fig. 12.18B)**. The spectrum consists of multiple frequencies within a sampling gate for a given time. It continuously updates in real-time spectral Doppler display. Video monitor displays spectrum below 2D B-mode image, as a *moving trace*. Doppler shift frequency in Y-axis vs time in X-axis displays the spectrum. It is worth to recollects that Doppler shift frequency is proportional to blood velocity. Doppler signal intensity at a given frequency shift at a given time is shown as *brightness* at a point in the display. Velocity in one direction is shown above the X-axis (positive), and velocity in reverse direction is placed below the X-axis (negative). As new data arise, the spectrum is updated and scrolled from left to right. Image appears as *choppy sinusoidal wave* of heartbeat cycle that represents pulsatile blood.

Blood flow may be laminar, blunt, or turbulent depending on the vessel wall characteristics, size, shape, and flow rate. Spectrum display reveals presence of flow, direction of flow, and flow characteristics of blood. Small Doppler angle gives better determination of direction of flow. Fast laminar flow presents at the center of a large smooth vessel, and slower flow presents near the walls due to frictional forces. Normal flow spectrum represents the hemodynamic features of a given vessel.

Turbulent is caused by plaque and stenosis, the flow spectrum represents disease pattern, and curve is filled with wide distribution of frequencies of wide range of velocities. Hence, a large Doppler gate positioned to encompass an entire lumen will contain a large range of blood velocities. A smaller gate positioned at the center of the vessel will have a smaller, faster range of velocities. A Doppler gate positioned near stenosis in the turbulent flow pattern will measure the largest range of velocities. It is very difficult to identify the lack of flow, that is due to noise. Normal blood flow is represented by a specific characteristic spectrum. Disturbed and turbulent flow alters the spectrum proportional to disease pattern.

Doppler spectrum techniques can predict vascular impedance, pulsatile velocity changes relative to circulation. Pulsatility index (PI) and resistive index (RI) are the quantities that describe Doppler spectrum character as follows:

$$\text{Pulsatility index} = \frac{\text{Maximum flow} - \text{Minimum flow}}{\text{Average flow}}$$

$$\text{Resistivity index} = \frac{\text{Maximum flow} - \text{Minimum flow}}{\text{Maximum flow}}$$

Aliasing

Aliasing artifact is caused by insufficient sampling rate relative to high frequency Doppler signal **(Fig. 12.19)**. Minimum of 2 samples per cycle of Doppler shift frequency is required to overcome an aliasing and to determine velocity unambiguously. Aliasing signal appears wrap around negative signal and take an appearance of reverse flow. In that case, an velocity scale is adjusted to a wider range. If scale is already in maximum, spectral baseline (0 velocity) is shifted so that it covers higher forward velocity and lesser reverse velocity. Maximum, minimum, and an average Doppler spectral values are used to quantify PI and RI. However, the minimum and maximum Doppler shift cannot exceed ± PRF/2.

Power Doppler

Power Doppler is a signal processing method that relies on total strength of the Doppler signal (amplitude) and ignores directional (phase) information.

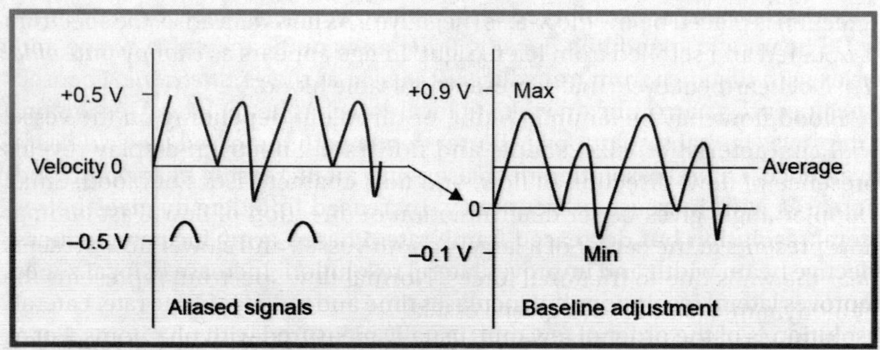

Fig. 12.19: Aliasing of signals and remedial measures.

Power mode of signal acquisition is dependent on amplitude of all Doppler signals, regardless of frequency shift. This improves sensitivity to motion (e.g., slow blood flow), at the expense of directional and quantitative flow information. Images are more sensitive to motion and are not affected by the Doppler angle.

Doppler uses the same levels of power as standard color flow procedure (no increased transmit power) and it is more sensitive than color Doppler flow imaging. The image signal does not vary with direction of flow. Aliasing is not a problem as only the strength of the frequency shift is analyzed, but not the phase. Greater sensitivity allows detection and interpretation of very subtle and slow blood flow. Frame rates are slower and flash artifacts may occur, which are related to color signals arising from moving tissues, patient motion, or transducer motion.

IMAGE QUALITY AND QUALITY CONTROL

Image Quality

Ultrasound image quality depends on (1) spatial resolution, (2) contrast resolution, and (3) noise. Spatial resolution is the ability to resolve two closely placed objects. It is divided into an *axial resolution, lateral resolution, and an elevational resolution.*

Axial Resolution

Axial resolution is an ability to separate two closely spaced interfaces along the axis of beam and it is determined by spatial pulse length. It is equal to 1/2 spatial pulse length and depends on pulse frequency and duration. Higher the frequency, shorter the pulse and better the axial resolution. Greater damping transducer (low-Q) gives short pulses which increases axial resolution. It deteriorates with increasing pulse length, decreasing frequency and increasing wavelength. Typical axial resolution is 0.5 mm for a sound wave of 0.3 mm wavelength which has three wave per pulse.

Lateral Resolution

Lateral resolution is an ability to separate two adjacent objects, determined by US beam width and line density. It depends on beam width, shape and varies with distance from transducer. It is best at the *Fresnel zone*. Focused transducer has narrow beam width at focal zone has better lateral resolution. It improves lateral resolution at shorter depth, with increased *far-field beam* divergence. Lateral resolution decreases with an increasing beamwidth and increases with increase of frequency. Increased line density gives better lateral resolution but decreased frame rate. Phased array focusing reduces effective beam width and improves lateral resolution. Increase of focal zones improves lateral resolutions but increases time and reduces frame rate. Lateral resolution is of the order of few mm, usually measured with phantoms. For a given axial resolution, the lateral resolution is 3–5 times larger.

Elevational Resolution

Elevational resolution is in slice thickness direction which is perpendicular to the image plane. It depends on transducer element height and is depth dependent. Hence, near field/far field controls elevational resolution. It is poor at adjacent to the transducer array and after the focal zone. Elevational focusing can be achieved with an acoustic lens shaped along the height of the elements. It can produce an elevational focal zone closer to an array surface. On the other hand, *1.5D transducer array* transducer can be used. It has several rows (5-7) of independent elements in an elevational direction. 1.5D indicates that the number of elements in an elevational direction is <than that of lateral direction (100-200). Phase delay can be performed on the elements of different rows so that the beam is focused on the slice thickness direction of a given depth. Multiple elevational transmit focal zones is possible but goes with time penalty.

Contrast Resolution

Contrast is generated by differences in signal amplitude that depends on difference of an acoustic impedance, density, and size of scatterer within tissues. Scattering creates additional signals from areas other than an echo from specular reflections and degrades contrast. Proper signal processing and attenuation differences give difference in grayscale. *Microbubble contrast agent* improves visualization of vasculature and helps tissue perfusion. *Harmonic imaging* improves image contrast, by degrading signals from low frequency echoes. Doppler ultrasound involves moving structures with good signal processing which improves contrast. Contrast resolution also depends on spatial resolution. In wider slice thickness, echoes from small structures are averaged over a minimum volume resulting lower signal or loss of signal. Structures larger than the minimum volume element gives better contrast. Increase of transmit power or PRF will improve contrast but there is trade-off between transmit power and bioeffects.

Temporal resolution is an ability to resolve events in time. It is very important in an examination of highly moving organs, e.g., echocardiography. Temporal resolution depends on pulse repetition frequency (PRF).

Noise

Noise is generated from electronic amplifiers, environmental sources (power fluctuation, equipment malfunction) and TGC which reduces contrast and increases noise with depth. A low noise, high gain amplifier is required for optimal low contrast resolution. Exponential attenuation of beam over depth reduces contrast and increases noise. It requires TGC to maintain depth uniformity. Signal processing reduce noise, so that temporal averaging improves signal-to-noise ratio (SNR). However, it results in lower frame rate and poor spatial resolution. Low power operation ultrasound systems (OG) need higher electronic amplification, to increase week echo amplitude resulting higher noise and lower SNR.

Quality Control

Quality control program is required for ultrasound equipment on pediatric interval. It needs tissue equivalent phantoms with acoustic targets of various sizes and an echogenic features embedded in it **(Fig. 12.20).** The phantom should evaluate the clinical capabilities of US equipment. General phantom consists of three modules, namely *(1) system resolution module, (2) elevational resolution module and (3) system uniformity module.*

In the system resolution module, phantom is filled with a *tissue mimicking gel* having tissue equivalent attenuation of 0.5–0.7 dB/cm per MHz. *Low-scatter targets, dead zone targets, horizontal accuracy targets, grayscale targets, axial resolution targets,* and *vertical accuracy targets* of various sizes are embedded in the gel. Spatial resolution, contrast resolution and distance accuracy are tested with this module. *Axial resolution* is tested with high contrast objects separated by 2, 1, 0.5 and 0.25 mm at three different depths. *Lateral resolution* is measured by lateral spread of high contrast targets/grayscale scale targets. *Vertical targets* are used to check vertical distance precision and accuracy and it should be within 5% of known distance. *Low-scatter targets* are kept at various depths to determine penetration depths.

Elevational resolution module consists of low contrast, *small diameter spheres of 2 mm and 4 mm* uniformly spaced with depth. It is used to check an elevational resolution with depth variation and partial volume effects. This finds much important while using 1.5D transducer array, 3D imaging, and multiple transmit focal zones to reduce slice thickness at various depths.

System uniformity module consists of an uniformly distributed *scattering materials.* It is used to test an image uniformity and penetration depth. Generally higher frequency has lower penetration depth. Evidence of

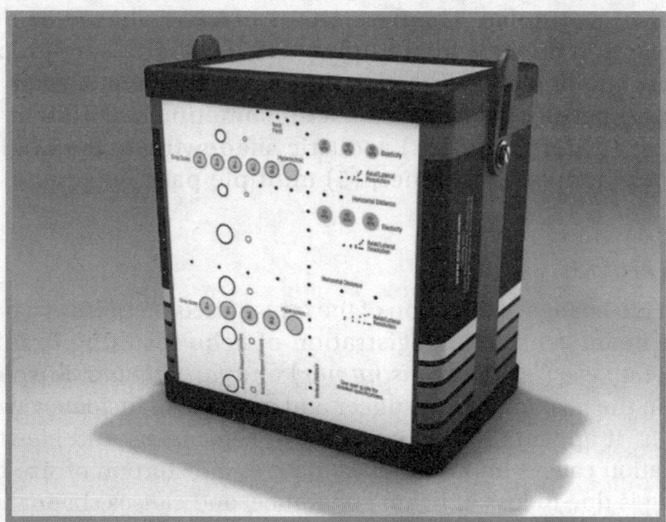

Fig. 12.20: Ultrasound quality assurance: Multi-purpose multi-tissue ultrasound phantom. (*Courtesy:* Sun Nuclear)

vertical-directed shadowing in linear arrays or angular-directed shadowing for phased array indicates malfunction of a transducer. Horizontal variation indicates insufficient handling of transitions between focal zones during the multifocal mode.

In addition, all probes should be tested as per manufacturer specifications initially and ongoing basis. Maximum depth is visualized by identifying the low contrast scatter in an uniformity phantom. For example, a depth of 18 cm for abdominal scans and 8 cm for small anatomical structures is an expectation for beam attenuation of 0.7 dB/cm in a medium for a single transmit focal zone. In the case of multi-frequency transducer, mid-frequency is used to access gray level and image uniformity by using an uniformity phantom module. *American college of radiology (ACR)* accreditation QC program have suggested various tests and frequency.

A black line on the screen suggests that the transducer has a dead crystal. A shadow on the screen indicates a week crystal in the transducer which affects crystal vibration. Cracks, if any in the crystal will cause noise in the image.

Before buying a probe, one must check, whether the probe is compatible to the system, penetration depth is better at low frequency (2.5 MHz–7.5 MHz) and at higher frequency (above 7.5 MHz). Image quality is poor in low frequency and better in high frequency.

ARTIFACTS AND BIOEFFECTS

Artifacts of Ultrasound

Artifact is an image formed by an echo which does not relates its location, intensity, or actual interfaces in the patient. It arises from incorrect display of an anatomy or noise. They are either machine-based or operator-based artifacts. It appears in multiples, and the sources are propagation, attenuation, equipment malfunction or design and operator error. Artifacts give misleading information but useful sometimes. Different types of artifacts are (1) refraction, (2) acoustic shadowing and enhancement, (3) reverberation, (4) side lobes, (5) multiple path reflection, (6) slice thickness, and (7) speckle.

Refraction Artifacts

Refraction is a change of direction of the transmitted US pulse at a boundary. Refracted beam causes misregistration of echo resulting in misplaced anatomy, e.g., *eye (lens-vitreous humor)* and *fatty tissues.* Misplacement depends on the position of transducer and an angle of incidence with tissue boundaries. It appears as *misregistration, defocusing,* and *ghost images.* Misregistration causes improper placement and distortion of size or shape. Defocusing is due to loss of beam coherence, and causes shadowing at the edges of large and curved structures **(Fig. 12.21A).** Ghost images are due to an altered sound beam path **(Fig. 12.21B).**

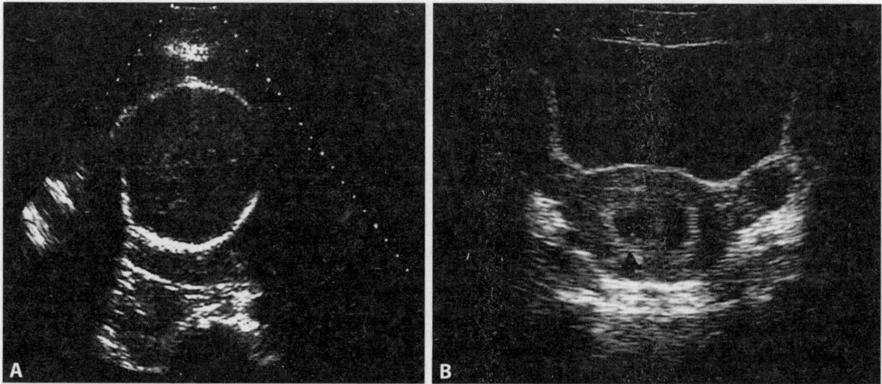

Figs. 12.21A and B: (A) Refraction artifacts, defocusing type, cause shadowing at the edges; (B) Refraction artifacts appear as Ghost images: Single gestational sac – duplicated. Second copy of the reflector, which is side-by-side at the same depth as the true reflector.

Acoustic Shadowing and Enhancement

Shadowing is a reduced echo intensity behind a highly attenuating or reflecting object. It is a hypointense signal area, distal to an object or interface. It is caused by objects with high attenuation or reflection of incident beam without return of echo. Highly attenuating objects reduce intensity of transmitted beam which can induce low intensity streaks in an image, e.g., *bone, and kidney stones.* As a result, the anechoic or hypoechoic region is seen deeper to a highly attenuating medium **(Figs. 12.22A and B)**. Reflection from a curved surface eliminates distal propagation of sound and causes streaks or shadowing.

Enhancement is an increased echo intensity behind a minimally attenuating object. It occurs in structures having very low US attenuation, e.g., fluid-filled cavity like flied bladder cysts. It is due to increased transmission of sound through these structures.

Shadowing or enhancement may prevent visualization of true anatomy and is considered as a beneficial artifact. It may be divided into *clean and dirty artifacts.* Clean artifact may appear posterior to calcification or bone due to high percentage of absorption and reflection with no transmission. Dirty artifacts appear posterior to air filled structures due to high percentage of reflection and small percentage of transmission.

Reverberation

Reverberation artifact is due to multiple echoes generated between two closely spaced interfaces. As a result, the US beam gets back and forth reflection during acquisition. Image contains an object at regular interval, but amplitude reduces due to reverberations. It is usually caused by reflections between transducer and a strong reflector such as metallic objects, e.g., *pullet fragments and air pockets/partial liquid anatomy.*

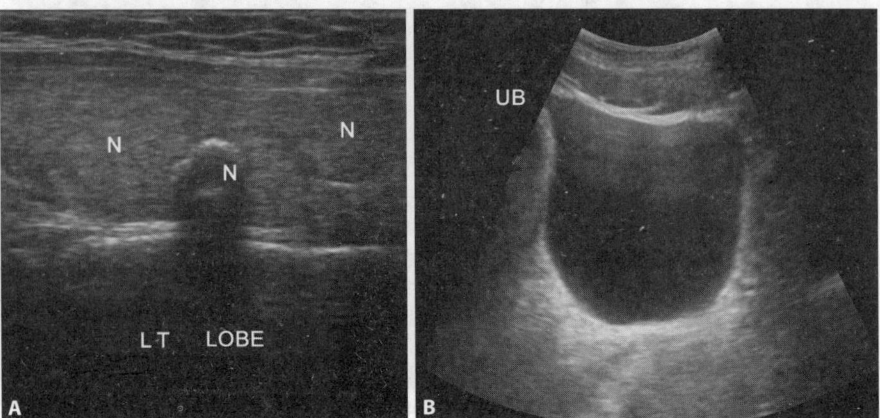

Figs. 12.22A and B: (A) Acoustic shadowing (thyroid); (B) Acoustic enhancement (bladder).

The reverberation artifacts appear as series of bright bands, parallel to sound beam's main axis with decreasing intensity and equidistant from each other. *It is also called ring down or comet tail artifacts* and commonly seen in images of bowel gas or sections of bladder wall **(Fig. 12.23A).** Comet tail artifact arises from reverberation whereas ring town arise from resonant vibrations within fluid trapped between a tetrahedron of air bubbles. The later creates continuous sound wave that is transmitted back and forth to the transducer and displayed as series of parallel bands.

Side Lobes

Emissions of US in the off-axis direction is called side lobe or grating lobe. It arises from the expansion of crystal elements orthogonal to main beam. Echoes of the side lobes are positioned in an image as if they arise from the main beam. Sidelobes artifact occurs near a strong specular reflector. It may mask weak echoes that are within the main beam's axis. Side lobes may redirect diffuse echoes from adjacent soft tissues into an organ which appear as hyperechoic, e.g., *gallbladder*. In gallbladder imaging, it produces artificial *pseudo sludge*. Side lobes are forward in nature and present in all single and multielement transducer array.

Grating lobes occurs in multielement array due to division of transducer's surface into large number of small elements. US energy is produced at large angle compared to main beam. This misdirected energy can give *ghost images* from off-axis high contrast structures. It can be avoided by keeping closely spaced elements in the transducer array. Linear array has larger width and spacing of their transducer elements hence, it is more prone to grating lobes than phased array probes.

Multiple Path Reflection

Whenever there is an oblique reflection, the beam reaches a second reflector and an echo return via first reflector to transducer. It usually occurs near highly reflective surface, e.g., *interface of liver and diaphragm.* Generally, transducer receives echoes from liver mass and diaphragm. Since, the diaphragm echo is much strong, it travels from the diaphragm to the liver mass gives another set of echoes which is directed back to the diaphragm. In turn, echoes reflected from the diaphragm travels to the transducer. The back and forth second echo from the liver mass gives an artifact in the image, which is like a mirror image of the mass, placed beyond the diaphragm. Thus, it causes ghost or apparent image, and an anatomy is misplaced on the beam axis distal to an actual position.

Slice Thickness

Off-axis echoes from outside the slice thickness appear in the region that is echo free. Slice thickness is determined by beam width, and it varies with depth. Sources of artifact are loss of signal from objects that are smaller than volume element due to partial volume averaging and inclusion of signals from highly reflective objects that are not in an imaging plane. It results in false echo, not controllable by the user, e.g., *lumens of large blood vessels and large cysts.* This artifact is significant at distance close and far from the transducer.

Speckle

If scattering surfaces are spaced at distances less than axial resolution, echoes undergo constructive and destructive interference, that increases noise and is seen as *speckle* (textured appearance). Echo pattern is random, unrelated to scattering structure but useful to differentiate tissues. Higher frequency transducers create finer speckle patterns than lower frequency transducers. Speckles are typically associated with *liver parenchyma, thyroid, heart muscle, skeletal muscle, spleen,* and *kidney* (**Fig. 12.23B**).

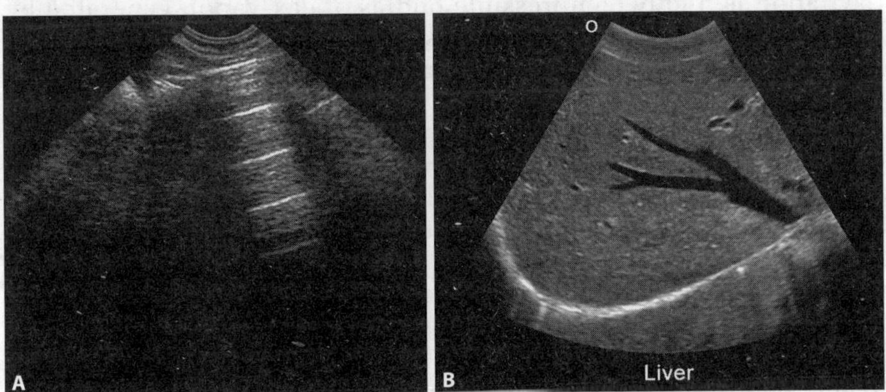

Figs. 12.23A and B: (A) Ring down artifact (reverberation) seen in bowel gas, (B) Speckle artifact—liver shows speckle pattern.

Bioeffects

Diagnostic ultrasound is a safe tool. Deleterious bioeffects on either patients or operators have not been reported. However, any harm can be caused by diagnostic US intensities. Hence, the user must consider issues of benefits versus risks. The main bioeffects are (1) thermal effects, (2) cavitations and (3) acoustic power.

Thermal Effects

Tissue absorbs ultrasound energy and converts into heat which is dissipated in all parts of tissue. Absorption of ultrasound energy causes thermal effects. It depends on heat deposition rate and how fast heat is removed by blood flow, and heat conduction. Heat indicators are I_{SPTA} (*SPTA stands for spatial peak temporal average intensity)*, and *thermal index (TI)*. Heat dissipation is found by an average US intensity at the focal zone and absorption coefficient of tissue. Absorption increases with frequency and varies with tissue type. Attenuation coefficient of bone is higher than soft tissue hence, tissue-bone interface absorbs more heat.

Thermal index is an acoustic power produced by a transducer to the power required to raise tissue temperature by 1°C in beam area. It is estimated by an algorithm that consider frequency (f), beam area, and acoustic output power. TI values are associated with intensity, I_{SPTA} and TI can be quantified for soft tissue (TIS), bone (TIB) and cranial bone (TIC). This is useful in obstetrics scanning of late term pregnancies and Doppler ultrasound.

In the diagnostic US, the rise in temperature is 1–2°C, which is well below the potential damage level. However, Doppler study may approach these levels with high PRF and long pulse duration. Nonthermal effects are mechanical movement of particles of a medium due to radiation pressure and an acoustic streaming, resulting a steady circulatory flow.

Cavitation

Cavitation is highly compressible bodies of gas/vapor, generated by ultrasound. It results from negative pressure, which induces bubble formation in medium. It can be subtle, readily observable, unpredictable, and sometimes violent.

Stable cavitations refers to pulsation of persistent bubbles in the tissue that occur at low/medium US intensities. *Transient cavitation* may occur at high intensity, bubbles respond nonlinearly to the driving force, causing a collapse, approaching speed of sound (bubbles may dissolve, and disintegrate or rebound). Free radicals such as H*, and OH* may perform chemical changes in DNA. Short pulses can form transient cavitations however, diagnostic intensity is below the threshold limit of 1 kW per cm^2.

Mechanical index (MI) is a value that estimates the likelihood of cavitations by ultrasound beam. MI is directly proportional to peak rarefactional pressure, and inversely proportional to square root of frequency (MHz). An attenuation of 0.3 (dB/cm) is assumed for an algorithm that estimates MI. As US output

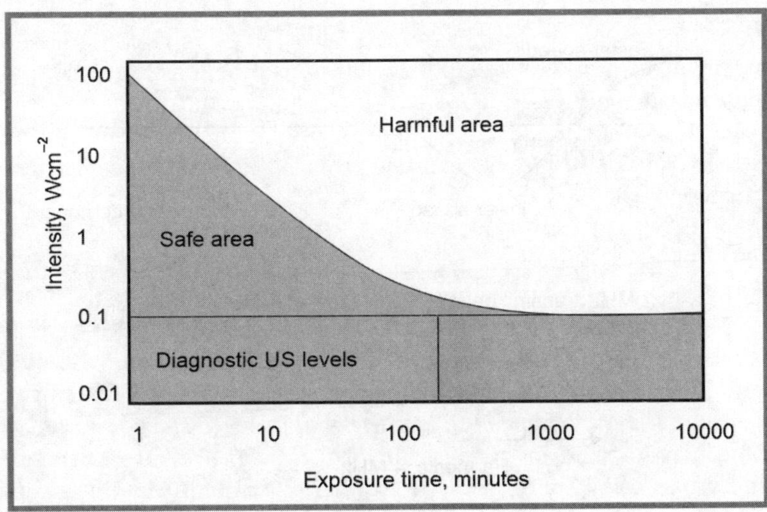

Fig. 12.24: Bioeffects of ultrasound showing the safe and harmful areas in terms of intensity vs exposure time.

power is increased, the MI increases linearly. An increase in transducer frequency decreases the MI by square root of 4 or by a factor of 2. MI values are associated with I_{SPTA}, the measure of intensity.

Acoustic Power

Acoustic power is a rate of energy production, and its unit is *Watt (W)*. Acoustic intensity is a rate in which sound energy flows through unit area, and its unit is Wcm^{-2}. Acoustic power level depends on operational characteristics of the system, namely *transmit power, PRF, f,* and *operation mode*. In diagnostic radiology, intensity levels are kept below the threshold for established bioeffects **(Fig. 12.24)**.

Biological effects are demonstrated at higher US power levels. It includes macroscopic damage (rupturing of blood vessels, breaking up of cells) and microscopic damage (breaking of chromosomes, changes in cell's mitotic index). No bioeffect is seen below an I_{SPTA}, of 100 mWcm^{-2}. The levels and durations for typical imaging and Doppler studies are well below the threshold for known adverse effects. Though it is safe, it should be used only in patients for whom there is an overall benefit. *American Institute of Ultrasound in medicine* recommends ALARA principles. FDA, US recommended mandatory display of TI and MI as acoustic output indices.

HARMONIC IMAGING AND ELASTOGRAPHY

Harmonic Imaging

Harmonic imaging is a nonlinear propagation of ultrasound which interacts with tissues that results in high frequencies. In nonlinear wave, high pressure

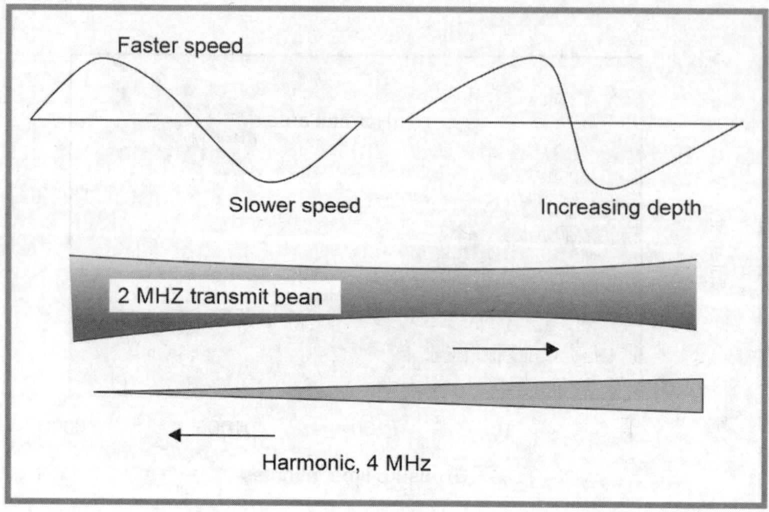

Fig. 12.25: Principle of harmonic imaging, sound wave gets distorted over depth. Double the fundamental frequency appear as harmonics concentrating at the center of beam.

part of the wave travels faster and low-pressure part travels slower and the wave gets distorted **(Fig. 12.25).** This distorted wave (change in wave) form leads to generation of harmonics from a tissue. It provides better quality images relative to conventional ultrasonogram. Harmonic frequency refers to integral multiple of frequencies of ultrasound pulse. For example, if the center frequency of ultrasound is f_o then harmonic frequencies are $2f_o$, $3f_o$, $4f_o$ etc. If a frequency centered at 2 MHz is transmitted, it will produce harmonic frequency bands at 4 MHz, 6 MHz, etc. In practice, up to second harmonics is used for imaging since other harmonics has decreasing amplitude not suitable for imaging. Harmonic wave generated with tissue increases with depth up to a point, and then decreases with depth due to attenuation. Hence, maximum harmonic intensity is available at an optimum depth below the surface.

The original frequency emitted by a transducer is called *fundamental frequency.* Transmitted pulse consists of range of frequencies around the central frequency. In a linear medium, an echo pulse is same as fundamental frequency but has lower energy. In a nonlinear medium, the harmonic waves of higher frequency and lower energy is emitted along with fundamental frequency. Amplitudes of harmonic waves are lower than the fundamental frequency wave. Sub-harmonic frequencies of f/2, 3f/2, 5f/2 of fundamental frequency is also emitted. These frequencies of 3f/2, 5f/2 are called *ultra harmonic frequencies* which are suitable for deep structure imaging. Production of harmonics is proportional to square of the fundamental intensity.

Harmonic Imaging Techniques

Various techniques are used to eliminate the fundamental frequency, namely (1) bandwidth receive filtering, (2) pulse inversion, (3) side-by-side phase cancellation, and (4) pulse-coded harmonics.

In bandwidth receive filtering, lower frequency of fundamental frequency is filtered, and higher harmonic frequency is used for imaging. It gives an enhanced image with noise elimination but reduces axial resolution.

Pulse inversion is a technique in which two pulses of 180°phase difference are emitted sequentially into the tissue. Summation of these received echoes cancels the fundamental echoes along with odd harmonic frequencies. Only even harmonic waves are used which has double the size of an amplitude. It is also called *phase cancellation or temporal cancellation technique*. It preserves axial resolution along with better tissue contrast. It depends on fixed frame rate and tissue motion, and lower frame rate degrade an image quality.

Side-by-side phase cancellation is like the phase inversion technique in which two pulses with opposite phases are transmitted along adjacent line of sight. These adjacent lines then added to cancel the fundamental frequency. It is also known as *spatial cancellation technique*. It preserves harmonic frequency bandwidth.

Pulse-coded harmonic technique transmits relatively complex pulse sequence into the body with a unique code and recognize the code imprinted on an each pulse. The unique code is also recognized in the echoes, so that fundamental echoes are identified and cancelled out.

Clinical Application

Harmonic imaging enhances contrast agent by sending low frequency pulse and receiving higher harmonics. It eliminates echo clutter from the fundamental frequency in the near field. Though signal gets attenuated, harmonics travel only half of the distance, hence have larger signal. Large pulse length with high transducer Q factor is employed. It makes it easier to separate harmonics from the fundamental frequency. Though it degrades axial resolution, the benefit of harmonic imaging overweighs the loss of axial resolution.

Super harmonic ultrasound imaging captures images from second harmonic resulting in greater contrast-to-tissue ratio (CTR). Up to fifth harmonic can be used in this imaging but require >130% bandwidth. Special phased array transducers are designed for this which contains two different elements arranged in an interleaved pattern. Its role in an ophthalmic tumor perfusion has been reported.

Tissue Harmonic Imaging

Based on harmonic imaging concept, *native tissue harmonic imaging (THI)* has been developed. It is a signal processing technique which improves contrast resolution. In this, low frequency sound is sent, and higher frequency harmonic produced by the tissue are received. The returning harmonic frequencies are used to form an image. Harmonic frequencies are generated by nonlinear distortion of wave, and it travels faster than the low frequency wave. The wave distortion increases with depth and concentrates at the central area of the beam. In imaging, the first harmonic is generally used since it has less attenuation and higher order harmonic may exceed the band width. Hence, band width is set for first harmonic, low frequency echoes are filtered, and reflections and scattering from adjacent tissues are eliminated. Removal of low frequency eliminates artifacts that leads to an improved image contrast.

Tissue hormonic imaging is used in an echocardiographic study to have an improved endocardial border resolution and detect regional wall motion. MI is >1 and transmit frequency should be < 2. It is useful to estimate 3D left ventricular ejection fraction. It is combined with M-mode to access value thickness and mass. It is useful to detect *shunts in transthoracic* direction and *bubbles in the left atrium*. It has higher sensitivity in detecting shunts and MI should be < 0.3.

Harmonic imaging gives an improved lateral resolution, reduced side lobe artifacts, absence of multi-reverberation artifacts. It has increased SNR and improved resolution in large body habitus. It has definite role in obesity, hollow structures, and deep-seated major vessels. Native tissue harmonic imaging is useful in abdominal imaging. It starts with low frequency for easy penetration and receives good quality high frequency harmonics with less clutter. It can differentiate cysts from solid mass which is more hypoechoic. It can be used to evaluate an implant and guided biopsy.

Advantages of THI are improved contrast resolution, beneficial effects of artifacts, reduced noise in the near field, improved imaging of deeper tissue and improved lateral resolution and reduced section thickness. Disadvantages include decrease of axial resolution due to narrow bandwidth. Conventional ultrasound is still having major role in diffuse fatty liver like structures. Bioeffects of ultrasound remains the same and role TI and MI is still relevant here.

Contrast-enhanced Imaging

Contrast agents are used in ultrasound to get better image quality. It enhances echo signal from the blood. The presence of contrast increases reflections from tissues. They should have low toxicity and be easily eliminated from body. First generation contrast agent used bubbles encapsulated in an *albumin*. Second generation has inert *perfluorocarbon gas* core like *perfluoropropane* (C_3F_8) encapsulated in *phospholipid shell*. It is insoluble in blood, shell is more deformable, and has an increased circulating half-life. Various type of contrast media are:

- Air-filled microspheres encapsulated in thin shell of an albumin
- Low-solubility gas encapsulated in a lipid shell
- Perfluorocarbon nanoparticles
- Gold-bound colloidal microbubbles

Contrast media are based on *microbubbles or nanoparticles of <1 μm*. Microbubbles are encapsulated usually in shells to prevent dissolve of gas in the blood. Since, the bubble diameter is less than the ultrasound wavelength, they easily resonate at ultrasound frequency and at harmonic frequencies. It scatters ultrasound strongly since there is difference of acoustic impedance between gas and soft tissue. Their fundamental resonant frequency is 2–4 MHz which is convenient and it depends on bubble radius and shell's property.

Harmonic imaging can be done with contrast media like *air filled microspheres*. It differentiates echoes produced by microbubbles from the echoes produced by tissues. It exploits nonlinear scattering property of microbubble. The bubbles are smaller than (3–6 μm) the blood cells. It is injected intravenously before ultrasound imaging. When US beam travels nonlinearly and incident on microbubbles in tissue, the microbubble vibrates and strongly reflect or reemits higher order harmonic sound waves. Spherical symmetry of microbubbles gives strong resonance. The echo is unique and characteristics of its origin. Cancerous or diseased tissues have higher blood flow that look lighter in the image. Thus, harmonic frequency is generated on reflection from microbubble, known as *contrast harmonics*. Ultrasound can destroy bubbles at high frequency. This principle is used to study refill dynamics with lower ultrasound power, especially in *reperfusion imaging*.

Elastography

Elastography is a non-invasive technique which estimate tissue stiffness, referred to as **Young's modulus (E)**. Tissue stiffness is a biomarker of tissue pathology. Ultrasound elastography measures mechanical properties of tissue by studying the response of the tissue to an acoustic energy. Young's modulus is a constant which relates the applied force per unit area (stress) and resultant relative change in tissue dimension (strain). Various methods of elastography are *(1) quasi static or strain elastography,* and *(2) dynamic or shear wave elastography*.

Strain Elastography

In this, force is applied by application of probe pressure or through endogenous mechanical force, then:

$$E = \frac{\sigma}{\varepsilon}$$

where, σ refers to an external applied force per unit area or stress and ε refers to strain and E is the Youngs modulus. Here, the Young's modulus is not computed. Due to an applied force, tissue stiffness changes which is called *strain*. More stiffer lesions deform less and have low strain. Strain ratio is the ratio between strain in a region to strain in a reference region. Knowledge of applied force is not required in this technique therefore it is used commonly. Strain elastography (SE) is further divided into two, based on method of tissue excitation *(1) excitation by manual pressure,* and

(2) excitation from natural physiological motion. The former is more suitable for superficial tissues whereas the later is good for deep lying tissues. Tissue displacement is calculated by radio frequency (RF) data before and after an elastography procedure. *Strain ratio, elasticity score, fat to lesion strain ratio,* and *elastography- to- B-mode size ratio* is used as quantification.

Shear Wave Elastography

In shear wave elastography (SWE), a tissue shear wave is induced by an imaging device. It computes **Young's modulus** (E) by using the relation:

$$E = 3\,\rho\,c_s^2$$

where, ρ is tissue density, and c refers to speed of shear wave. Systems has facility to convert stiffness values, kPa into m/s. In SWE, mechanical shear wave travels slowly,1–10 m/s and wave propagation velocity depends on tissue stiffness (velocity of ultrasound in tissue is 1540 m/s). Vendor uses compressive acoustic waves which induce and track shear waves. Induced shear wave travels perpendicular to compressive wave, and involvement of tissue motion is monitored at multiple locations by the probe. Velocity can be estimated, in turn the Young's modulus. SWE can be used in variety of tissues for various applications. Various method of shear wave elastography are *(1) transient elastography, (TE), (2) point shear wave elastography, (3) 2-D shear wave elastography,* and *(4) supersonic shear wave elastography.*

In transient elastography, 3.5 MHz probe is used with a vibrator. Mechanical pulse is induced at the skin surface by the vibrator and a transient wave is generated which goes in longitudinal direction. The velocity of wave is measured and is converted into pressure unit, kilopascal (kPa) that reflects the tissue stiffness. In transient hepatic elastography, a *Fibroscan* device sent 50 MHz sound into the liver by a small transducer. The shear wave velocity is measured and converted into kPa. It is a gold standard to stage *fibrosis,* it is noninvasive, offer quantification, fast, and good reproducibility. Limitation includes application in obese and ascites patients.

Point shear wave elastography (pSWE) uses focused ultrasound which leads to tissue displacement. The resultant shear waves are monitored and speed of sheer wave is estimated. It is an algebraic function of tissue stiffness. This process is referred to as *acoustic radiation force impulse (ARFI)* imaging.

In 2-D shear wave elastography, an acoustic radiation force is used to displace tissue at multiple points. The resultant shear wave is easily detectable with high frame rate imaging. Real-time monitoring of shear wave propagation at multiple point is possible.

Supersonic shear wave elastography involves generation of multiple shear waves along same longitudinal axis leading to propagation of plane shear wave. Velocity of this plane at each point of image in real-time can be measured. It gives real-time image, goods reproducibility, quantification, and short acquisition time. Its limitations are expensive and complex software.

Elastography has application in liver, kidney, breast, prostate, thyroid, pancreas, and spleen.

BIBLIOGRAPHY

1. Allisy-Roberts PJ., Williams, J. Farr's Physics for Medical Imaging, 2nd edn. Elsevier, 1996.
2. Bushberg JT, Seibert JA, Leidholdt EM Jr., Boone JM. The Essential Physics of Medical Imaging, 3rd edn. Lippincott Williams and Wilkins; 2012.
3. Dance DR, Christofides S, Maidment ADA., McLean ID, Ng, KH. Diagnostic Radiology Physics: A Handbook for Teachers and Students, IAEA; 2014.
4. Grogan SP, Mount CA. Ultrasound Physics and Instrumentation, Madigan Army Medical Center, National library of Medicine; 2023.
5. Huda W, Slone RM. Review of Radiological Physics, 2nd edn. Lippincott Williams and Wilkins; 2003
6. Lang RM, Goldstein SA, et al. ASE's Comprehensive Echocardiography, 2nd edn. Elsevier; 2015.
7. Ozturk A, Grajo JR, Dhyani M, Anthony BW, Samir AE. Principle of Ultrasound Elastography. Abdom Radiol(NY); 2018; 43(4): 7773-785
8. Thayalan K. Basic Radiological Physics, 2nd edn. Jaypee Brothers Medical Publishers (P) Ltd, New Delhi; 2017.
9. Uppal T. Tissue Harmonic Imaging. Australas J Ultrasound Med; 2010;13(2): 29-31.

Magnetic Resonance Imaging

MRI: THE BASICS

Magnetic resonance imaging (MRI) was discovered by a chemist, **Paul C Lauterbur** (1970), Stony Brook, at New York. Initially, it was named as *zeugmatography* by a Greek word. He jointly used radiofrequency (RF) and spatial magnetic field gradients to generate images that display magnetic properties of the proton, reflecting clinically relevant information. Basically, it is a nuclear magnetic resonance (NMR) technique, applied for human imaging. *Nobel Prize* in medicine in physiology and medicine was awarded to **Paul C Lauterbur** and **Sir Peter Mansfield,** for above discovery (2003). Sir **Perter Mansfield** is a solid-state physicist who developed an echo planar MRI at the same time.

Nuclear magnetic resonance (NMR) is a spectroscopic study of magnetic properties of nucleus in an atom (1940). Protons and neutrons of the nucleus have magnetic field associated with their nuclear spin and charge distribution. *Resonance* is an energy coupling that causes an individual nucleus, when placed in a strong external magnetic field, to selectively absorb and later release an energy unique to those nuclei and their environment.

Special feature of MRI includes (1) high contrast sensitivity to soft tissue difference, (2) inherent safety to patient since it is not using an ionizing radiation, (3) to examine anatomic and physiologic properties of patient, and (4) imaging of blood flow without contrast. Limitations include (1) high equipment cost, (2) scan acquisition complexity, (3) long imaging time, (4) image artifacts, and (5) patient claustrophobia.

Magnetism

Magnetism is a fundamental property of matter, generated by moving charges. Every matter possesses *magnetic susceptibility*. Based on susceptibility, material may be divided into *(1) diamagnetic, (2) paramagnetic, and (3) ferromagnetic*. Diamagnetic materials have negative susceptibility, which will oppose the applied magnetic field, e.g., *Calcium, and water*. Paramagnetic material has slightly positive susceptibility, that will enhance the applied magnetic field, e.g., *Gadolinium contrast agent*. Ferromagnetic material has higher positive susceptibility, that will enhance an external field significantly, e.g., *Iron, Cobalt, and Nickel*.

Magnetic field has direction that depends on the sign and direction of charge motion. *Magnetic field strength (B) or magnetic flex density* is the number of magnetic lines of force per unit area and its SI unit is *tesla (T)*. Alternate unit is *Gauss (G)* and 10000 G =1T or 10 G =1mT.

Hydrogen Characteristics

Human body is abundant in water and consists of 80% Hydrogen which behaves like a tiny bar magnet. Atomic nuclei consists of protons and neutrons. They spin continuously like a top, their spin and charge distribution have magnetic field by *magnetic dipole*. Since, proton has positive charge and a spinning nuclei have *nuclear spin* and exhibits an *angular momentum and magnetic moment*.

Magnetic moment is a vector quantity that refers to strength and an orientation of a magnetic dipole. Neutron also has charge distribution though their net charge is zero. Its charge in-homogeneities on subnuclear scale gives magnetic field to the neutron. Neutron magnetic field is equal to that of proton but in an opposite direction. Hence, proton and neutron pairing occurs within the nucleus and cancels their net magnetic moment. Presence of unpaired spins only determines nuclear magnetic moment of the nucleus **(Fig. 13.1)**.

If the total number of protons (P) and neutrons (N) in the nucleus is even, the magnetic moment is zero. If N is even and P is odd or N is odd and P is even, the noninteger nuclear spin generates a magnetic moment. Hence, ^{1}H, ^{17}O, ^{23}N, and ^{31}P are the nuclei in the human body suitable for MR imaging. However, Hydrogen scores over other nuclei in terms of its isotopic abundance, magnetic moment, relative physiologic concentration, relative

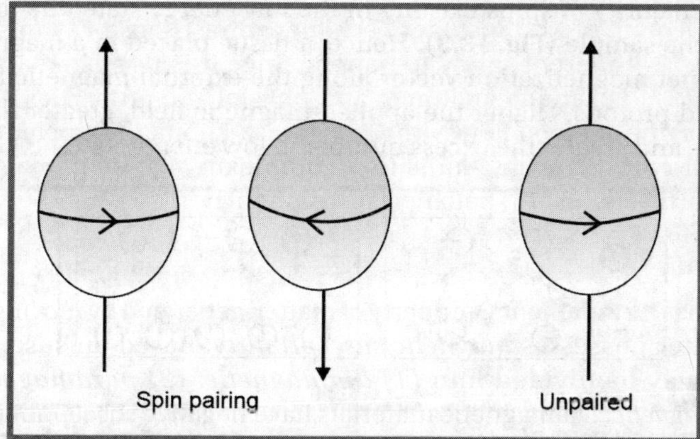

Fig. 13.1: Spin pairing in the nucleus, unpaired spins give the magnetic moment.

Table 13.1: Physical properties of various nuclei suitable for MR imaging.

Nucleus	% Isotopic abundance	Magnetic moment	Relative physiological concentration, %	Relative sensitivity	Gyromagnetic ratio, γ/2π, (MHz/T)
^{1}H	99.98	2.79	10	1	42.58
^{13}C	0.011	0.70	18	–	10.7
^{17}O	0.04	−1.89	65	9×10^{-6}	5.8
^{19}F	100	2.63	<0.01	3×10^{-8}	40.0
^{23}Na	100	2.22	0.1	1×10^{-4}	11.3
^{31}P	100	1.13	1.2	6×10^{-5}	17.2

(*Courtesy:* Jerrold T Bushberg et al, 2012)

sensitivity, and gyromagnetic ratio **(Table 13.1)**. Hence, Hydrogen nucleus forms the basis for most clinical MR imaging.

Proton and External Magnetic Field

Spinning proton often referred as a spin that behaves like a bar magnet. The magnetic moment of a single proton is very small, not detectable, whereas billions of nuclei give measurable MRI signal. Generally, spins are randomly distributed in the tissue, which are due to thermal energy agitation, results in no tissue magnetization. Hence its magnetization vector is zero. Under the influence of an external magnetic field (B_0), the spins get aligned and have an orderly orientation **(Figs. 13.2A and B)**. The protons have either *spin up or spin down orientation* under an external magnetic field and spin down has more energy, less population and spin up has more population and less energy.

Thus, spins are distributed in two energy states, namely, low energy level and high energy level. Spins having low energy align parallel to an external magnetic field and spin up wards (parallel). Spins having high energy oppose the external magnetic field and spin downwards (antiparallel). However, there is a slight majority of spins existing in the low energy state due to thermal energy of the sample **(Fig. 13.3)**. Hence, a tissue placed in a magnetic field has small net magnetization vector along the external magnetic field, due to unpaired protons. Higher the applied magnetic field, greater the energy separation, and greater the excess number in low energy state.

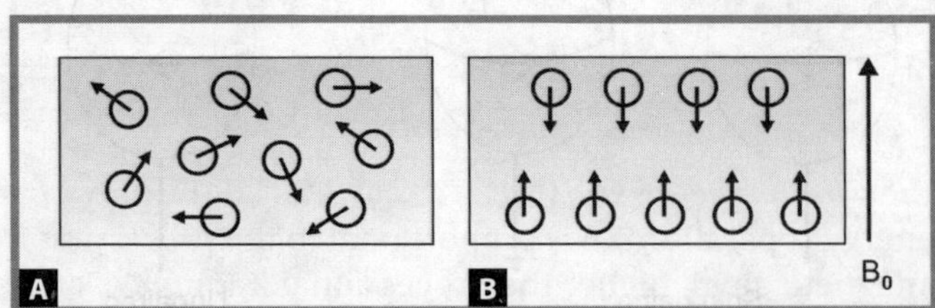

Figs. 13.2A and B: (A) Random orientation of spins and their magnetic moment; (B) Orderly orientation of spins in the presence of an external magnetic field.

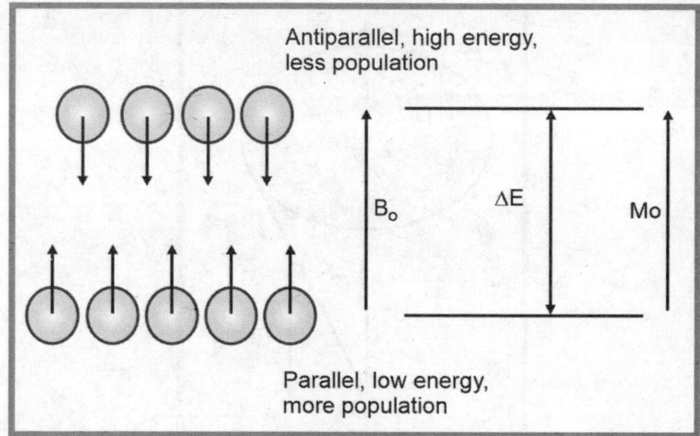

Fig. 13.3: Orderly orientation and energy separation of spins, under an external magnetic field.

Number of excess protons is about 3 spins per million at 1.0 T magnetic field strength. In a typical MRI voxel volume, there are about 10^{21} protons in one cm^3 of tissue resulting in 3×10^{15} more spins ($3 \times 10^{-6} \times 10^{21} = 3 \times 10^{15}$) in the low energy state, that gives an observable magnetic moment and MR signal. Generally, MRI signal is week and efforts are made to maximize the signal-to-noise ratio (SNR).

Precession

External magnetic field not only separates spin energy states it also exerts a force on the proton in a perpendicular direction so that proton undergoes *precession* **(Fig. 13.4).** Precession is an interaction between mass of spinning proton and mass of the Earth, that has gravitational field. Hence, proton not only spins but also precess in the presence of an external magnetic field. The direction of the spin axis tilts and rotates around an external magnetic field with fixed frequency. It is like a spinning top that wobbles due to force of gravity. This precession occurs at an *angular frequency* (ω_o) that is proportional to magnetic field strength (B_o). **Larmor equation** gives the relation between magnetic field strength and an angular frequency (ω_o):

$$\omega_o = \gamma \times B_o$$

$$2\pi f = \gamma \times B_o$$

$$\text{or } f = \frac{\gamma}{2\pi} \times B_o$$

where, γ is the *gyromagnetic ratio* (MHz/Tesla), and f is the *linear frequency* in MHz. The energy separation ΔE is proportional to the precession frequency. Larger the magnetic field, higher the processional frequency, and higher an energy separation. The gyromagnetic ratio is unique to each element its value for Hydrogen is 42.58 MHz @ 1 T as shown in **Table 13.1.**

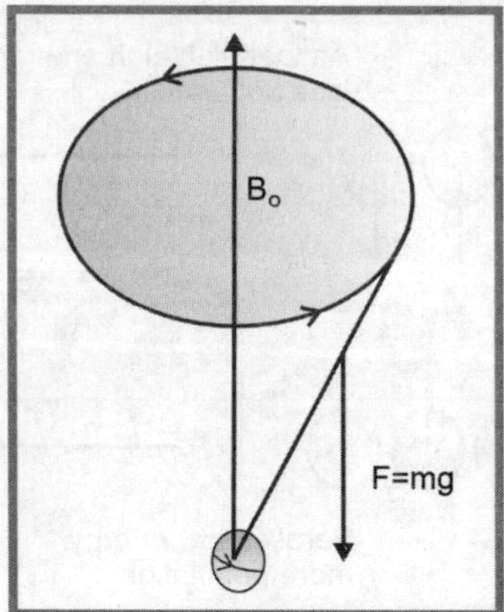

Fig. 13.4: Proton undergoes precession with Larmor frequency (B$_o$), under the influence of an external magnetic field.

Precession is a form of change in a magnetic field. Any change in magnetic field induces an electric current in a coil placed nearby. This induced current appears as signal, that can be detected, measured, and stored.

Magnetization Vector

Sum of all nuclear moments is called net magnetization (M) and it is a vector having magnitude and direction. It behaves like an individual nuclear moment behaves. The M has three components, namely, *(1) longitudinal (M$_Z$), (2) transverse (M$_{XY}$), and (3) equilibrium (M$_O$).*

The M$_Z$ is longitudinal magnetization, which is component of the net magnetization, parallel to an applied magnetic field, along Z-axis. It is invisible and not directly measurable, because it is so small relative to B$_o$. To observe M$_Z$, it should be rotated and separated from B$_o$. If it is rotated, it precess about the Z-axis with same frequency as that of the individual nuclear magnetic moments which precess at *Larmor frequency*. To rotate the Z-axis, another magnetic field is required from a perpendicular direction. Radiofrequency pulse (RF) offers this magnetic field along the X-axis. Rotation of any angle is possible by time/intensity RF pulse.

Rotation of M$_Z$ into the XY plane is called *Flipping*. M$_{XY}$ is transverse magnetization, component of net magnetization in XY plane and perpendicular to an applied magnetic field along the Y-axis **(Fig. 13.5)**. M$_X$ and M$_Y$ are collectively represented by M$_{XY}$ which can be measured.

Equilibrium is a condition in which M$_Z$ or M$_Y$ is maximum. When M$_Z$ is maximum the transverse magnetization is zero and the M$_Z$ is said to be equal to M$_O$. When M$_Y$ is maximum the longitudinal magnetization is zero and the M$_Y$ is said to be equal to M$_O$. It is determined by the excess number of protons that are in the low energy state. At equilibrium, the vector component of the spins is oriented randomly in the XY plane and cancels each other's magnetic moment hence transverse is zero.

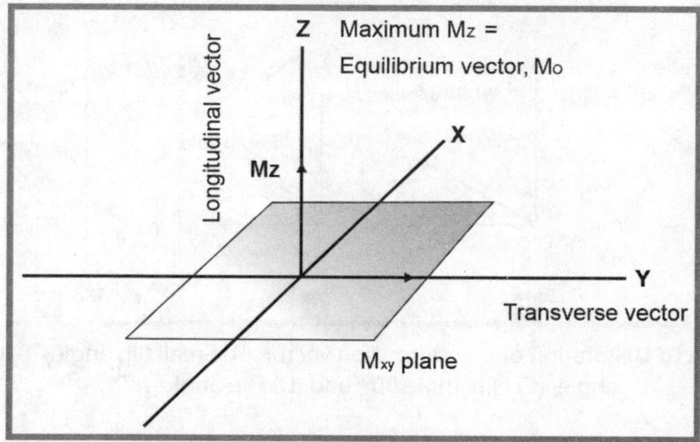

Fig. 13.5: Longitudinal magnetization vector and transverse magnetization vector of a proton.

Radiofrequency and Resonance

If an RF pulse having frequency equal to Larmor frequency of tissue (42.58 MHz) is applied perpendicular to the magnetic field, then it is absorbed by the proton nuclei and resonance occurs. Resonance is a condition at which two frequencies are equal so that an energy absorption take place. At resonance, RF does two things:

1. Converts spins from low energy—parallel direction to the high energy—antiparallel direction, and spins are said to be excited.
2. Resonance pulls the protons and make them in phase from out of phase, but they continue precession.

Two types of RF pulses are used in MRI, namely 180° RF pulse and 90° RF pulse. The 180° RF pulse has total energy, so that it gives required energy to each proton and tilt them by 180°. All the excess protons in the low energy move to higher energy state during resonance. Thus, application of 180° RF pulse set greater number of protons in spin down and a smaller number of protons in spin up position. This reverses the magnetic vector M_z to $-M_z$ direction. This is said to be *flip* towards -Z axis, refers to proton movement from one energy state to another.

A 90° RF pulse is one that has an energy equal to half of the total energy, which tilts half of an excess proton dipoles. Now the number of spins in lower and an upper energy are equal. Thus, application of 90° RF pulse will bring an equal number of protons in spin up and spin down position, they are still in phase and continue their precession. Now, the M_z is reduced to zero and the phase coherence of the dipole produces a transverse magnetism, M_{xy}, which is equal to tilting the M_z to 90°. Application of radiofrequency is generally referred as 180° RF pulse and 90° RF pulse in MRI physics.

Strength of the magnetic field determines the tissue resonant frequency. Frequency increases or decreases linearly with an increase or decrease of

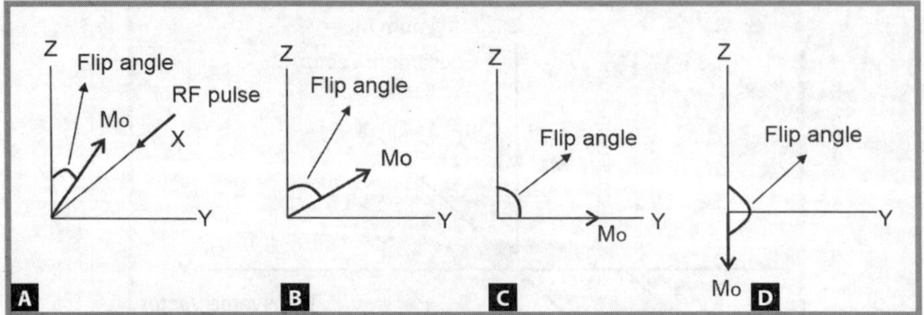

Figs. 13.6A to D: Rotation of magnetization vector: (A) Small flip angle; (B) Large flip angle; (C) Flip angle 90°; and (D) Flip angle 180°.

magnetic field strength. Typical magnetic field strength for imaging is 0.3 to 4.0 T range. In the case of Hydrogen, the protons precessional frequency is 21.29 MHz, 42.58 MHz, 63.87 MHz, and 127.74 MHz, for 0.5 T, 1.0 T, 1.5 T and 3 T magnetic field strength, respectively.

Flip Angle

Flip angle describes the rotation through which the longitudinal magnetization vector is displaced to generate a transverse magnetization during resonance **(Figs. 13.6A to D)**. Common flip angles are 90° and 180° (proportional to time). A 90° angle provides largest possible transverse magnetization for a RF pulse application of 10–100 msec duration. Such RF pulse is referred as 90° RF pulse. Fast MRI technique uses smaller flip angle (30°) and generates lesser signal in the transverse but offer greater transverse magnetization per exciting time. Instead of 90° flip angle, 45° flip angle needs only half the time, but sin 45° = 0.707, that means it gives 70.7% of the signal, which is quite sufficient for an image processing.

MRI Signal

As 90° RF pulse is withdrawn, the perturbed system goes back to its equilibrium state. Now the resonance is over, and the transverse vector continues to rotate in the M_{XY} plane and induces an AC voltage in the RF receiver coil. This is the MR signal called *free induction decay (FID)*. This signal is also a RF having voltage in the order of mV. The time constant that describes this process is referred to as *relaxation time*. MR signal is greater when 90° RF is switched OFF.

After the resonance, an individual spin go out of phase, and return to their original orientation. As a result, longitudinal vector, M_Z grows and transverse vector, M_{XY} decreases. Hence, the induced MR signal undergoes decay, but frequency remains the same **(Fig. 13.7A)**. This signal is not used MR imaging, but its mirror image is used which is obtained by further application of 180° RF pulse or changing the magnetic gradient field as in gradient echo **(Fig. 13.7B)**. The FID signal is a plot of signal intensity vs time. If a *Fourier transform (FT)* is performed on the FID, it is converted into a plot of signal

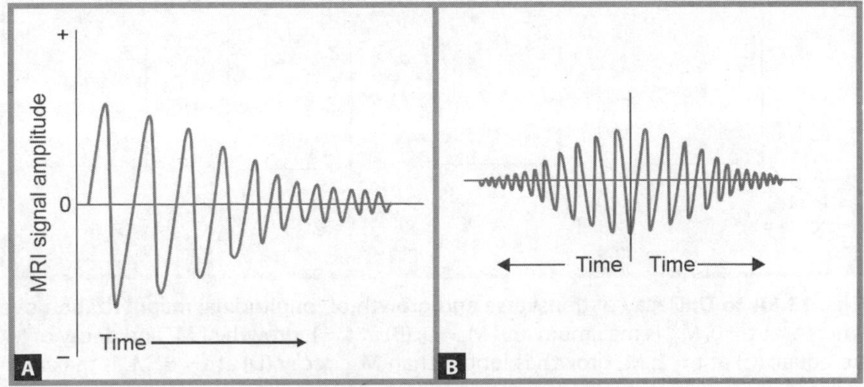

Figs. 13.7A and B: (A) MRI signal: Free induction decay (FID) after the withdrawal of 90° RF pulse; (B) Actual MR signal used for image processing.

intensity vs frequency or an inverse of time. Each peak in the plot indicates the characteristics of the tissue.

Thus, MR signal from an each voxel can be identified to produce their gray shades in the final image. The signal produced by the 90° pulse depends upon M_z immediately before the RF pulse is applied. The signal is proportional to (1) proton density (p/mm³), (2) gyromagnetic ratio of the nucleus, and (3) magnetic field strength (B_o).

Only mobile protons give MR signal and major part of the signal is due to water. Large molecule or bound molecule (bone) do not give MR signal. The air in sinuses does not have Hydrogen, hence appear black. The proton density is higher in fat than soft tissue, higher in grey matter than white matter.

RELAXATION TIMES

When the RF pulse is switched OFF, the magnetization vector returns to an equilibrium position and the spins undergo loss of phase coherence. As a result, transverse magnetization vector decays and longitudinal magnetization vector grows **(Figs. 13.8A to D)**. Hence, two signals are obtained, namely, T1, the longitudinal time constant and T2, the transverse time constant. This process is known as relaxation, above time constants are called T1 relaxation time and T2 relaxation time, respectively. Both are affected by tissue molecular structure and chemistry. Normal and abnormal tissue can alter T1 and T2 relaxation times. Pixel intensity is not a simple relation with T1 and T2 relaxation time. Bright or dark appearance of pixel is due to RF pulse sequence.

T1 Relaxation Time

After the resonance, the dipoles constantly jostled by thermal energy of the surrounding molecules. Protons loss energy to the molecular lattice and dipoles return to parallel to the Z axis one by one. Thus, M_z slowly reappears

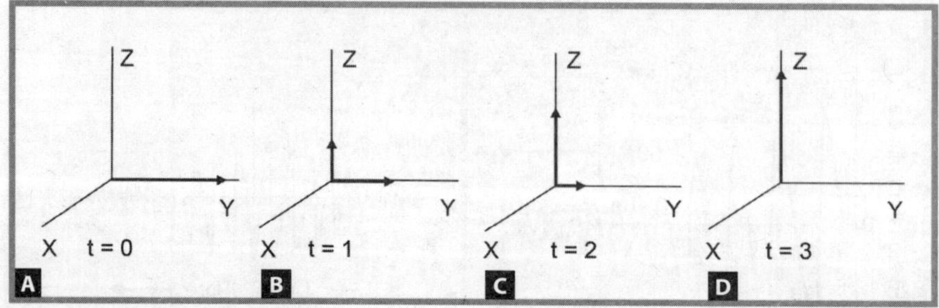

Figs. 13.8A to D: Decay of transverse and growth of longitudinal magnetization over time: (A) at t = 0, M_{XY} is maximum and $M_Z = 0$; (B) at t = 1, growth of M_Z and decay of M_{XY} are equal; (C) at t = 2, M_Z growth is longer than M_{XY} decay (D) at t = 3, M_Z is maximum and is M_{XY} zero.

after the resonance. Return of M_Z to equilibrium value of M_O, requires exchange of energy between spin and tissue lattice, which is called *spin-lattice relaxation*. It is an exponential event and measured by a time constant, T1. T1 is a time required to recover 63% of the longitudinal magnetization, M_Z **(Fig. 13.9)**.

Recovery of M_Z versus time is given by a relation:

$$M_z(t) = M_o(1 - e^{-\frac{t}{T1}})$$

where, M_Z is the longitudinal magnetization that recovers after a time *t*, with relaxation constant *T1*. When t = T1, then $1 - e^{-1} = 0.63$ and $M_Z = 0.63$ M_o. Full longitudinal recovery depends on T1 time constant. In time equal to 3 × T1 times after the 90° RF pulse, 95% of equilibrium magnetization is established. Return of 100% equilibrium magnetization takes about 5 × T1 times.

T1 time is not measured directly, it is measured for a specific tissue with sequence of 90°RF pulses. It is done by using various delay times (ΔT), between two 90° RF pulses. After an initial RF pulse, another RF pulse is applied with a delay time. The longitudinal magnetization recovered during the delay time is converted into transverse magnetization. The resulting peak amplitude is recorded, and the sequence is repeated with different delay times. The maximum amplitude of the resultant FID is plotted as a function of delay time. The plot fits to an exponential recovery function from which T1 is determined.

T1 Relaxation and Tissue

Protons lose energy to the surrounding molecules (*lattice*) and the rate of energy loss depends on tissue composition. T1 depends on dissipation of absorbed energy into the surrounding molecular lattice. Relaxation time varies substantially for different tissue structures and pathologies. Energy loss is more rapid in tissues that are more complex, and T1 is short, 100 msec. Energy loss is slower in simple molecule like water, and T1 is long,

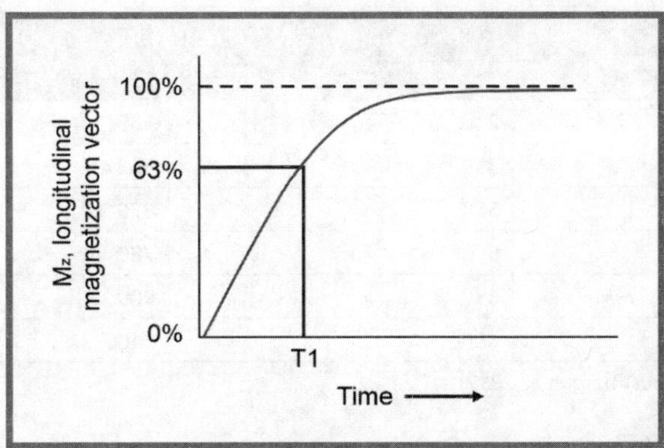

Fig. 13.9: Spin-lattice relaxation time. Longitudinal magnetization undergoes exponential growth with time. T1 corresponds to the time, that have 63% growth of M_z.

2500 msec. Energy transfer is efficient, if the precession frequency of an excited proton overlaps the vibration frequency of molecular lattice. Large and stationary molecules have low vibration frequencies, little overlap, results in longest T1.

Large molecules with slow moving and near the resonant frequency share more energy from protons. Fat absorbs energy effectively and have short T1. Moderately sized molecules like lipids, proteins and fats have more structured lattice. They have an increased overlap and most conducive for spin-lattice relaxation with short T1.

Small size, an aqueous molecule have wide vibration frequencies (low, medium, and high), have little overlap, result in long T1. They have little inertia and ineffective in removing energy from the protons. *Free water, urine, amniotic fluid, cerebrospinal fluid (CSF), and salt solutions* have long T1. Tissue having higher % of water always have long T1. Solid atoms and rigid macromolecules are relatively fixed, least effective in removing energy from protons. Thus, *compact bone, teeth, calculi,* and *metallic clips* have long T1, since they are solid and rigid. T1 relaxation increases with higher field strengths. However, this increases *Larmor frequency,* and reduces the spectral overlap, resulting in longer T1 time **(Table 13.2)**.

In general, the inability to release energy to the lattice results in relatively long T1 relaxation. Water has an extremely long T1, addition of water-soluble proteins (Hydrogen layer bound the molecule) slows the molecular motion. The vibrational frequency changes from high to low, increases an overlap and shortens the T1. Biologic tissue's T1 ranges from 0.1 to 1 second in soft tissues and 1–4 seconds for aqueous tissues (CSF) and water.

Contrast agent deceases T1 relaxation, by allowing free protons to become bound. This creates a Hydrogen layer, which is known as *spin lattice energy sink.* Even a small amount of *Gadolinium contrast* in pure water (*e.g., diethylenetriaminepentaacetic acid-DTPA*) has a dramatic effect on T1 shortening from second to millisecond.

Table 13.2: Variation of T1 time with magnetic field strength, for various biological tissues.

Tissue	T1, ms @ 0.5T	T1, ms @1.5T
Fat	210	260
Liver	350	500
Muscle	550	870
White matter	500	780
Gray matter	650	900
Cerebrospinal fluid	1800	2400

(*Courtesy:* Jerrold T Bushberg et al, 2012)

T2 Relaxation Time

Decay of transverse magnetization, M_{xy}, requires an exchange of energy between spin and spin. Energy transfer between nuclei creates loss of phase coherence, resulting an exponential decay of transverse magnetic vector based on tissue type. Most of the dephasing effect is due to field inhomogeneity of the magnet. Some spins rotate faster, and some rotate slower. The net strength of transverse magnetization decreases, and an induced FID signal also decreases. This is called *spin-spin relaxation*, which is an exponential decay. It is measured by a time constant T2. It is the time taken to reduce the transverse magnetization vector to 37% of the peak value **(Fig. 13.10)**. Only 5% remains after three time constant. T2 mechanisms are determined by the molecular structure of the sample and T2 is few tens of milliseconds. Transverse and equilibrium vector are given by the relation:

$$M_{xy}(t) = M_o e^{-\frac{t}{T2}}$$

where, M_{xy} is the transverse magnetic moment at time *t*. When t = 0, $M_o = M_{xy}$, the transverse magnetization. When t = T2, then $e^{-1} = 0.37$, and $M_{xy} = 0.37\, M_o$.

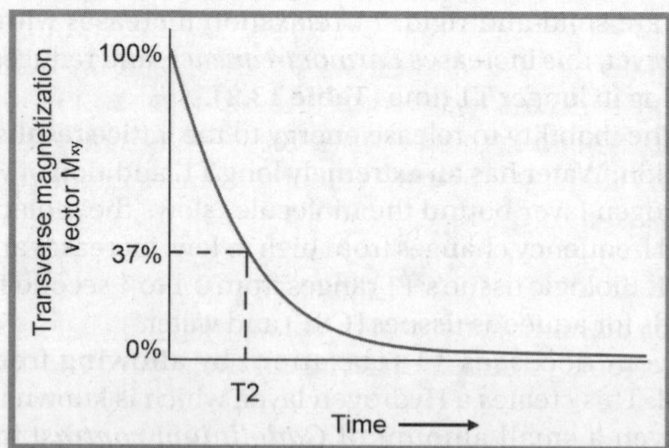

Fig. 13.10: Spin-spin relaxation: Transverse magnetization undergoes an exponential decay. T2 corresponds to time that have 37% of M_{XY}.

T2 Relaxation and Tissue

The causes of spin-spin relaxation are interaction of proton magnetic field with that of neighboring proton. During dephasing, spinning proton experiences a tiny magnetic field from a neighboring proton. Though the proton is affected slightly, the external magnetic field is affected little, and its field varies from place to place in microscopic scale. Hence, it influences the spinning proton some; rotates faster and some slower.

Nonsymmetric shape of humans and interfaces can distort magnetic fields resulting magnetic inhomogeneities. It is known as *intrinsic magnetic inhomogeneities*, which is based tissue character and patient related. *External magnetic inhomogeneities* due to imperfections in the magnet, which accelerate the dephasing process is a machine related one. T2 decay time constant addresses only an intrinsic inhomogeneity.

Variation of magnetic field is higher in solids and rigid molecules where atoms are relatively fixed. Large, nonmoving structures with stationary inhomogeneities dephase quickly and have a very short T2, e.g., *compact bone, teeth, calculi,* and *metallic clips.* Water bound to the surface of proteins or other large molecules, moves slowly, hence shorter the T2, e.g., *Hydrogen in fat.*

Small, mobile molecules in an amorphous liquid exhibit long T2, e.g., *free water.* Their fast and rapid molecular motion reduces or cancels intrinsic magnetic inhomogeneities of the spins. Lighter molecules are in rapid thermal motion, it smoothens the local field variation, hence long T2. Thus, *free water, urine, amniotic fluid, CSF, solutions of salt* have long T2. Greater the percent of free water in tissue, longer the T2, e.g., spleen > liver, renal medulla > cortex. As the molecular size increases, its motion is constrained, the intrinsic inhomogeneity is higher, and T2 decay is more rapid.

T2* Relaxation Time

Magnets has field inhomogeneity of few parts per million (PPM) or few μT @ 1 T external magnetic field. This causes extrinsic magnetic inhomogeneities that make loss of phase coherence more rapidly than from spin-spin interactions. If an intrinsic and extrinsic inhomogeneity is considered, the spin-spin decay constant T2 is reduced to T2* **(Fig. 13.11)**. Spins at higher field rotates faster than that in lower fields. Dephasing decreases transverse magnetization intensity. The MRI signal decreases exponentially with T2* decay rate constant:

$$\text{FID signal} = \frac{e^{-1}}{T2^*}$$

T2* depends on homogeneity of the main magnetic field and presence of susceptibility agents (contrast material) in the tissue. The T2* is related to T2 as follows:

$$\frac{1}{T2^*} = \frac{1}{T2} + \frac{1}{T2_{\text{inhomogeneity}}}$$

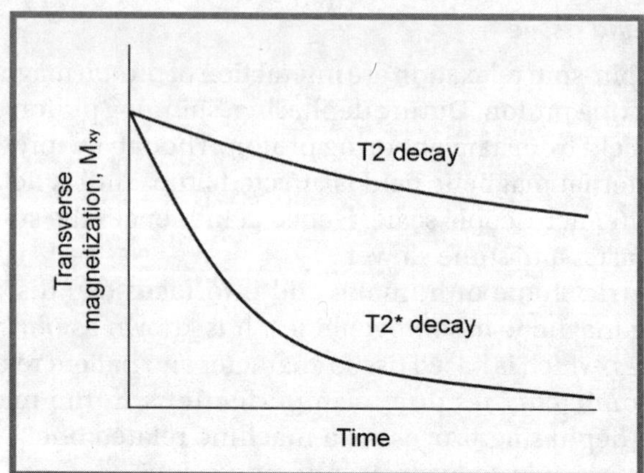

Fig. 13.11: T2 decays with intrinsic magnetic inhomogeneities and T2* decays with both intrinsic and an extrinsic magnetic inhomogeneities.

T2* is few msec and always <T2. Influence of T2* on dephasing can be eliminated by spin echo sequence imaging. Paramagnetic and ferromagnetic contrast agents disturb the local magnetic field homogeneity and shorten T2*.

Comparison of T1 and T2

T1 is significantly longer than T2, and T1 time of 500 msec has a corresponding T2 time of 50 msec (5–10 times shorter). Molecular motion, size and interactions influence T1 and T2. Small molecules exhibit long T1 and long T2 **(Fig. 13.12).** Intermediate sized molecules have short T1 and short T2. Large, slowly moving, or bound molecules have long T1 and short T2 times. Most tissues of interest in MRI involve intermediate and small sized molecules.

Hence, a long T1 usually refers to long T2, and short T1 infers to short T2. The differences in T1, T2 and T2* provides high contrast in MRI. Magnetic field

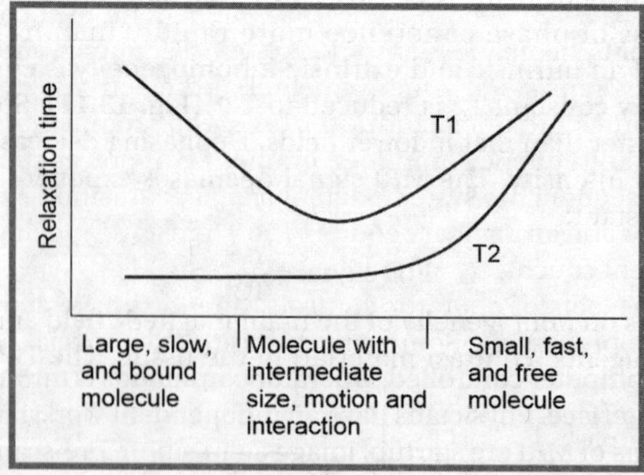

Fig. 13.12: Molecular size, motion, interaction affects the relaxation times T1 and T2.

Table 13.3: T1 and T2 time for various body tissues.

Tissue	T1, msec	T2, msec
Bone, teeth	Very long	Very short
Water	3000	3000
CSF	2000	150
Gray matter	800	100
White matter	650	90
Spleen	400	60
Kidney	550	60
Liver	400	40
Fat	250	80

(*Courtesy:* Allisy-Roberts PJ et al, 2008)

strength influences T1 (Larmor frequency) but has an insignificant impact on T2 decay. Abnormal tissue tends to have higher proton density (PD), T1 and T2, than normal tissue due to an increased water content or vascularity. T1 and T2 show greater variation than proton density. The range of T1 and T2 values are higher for brain, compared to CT, hence MRI has superior soft tissue contrast.

Agents that disturb the local magnetic field are either paramagnetic blood degradation products, or an element with an unpaired electron spin (*e.g., Gadolinium DTPA*) or any other ferromagnetic materials, cause significant decrease in T2*. The T1 and T2 values for various body tissue is given in **Table 13.3**.

MRI EQUIPMENT

Magnetic resonance imaging equipment is either closed bore or open bore or standing/sitting type MRI. Closed bore MRI gives high quality images, whereas open MRI offers more comfort to the patient. MRI contains three major components, namely (1) gantry, (2) system electronics, and (3) operator console. Gantry consists of a main magnet and electromagnetic devices. System electronics includes computer for signal acquisition, frequency synthesizer, radiofrequency amplifier, gradient coil power supply, magnet power supply, sequencing system, digital signal acquisition system, digital image processor and an ancillary equipment. There is no moving part in MRI except the patient couch.

There are two sets of operator controls, one for image acquisition and other for image processing. Some controls are under special function keys and other are computer controlled. Operator commands is through mouse or touch screen interface. Physicians have an independent workstation. Various control functions of MRI are startup, image acquisition, pre-scan calibration, image scanning, and image processing, display, and manipulation. For

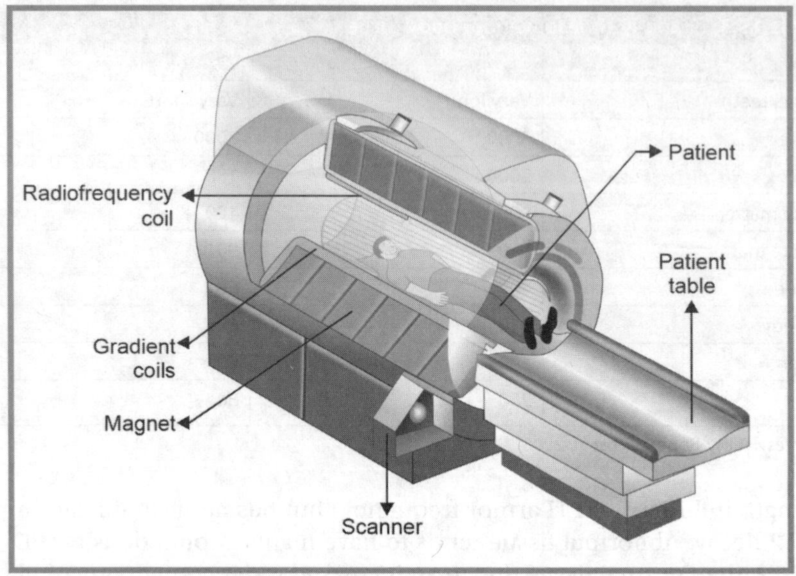

Fig. 13.13: Anatomy of a typical magnetic resonance imaging equipment.

better understanding, its components are discussed as follows: (1) magnet, (2) shim coil, (3) gradient coils, (4) radiofrequency coils, and (5) patient table **(Fig. 13.13).**

Magnet

Magnet is the heart of MR system, and it requires a strong, stable magnet with spatially uniform magnet field. Magnetic fields are measured in tesla (T), after the scientist **Nikola Tesla**, and 1 T=10,000 gauss (G). Earth has its magnetic field which is about 50 µT. Clinical MRI requires high homogeneity of the order of few parts per million (ppm). A homogeneity of ±5 ppm is a variation of ±7.5µT throughout an imaging volume of 1.5 T magnet. The required homogeneity over a spherical volume of 20 cm is ±1 ppm in a super conducting magnet.

Shim coils address this issue and work with direct current and make the main magnetic field an uniform throughout the imaging volume. The patient is placed inside core of magnet, surrounded by set of coils connected to a RF generator. This coil is known as *body coil* which can transmit and receive RF signal. Magnet is also surrounded by three *gradient coils* to offer field gradients. Type of magnet includes *(1) permanent magnet, (2) resistive electromagnet (3) superconducting magnet.* The fringe fields are negligible in permanent magnet, and greater in resistive and superconducting magnets.

Permanent Magnet

Permanent magnet consists of brick size ferromagnetic ceramic materials as array of 2–5 layers with 1 m wide **(Fig. 13.14).** Two arrays are positioned

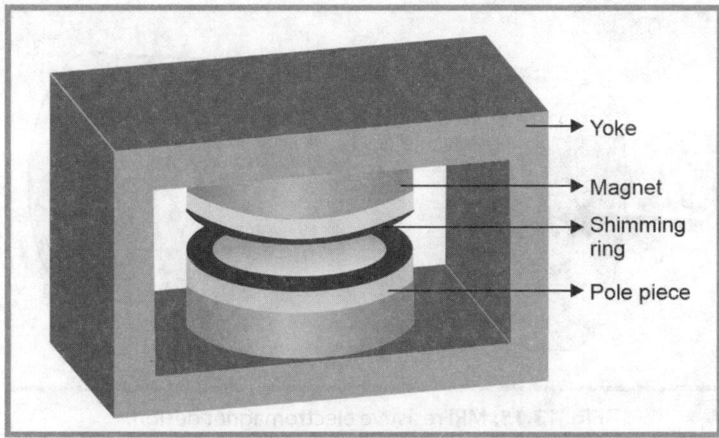

Fig. 13.14: Permanent magnet small open MRI scanner.
(*Courtesy:* Yiyuan Cheng et al, 2011)

opposite to each other with 0.5 m/1.0 m gap. Two Iron slaps are positioned on the magnet to form *pole pieces.* Screws or mechanical shimming is provided to vary the homogeneity. They are attached to a heavy *Iron yoke* which provides return paths for the magnetic lines. It provides stability, contains fringe fields and intensifies (B_o) in an imaging aperture. There are two shim coils in the permanent magnet. An open type of MRI system can go up to 0.3 T, suitable for children, aged, and an interventional work. It will facilitate large patients or claustrophobia or anxious patients. Off-axis body parts can be positioned at the center of the FOV. The weight of the magnet is about 90 ton with vertical field system. Though they find limited application, still the choice for extremity imaging.

Advantages of permanent magnets are insignificant fringe field, low electric power consumption, and absence of cooling system. Disadvantages include poor magnetic field homogeneity, limited field strength, and reduced spatial and contrast resolution.

Resistive Electromagnet

Current flowing in a coil will induce magnetic field is the principle used in an electromagnet. Coil also resists the flow of current, hence the name resistive electromagnet. Most common is the *solenoid resistive electromagnet with Aluminum (Al)* trips. It is wound spirally around a tube with several thousand layers and four coils are used **(Fig. 13.15)**. Though *Copper* is superior in terms of conductivity, Al is cheaper. It can offer magnetic field strength of 0.3 T with 0.5 mT fringe field of at 2 m. It weighs about 4 ton and requires 80 kW electric power consumption.

Advantages are less expensive at startup, and magnetic field is easily turned OFF. This eliminates hazards of ferromagnetic projectiles during nonimaging time. However, the running cost is more since it consumes high electric power

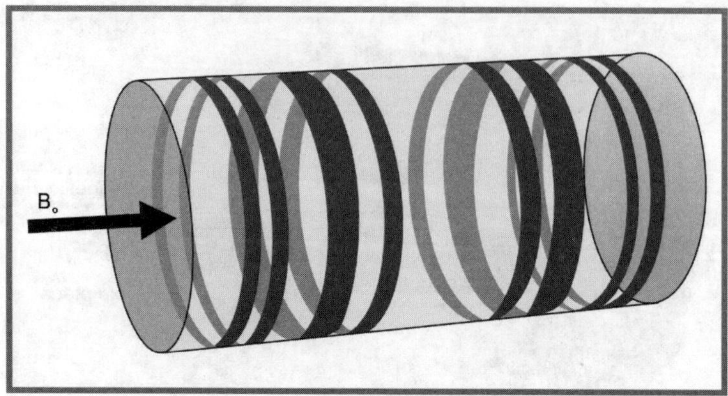

Fig. 13.15: MRI resistive electromagnet design.

and need water cooling and heat exchanger for the magnet. The siting cost of a resistive electromagnet MRI is cheaper than the super conducting magnet MRI.

Superconducting Electromagnet

To produce best clinical images high magnetic field strength is required. Superconducting electromagnet offers such high magnetic fields greater than the resistive electromagnets. Superconductivity is the property of certain materials to conduct electricity without resistance. Such material attains superconductivity at temperature below a *critical temperature*. Once an electric current begin to flows in the superconductor, it will flow indefinitely.

Superconductor is made by a *Niobium-Titanium (NbTi) wire in a Copper matrix,* and its critical temperature is 9 K. It is in the form of a solenoid in which direct current flows. *Liquid Helium (cryogen)* vaporizes easily at 4 K(–269°C) and maintains the NbTi wire below its critical temperature. *Liquid Nitrogen* which vaporizes at 77 K is used to insulate liquid Helium. Typical design is a six-coil superconducting magnet. The container housing the super conducting wire and cryogens is called *cryostat.* Superconducting magnet is basically an air core cylinder of 1 m diameter and 2–3 m depth with one side closed **(Fig. 13.16)**. Magnet weighs about 10 ton, needs 20 kW electric power for operation and require cooling.

Superconducting magnet has fringe fields and 0.5 mT fringe field is at 10 m. Fringe fields can be reduced by *passive or active shielding*. Passive shielding is a placement of ferromagnetic material in the walls of the MRI room. It is much heavy and costly and rarely used. Active shielding provides second set of superconducting coils kept outside the primary coil but within the cryostat. Since, it carries current in an opposite direction and it opposes the primary current and reduces fringe fields. It is highly expensive but shorten the length of magnet and commonly used. Generally, two active-shielded coils are used in superconducting magnet to reduce fringe fields.

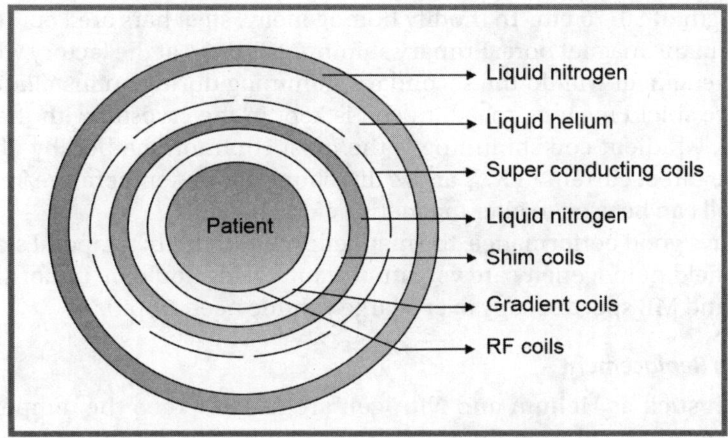

Fig. 13.16: Cross-sectional view of MR gantry design.

If temperature raises, magnet loses superconductivity, and the stored energy is converted into heat. Such sudden raise in temperature in magnetic coil windings is called *quenching*. To shut down the system, the stored electromagnetic energy in the coil must be removed carefully. Quenching introduces resistivity in the coils which reduces the magnetic field in coil windings and produces heat. This heat rapidly converts the liquid Helium into gaseous form which has some bioeffects.

Modern magnet design has an open architecture, reduces Helium boil-off and eliminate liquid Nitrogen component. *Cryocooler* is used to cool the radiation shields of the main magnet and to recondense the Helium present in the magnet. It reduces the consumption of Helium by a factor 5 and advanced cryostat and actively shield magnet can avoid helium refill for up to 3 years.

Advantages of superconducting magnet are large current can be used without overheating. It provides horizontal fields from 0.5 T to 4.0 T with high field homogeneity of 0.1–5 ppm over a 40 cm FOV. High magnetic field strength is useful for MR spectroscopy. Since, it gives high SNR, the spatial and contrast resolution is high with shorter scan time. Magnetic field is better homogenized or shimmed to achieve 1 ppm in a 40 cm FOV.

Disadvantages of superconducting magnet include high initial capital and sitting cost, cryogen cost, difficulty in turning OFF the magnetic field, extensive fringe field, and uncontrolled quenching due to boiling of helium.

Shim Coil

Shimming is a process of making an external magnetic field uniform throughout the volume. Hence, *shim coil* is provided which supcrimpose magnetic field and provides small differences on the main field to improve field uniformity. Imaging volume in MRI is a cylindrical diameter of 60 cm and length of 50–70 cm. To modify homogeneity, steel bars are kept in trays located in the magnet bore. Primary shimming is done at the factory whereas the site engineer will do the secondary shimming during an installation. In an active shield magnet, the shim coil is kept in the cryostat with the main magnet. Gradient coil shimming is the most common method by offset of baseline direct current in X, Y and Z directions. Room temperature/resistive shim coil can be used to alter magnetic field in patients.

To have good performance, the magnetic field strength, temporal stability, and its field homogeneity are very important. Field should be uniform up to 5 ppm and MR spectroscopy over a large volume need 1 ppm.

Cryogen Replacement

Cryogen such as Helium and Nitrogen are used to keep the temperature below certain level to maintains superconductivity in MRI. It levels will decrease due heat and boiling and requires regular replacement. Liquid Nitrogen is stable and vaporizes at 77 K, whereas Helium is unstable and vaporizes at 4.2 K. Helium is obtained from natural gas and separated by freezing out the low volatile components and liquefying Helium. Due to boil-off the Helium levels reduced to 1–2% and Nitrogen levels up to 5–7% per day in a stationary magnet. It may be higher for a mobile magnet. Critical cryogen level is 50% of the total volume below which quench occurs.

Certain magnets are designed as Nitrogen free, and only Helium is used. The boil-off Helium is captured, condensed to liquid, and reused, which require less frequent replacement. Cryogenic gases are supplied to MRI in vessels called *Dewars*. MRI user must have contract for cryogen supply and refilling with vendors. Cryogen is filled in dewars and transported to the hospital site. Only specially trained personnel can handle Dewars, and cryogen refill as it involves skin hazards **(Fig. 13.17).** He should wear safety glasses for eye production and heavy gloves for hand protection. All connecting tubes are precooled before refilling to avoid thermal effects.

Nitrogen is replaced regularly, and Helium needs annual replacement. They easily vaporize during filling the cryostat and transport. Cryogens cannot be stored in dewars and kept for several days.

Gradient Coils

Gradient coils are used to offer varying magnetic field in X, Y and Z directions. Their magnetic field is measured in mT/meter. It differentiates positions of the signal in a 3D patient and localizes MRI signal which is important for computing images. These field gradients are obtained by superimposing the magnetic fields of one or more coils. In true sense, they are not coils, but they are broad, thick, *Copper conducting bands* of 10 mm wide and 4 mm thick. They are embedded in a strong *epoxy resin casing* to prevent movement. Since, low resistance coils are designed, production of heat is minimal, occasionally water cooling is used.

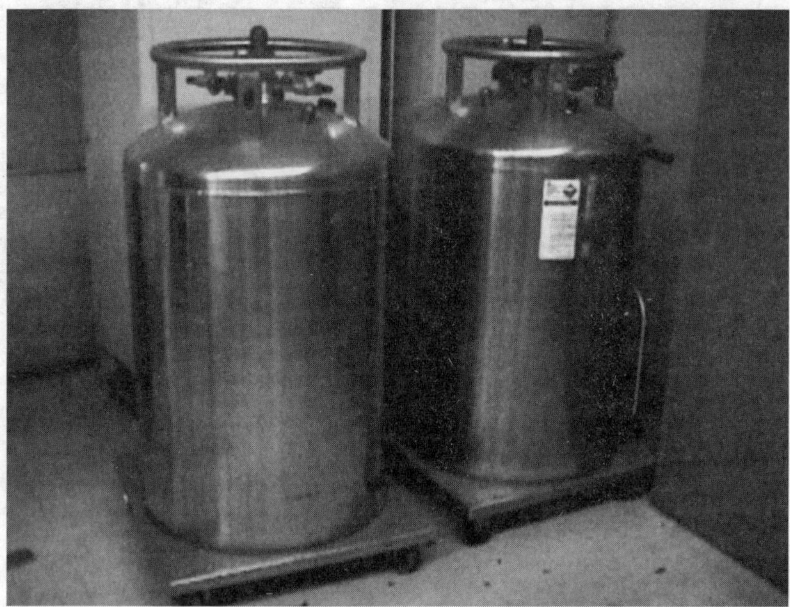

Fig. 13.17: Cryogen filled dewars.

Peak amplitude of the gradient field determines the steepness of the gradient magnetic field strength, and it varies from 1 to 60 mT/m. *Slew rate* is the time required to achieve the peak field amplitude. Shorter slow rate is always better, and it ranges from 5 to 250 mT/m/msec. High slew rate coils induce an eddy current in other coils or metals nearby. It may impair scan performance and create artifacts hence, shielded gradient coils are required. They are kept near the magnetic bore, produce an eddy current that oppose an eddy current produced by gradient coils. Self-shielding gradient coils offer large imaging volume. They can provide magnetic field up to 40 mT/m. Gradient coils are switched ON and OFF rapidly within 500 μs, which makes *thump, thump, thump* noise which is heard by the patient.

Three sets of gradients coils carrying direct current are used along Z, Y and X-axis and they are named as *slice selection gradient (SSG), phase encoding gradient (PEG)* and *frequency encoding gradient (FEG)*. They are orthogonal to each other and offer gradient field in any direction. All coils are connected to an amplifier, which control the rise time and maximum value of the gradient.

Slice gradient is an axial gradient in Z direction produced by *Helmholtz coils*. Gradient produced in X and Y direction are called *saddle coils*. If independently energized, each gradient produces a linearly variable magnetic field across FOV. Gradient polarity reversal is also possible. Usually, gradients are sequenced in a specific order and sometimes gradients overlap partially or completely. A positive gradient field increases an external magnetic field (B_0), and negative gradient field reduces B_0 **(Fig. 13.18).**

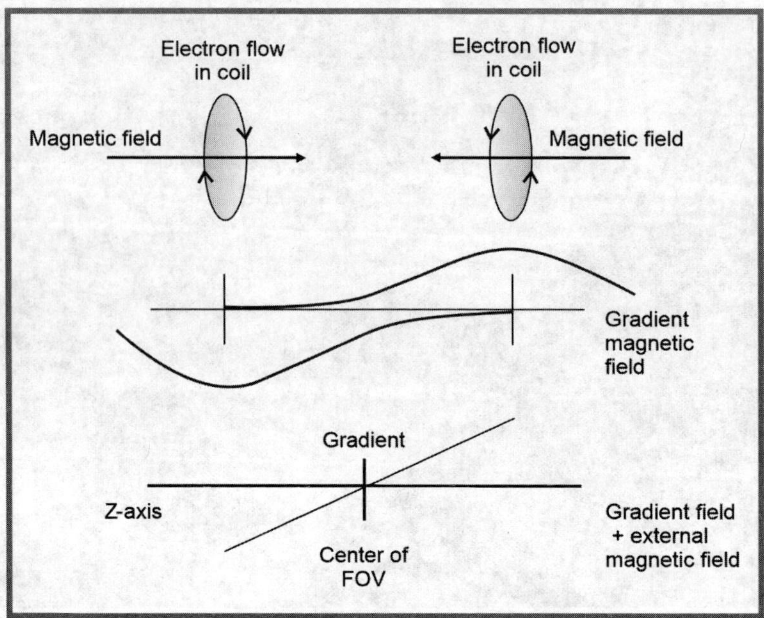

Fig. 13.18: A pair of coil in the Z-axis is energized with DC current to produce gradient magnetic field.

Slice Selection Gradient

Z-gradient is a pair of circular coils wound on a cylinder, withstand DC current up to 20 A and offer a gradient field of 10–40 mT/m. This produces a controlled magnetic field gradient along Z-axis (cranial-caudal). Change of magnetic field permits selection of slice, hence it is referred as slice *selection gradient (SSG)*. This coil is superior then other coils because all segment gives gradient field, and gradient per ampere-turn is greater.

MR image is made up of series of parallel slices, e.g., transverse slices, which are imaged in turn. Along with 90° pulse, the pair of Z coil is energized with a DC supply **(Fig. 13.19).** The total magnetic field decreases at the head side and increases at the toe side, remains the same at an isocenter. It varies from head to toe with constant increment of mT per meter. Protons at the head side precess slowly, and are faster at the toe side, and have moderate precession at the middle (*null point*) **(Fig. 13.20).** The protons in the selected slice precess with narrow range of frequency.

A narrow band RF pulse is applied to the whole volume and only protons in the thinner slice are excited. The spins along the gradient that have a precessional frequency equal to RF will absorb energy due to resonance. The magnetic vectors of the above spins will tip and gives MR signal.

Slice thickness depends on (1) RF bandwidth, and (2) gradient strength across FOV. Slice thickness is reduced either by increasing the gradient magnetic field or decreasing the RF band width. Thinner slice gives better

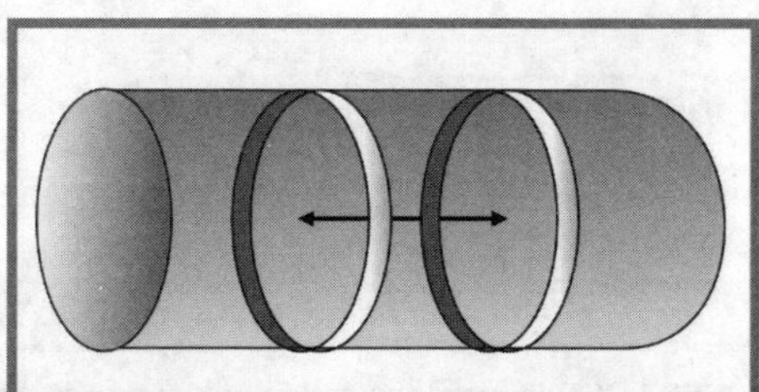

Fig. 13.19: Z-axis gradient coil for slice selection.

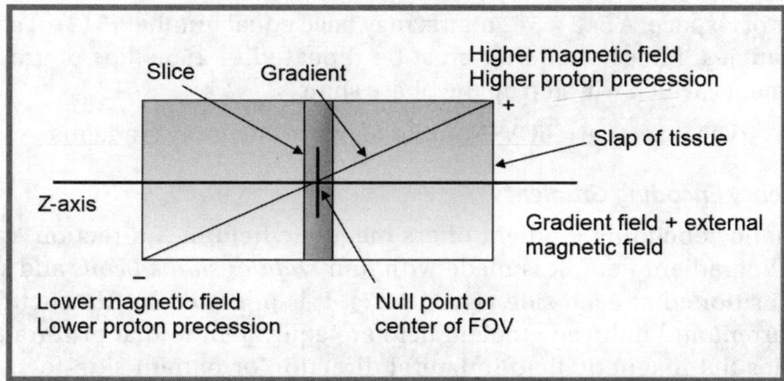

Fig. 13.20: Gradient magnetic field makes the proton faster at the toe side and slower at the head side and moderate precession at the middle (null point).

anatomical detail with lesser partial volume effect, but takes longer time and typical slice thickness range is 2–10 mm. The RF may excite tissues on either side of the selected slice, since it has higher or lower frequency about the band width and generate signal. This is called *cross talk,* which affects an image slice. Hence, a gap equal to 10% of slice thickness should be kept in between slices. This is not required in an interleaved scanning.

Phase Encoding Gradient

Phase encoding gradient offer magnetic gradient field in Y-axis, in an anterior-posterior direction. It is like a X-gradient and does slice selection in the *coronal plane.* Gradient X and Y precisely localize the voxel's origin of MRI signal. It is operated with a direct current.

Protons are excited initially by 90° pulse, which are in phase coherence. Now, the Y gradient coil is switched ON for few msec **(Fig. 13.21)**. Spins in the upper (front) voxel precess slowly, and that are at the bottom (back) precess faster. Thus, spins in an upper voxel lags that of bottom voxel. Even if the gradient pulse is over, all precess at the same rate, but phase differences exist, depending on the position. Thus, MR signal has phase variation from different pixel of tissue, in the selected slice.

Steep gradient gives an even distribution of spins, and the total signal is zero. No gradient means, all spins are in phase, which gives maximum

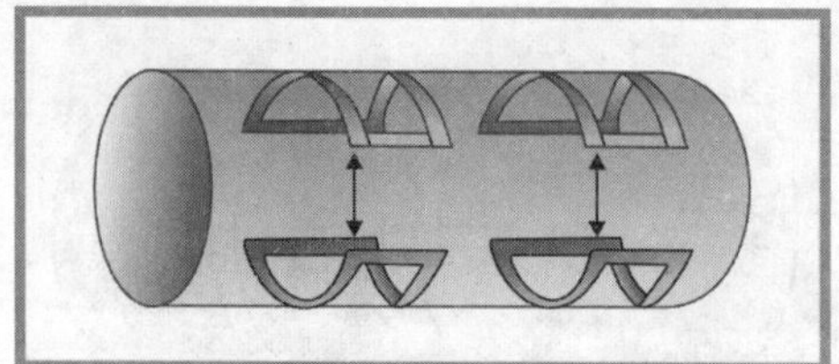

Fig. 13.21: Y-axis gradient coil for phase encoding.

signal. This is known as *zero spatial frequency*, and data are stored at the center of k-space. A 512 × 512 matrix may have equal number (512) of spatial frequencies. Phase encoding must be repeated in 256 steps of gradient increments, which will step up the phase shifts:

The pixel size = FOV/Number of phase encoding gradients

Frequency Encoding Gradient

Frequency encoding gradient offers magnetic field in X direction, called *readout* gradient field. It is made with four *saddles shaped coils* and set of two positioned at each side **(Fig. 13.22)**. It is operated by direct current, the current and induced gradient field are equivalent to that of Z gradient. It varies the magnetic field in lateral direction or patient side-to-side. It provides spatial localization in X-axis and useful to select slices in sagittal images.

When phase encoding gradient is applied, the X-gradient coil is energized and applied in the orthogonal direction. Protons in a vertical column experience same magnetic field and emit MR signal of same frequency. Spins in the left side precess slowly, and that in right precess faster, resulting in a frequency gradient from left to right. The MR signal from a given slice consists of range of RF frequencies, on either side of the applied pulse.

Radiofrequency Coils

MRI machine has radiofrequency (RF) coils which can carry an alternate current of 10–20 MHz. Coils that only send RF waves are called *transmitter coils*, whereas that transmit and receive RF waves are called *transmit/receive coils or body coils*. Similarly coils that receive only RF wave is called *receiver coils which* provide larger signal, lesser noise, and improve SNR.

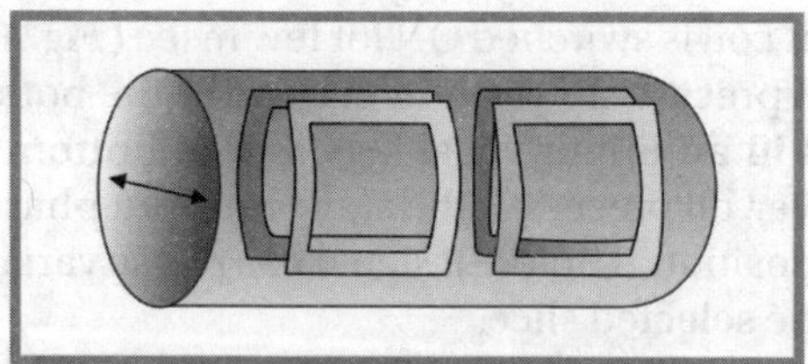

Fig. 13.22: X-axis gradient coil for frequency encoding.

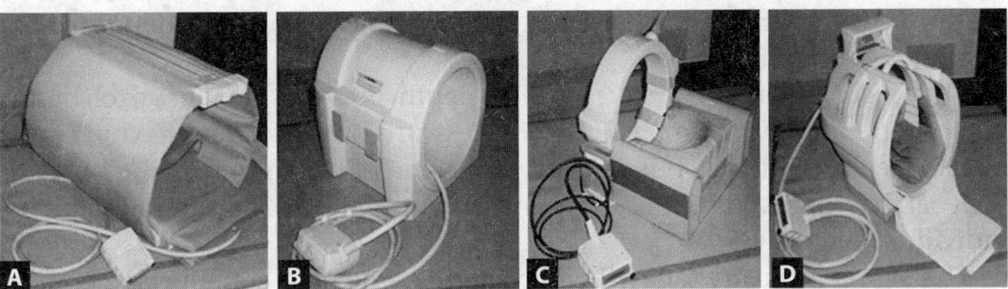

Figs. 13.23A to D: (A) Body coil; (B) Knee coil; (C) Head and shoulder coil; (D) Head coil.

RF is a part of an electromagnetic radiation and produces magnetic field perpendicular to the main magnetic field. The signal comes from the *frequency synthesizer* to the RF probe. This frequency band is amplified and feed the RF energy to the coil. Coil design is either *saddle or quadrature* type. In saddle design, the intensity of RF emission and sensitivity of received signal are uniform. Quadrature coils receive signal from multiple directions that improves SNR. It can be constructed more homogeneously for RF transmission.

RF probe is also be classified as (1) homogeneous volume coils, and (2) inhomogeneous coils. Homogeneous coils transmit RF and receive MR signal. It includes *body coils* and *head*/extremity *RF coils*. Inhomogeneous coils are only-receive coils and does not transmit RF energy. Generally, MRI signal has both signal and noise. Signal comes from the slice that is being excited and noise comes from all the tissues within the sensitive volume. All the coils, except the body coil improves SNR by reducing noise. Based on clinical application, RF coils are divided into *(1) body coils, (2) head/extremity coils, (3) surface coils, and (4) phased array and matrix coils* (**Figs. 13.23A to D**).

Body Coils

Body coil is a standard one permanently fixed in the gantry. It transmits RF and receive MR signal, e.g., chest and abdomen imaging. It is a robust coil that can be used to image any part of a body. It is kept inside the gradient coils and appear as wound on a patient or an anatomy. It is also possible design coils for specific imaging which gives better SNR.

Head/Extremity Coils

Head coil is used for brain imaging, and it transmits and receives the signal. A quadrature *birdcage head coil* is attached to a neck coil and thoracic/lumber surface spine coil to get complete spine. An extremity coil is used to image lower extremity with high resolution.

Surface Coils

Surface coils are basically only-receive coils, and kept closer to an imaging site, e.g., *lumbar spine, knee, and orbit*. They are usually placed on patient's the surface of an anatomical interest. It can be encased in a rubber or plastic to give more stability.

They receive signals effectively from a depth, provides smaller voxel, better resolution, but have smaller FOV with less uniformity. They maximize the SNR of week FID signals but restricts the region of the volume being imaged. SNR can be improved by incorporating *quadrature* coils. It is designed for an individual anatomy.

The signal intensity falls off with distance from the coil. Surface coils is available in many shapes and sizes or individually fabricated. It includes extremity, joints, orbits, breast, and prostate. The design can be either flat or circular of varying diameter. Generally, body coil transmits RF energy and surface coil receives the MR signal. The body coil is decoupled while the signal is received by the surface coil. In such cases, the surface coil is kept inside the body/head coil and insulated from the skin. Lack of decoupling may damage surface coil and may burn the patient.

Advantages of surface coils include better SNR and an improved resolution. It is due to the coil is closer to the body part and reduced noise. Disadvantages include limited FOV and take longer time for coil placement.

Phased Array and Matrix Coils

One of the limitations of surface coils is reduced FOV, hence phased array or multi-coils are designed to overcome this. In phased array, several surface coils are coupled to produce single large image. Each coil is having its own receiver channels for processing, and they receive signal individually and then combine the signal. This makes the signal with lesser noise, high SNR with large FOV. All the individual signals are combined to have the composite signal. The composite signal addresses the spatial resolution and SNR. For example, to image the thoracic and lumbar spine, four surface coils of each having 10 cm FOV are used, and the composite signal comes from 40 cm FOV. Advantages of phased array coils include an uniform image over large volume, either linear or quadrature concept can be used, leads to an increased SNR, and enable parallel imaging.

Transmit phased array coils produce current on each element and have special amplifiers. The control of an amplitude and phase make them independent. It employs reduced pulse duration, with higher SNR, an improved field homogeneity, reduced specific absorption rate and it is useful in parallel MRI (SENSE).

Matrix coils are large phased array coils that contains 32 or more individual coils, and it can be used for general purpose. It has an electronic switching which can be interfaced to MRI electronics. It finds application in parallel MR imaging.

Patient Couch

MRI patient table is made with *stainless-steel and Carbon fiber* tabletop which support and position patients up to 150 kg weight. The lift speed and translation speed are 1 cm/sec and 10 cm/sec, respectively. Table should move to the imaging position with a positional accuracy of ±1 mm. Two or three-room lasers for patient positioning which intersect at an isocenter. It should accept patients from the ground floor and raise the patient up to an isocenter level. The couch must move in coordination with an imaging protocol with precision. Tabletop rotates 180° and offers Trendelenburg, reverse Trendelenburg, adjustable elevation, left/right lateral tilt, and optional reset function. A handheld remote-equipped with a safety lock to prevent an unintentional table movement. Couch position is visually displaced with the help of an electronic counter.

MRI patient transport table is used for shifting patient from the ward to MRI room. These tables are made with much slight magnetic *stainless-steel material.*

Signal Localization

Production of image involves: (1) collection and analysis of signal in terms of an amplitude, frequency, and phase, and (2) reconstruction of an image by using *Fourier transform algorithm.* For signal localization, gradient magnetic field is added onto an external magnetic field. This magnetic field strength is unique to each location that corresponds to specific *Larmor frequency.* The composite signal emitted by a whole slice comprise of spectrum of phases and frequencies. Signal amplitude depends on spin density, T1, and T2 parameters. Computer is used to analyze the signal for frequency and phase. Frequency analysis helps to identify an origin of each detected signal. Frequency analysis is performed by either 2-D or 3-D *Fourier transform algorithm.* Fourier transform is a mathematical process which converts a signal of amplitude vs distance, into a signal of amplitude vs frequency. This step makes the signal easy to store and digitize further.

Sinc Pulse, and K-space

Tissue slice is considered as rectangular shape. To excite a rectangular slice, RF pulse requires synthesis of a specialized waveform called *sinc pulse.* Its width determines the output frequency bandwidth (BW). A narrow sinc pulse and high frequency produce a wide BW. A broad and low frequency sinc pulse gives narrow BW, resulting in an increased SNR. Narrow BW is not always good, it results in *chemical shift artifact* and other undesirable image characteristics. There is trade-off in image quality hence, an optimal RF bandwidth and gradient field strength is required.

The k-space is a spatial frequency domain in computer, used to store an image. Each MR signal is Fourier transformed and fill a single line in k-space. K-space stores signal spatial frequencies and their origin. Spatial frequency corresponds to an image brightness. The number of lines filled in K-space is equal to the number of encodings in the sequence. High-amplitude phase encoding gradients fill the periphery of k-space (steeper gradient data), that contributes spatial resolution. Low-amplitude phase encoding gradients fills the center of the k-space (shallow gradient data), that contribute to contrast resolution. Zero phase encoding gradient fills the central line of the k-space, gives the highest intensity line of k-space.

Once k-space is filled, the matrix contains array of cells each containing real and an imaginary number which gives a map of magnitude and phase. There is an inverse relation between matrix of k-space and image. Bigger the size of k-space sampled, smaller the structures to be resolved. Each cell in the matrix k-space contain an information about all the image pixels. Each image pixel collects information from every matrix cell.

2-D Image Formation

MRI image is formed with pulse sequence which refers to strength, order, duration, application of gradient fields, and repetition and detection of RF pulse. It is repeated *n* times with an interval called *repletion time interval (TR)* to get phase encoding. This decides the number of pixels in the Y direction, where $n = 128$ or 256. The number of pixels is related to number of samples in the FID signal, that is 128 or 256. For a given FOV, the increase of pixels will increase the resolution but reduces signal strength. Time taken to complete an image sequence depends on number of repeat acquisition (N_{ex}), number of phase encoding steps (n), and TR value:

$$\text{Imaging time} = N_{ex} \times n \times TR$$

Higher the repeat acquisition steps lesser the noise but higher an imaging time. For example, if $N_{ex} = 4$, $n = 128$ and $TR = 500$ msec, then:

$$\text{Imaging time} = 4 \times 128 \times 0.5 \text{ s} = 256 \text{ s}$$

In practice, an image acquisition collects multiple images from several slices in each TR interval in an interleaved method. Number of pulse sequences are used to generate signal intensity from a given site. Imaging sequences are explained in subsequent paragraphs.

BIO-EFFECTS AND SAFETY

Magnetic resonance imaging (MRI) is a diagnostic procedure without any ionizing radiation. It uses a powerful magnetic field, radio waves, rapidly changing magnetic field for scanning. It causes no pain and system makes loud noise during the procedure. Patient is always monitored during an examination. Patient can communicate to the technologists while the scanning is going on. Hazards arise from *(1) static magnetic field, (2) gradient magnetic field, (3) radiofrequency field,* and *(4) cryogenic liquids.*

Static Magnetic Field

Magnetic resonance (MR) uses magnets which generate high static magnetic field. Clinical imaging systems typically have field strengths up to 3T (1T = 10,000 Gauss, the Earth's magnetic field is ≈ 0.5 Gauss) while MRI for spectroscopic research applications go up to 17.5 T. There is an evidence of biological effects by static magnetic field >1 T and it includes *(1) projectile missile hazards, (2) medical device displacement, (3) medical device disruption* and *(4) bioeffects.*

There may be force orientation effects on biological molecules (*hemoglobin, free radicals*) and some sensory effects like *nausea, vertigo,* and *metallic taste.* Recent studies have come out guidelines for an occupational exposure: 2T for occupational exposure of head and trunk, 8 T for occupational exposure of limb, and 400 mT for the public addressing all parts of the body. This exposure will not be applicable to patients undergoing MRI scan for diagnosis and therapy.

Studies on humans reveals that there are no confirmed results about the health effects of static magnetic field. *World Health Organization (WHO)* stated that there is no evidence on short-and long-term adverse effects of MRI static magnetic field on human health (2015).

In vitro studies have shown there is no MRI effects on cell growth, cell proliferation and cell cycle and an apoptotic cell death up to 10T. However, blood oxygenation dependent increase in blood velocity has been observed for an exposure of 1.5 T MRI magnetic field. In vivo studies on animals infer that there is no consensus to draw any conclusion relative to the *genotoxicity or carcinogenicity* of static magnetic field.

Projectile Effect

Powerful magnetic field of the MRI magnet can attract metal objects made with ferromagnetic (e.g., Iron) and make them to move with sudden and greater force. It will create risk anyone including patient who is present in an object's flight path. Attraction of ferromagnetic object varies with square of the magnetic field and inversely with cube of the distance. Hence, great care is taken while bringing an external object to the MRI room. Ferromagnetic *screwdrivers, Oxygen tanks* should not be brought into the MRI room. MRI system can pull the gadgets like *medical implant, aneurysm clips, medication pumps* from the patient body. *Scissors, scalpels* become lethal projectiles in MRI room. Oxygen cylinder, patient bed, and fire fitting apparatus have caused major injuries in the past.

Fringe Field

Fringe field is a peripheral magnetic field around a powerful magnet in MRI, e.g.,1.5 T magnet has 1 mT, and 0.5 mT fringe field at 9.3 m and 11.5 m, respectively **(Fig. 13.24).** The stary magnetic field around the magnet is 3-dimmentional field measured in Gauss (G) or milli tesla (mT). Plot of fringe field is available from the manufacturer, and it is longest along the direction of an axis. The strength of magnetic field decreases with distance from the core of the magnet. The magnetic field is inversely related to third power of the distance ($1/r^3$) from an isocenter. It means that the magnetic field decreases more slowly as one move away from the center of magnet. If one moves twice the distance from the scanner, fringe field will decrease by a factor of 1/8.

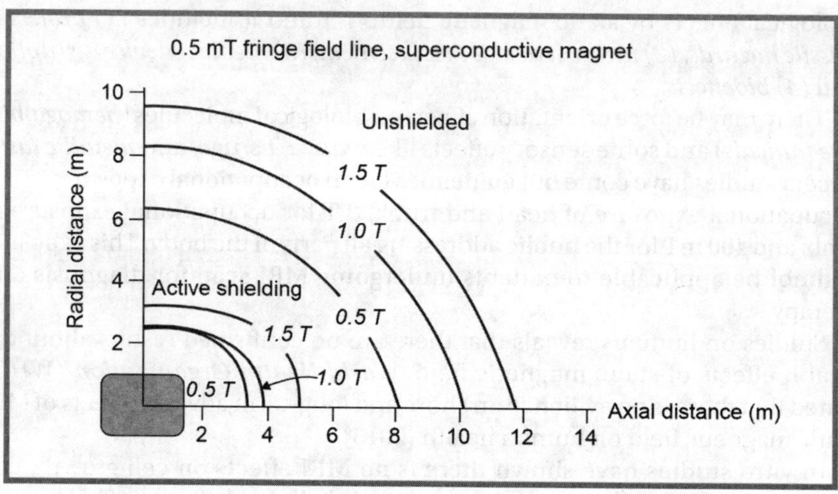

Fig. 13.24: Fringe field measured in mT for shielded and unshielded magnet. Fringe field decreases with distance.

Fringe field has an elongated tail which can extend beyond the MRI scanning room however, it depends on the magnet design and geometry.

Extensive fringe fields create hazardous condition in adjacent areas and cause an interference with an electronic device like pacemaker. Areas above 0.5 mT or 5 gauss (G) requires restricted access with warning signs as per FDA, US. Disruption of the fringe fields can reduce an homogeneity of an imaging volume (automobile, elevator, etc.). Smaller field of 3 G may affect nearby *CT* and *MRI scanners, gamma cameras, image intensifiers,* and *color TVs.* Fringe field of 10 G may affect *computers* and field of 30 G may magnetize the watch and erase *CDs and credit cards* and promote projectile effects.

MRI system is shielded to contain fringe field within the MRI room. Mostly 5 G field is contained within the room. The 5 G and 30 G position must be indicated on the floor with special marking with colored taps so that it gives not only warning but also restriction of personnel.

Gradient Magnetic Field

Gradient magnetic fields are often switched ON and OFF and considered as varying magnetic field ranging between an extremely low frequency (ELF) and intermediate frequency (IF). Primary safety concern includes *(1) peripheral nerve stimulation, (2) acoustic noise,* and *(3) interference with auxiliary equipment.*

There is a possible relation between FLF and cancer. Decreased survival of children with leukemia after an exposure to ELF magnetic fields has been observed. Gradient magnetic field produces an eddy current field in the patient that could stimulate *nerves* and *muscles* and in turn generate cardiac stimulation and ventricular fibrillation.

Study of gradient magnetic field effect on humans reveals that *cardiac stimulation* is unlikely but cause of patient discomfort due to peripheral nerve stimulation. There is a potential health risk beside peripheral nerve and cardiac stimulation to the patient due to an exposure of varying magnetic field.

In vitro studies have reported an increase of *DNA strand break* after exposure to ELF. It also revealed an increase of *micronucleus frequency in human fibroblasts* exposed to 50 Hz power line signal. However, there is no evidence of *teratogenic effects* due to an exposure of such magnetic field.

Acoustic Noise

Magnetic gradients are used to get positional information in MRI and an electric current is passed through the specially made solenoid, known as *gradient coils.* Switching the gradient fields changes the **Lorenz force** experienced by the gradient coils, resulting minute expansion and contraction of the coils. Since, the gradient coils are inside the MRI, there is large force between gradient coils and the main magnet. It creates a noise (*clicking or beeping*) that is heard by the patient. Noise is more with high tesla machines and rapid imaging techniques. It may reach 120 dB which is a threshold limit for causing sensation in human *ear canal.* Threshold limit for ear pain is about 140 dB. Since, dB is logarithmic, a 10-fold increase in dB leads to 100–fold increase in an intensity. Ear plugs are provided for ear protection during MRI scanning. Some vendors have come with silent MRI in which sound absorbers are used.

Radiofrequency Field

Radiofrequency (RF) electromagnetic field consists of frequency in the range 100 kHz–300 GHz. This type of RF is used in cell phones. Primary safety concern arises from *(1) tissue heating, (2) medical device heating, (3) medical device disruption* and *(4) interference with patient monitoring auxiliary equipment.*

Patient is exposed to varying RF electromagnetic field which can induce effects via *multiphoton absorption* due to direct heating. There are two types of biological effects by RF: *(1) nonthermal effects,* and *(2) thermal effects.* Nonthermal effects are due to direct interaction of magnetic field with tissues. Above adverse effect arises from direct energy transfer from magnetic field to the living organs. It is nonlinear and depends on field frequency.

Raise in temperature depends on electrical and geometrical tissue properties, the type of RF pulse used, its repetition time and the frequency of the radiation. The frequency range used in MRI is sufficient to offer high absorption of energy to the human body. *Eyes* and *testis* are sensitive to heating due to lack of perfusion, it is considered as dangerous on patient safety point of view. *Tattoos and permanent cosmetics* realized with *Iron oxide or other metal-based pigments,* can cause reactions or adverse events.

A measure of *specific absorption rate (SAR)* is defined for RF absorption which is the RF energy deposited per unit mass. Measurement of heat is not possible in patients during scanning, but SAR can be used as an index that controls raise in temperature. MRI scanner's software records SAR value as a whole-body measure and it should be within the limits recommended. Threshold limit of SAR is 4 W/kg for a whole-body scanner, calculated for a body temperature increase up to a 0.6 °C and a scanning period of 20–30 min. SAR is higher for large body site, higher magnetic field, and high conductivity tissue (*brain, blood, liver, and CSF*). It is also higher for a 180° pulse, than 90° pulse, spin echo sequence than GRE.

In vitro studies have found no evidence of *genotoxicity or cytotoxicity*. RF exposure does not cause an increase in *gene mutation, in chromosome aberration frequency or in sister chromatid exchange frequencies*, suggesting that RF exposure during a MR procedure is unlikely to be *genotoxic*.

Human studies with SAR limit of up to 4 W/kg showed no abnormal increase of temperature and no physiological changes. Raise of body temperature up to 0.6 c is found to alter *heart rate, blood pressure* and *blood flow*. Physiological alterations in *visual, auditory, endocrine, neural, cardiovascular, immune, reproductive,* and *developmental functions* were reported for high level RF exposure. No epidemiological studies are available regarding RF fields association with MRI. To conclude *interaction between RF* and *biological tissues during MR procedures could be unsafe for patients.*

Cryogenic Liquid

Liquid Helium is kept in a *cryostat* and must be replenished periodically based on workload. A refrigerator system is used to reduce Helium losses. The air entering the system may solidify and the coolant level must be checked daily. If level is too low, quenching may occur, which rises temperature and superconductivity of the magnet will be lost. As superconductivity fails, Copper does the conductivity of an electric current. As temperature rises, liquid Helium boils rapidly, vented outside the building causing hazards. Cryogen related safety concern arises *from (1) bodily harm, (2) asphyxiation,* and *(3) nephrogenic systemic fibrosis (NSF).*

Quenching may happen manually during emergency or accidentally. It may cause severe damage to the superconducting coils which is common in an accident quenching. A fire in the MRI room can cause quenching and proper fire-fighting system is provided in the site. A *Helium vending machine* is provided so that the gaseous Helium is vented out to environment. Otherwise, Helium fills the MRI room and replace Oxygen, hence an *Oxygen monitor* is must in MRI room. If Oxygen falls below certain limit, immediate evacuation of patient and personnel is necessary. During Helium or Nitrogen leak one may hear a *hissing noise* and get alerted, and everyone should be evacuated. Both gases displace Oxygen and cause an *asphyxiation*.

When quenching occurs if the scan room door is closed, depletion of Oxygen in the room increases room pressure, relative to control console. This may prevent opening the scan room door. In such case, the glass partition between the scan room and console must be broken to reduce room pressure. It is easy to open the door now and the patient is evacuated immediately. The patient is evaluated for *asphyxia, hypothermia,* and *ruptured eardrums.*

Implants and Foreign Bodies

Pacemaker is contraindication for MR imaging and several cases of *arrhythmia or death* have been reported in patients with pacemakers. The risk comes from the induction of RF by the pacemaker electronics and wires, resulting inappropriate pacing of the heart. Proper protocol is needed while handling patients with peace makers. Risk mainly arises from pacemaker malfunction rather than RF field.

Ferromagnetic foreign bodies like *metal fragments or metallic implants like surgical prothesis* and *aneurysm clips* are also having potential risk. Interaction of magnetic RF in such objects can lead to *trauma* due to movement of these objects in the magnetic field, thermal injury due to RF induction heating or failure of an implanted device. Physical examination of the patient is difficult hence, an orbital X-ray can be done in any suspected patients to verify whether they have metal fragments. *Titanium* is nonferromagnetic material suitable for an implant. It is safe under MRI from movement point of view and gives less artifact around the implant, even lesser than that of *stainless steel.* Artifacts create empty space around the implant called *black-hole artifact.* For example, a 3 mm *Titanium coronary stunt* may appear as 5 mm area of an empty face, whereas stainless steel may produce 10–20 mm empty space.

Patient should be completely screened before the MRI procedure. Patient should remove *hearing aids, watches, jewelry, cell phone, and certain clothes that have metallic threads or fasteners.* In addition, *makeup, nail polish or other cosmetics* may contain metallic particles should be removed before the MRI procedure. Athletic wear including *pants, shirts, socks, braces* and *metal-based fabrics or metal-based anti-bacterial compounds* may create hazards.

Claustrophobia

MRI scanners are made with long closed tunnels and patient position lies at the center of the magnet or tunnel. Patient cannot tolerate claustrophobia in such situations with long scanning time. Modern scanners are designed with wider bore with short scanning time. Claustrophobia is less an issue and majority can tolerate it. Open MRI scanners has no claustrophobia issue however, their image quality is poor. Of late 1.5 T open MRI with good quality image is made available.

Contrast Agent

Commonly used contrast agent is *Gadolinium (Gd)* chemical compound. It is much safer than the contrast agents used in radiography and CT scans. *Anaphylactoid reactions* less at the rate of 0.03 to 1%, it also has lower incidence of *nephrotoxicity* compared to an Iodine contrast. Though it is recommended as safe tool for renal impairment, there is risk in patients with severe *renal failure* and patient undergoing *dialysis.* It may lead to serious illness and *nephrogenic systemic fibrosis.* Hence, current guideline state that dialysis patient receives Gadolinium agents only where it is essential and clinically warranted, after the MRI scan patient should undergo dialysis. Contrast agents may be injected intravenously which will enhance the appearance of *blood vessels, tumors, or inflammation or determine active disease progression.*

Pregnant Patient

No bioeffects on fetus due to MRI scan has been proved. However, current recommendation state that MRI should be taken only if essential, as a precaution measure. It is very important during first trimester in which an *organogenesis* takes place. The biological effect of MRI is same for pregnant women and fetus however fetus is more sensitive. Use of contrast agent may cross the *placenta* and enter the fetal blood stream. Hence, contrast agent like *Gadolinium* compounds should be avoided during pregnancy. However, of late MRI is being used for diagnosing congenital abnormality of fetus. This is accepted based risk vs benefit concept and provides more diagnostic information than an ultrasound and CT scan.

Room Design and Shielding

MRI room requires adequate space with four zones as per *American college of radiology* (**Fig. 13.25**). Zone one is main reception and patient waiting, accessible to all public and it connects the main corridor for patient movement. Zone two is a controlled area where patients and visitors are controlled. It serves as patient preparatory room and waiting area through which patient travels to the MRI room.

Zone three is potential for an injury by ferromagnetic materials. Access to the zone three is strictly controlled and it is under supervision. It is basically the control room for MRI where the computers, UPS and battery are housed.

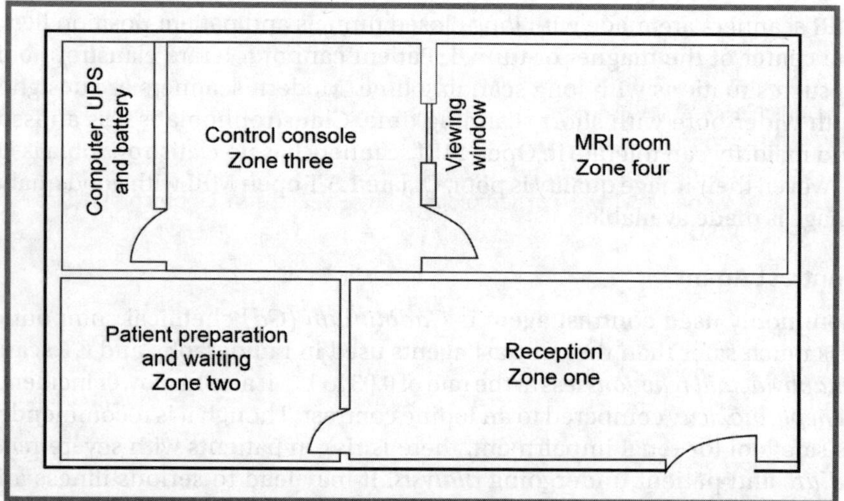

Fig. 13.25: Model layout for housing MRI equipment, shows zones for different works (about 100 sq m area).

Physical restriction, pass-key locking system is mandatory for this zone. Area in which fringe fields > 0.5 mT is clearly marked by pasting yellow taps on the floor. It is restricted for public access with reliable methods.

Zone four is MRI equipment room which is marked with warning sign and light, stating that—*The Magnet Is ON*. Unauthorized and unscreened entry is restricted even at an emergency. The room is always locked when unattended. Only MR compatible items should be brought to the room. The entrance should be designed so that the technologist able to see the door directly and observe and control access by line of sight. MRI personnel should be trained and able to handle an emergency situation, if any. During emergency, the patient is stabilized with basic life support and shifted to zone two immediately.

Magnetic flux lines from the magnet go beyond the room which decreases with distance. Such peripheral magnetic field is called *fringe field*. Any *metallic object, elevator and ferromagnetic material* nearby can disrupt magnetic field uniformity and degrade the image quality. Hence, magnetic shielding is provided with *steel plates* around the MR magnet. MRI room also requires RF shielding to prevent RF signals both entering the room and going out of the room. RF shielding is done with *faraday cage*, that consists of *copper metal sheet*. RF shielding also addresses an outside RF signal arising from radiobroadcasting.

BIBLIOGRAPHY

1. Allisy-Roberts PJ, Williams, J. Farr's Physics for Medical Imaging, 2nd end. Elsevier; 2008.
2. Bushberg JT, Seibert JA, Leidholdt EM Jr., Boone JM. The Essential Physics of Medical Imaging, 3rd edn. Lippincott Williams and Wilkins; 2012.
3. Bushong SC, Clarke, G. Magnetic Resonance Imaging: Physical and Biological Principles, Elsevier; 2015.
4. Cheng Y, Xia L, Crozier S. Design and Optimization of a Permanent Magnet for Small-sized MRI Based on Particle Swarm Optimization Algorithm, Engineering; 2011.
5. Hartwig V, Giovannetti G, Vanello N, Lombardi M, Landini L, Simi S. Biological Effects and Safety in Magnetic Resonance Imaging: A Review. Int J Environ Res Public Health. 2009; 6(6): 1778–1798.
6. https://my-ms.org. MRI safety
7. Huda W, Slone RM. Review of Radiological Physics, 2nd edn. Lippincott Williams and Wilkins; 2003.

MR Imaging Sequences and Image Quality

IMAGE SEQUENCES

Sequences in MRI refers to strength, order, duration, application of gradient fields, and repetition and detection of RF pulse. It is an orderly combination of RF and gradient pulses designed to acquire data from an echo. Data to create an image is obtained in series of steps. Tissue is excited by an RF pulse in the presence of slice select gradient. Then phase-encoding and frequency encoding (readout) gradients are required to spatially localize the protons in the order of 2-Dimensions (2D). After the data is collected and the process is repeated for a series of phase-encoding steps. MRI sequence and parameters are so selected to suit an individual clinical application.

In MRI, the signal, free induction decay is not usually measured, since, it decays within millisecond. It is due to imperfection of magnet, distortion of static magnetic field by patient, application of field gradient across the voxel and spin-spin interaction in the tissue. As a result, some spins precess faster, and some are slower after the 90° pulse. Further one or more steps are needed to cancel external magnetic field variation and make the MR signal measurable. They are referred as sequences that vary with an imaging application. The main sequences are (1) *spin echo pulse sequence (SE)*, and (2) *gradient recalled echo (GE)*. Different vendors use different nomenclature for their imaging sequences **(Table 14.1)**.

SPIN ECHO PULSE SEQUENCE

Spin echo pulse sequence nullify an external magnetic field variations due to an imperfection of magnet, distortion due to patient (susceptibility), and gradient across the voxel **(Hahn,1950)**. It was further modified by **Carr-Purcell-Meiboom-Gill (CPMG)**. Advantages of spin echo imaging are high SNR, true T2 weighting and lower susceptibility effects. Disadvantages are long scan times and use of more RF power.

Table 14.1: Terminology of MR imging sequences used by different vendors.

Sequence	Philips	Siemens	GE	Hitachi	Toshiba
Spin echo (SE)	SE	SE	SE	SE	SE
Multi-echo SE	Multi-SE	Multi-echo MS	SE	SE	Multi-echo
Fast SE	Turbo SE	Turbo SE	Fast SE	Fast SE	Fast SE
Ultrafast SE	SSH-TSE UFSE	SSTSE HASTE	SS-FSE	FSE-ADA	(Super) FASE DIET
IR	IR IR TSE	IR/IRM Turbo IR/TRIM	IR FSE-IR	IR FIR	IR Fast IR
STIR	STIR STIR TSE	STIR Turbo STIR	STIR Fast STIR	STIR Fast STIR	STIR Fast STIR
FLAIR	FLAIR FLAIR TSE	FLAIR Turbo FLAIR	FLAIR Fast FLAIR	FLAIR Fast FLAIR	FLAIR Fast FLAIR
Gradient Echo (GE)	FFE	GRE	GRE	GE	FE
Spoiled GE	T1-FFE	FLASH	SPGR MPSPGR	RSSG	RF-Spoiled FE
Ultrafast GE	T1-TFE T2-TFE THIRVE	Turbo FLASH VIBE	FGRE Fast SPGR FMPSPGR VIBRANT FAME LAVA	SARGE	Fast FE RADIANCE QUICK 3D
Ultrafast GE with magnetization preparation	IR-TFE	T1/T2-Turbo FLASH	IR-FSPGR DE-FSPGR	–	Fast FE
Steady state GE	FFE	FISP	MPGR GRE	TRSG	FE
Contrast enhanced steady state GE	T2-FFE T2	PSIF	SSFP	–	FE
Balanced GE	Balanced FFE	Turbo FISP	FIESTA	BASG	True SSFP
SE-Echo planar	SE-EPI	EPI SE	SE EPI	SE EPI	SE EPI
GE-Echo planar	FFE-EPI TFE-EPI	EPI Perf EPIFI	GRE EPI	SG-EPI	FE-EPI
Hybrid echo	GRASS	TGSE	–	–	Hybrid EPI

(*Courtesy:* e-MRI IMAIOS Inc)

In the spin echo pulse sequence, 90° RF pulse is followed by a 180° RF pulse. The 180° RF pulse is applied halfway (TE/2) between an excitation pulse and echo. After the 90° RF pulse, the magnetization vector goes in the transverse plane. Due to T2* dephasing, some spins are faster, and some are slower. The 180° RF pulse helps to flip the spins vector so that slower spins become faster and faster spins become slow. Thus, the 180° RF pulse eliminates systemic magnetic field inhomogeneities.

Time of Echo and MR Signal

After time delay of TE/2 a *spin echo* signal is formed (**Fig. 14.1**). It appears as an echo of initial FID signal which consists of two FID signal back-to-back or mirror image of an echo. The signal amplitude is reduced by a factor of T2 decay. *Time of echo (TE)* is the time between midpoint of 90° RF pulse and production of spin echo signal. The time delay (TE/2) is the time between 90° RF and 180° RF pulse application, and TE ranges from 5–140 milliseconds (msec). Longer the TE the smaller the signal amplitude. The MR signal (S) depends on:

❑ Spin density (ρH)
❑ Signal from fluid flow, f(v)
❑ T1 and T2 (tissue properties)
❑ TR and TE (machine parameters)

In general, MR signal is given by an equation:

$$S \propto \rho H\, f(v)\left[1 - e^{-\frac{TR}{T1}}\right] e^{-\frac{TE}{T2}}$$

Signal data is stored as line of k-space and each line of data is *Fourier transformed* to extract frequency information from the signal. The process is repeated for different phase-encoding steps.

Rephasing Pulse and Time of Repetition

The 180° RF pulse is called *rephasing or refocusing pulse*. It achieves spins rephasing and generates an echo and it is repeated to get multiple echoes. The sequence is repeated with a *repetition time (TR)* which is the time interval between two successive 90° RF pulse and its range is 300–3000 msec. Time required for full recovery of longitudinal magnetization is 4 × T1 after 90° RF pulse. Hence, subsequent 90° RF pulse is applied before the completion of longitudinal magnetization recovery of tissues. Spin echo sequences can be modified to differentiate:

❑ T1 differences of tissues, referred to as *T1 weighted image*.
❑ T2 differences, referred to as *T2 weighted image*.
❑ Proton density differences, referred to as *proton density (PD) weighted image*.

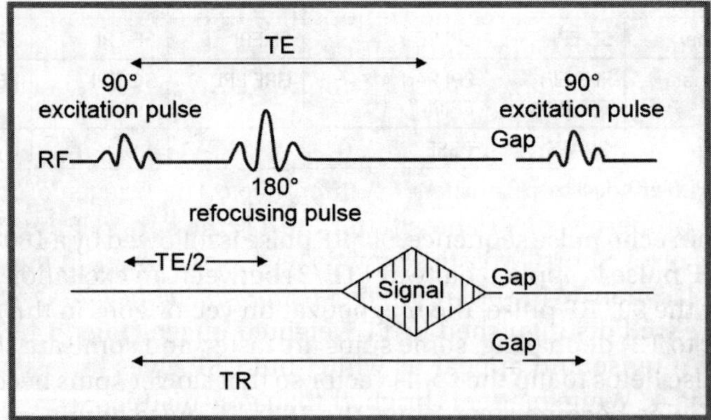

Fig. 14.1: Pulse echo sequence principle and one cycle events.

Imaging Cycle

First 90° RF pulse and slice selection gradient are simultaneously applied to excite a slice of tissue. FID signal is not measured, and the phase-encoding gradient is switched ON. Though all the spins have same frequency but have phase shift that depends on the position along the Y-axis. Thus, phase-encoding gradient helps to locate the signal in the patient, it is followed by application of frequency gradient in X-direction. After time interval of TE/2, 180° RF pulse and slice selection gradient is applied. Now an echo is emitted which is a mirror image of the FID which is measurable. Now the frequency encoding gradient is switched ON while an echo is emitted. The above is said to be *one cycle*. After a gap, again 90° RF pulse and 180° RF pulse is repeated, and second echo is formed. Hundreds of such repeated cycles gives one MR image frame. Events that are happening in one cycle are:

❑ The 90° RF pulse rotates the magnetization vector into transvers plane. Just after the 90° RF pulse, dipoles are in phase, the transverse magnetization is maximum, and the FID signal is not measured since it decays fast.

❑ After the removal of 90° RF pulse, dephasing occurs, some spins precess faster and some precess slower, and FID signal decays with T2*.

❑ When 180° RF pulse is applied, all the dipoles tip from spins up to spin down position. It turns the individual magnetization vector to rotate by 180° in X-direction. Fast spin becomes slow and slow spins become fast, and rephasing takes place and signal grows.

❑ After a time (TE/2), spins are in phase momentarily and the MR signal is at its peak. Thereafter spins goes out of phase and MR signal decays.

T1 Weighted Image

T1 weighted image is one where the contrast is based on differences of T1 characteristics between tissue and de-emphasizing T2 differences, e.g., *fat and water*. To get T1 weighting, TR must be short enough so that either fat or water will not have to fully return to B_o. If TR is too long, they return to B_o and recover their longitudinal magnetization fully. If this happens, T1 relaxation is complete in fat and water and their differences in their T1 time cannot be demonstrated on an image. Thus, TR controls how far each vector recovers before it is excited by the next RF pulse.

Hence, it employs short TR (<600 msec) to maximize the contrast and short TE (<20 msec) to minimize T2 differences. The image contrast is due to recovery properties of T1 and shorter the T1, the stronger the signal, and brighter the pixel. Short T1 tissues provide high signal intensity since they got complete relaxation. In the brain, *cerebral tissues, fat, white matter, grey matter,* and *CSF* are well distinguished in T1 weighted image **(Figs. 14.2A and B)**. Fat is most intense and appear as white, but CSF gives lowest signal and appear as black. White matter is brighter than grey matter.

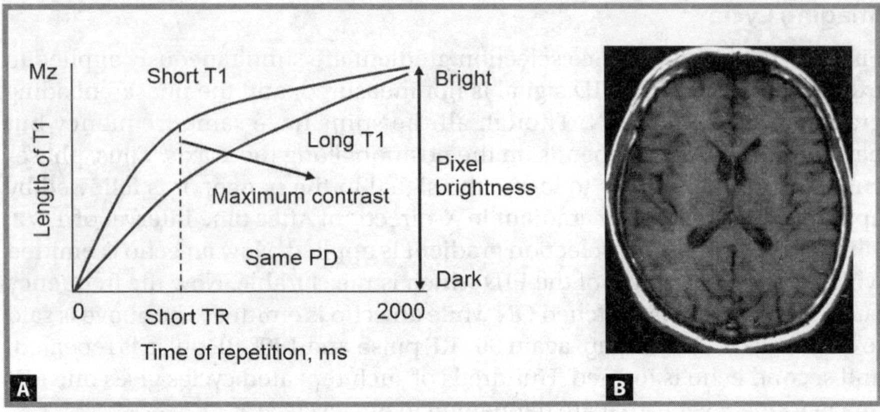

Figs. 14.2A and B: T1 weighted image. (A) T1 contrast vary with TR, maximum contrast for short TR, for a constant PD; (B) T1 weighted image of brain, short TR = 500 msec, and short TE = 8 msec.

T2 Weighted Image

T2 weighted image is one where the contrast dominantly depends on the differences in T2 times between tissues and de-emphasizing T1 difference, e.g., fat and water. The TE controls the T2 decay that is allowed to occur before the signal is received. To get a T2 weighted image, TE must be long so that fat and water will have enough time to decay. If TE is too short, they have no time to decay and their T2 differences cannot be demonstrated in the image.

It employs long TR (1000–2000 msec) to reduce T1 contrast and long TE (>60 msec) to maximize T2 contrast. Longest TE offers greater image contrast of differences between T2 tissues. However, TE should not be too long, it may produce small signals, may get masked in the background. An image contrast is due to recovery properties of T2, and longer the T2 the stronger the signal and brighter the pixel. In T2 weighted brain image, *water* and *CSF* is brighter than fat. Since grey matter has longer T2 and higher PD, appear brighter than white matter **(Figs. 14.3A and B).**

Proton Density Weighted Image

Proton density weighting is one in which the differences in the number of protons per unit volume in tissue is a dominant factor by which an image contrast is achieved. Greater the spin density, larger the longitudinal magnetization, e.g., *lipids, fats.* Proton density always present in tissue at certain level. To have proton density weighted image, the T1 and T2 contrast must be de-emphasized so that proton density dominates with its contrast. Long TR permits fat and water to fully recover their longitudinal magnetization, in turn diminishes T1 weighting. A short TE does not permit fat and water to decay, in turn diminishes T2 weighting.

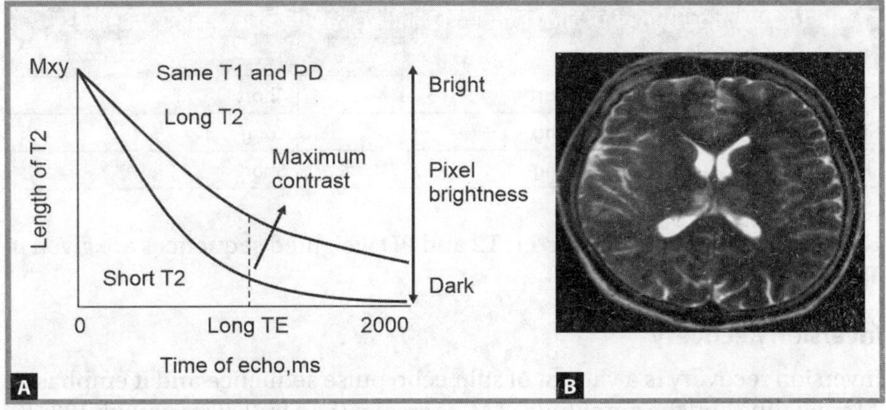

Figs. 14.3A and B: T2 weighted image. (A) T2 vary with time of echo, long TE gives maximum contrast, for constant T1 and PD; (B) T2 weighted image of brain, long TR = 2400 msec, and long TE = 90 msec.

It employs long TR (>1000–3000 msec) to minimize T1 contrast and short TE (15 msec) to minimize T2 effects. It gives greatest signal strength with less noise **(Fig. 14.4)**. Higher the PD stronger the signal and brighter the image. Hence, *CSF, fat* appears white but *white matter* appears black. *Grey matter* appears brighter than *white matter*. Though the signal to noise ratio (SNR) is higher, the image contrast is poor.

Overall, tissues with large T2 and large PD gives large signal with bright pixel. Tissues with long T1 and arterial blood flow gives small signal with dark pixel. *Air* and *cortical bone* have no Hydrogen, always appear as black. The TR controls over T1 weighted image whereas TE controls T2 weighted image.

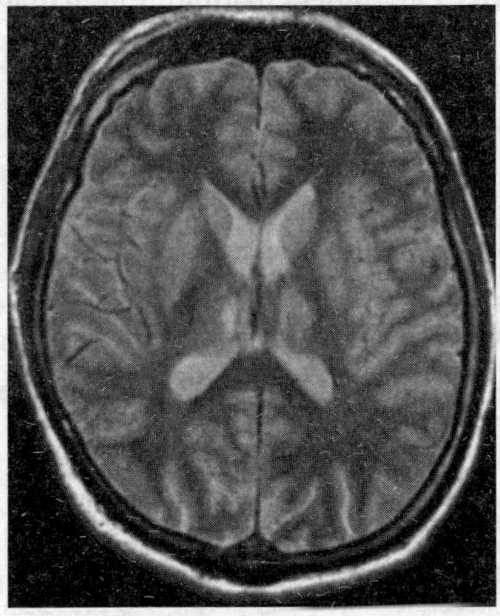

Fig. 14.4: Proton density weighted brain image with long TR = 2400 msec and short TE = 30 msec.

Table 14.2: Comparison of TR and TE for T1, T2 and PD weighted imaging sequences.

Weighted sequence	TR	TE
T1	Short	Short
T2	Long	Long
PD	Long	Short

Comparison of TR and TE for T1, T2 and PD weighted sequences are given in **Table 14.2**.

Inversion Recovery

Inversion recovery is a variant of spin echo pulse sequence and it emphasize T1 weighting and the amplitude of M_z is greater than by 2. It starts with 180° RF pulse which inverts the longitudinal magnetization vector through 180° that is M_z become $-M_z$. Once the 180° pulse is removed, the magnetization vector begins to relax and back to B_o. The spins return parallel to Z-axis, by *spin-lattice relaxation*, and M_z recovers after a time 0.69 × T1. Complete recovery consumes 4 × T1 duration.

After a delay time, *Time of inversion (TI)*, a 90° RF pulse is applied (readout pulse), which tilts the available M_z into the transverse plane and an FID signal is produced. A second 180° RF pulse at time TE/2, produces an echo signal at time TE which forms final signal intensity **(Fig. 14.5A)**. Image contrast depends on TI, TR, and TE and primarily on longitudinal magnetization and TI.

One cycle in an inversion recovery is 180° RF pulse, 90° RF pulse, and 180° RF pulse and the cycle is repeated after, time of repetition (TR), e.g., 1000 msec. It employs short TE (20 msec), to minimize T2 dependency. Basically, an inversion recovery gives T1 weighted images and tissue with longer T1 is suppressed **(Fig. 14.5B)**. Differences in longitudinal magnetization is larger in

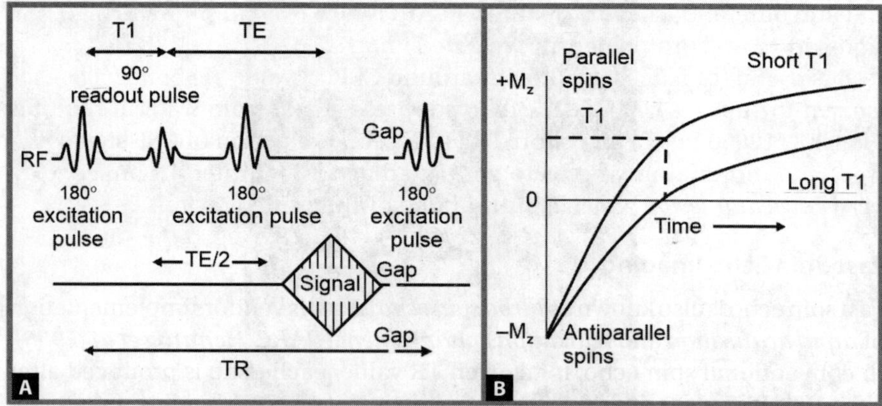

Figs. 14.5A and B: (A) Inversion recovery sequence principle and one cycle events; (B) Tissue with short T1 gives large MR signal for a given TI. Tissue with long T1 yet to recover, and get suppressed.

an inversion recovery and this is used to increase T1 weighted image contrast. Longer the TI or shorter the T1, greater the MR signal and thus TI controls the tissue contrast.

Inversion recovery is a heavily weighted T1 recovery, 180° RF pulse produce large contrast differences between fat and water. It is time consuming but gives better grey and white matter discrimination. Inversion recovery sequence forms the basis for many more sequences:

❏ STIR: Short Tau or Time Inversion Recovery
❏ FLAIR: Fluid-attenuated Inversion Recovery

STIR

STIR stands for *short-time inversion recovery* and its important clinical application is fat suppression. Fat produces bright intense signal which obscure contrast in other tissues. Fat has short T1 relaxation time, selection of short TI permits fat to recover from full inversion to the transvers plane so that there is no longitudinal magnetization for fat. If a 90° RF excitation pulse is applied after a delay time TI, the fat signal is nullified. Thus, it eliminates high signal from fat and enhances the surrounding image contrast so that true abnormalities can be detected, e.g., detection of an *optic neuritis*.

STIR is used to suppress fat signal in a T1 weighted image and a short TI of 150–175 msec achieves fat suppression. TI values varies with magnetic strength, a 1.5 T scanner need 140 msec.

FLAIR

FLAIR stands for *fluid-attenuated inversion recovery,* and it is another variant of spin echo pulse sequence. By selecting a suitable TI value, signal from long T1 can be suppressed, e.g., *cerebrospinal fluid (CSF)*. This TI time corresponds to the time of recovery of CSF from 180° inversion to the transverse plane. CSF has relatively long T1, selection of an optimal TI, nullify the signal from CSI and other fluid-filled structures. FLAIR is also used to suppress high CSF signal in T2 and proton density weighted images.

It is useful to visualize pathology around CSF. TI value of about 2000 msec is used to suppress CSF at 1.5 T. To suppress signal from water it requires longer TI (2000 msec) and short TR (10 msec). Reduction of CSF signal and water-bound anatomy helps to get true diagnosis in the MR image, e.g., *periventricular lesion* which is surrounded by fluid-filled regions.

Fast Spin Echo Imaging

Fast spin echo is also known as *turbo spin echo (TSE)* is vendors implementation of *rapid acquisition* and *relaxation enhancement (RARE, **Henning et al, 1986**)*. In conventional spin echo, for a given TR value, each echo is produced after each 180° RF pulse with single step application of phase-encoding. Each echo has its own k space, every new echo adds one line of k-space. Since, one TR for a line of k-space is used, it repeats the TR, 256 times for a matrix of 256 × 256.

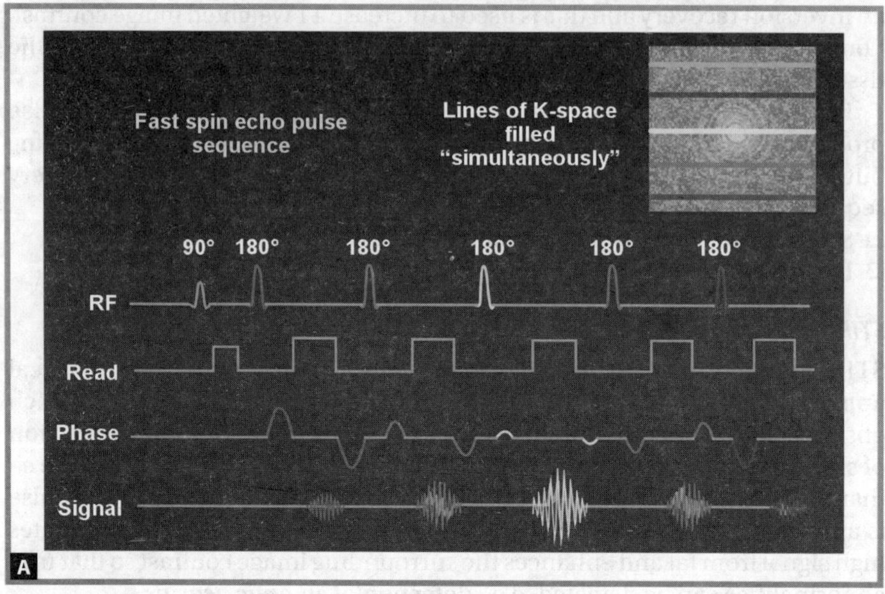

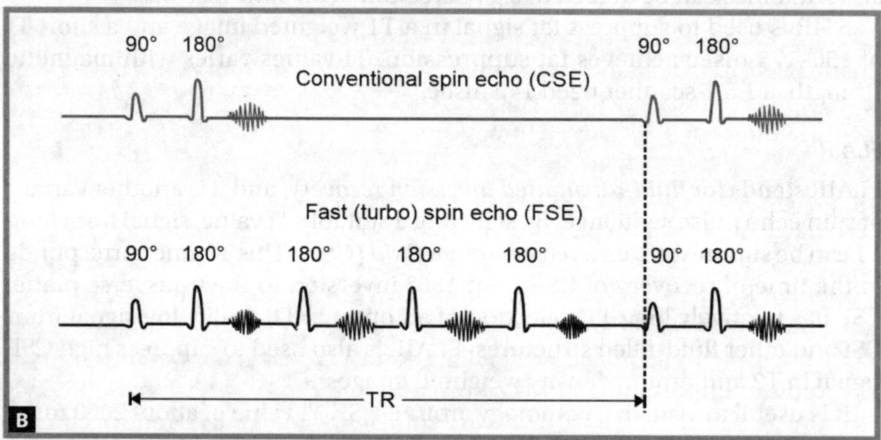

Figs. 14.6A and B: (A) Fast spin echo pulse sequence; (B) Comparison with conventional spin echo sequence.
(*Courtesy:* AD Elater, Elster LLC, 2023)

Fast spin echo manipulates the conventional spin echo to save time. It produces train of 3 echoes in one line of k-space (**Figs. 14.6A and B**):

90º – 180º – echo – 180º – echo – 180º – echo – 180º – echo................
.... 90º – 180º – echo......

The phase-encoding gradient changes after each echo, multiple lines of k-space can be obtained for a given TR time. Instead of allotting one k-space for each echo in this, three echoes are filled in one k-space. Since, it fills 3 lines into a single k-space, time is reduced by a factor 3 compared to conventional spin echo. The TR must be repeated only 86 times (256/3 = 86), instead of 256 to fill 256 lines of k-space. The number of echo's produced in a TR interval is called an *echo tarin length (ETL) or turbo factor*. It ranges from 4–32 for general imaging and 200 for rapid imaging like an echo planar.

Even though scan time is reduced, the SNR is retained as there are 256 phase-encoding steps. Advantages are higher spatial resolution, less susceptibility induced signal loss and lengthening of TR. Motion artifact is less severe and able to manage poorly shimmed magnetic field. It is superior then the conventional SE sequence. Disadvantages includes, unable to detect small calcification area and hemorrhage and not suitable for infants and children due to tissue heating. Vendors names of the sequence are *fast spin echo (FSE), GE Healthcare and turbo spin echo (TSE), Siemens/Philips.*

Image Contrast

Contrast distinguishes soft tissues by the differences observed in MR signal intensities. For example, differences between grey and white matter in neuroimaging. MR image contrast is influenced by both tissue and machine parameters. Tissue parameters are PD, T1, T2, tissue susceptibility and dynamics. Machine parameters are TE, TR, TI which are an operator-controlled. Tissue pathology, type of sequence and contrast media can also influence contrast.

Brightness of a pixel in an imaging volume depends on (1) proton density, (2) recovery of M_z (length of T1, compared to TR), and (3) decay of M_{xy} (length of T2, compared to TE). Hence, the selection of TR and TE is critical, so that an image brightness depends on any one of the tissue parameters T1, T2, PD. Images can be obtained as T1 weighted image, or T2 weighted image and or PD weighted image. To acquire T1, PD, and T2 image contrast, specific values of TR and TE are chosen for a given pulse sequence. Selection of suitable TR and TE values weighs an image so that one contrast is dominant over the other two.

Another important factor is *contrast-to-noise ratio (CNR)* that influences the image contrast. If noise levels are sufficiently high, it will reduce contrast. Two images may have same contrast but with different noise levels. Image with lower CNR always goes with lower contrast. If signal intensity of two tissues is S1 and S2, then the CNR of two tissues is related by:

$$CNR12 = \frac{(S1 - S2)}{Noise}$$

GRADIENT RECALLED ECHO

Gradient recalled echo (GE) is the simplest form of MR sequence and uses a magnetic field gradient to induce an echo, instead of 180° RF pulse. It consists of series of excitation pulses, and each pulse is separated by a specific *time of repetition (TR)*. After a time, TE, an echo is acquired, and data is processed. TE is called *time of echo*, is the time between the mid-point of an excitation pulse and the mid-point of data acquisition.

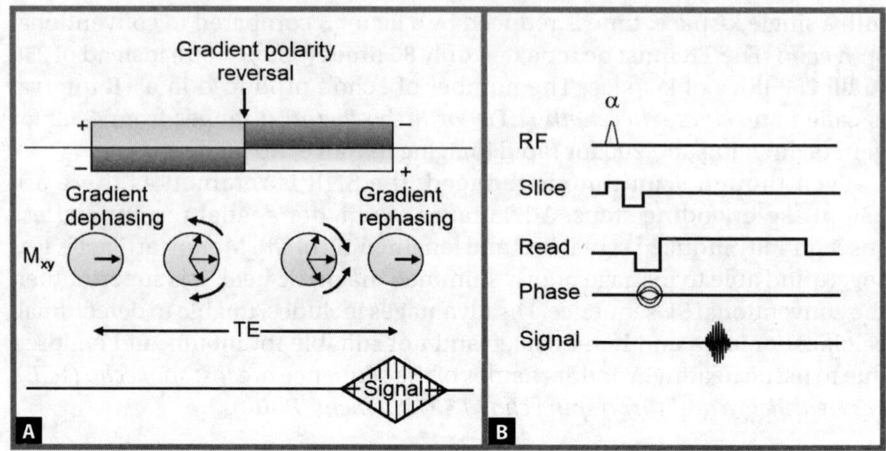

Figs. 14.7A and B: (A) Gradient recalled echo (GE) imaging principle; (B) Basic GE sequence.

It employs short TR, short TE, and low *flip angles* (α). After a α-excitation in the presence of slice selection gradient, the FID signal is generated. Magnetic field gradient polarity is reversed so that the spins are in phase and precess at the same frequency. The phase-encoding and frequency encoding gradient magnetic field are applied simultaneously. As a result, spins rephase and generate an echo of FID signal **(Figs. 14.7A and B)**. It is called *gradient-refocused echo or gradient echo or simply GE.*

GE will not compensate for an external magnetic field inhomogeneity. There is an increased sensitivity to T2* decay. If the frequency encoding gradient magnetic field is applied after the phase-encoding gradient magnetic field, the spins dephase with T2* relaxation time. It allows fast acquisition and facilitate 3-D imaging. For example, 256 phase-encodings steps can be acquired in 1.3 s for a given TR of 5 msec.

GE is not a true spin echo technique but a purposeful dephasing and rephasing of FID. The magnetic field inhomogeneities and tissue susceptibilities are emphasized in GE and hence the image is T2* weighted. Manipulation of parameters can give blood flow and an angiographic image.

Advantages of GE are fast imaging, low flip angle and less RF power, Disadvantage includes difficult to generate good T2 contrast, sensitive to B_o inhomogeneity and sensitive to susceptibility effects. GE has number of advanced specialized sequences:

❑ FLASH: Fast Low-Angle Shot
❑ FISP: Fast Imaging with Steady-state Precession.
❑ SSFP: Steady-state Free Precession or PSIP (FISP letters are reversed)

Flip Angle and Ernst Angle

Selection of flip angle (α) is much vital to achieve a T1 weighted image. GE sequence generally uses α <90° and very short TRs, say 150 msec based on

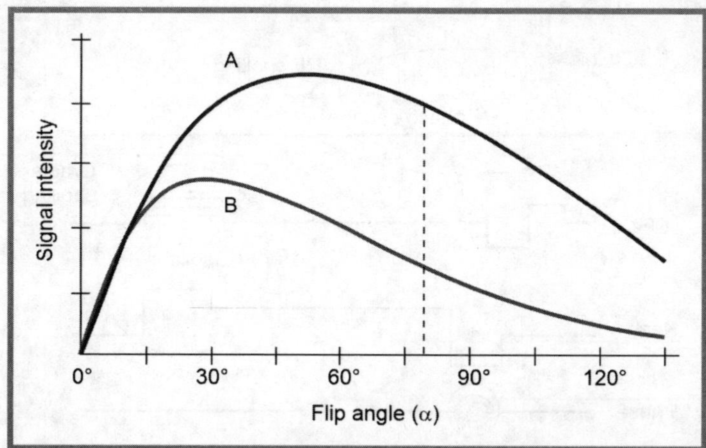

Fig. 14.8: Filp angle (α) verses MRI signal intensity, for 30°–70° flip angle, maximum intensity for a single tissue, however, the maximum contrast for different tissue A and B occur only at greater Ernst angle as shown in dotted lines.
(*Courtesy:* AD Elater, Elster LLC, 2023)

required contrast. More transverse magnetization is generated with smaller α, due to quick buildup of magnetization in tissue. Optimal α depends on the T1 value of the tissue. A short T1 value goes with large α angle. For a given T1 value, there is an optimum α that will the give most intense signal from a sequence is called *Ernst angle:*

$$\cos \alpha = \left[\exp \left(-\frac{TR}{T1} \right) \right]$$

When TR >> T1, the Ernst angle approaches to 90° only. For example, with a scan parameter of T1 of 800 msec, and TR of 3000 msec, the flip angle is calculated as 89°<90° from the above equation. Short TR (< 0.2 seconds) uses smaller α angle, < 45°, and long TR (> 0.2 seconds) uses large α > 45°. Use of α between 30°–70° makes the flip angle nearer to an Ernst angle **(Fig. 14.8)**. Ernst angle is estimated in *time of flight (TOF) angiography* which considers both relaxation of blood and tissue.

Tissue contrast in GE depends on TR, TE, and α. Shorter the TR smaller the α that gives maximum signal intensity. Long TR imaging will differentiate T2 and T2* and the moving blood appears bright. Though an Ernst angle gives maximum intensity for a single tissue, it may not give contrast between two different tissues. Contrast is obtained at an angle even greater than the Ernst angle. Ernst angle is used to maximize signal in commonly used Spoiled-GE sequences like FLASH, SPGR, VIBE, T1-FFE, MPGR, MP-RAGE.

FLASH

Flash is a prototype sequence first developed, also known as *Spoiled gradient recalled echo (SPGR).* The term spoiling refers to an elimination of steady-state transverse magnetization. It can be done by (1) variable gradient spoilers,

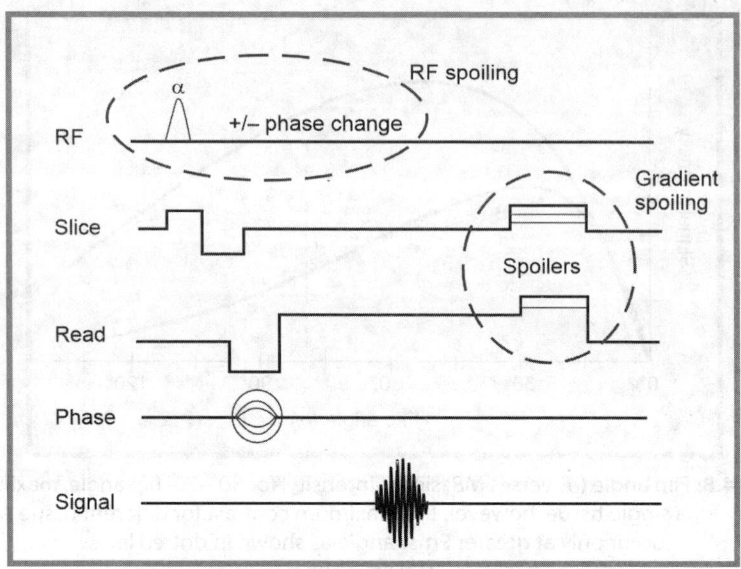

Fig. 14.9: FLASH/spoiled GE sequence.

(2) applying RF spoiling, and (3) lengthening TR **(Fig. 14.9)**. Since, transverse magnetization is eliminated, only longitudinal magnetization influences the signal in FLASH technique. When α angle is large, it offers increased T1 weighting and reduced T2* weighting. When α angle is small, it offers an increased PD weighting and reduced T1 weighting.

In the gradient spoiling, slice select gradient is applied with variable amplitudes at the end of each cycle just before the next RF cycle. Spoiler gradient strength is varied either linearly or semi randomly from view to view. Variable gradient spoilers destroy the phase coherence of M_{xy} after the GE signal digitized. It employs steady-state for longitudinal component of microscopic magnetization, M_z. The steady-state refers to constant longitudinal magnetization after repeated small flip angles α. In this method, spoiling is spatially nonuniform since the gradients produce spatially varying fields, hence it is not an adequate method.

In RF spoiling, the phase of the RF-carrier is changed according to a predefined formula from view to view. It increments the phase quadratically by using a recursive formula. Completely randomized pattern of phase change should be used since spin clustering may occur. RF spoiling is superior to gradient spoiling because it does not create an eddy current, and it is spatially an invariant. *Vendors sequences are SPGR, FSPGR (GE Healthcare), FLASH, and VIBE (Siemens healthineers), and T1-FFE in Philips, respectively.*

In long TR spoiling, TR >>T2*, the transverse magnetization become zero at the end of the cycle. TR time of several hundred msec are used to spoil the transvers magnetization. Spoiling can be enhanced by operating in 2-D multi-slice mode. However, off resonant effects from RF pulses for other slices and their associated imaging gradient may disrupt the transverse coherences. Vendors sequences are MPGR, MERGE (GE Healthcare), MEDIC (Siemens healthineers), and multi FFE (Philips), respectively.

FLASH sequence produces T1 weighted image that is controlled by TR and α. Repetition of low α angle generates both FID and SE signals. Sum of the FID and SE forms the total signal.

FISP

FISP stands for *Fast Imaging with Steady-state Precession*. Generally, either in spin echo (SE) or gradient echo (GE), there is a residual transverse magnetization at the end of each cycle, and it remains for the next cycle. After a few cycles, this residual *magnetization reaches a steady state value (MSS)*. In FISH technique, the above steady-state magnetization is added to the transvers magnetization, created by a small angle, α RF pulse **(Fig. 14.10)**. Thus, it helps to lengthen the transverse magnetization vector in the X-Y plane. Tissues with longer T2 may have longer MSS than tissues with shorter T2. It also provides more T2* weighted images. At the end of each cycle a *rewinder gradient* is applied along the phase-encoding direction. It will reverse the effects of an earlier phase-encoding gradient applied at the beginning of the cycle.

FISP is a basic type of refocused GE pulse sequence. Refocusing principle is one in which two or more signals can be obtained simultaneously to maximize SNR. It is done by re-encoding and reusing signals from the previously measured k-space line. FISH acquires signal from both FID and simulated

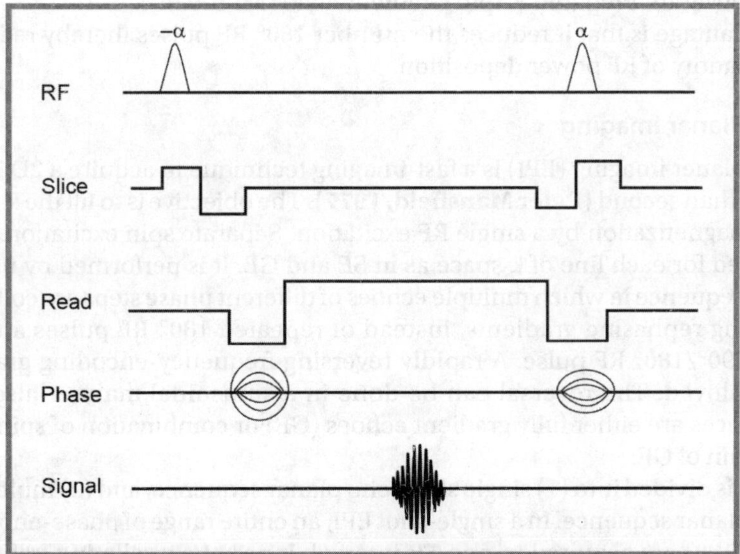

Fig. 14.10: FISP with balanced steady-state sequence, showing symmetric gradients along all three axis and echo formation at the middle of the sequence, hence the name true FISP.

echo (STE). Refocused GE finds application in an *orthopedics*, and dynamic studies of *heart* with breath hold imaging methods.

Hybrid Fast Imaging Techniques

Hybrid imaging refers to mixture of spin echo and gradient echo techniques. It is understood that 180° RF rephasing pulse is used in spin echo to create a spin echo train whereas several gradient echoes exist between each 180° RF pulse. Speeding the GE technique by reducing TR with α angle leads to loss of contrast in an image. Hence, an inversion recovery of spin echo is combined with GE techniques to overcome this. It is referred as *hybrid fast imaging techniques or simply turbo*. Such methods are called (1) *turbo FLASH, (2) snapshot FLASH, (3) snapshot-GRASS* and *(4) insta.*

Turbo spin echo imaging starts with a single 180° RF excitation, and an inversion pulse in a selected slice. Then several α pulses are applied resulting multiple spin echoes. They are progressively phase encoded and simultaneously the readout gradient is reversed alternatively. Inversion recovery generates T1 weighted image and each line in k-space encounters slightly different T1 weighted image. The k-space obtained with low amplitude phase-encoding gradient is important for contrast. Turbo technique gives an image one slices at a time with reduction of motion artifacts.

Turbo is capable of (1) controlling contrast within an image, e.g., liver and the breast or brain perfusion, (2) filling of k-space is selectable, and (3) changing flip angle of RF excitation pulse from one Fourier to another. Vendors hybrid sequences are GRACE (Philips), TGSE (Simens healthineers), and hybrid EPI (Toshiba). The 3-D version of the turbo technique is called Magnetization Prepared RApid Gradient Echo (MPRAGE).

Advantage is that it reduces the number 180° RF pulses thereby reducing the quantity of RF power deposition.

Echo Planar Imaging

Echo planer imaging (EPI) is a fast-imaging technique to acquire a 2D image in less than second **(Peter Mansfield, 1977)**. The objective is to fill the k-space with magnetization by a single RF excitation. Separate spin excitation is not required for each line of k-space as in SE and GE. It is performed by using a pulse sequence in which multiple echoes of different phase steps are collected by using rephasing gradients, instead of repeated 180° RF pulses after an initial 90°/180° RF pulse. A rapidly reversing frequency-encoding gradient is employed. The reversal can be done in a sinusoidal manner also. EPI sequences are either fully gradient echoes (GE) or combination of spin echo and train of GE.

EPI is divided into (1) single shot echo planar sequence, and (2) multi-shot echo planar sequence. In a single-shot EPI, an entire range of phase-encoding steps (128) are acquired in one TR interval. It permits oscillating frequency encoding gradient pulses and fill the k-space after a single RF pulse. In a multi-shot EPI, the phase steps range is divided into several shots or TR periods. For example, an image of 128 phase steps is divided into 2 shots of 64 steps each. Image can be obtained in 20–100 msec with high temporal resolution which is suitable for cardiac imaging. Data processing speed is higher hence, EPI become a much popular technique as fMRI.

EPI sequence starts with 90°, and 180° RF pulse along with slice selection gradient like the spin echo **(Fig. 14.11)**. Then frequency encoding gradient oscillates rapidly from positive to negative amplitude, resulting train of gradient echoes. Each echo is phase encoded differently along the Y-axis. Simultaneously, the readout gradient is reversed from positive to negative over entire length of an echo. Each oscillation of frequency-encoding gradient is related in one line of k-space image data. The data is collected and stored in k-space and 2D *Fourier transform* is applied to create an image.

Proton density or T2 weighted image is also possible, GE-EPI hybrid provides T2* weighted image. T1 weighted image is possible by applying an inverted pulse before an excitation pulse to produce saturation.

It is sensitive to motion, but motion related artifacts are rare due to short imaging time. Its SNR is low, contrast is like spin echo technique, and resolution is limited by the SNR. Advantages are shorter imaging time, decreased motion artifact, and rapidly changing physiological process like *blood flow and kinetic activity*. It provides precise image of the brain and other internal organs. Limitations include sensitivity to susceptibility

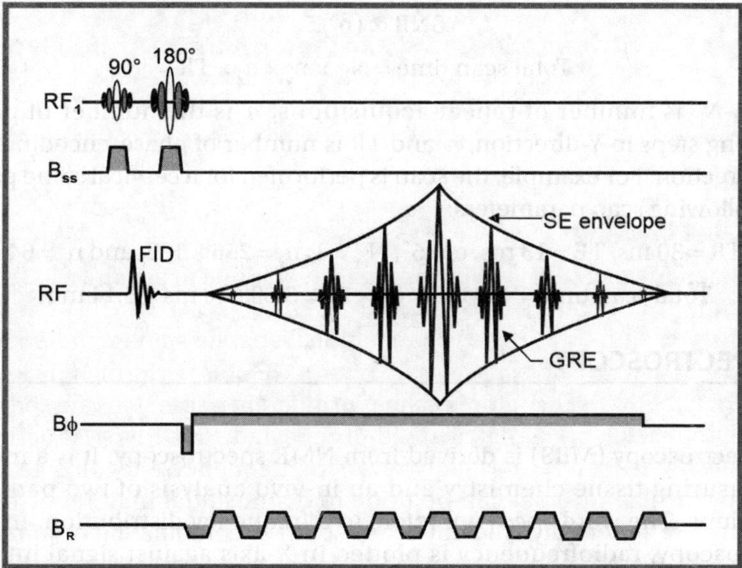

Fig. 14.11: Echo planar imaging pulse sequence: RF₁ is the RF pulse, Bss is the slice selection gradient, Bφ is the phase-encoding gradient and BR is the readout gradient. After one excitation, the readout gradient is reversed from positive to negative shows generation of GE signal at each time.
(*Courtesy:* Radiology key)

effects and inhomogeneity of the external magnetic fields. Long echo tarin length causes greater T2* weighting which needs high performance gradients.

EPI finds application in cardiac imaging, abdominal imaging, diffusion imaging, perfusion imaging and functional imaging.

3D Volume Imaging

In 3D imaging two sets of orthogonal phase-encoding gradients are used along with frequency-encoding gradient. A nonselective RF pulse excites simultaneously the spins in the volume and 3D Fourier transform is applied in all three axes. Once the volume data is reconstructed, 2D image in any plane can be obtained. The duration of time in 3D imaging is:

$$\text{Imaging time} = N_{ex} \times n_1 \times n_2 \times TR$$

where, n_1 is number of phase-encoding steps in one plane, and n_2 is number in the orthogonal plane. Advantages of 3D imaging is high resolution in all orientations and generation of an arbitrary oblique slices by post processing. Disadvantag include longer imaging time and prone to motion artifacts.

GE techniques can be used for 3D volume imaging with contiguous thin slices. It requires an addition of phase-encoding steps in the slice-selection, along Z direction. Advantage is the absence of cross talk and an increased SNR:

$$SNR \propto (n_z)^{\frac{1}{2}}$$

$$\text{Total scan time} = N_{ex} \times n_y \times n_z \times TR$$

where, N_{ex} is number of repeat acquisitions, n_y is the number of phase-encoding steps in Y-direction, n_z and TR is number of phase-encoding steps in Z-direction. For example, the scan is performed for a cervical spine patient with following scan parameters:

$$TR = 30 \text{ ms}, TE = 13 \text{ ms}, \alpha = 5°, N_{ex} = 1, n_y = 256 \times 192, \text{ and } n_z = 64$$

$$\text{Total scan time} = 1 \times 192 \times 64 \times 30 = 3,68,640 \text{ ms} = 6.14 \text{ min}$$

MR SPECTROSCOPY

Physics

MR spectroscopy (MRS) is derived from NMR spectroscopy. It is a method of measuring tissue chemistry and an in-vivo analysis of two pathology conditions. The word *spectrum* refers to a frequency distribution. In NMR spectroscopy, radiofrequency is plotted in X-axis against signal intensity in Y-axis. In MRI, the FID signal is a plot of signal time vs signal intensity. After the Fourier transform (FT), the plot is transformed to frequency vs signal intensity. The MR signal depends on gyromagnetic ratio of the nuclei. Since, Hydrogen has largest gyromagnetic value, its signals can be obtained completely and separately, from the nuclides.

Chemical Shift

Electron moving with charge generates its own magnetic field. This field is either added or subtracted with an external magnetic field. Due to the electron magnetic field effect, the resonance frequency gets altered slightly. However, an electron magnetic field is so small compared to an external magnetic field and have lesser impact, but it is sufficient to generate NMR spectrum that have peaks.

Every nuclear species produces more than one peak in the spectrum. For example, an *ethanol (CH₃CH₂OH)* gives three group of peaks in the NMR due to chemical structure of the molecule in which the nucleus is bound **(Fig. 14.12)**. There is a difference in resonance frequency in a single nuclear species. This pattern of difference in resonance frequency (Larmor frequency) is called *chemical shift*.

For example, Hydrogen in fat has an abundance of electrons and resonate at 150 Hz which is <water. There are three types of Hydrogen atom, two types of Carbon atom and one type of Oxygen atom resulting three, two and one NMR spectrum. Chemical shift is measured in frequency units which is based on magnetic field strength. Simplest way of measuring chemical shift is parts *per million (PPM)*. It refers to frequency difference $(f - f_o)$ divided by resonant frequency (f_o) of one of the peaks multiplied by million:

$$PPM = \frac{f - f_o}{f_o} \times 10^6$$

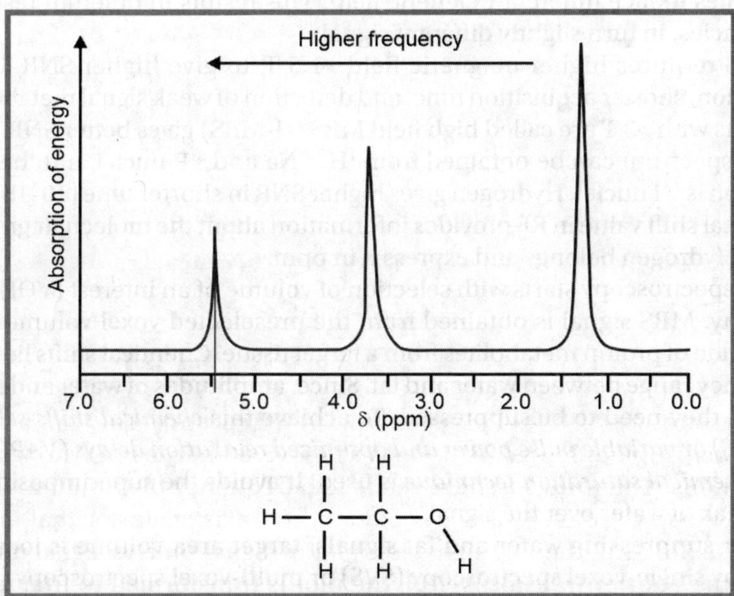

Fig. 14.12: NMR spectrum of Ethanol, shows three peaks: Smallest peak refers to single H in the OH group, highest peak refers to H in CH₃ group, and middle peak refers to H in CH₂ group.

For example, if the resonance frequency is 100,000,000 and 100,000,500, they differ by 500 parts in 100 million, or simply 5 ppm. Resonance peak range of ^{1}H, and ^{13}C is 10 ppm and 200 ppm, respectively. The difference in ^{1}H resonance frequency between fat and water is 3.5 ppm. Chemical shift is either positive or negative based on frequency. Higher frequency resonant peaks are down filed whereas lower frequency is up field.

Other parameters to analyze the spectrum is signal intensity and *J-coupling*. Signal intensity is an area of curve which identify chemical composition and structure. It helps to have both qualitative and quantitative analysis in chemistry and biomedical research. J-coupling is an indicator of molecular structure and appears as an additional lines in the spectrum. It is due to interaction of spins within the same molecule. It is expressed in Hz and independent of magnetic field. Differences seen in the spectrum is proportional to separation in chemical shift between the coupled nuclei.

Spectroscopy

Magnetic resonance spectroscopy (MRS) is an analytical method in chemistry that gives identification and quantification of metabolites in a sample. Its spectrum provides physiological and chemical information instead of an anatomy. It makes use of slight difference in resonance frequency of protons (chemical shift) that exists in metabolites. It is due to an electron cloud shielding around the nuclei, resulting slightly different resonance frequencies. Distribution of electrons within an atom causes the nuclei in different molecules to face different magnetic field. This results in different resonant frequencies, in turn slightly different signal.

MRS requires higher magnetic field >1.5 T, to give higher SNR, better resolution, shorter acquisition time, and detection of weak signal metabolites. Magnets with >3 T are called high field MRS (H-MRS) gives better SNR.

MR spectrum can be obtained from ^{1}H, ^{23}Na and ^{31}P nuclei and the most common is ^{1}H nuclei. Hydrogen gives higher SNR in shorter time (10–15 min). Chemical shift value in RF provides information about the molecular group to which Hydrogen belongs and express it in ppm.

MR spectroscopy starts with selection of volume of an interest (VOI) in an anatomy. MRS signal is obtained from the preselected voxel volume as an amplitude of proton metabolites from a target tissue. Chemical shifts lie in the frequency range between water and fat. Since, amplitudes of water and fat are greater, they need to be suppressed. To achieve this *chemical shifts-selective (CHESS) or variable pulse power and optimized relaxation delays (VAPOR) or STIR chemical saturation technique* is used. It avoids the superimposition of high peak of water over the signal.

After suppressing water and fat signals, target area volume is localized either by single-voxel spectroscopy (SVS) or multi-voxel spectroscopy (MVS) techniques. Single voxel MRS uses *stimulated echo acquisition mode (STEAM) or point resolved spectroscopy sequence (PRESS) sequences*.

Single voxel uses both long and short TE parameters. It doubles SNR, gives better spectral quality, has more artifacts but commonly used. It gives good quality spectrum, good field homogeneity with short TE. Short TE of 20–40 msec is used which gives higher SNR, less signal loss, more metabolites peaks. Long TE of 135–288 msec gives less SNR, less noisy spectra, and limited number of sharp resonances. After collecting an voxel data, *Fourier transform* is applied to separate composite signal into individual frequencies. Then it is plotted as trace for normal spectrum.

In a multi-voxel spectroscopy, many voxels are imaged simultaneously, and spatial distribution of metabolites are obtained in a single sequence. *Multi-voxel MRS* is followed by *magnetic resonance spectroscopic imaging (MRSI)* in which signal intensity of a single metabolite in an each voxel is color encoded. MRSI determines better spatial heterogeneity. It is according to concentration, and the generated parameter maps is superimposed on an anatomical MR image. Generally, single-voxel technique is used to make an initial diagnosis followed by multi-voxel acquisition.

Magnetic resonance spectroscopy imaging is a noninvasive method that provides spectroscopy information along with generated MR image. It provides frequency spectrum (frequency shift vs relative amplitude) of a tissue based on molecular motion and composition. Peak intensities and position in the spectrum indicate how an atom is bounded to molecule. A raw signal is normally dominated by water spectra that could make all other spectra invisible. Hence, water suppression is needed which is part of MRS technique. It generates regular black and white image whose brightness is based on T1 and T2 relaxation time. Add on spectroscopy infers cellular activity which has applications in oncology.

MRS is prone for artifacts due to motion, poor water or lipid suppression, field inhomogeneity, eddy current, and chemical shift. MRS has application in brain tumors, radiation injury, degenerative changes, hepatic encephalopathy, and cerebral ischemia.

Peaks

Peaks are plotted from right to left along the X-axis, and Y-axis represents the chemical shifts, in ppm unit **(Fig. 14.13)**. Normal choline (Cho), creatine (CR) and *N-acetylaspartate* (NAA) peaks forms a straight line that distended at an angle of 45° from the X-axis. This is known as *Hunter's angle*, which is useful to differentiate normal and an abnormal MRS. Metabolites peaks, caused by frequency shifts relative to a standard frequency can be analyzed. Combination of gradients and RF pulses are used to get signal of a localized rectangular volume. Cho normally comes from certain choline containing compounds which are vital for *membrane synthesis* and *degradation*. Brain tumors usually shows high choline peak due to an increased *membrane turnover*. NAA comes from normal neuronal or an axonal tissue, in brain tissue there is a *loss of neuronal tissue*, leads to reduced NAA.

Spectra obtained from the lesion and surroundings are interpreted based on certain criteria which includes (1) presence of or absence of pathologic metabolites, (2) relationship between concentrations of *Cho, CR, NAA,*

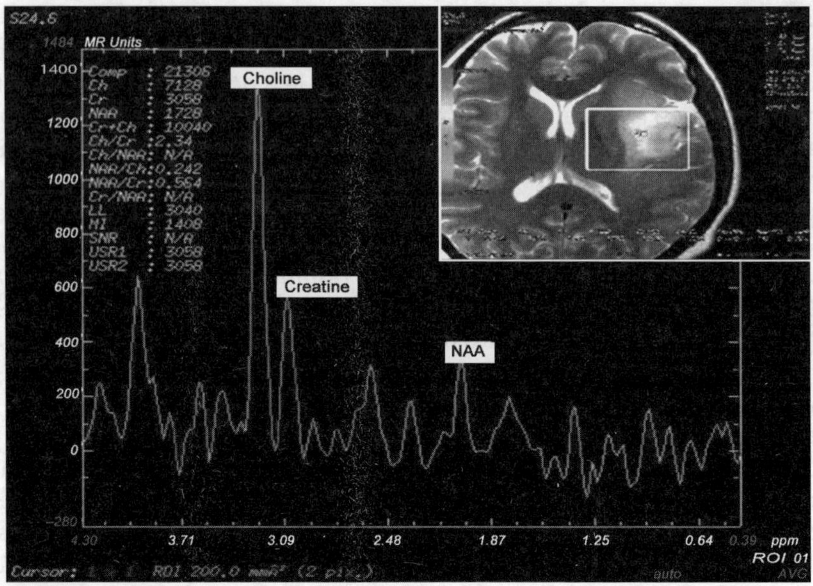

Fig. 14.13: MR spectroscopy of glioma with high T2 signal lesion of insular cortex shows raised choline peak, choline/creatine ratio with decreased N-acetylaspartate (NAA) peak.

(For color version, see Plate 1)

and *lactate* as ratios, e.g., NAA/Cr, NAA/Cho, Cho/Cr. Their normal and an abnormal values are 2, 1.6,1.2 and <1.6, <1.2 and <1.5, respectively. Increase of Cho with depression of NAA peak is seen in *malignancy*. CR peak is also reduced and serve as reference to calculate *metabolites ratio*. Presence of lipid peak indicates *hypoxia* and chances of *high-grade tumor*. Magnet of 3T gives better SNR, faster scans, and improved spectral resolution.

Thus, MRS is useful to identify *metabolic disorders, infections,* and *treatment evaluation.* To study an individual metabolism, sequential imaging with phase-encoding gradient is used. High magnetic field (3 T) is required for good spectral resolution and the field must be an uniform of about 1 ppm. To reduce imaging time, larger pixels (1 cm) are used.

Dixon Method

Dixon method or Dixon technique is an MRI sequence based in chemical shift principle **(W Thomas Dixon, 1984)**. The advantage of this technique is that it is designed to achieve an uniform fat suppression, can be combined with other sequences and weighted sequences, provide images with or without fat suppression from single acquisition, and quantification of fat.

Dixon technique believes that water and fat molecules precess at different rates. It is also believed that they are in-phase and opposed-phase over time. Reasons for this is that circulating electrons in nearby atoms influence the spinning proton and affects proton resonance frequency. For example, H-O bond in water gives small magnetic field relative to H-C bond in lipids. The resonant frequency in fat is 3 ppm is higher in fat than water. Measuring this difference in frequency or *chemical shift* is helpful to study an environment. This difference is enough to separate images of fat and water.

In this method, two spin echo images are obtained with slightly different echo times. The first image contains fat and water in-phase signals at the center of an echo and the second with fat and water out of phase signals after adjusting TE by msec. Both in-phase and opposed-phase images are combined mathematically, resulting four sequences:

1. In-phase image = water + fat
2. Opposed-phase image = water-fat
3. Fat only = in-phase image-opposed-phase image = (Water + fat) – (Water – fat) = 2 × fat
4. Water only = in-phase image + opposed-phase image = (Water + fat) + (Water – fat) = 2 × Water

However, Dixon method requires perfect external field homogeneity and no local susceptibility effects. The current Dixon method combines three echoes produced at different TE times, to get fat only and water only images which helps the quantification of fat. Limitations of modern Dixon is an increased TR time and *fat-water swap* artifact. Dixon technique finds application in abdominal, extremity and spine imaging. Vendors names are IDEAL and Flex (GE Healthcare), DIXON (Siemens), modified Dixon (Philips).

PARALLEL IMAGING MRI

Acquisition time of MRI is proportional to number phase-encoding steps. To reduce time, the phase-encoding steps must be reduced which leads to an *aliasing or wrap around artifacts*. To overcome this, parallel imaging principle is introduced. Parallel imaging is a group of MRI techniques that employs an acquisition that under sample k-space in the phase-encoding direction and eliminates aliasing artifacts. All techniques employ *multi-channel phased array coils* that have multiple independent receiver elements. Each element has an unique location and sensitivity profile which can help MRI signal spatial localization. This will offset the spatial information that is lost with skipped or missed phase-encoding lines.

For example, if four receiver coils are placed around the head, each coil is at different distance from the pixel **(Fig. 14.14)**. The signal received by each pixel varies with function of position. By studying the relative intensity of each coil, it is possible fix the source of MR signal. Thus, one can localize the signal without phase, frequency, and Fourier transform, e.g., from left parietal lobe. The signals from the individual coils are amplified, digitized, and processed simultaneously in parallel along separate channels, retaining their identities up to end. In contrast, in earlier method multiples surface array coils are used. Their individual output is combined in the final signal that is digitized and processed to get an image. Parallel imaging reduced the RF digital processing systems. Modern MRI offers 200 + coils and 128 + receiver channels.

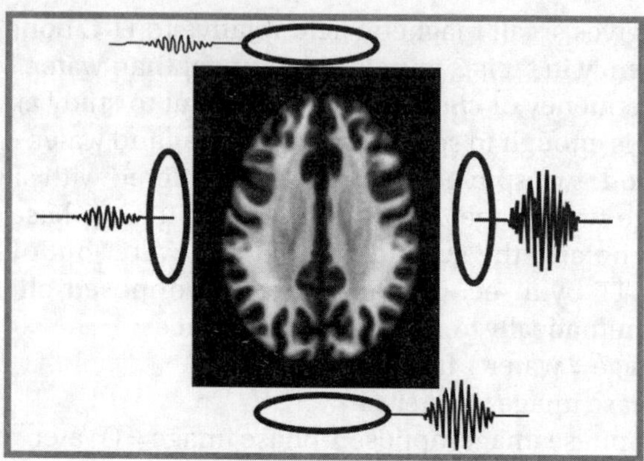

Fig. 14.14: Principle of parallel imaging which assist spatial localization.
(*Courtesy:* AD Elater, Elster LLC, 2023)

There are two concepts in parallel imaging *(1) image domain reconstruction and (2) k-space domain reconstruction.* In the former, aliased pixels are corrected in an image domain after Fourier transformation. It starts with a low-spatial-resolution full FOV acquisition which generates coil sensitivity map from each receiver coil element. The under sampled main pulse sequence is then applied, resulting in an aliased image from each receiver element. The information from the coil sensitivity map is applied to a reconstruction matrix inversion process which unwraps and combine these separate images to form a nonaliased full FOV image. Commercial names of these sequences are: (1) Sensitivity Encoding (SENSE, Pillips), (2) modified Sensitivity Encoding (mSENSE, Siemens Healthineers), and (3) Array Spatial Sensitivity Encoding Technique (ASSET, GE Healthcare).

In k-space reconstruction, an aliasing artifact is corrected in the k-space domain before an image reconstruction. The principle behind is that use of an acquired k-space data to estimate the missing under sampled data with the help of coil sensitivity profiles. First it performs under sampled pulse sequence and acquires an autocalibration signal data near the center of the k-space, as an additional data. This signal has same FOV as in the final image but with lower resolution. This autocalibration signal is used to generate weighting factors for each coil. Application of these weighting factor to an acquired data gives an estimation of the missing under sampled k-space data, for each coil acquisition. Fourier transform creates single coil images, that are combined to form the final image. Commercially available products are: *(1) GeneRalized Autocalibrating Partial Parallel Acquisition (GRAPPA, Siemens Healthineers),* and *(2) Autocalibration Reconstruction for Cartesian imaging (ARC, GE Healthcare).*

Parallel imaging reduces an imaging time by an accelerating factor of 1.5–2. It can be combined with other imaging time reduction techniques to reduce time still further. The number of independent receiver elements used in the multi-channel phased array coil is directly proportional to the acceleration factor. Limitation of parallel imaging is the reduction of SNR with an increasing acceleration factor. It is due to decreased signal acquired in the pulse sequence, geometry of the receiver elements, and reduced sensitivity at the center of the body. SNR can be improved by higher magnetic field, but residual aliasing appears as ghosts inside or outside an image. Residual aliasing arises from inaccurate coil sensitivity maps or errors in the generation of coil weighting factors.

MAGNETIC RESONANCE ANGIOGRAPHY

Magnetic resonance angiography (MRA) is used to study blood flow enhancement in human body. It is alternative to conventional angiography, without an ionizing radiation. It can be done in two ways:
- Noncontrast enhanced MR angiography (NC-MRA)
- Contrast-enhanced MR angiography (CE-MRA)

Noncontrast MR angiography does not use *Gadolinium contrast agent* for an imaging. The mechanism used includes flow-and inflow-related enhancement, suppression of stationary nonvascular background tissue, and use of imaging sequences involving T1 and T2 relaxation time of blood or the phase of MRI signal. NC-MRA can be done in several ways so that blood can appear either white or black **(Figs. 14.15A and B)**.

Dark blood MRA is done with *fast spin echo* acquisitions coupled with dual inversion-recovery magnetization or by other acquisitions. Bright blood NC-MRA is performed by: *(1) Flow independent (Balanced Steady-state Free Precession (bSSFP), (2) Nonsubtractive inflow-dependent-Time of flight (TOF), InFlow-Dependent Inversion Recovery (IFDIR), Quiescent Interval Slice-Selective (QISS), (3) Phase contrast angiography (PC), includes 2D/3D phase*

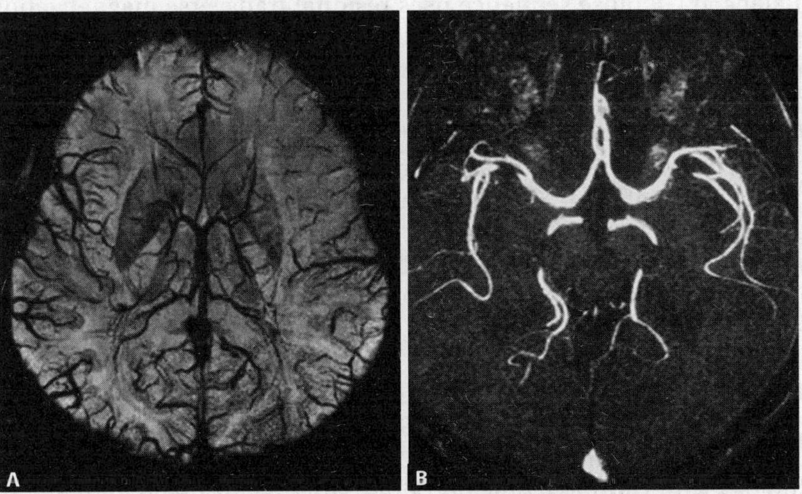

Figs. 14.15A and B: MR special angiogram sequences of brain: (A) Black blood MR angiogram; (B) Bright blood MR angiogram.

contrast and *4D phase contrast, and (4) Subtractive 3D MRA (cardiac gated 3D Fast Spin Echo (3D FSE) or fresh blood imaging, Flow-Sensitive Dephasing (FSD), and Arterial Spin Labeling (ASL).*

The above techniques can visualize an arterial bed of interest or quantifying blood flow. Few techniques are more sensitive to slow or complex flow and others are prone to motion artifacts of limited FOV. TOF is used to access an arteries of head and neck and bSSFP is used in imaging of an aorta and thoracic vessels. Renal arteries are imaged by IFDIR and PC is used to quantify blood flow. Generally above techniques are time consuming relative to contrast enhanced MR angiography.

Contrast-enhanced MR angiography employs T1 weighted 3D spoiled gradient-echo (GE) sequences, with flip angle 25°–50° by administrating *Gadolinium-based contrast agents.* Central k-space acquisition corresponding to an arterial phase of study maximizes visualization of an artery. Use of contrast agent shorten T1 interval of blood, and it appears as white. It is used to access vascular structure of any part of the body.

Flow Independent [Balanced Steady-state Free Precession (bSSFP)]

GE pulse sequence employs gradient refocusing of excited spins to produce signal. After each excitation and gradient refocusing cycle, there will be some residual magnetization that remains in the transverse plane. It is not desirable since it can alter the T1 and T2 weighting of the signal in the next excitation cycle. Hence, techniques are used to remove or spoil the residual magnetization so that the next cycle contains only recovered longitudinal magnetization. This method controls the T1 and T2 weighting of the final image. However, it reduces SNR because the loss of residual transvers magnetization.

Balanced GE pulse sequence uses residual transverse magnetization in the subsequent cycle. Since, the TR is minimized, the residual transvers magnetization is not decay completely before the next excitation. In the subsequent cycle, the recovered longitudinal magnetization is added to the residual transverse magnetization. After several such cycle a steady-state is achieved between longitudinal and residual magnetizations. The outcome signal consists of (1) free induction decay of newly excited longitudinal magnetization, T1 and T2 weighted, and (2) refocused residual transverse magnetization, T2 weighted. In bSSFP or fully refocused GE, longitudinal magnetization, T1 weighted and residual transvers, T2 weighted are recorded. It is a mixture of T1 and T2 weighting.

Application of bSSFP gives bright blood flow effect in MR angiography. Blood inherently possess an increased signal intensity unrelated to flow or contrast injection. Techniques are bSSFP sequences with T1 and T2 weighted and balanced gradient along all three X, Y and Z axis. Image predicts vascular pathology with shorter acquisition time, suitable for pregnant patients, or patient with compromised renal function.

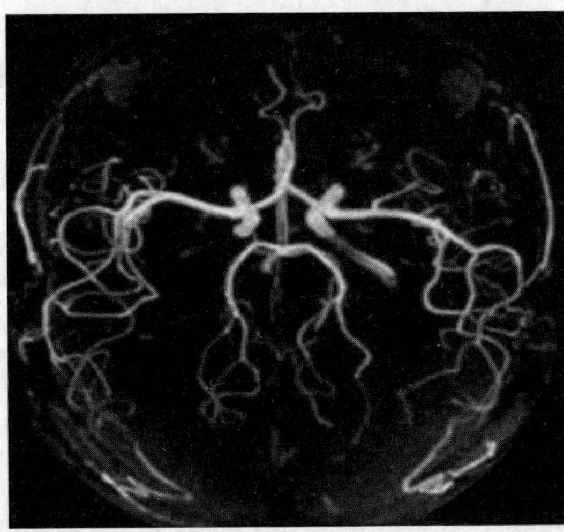

Fig. 14.16: Time of flight (TOF) angiography image to visualize flow within vessels without contrast media.

Time of Flight

Time of flight is an MRI technique which visualize flow within the vessel without contrast administration. The principle is based on flow related signal hyperintensity of spins entering an imaging slice. Since, the spins are unsaturated, they give more signal than surrounding stationary spins. It tags blood in one region and detects it in another region of body to differentiate moving blood from the surrounding. Penetration of tagged blood depends on T1, velocity, and direction of blood. GE techniques like GRASS or FISP are employed to detect unsaturated protons moving into the volume, resulting in high contrast bright blood signal. Image plane is kept perpendicular to flow direction.

In 2D acquisition, multiple thin slices are acquired with flow compensated GE sequence. The images can be combined by *maximum intensity projection (MIP)* algorithm, to get a 3D image of an vessel. MIP extracts highest signals in stack of images along a specific direction in a volume, and project images as function of an angle. This is superimposed on a residual stationary anatomy, to suppress an undesirable signal. The final image is shown as 3D vascular anatomy for various angles around the stack volume **(Fig. 14.16).** In 3D TOF, a volume of an image is obtained simultaneously by phase-encoding in the slice-select direction. MIP is used to get an angiography image.

Limitation of this technique is: (1) signal loss from the vessel due to (1) slow flow or flow from a vessel parallel to the scan plane which may gets saturated like stationary tissue and turbulent flow involving spin's dephasing and unexpected short T2 relaxation, (2) long acquisition time, (3) retrograde arterial flow may be obscured if the venous saturation bands have been applied, (4) ghosting and susceptibility artifacts.

Phase Contrast Angiography

Phase contrast MR angiography is used to visualize and quantify velocity. It is based on phase change that happens in moving protons in the blood. It uses bipolar gradients to produce phase changes in moving blood which are intrinsic to all MR signals. By using bipolar gradient, the degree of phase shifts are encoded and correlated with an velocity of proton.

If an equal and opposite gradient is applied, there is no phase shift in protons. However, the protons that are moving will undergo varying degree of phase shift since their location along the gradient is changing constantly. This principle is used to evaluate protons that are moving through a plane in 2D or space in 3D imaging.

It employs bipolar gradient before the phase-encoding and readout gradients. Consecutive excitations are performed, one gradient with positive polarity and a second gradient with negative polarity, with time delay (bipolar gradient encoding). Protons that are in plane undergo an uniform phase shift during the first gradient application. Protons moving in the direction of the gradient, will encounter different field strength, hence undergo different phase shift. Opposite gradient is applied to remove the phase shift applied to the stationary protons and changes the phase of the protons moving in the direction of the gradient. Faster protons experience a greater difference in an applied gradient than slower protons. Hence, greater phase shift is seen in faster protons. Visual inspection of phase shift map directly gives velocity information. Phase change signal information depends on the time of receipt of echo.

This is helpful to find a correlation between signal intensity and blood flow velocity. MRA is noninvasive, helpful in patients who cannot tolerate an iodinated contrast agents.

PERFUSION WEIGHTED IMAGING

Perfusion refers to delivery of blood at the level of capillaries and it is measured in ml per 100 gram per minute. Perfusion helps delivery of Oxygen, nutrients to the cells and removal of waste (CO_2) from them. It reveals the rate of blood delivery to capillary bed, and it is a measure of metabolic activity. Perfusion is different from bulk blood flow in major arteries and veins. MRI is a powerful in visualizing tissue perfusion in the brain and other parts of the body. *Dynamic Susceptibility Contrast (DSC)-MRI,* and *Dynamic Contrast-enhanced (DCE)-MRI* are exogenous techniques, whereas *Arterial Spin Labeling (ASL)* is an endogenous technique. In an exogenous techniques, contrast agent arrives from outside of tissue, whereas contrast is manipulated by Hydrogen spins within the tissue in an endogenous.

DSC-MRI is an exogeneous contrast-based technique. It involves an intravenous injection of a paramagnetic contrast agent like *Gadolinium chelates* to generate a bolus. *Gd-diethylenetriaminepentacetate* is a non-diffusible blood pool tracer. It performs rapid imaging to capture first pass of the contrast agent. After the injection, T1 and T2 relation time decreases due to an increased superstability effect.

DCE-MRI is another exogeneous-contrast enhanced angiography technique **(Figs. 14.17A and B).** It relies on an injection of a contrast agent, but after the injection the hemodynamic signals depends on T1 and it increases due to T1 shortening effect by contrast. DCE-MRI uses rapid and repeated T1 weighted images to measure signal changes induced by the paramagnetic tracer in tissue as function of time. The contrast agent is also injected intravenously to generate bolus. Extracellular contrast media diffuse the blood into an extravascular extracellular space of tissue at the rate decided by tissue perfusion and permeability of capillaries and their surface area.

Arterial spin labeling (ASL) is an endogenous technique that gives an absolute values of perfusion of tissue by blood. It utilizes an arterial water as an endogenous diffusible tracer which is normally achieved by magnetically labeling the incoming blood. ASL is a noninvasive without an injected contrast. It can be repeated in normal and an abnormal physiology with variation in time. It involves subtraction of two images, one is incoming blood labeled and the other has no labeling. The difference in signal removes the static tissue signal which is about<1%. ASL signal difference depends on blood T1 relaxation time and labeling decay after a long delay time.

Contrast based perfusion needs high temporal resolution. These methods permit an estimation of blood flow, blood volume, and mean transit time (MTT), especially in an acute stroke and tumors. Measurement of contrast

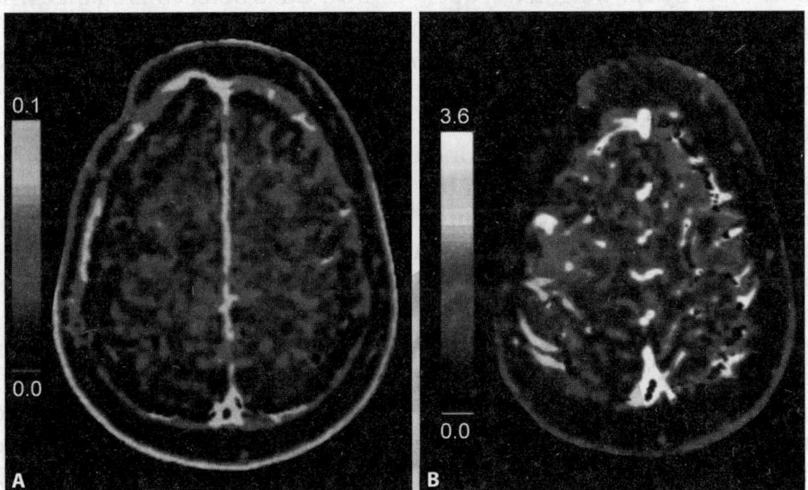

Figs. 14.17A and B: MR perfusion weighted imaging-Dynamic contrast-enhanced perfusion: (A) Axial volume transfer coefficient; (B) Plasma volume map shows mild increase in perfusion in recurrent metastasis in right frontal lobe.
(Courtesy: David Fussell, 2013)

(For color version, see Plate 2)

agent permeability-surface area and fractional volume of an extravascular extracellular space is useful to evaluate diverse diseases. They can be used as biomarkers to access medical or surgical therapy outcomes.

Perfusion weighted MR imaging finds application in the evaluation of an ischemic condition, neoplasm and neurogenerative diseases.

Functional MRI (fMRI)

Functional MRI imaging (fMRI) is used to get functional information about cortical activity. It detects subtle alteration in blood flow against to stimuli or task. Commonly used technique is *blood oxygen level dependent (BOLD) imaging*. It is based on blood oxygenation, blood volume or blood flow changes in brain along with mental activity **(Linus Pauling,** 1936**)**.

Blood flow in brain is controlled in response to Oxygen and Carbon dioxide (CO_2) tension of cortical tissue. When a certain part of cortex increases its activity, an extraction fraction of Oxygen from local capillaries initially drops the *oxygenated hamoglobin (oxy Hb)* and increase in local CO_2 and *deoxygenated haemoglobin (deoxy Hb)*. After a lag of 2–6 seconds, cerebral blood flow (CBF) increases, in turn it supplies surplus oxygenated hemoglobin. Thus, the local tissue oxygenation gets rebound which is being imaged.

There is a fundamental difference between oxy Hb and deoxy Hb. Oxyhemoglobin is diamagnetic and has no effect on signal. Deoxyhemoglobin is a paramagnetic agent, due to an unpaired electrons and produce local dephasing of protons. Thus, reduces the signal from tissues in the immediate vicinity. Heavily $T2^*$ weighted sequences are used to detect this change which is about 1–5%. Since, the effects are short lived, rapid imaging sequences like an *echo planar imaging (EPI) with $T2^*$ weighted (fast GRE)* is used. Thus, deoxyhemoglobin serves as an in-vivo *positive contrast agent* in fMRI study. Its concentration is influenced by variation in an oxygenation and tissue metabolism and signal intensity increases with magnetic field strength.

Blood oxygen level is compared between stimulus and rest, to study brain function. At rest oxyhemoglobin (fully oxygenated blood) and deoxyhemoglobin levels are equal. During activity, more Oxygen is extracted from capillary, resulting increased blood flow that causes change in deoxyhemoglobin.

In BOLD sequence, multiple $T2^*$ weighted images of brain are produced at rest. Later, the patient is subjected to stimulus and again multiple BOLD images are obtained **(Fig. 14.18)**. Rest image data set is subtracted from stimulus data, by voxel. Since, BOLD image depends on blood Oxygen levels, an area of high metabolic activity will show a change in signal. Voxels that define change in signal indicates brain activity due to stimulus/task. The stimulus may be physical, sensory, or cognitive, e.g., finger movement, light lashes or sound, problem solving.

BOLD images are obtained continuously with repeated application of stimulus at periodic intervals. Brain areas show time dependent activity that

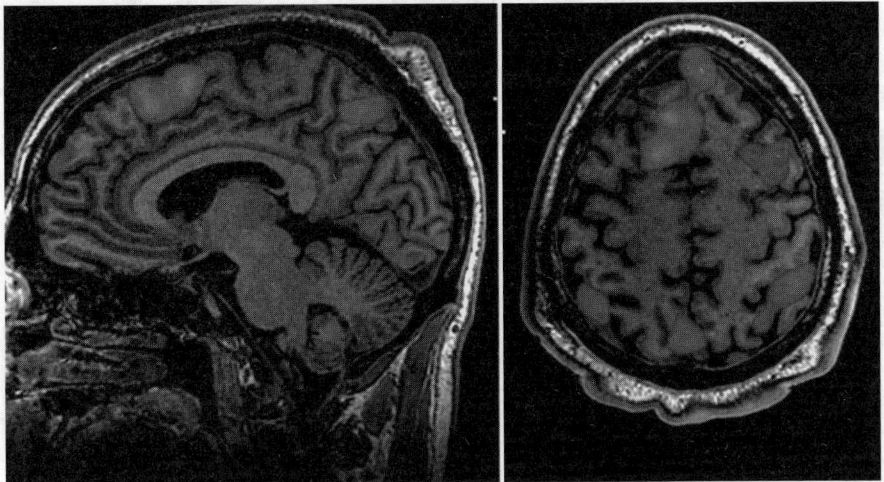

Fig. 14.18: fMRI shows activity of brain.
(For color version, see Plate 2)

correlate with time dependent application of stimulus. This is statistically analyzed by a computer and coded in color scale to generate functional map. It is superimposed on a high-resolution greyscale brain image, to get color overlay.

Limitations of BOLD technique include CBF is only an indirect marker of an activity, smallest area that brain have its blood flow individually regulated is mm dimension, and CBF increases against an increased activity with lag of 2–6 seconds. Technique related limitation includes T2* sequence is susceptible to field inhomogeneity arises from bone-gas interface, hemosiderin/blood products, rapid flow in large veins, and metal. Since, the detected change is so small (1–5%), an artifact may interfere with an image.

DIFFUSION WEIGHTED IMAGING

Diffusion refers to random motion of water molecule due to thermal energy in tissue, referred to as *Brownian motion*. In homogeneous medium, diffusion is random and an isotropic, that is motion is equal in all directions. Hence, in normal state water motion is an isotropic in tissues. In a complex environment, water exhibits directionally dependent diffusion and an anisotropic, that is the motion is not equal in all directions.

In a complex environment, water divided between cells and extracellular compartments. The relative proportion of water distribution between the compartments is affected by pathology process. In such cases, restriction of molecular motion is there due to local cellular structure interactions. Intracellular components offer more restriction than extracellular. Hence, water molecular motion is an anisotropic and direction dependent, e.g., white matter.

Different tissues of human body have characteristic cellular architect and proportion of an intra-and extracellular components hence, they exhibit characteristic diffusion properties. Highly cellular tissues or those with cellular swelling exhibit lower diffusion coefficients. In human body, water diffusion occurs in several compartments: (1) diffusion within an intracellular fluid, within cytoplasm generally and within organelles, (2) diffusion within an extracellular fluid, interstitial fluid, intravascular, lymph, various biological cavities-and extracellular of the brain, and (3) diffusion between intra-and extracellular compartments. Contribution of each one depends on tissue and pathology. Diffusion is more useful in tumor characterization and cerebral ischemia.

Diffusion weighted imaging (DWI) is an MRI technique by which random Brownian motion of water molecule is measured within the voxel of tissue. Diffusion weighted imaging provides both qualitative and quantitative information about diffusion properties. Imaging technique involves two diffusion sensitive gradients, one on either side of 180° refocusing pulse. The gradients are same magnitude but are in an opposite direction. The first gradient lobe is called *dephasing gradient* which will dephase the spin of water molecules. Second gradient is called *rephasing gradient* which will rephase the spins to an original value **(Fig. 14.19)**.

Basic principle of DWI is attenuation of T2* signal based on how water molecules diffuse in that region. DWI involves *spin-echo-echo planar sequence (SE-EPI) or non-EPI techniques (turbo spin echo)*. If the water molecule diffuses easily, lesser initial T2* signal remains. For example, in CSF water can easily diffuse, lower the signal, and the ventricle appear black. In brain parenchyma, diffusion is difficult due to cell membrane, T2* is less attenuated,

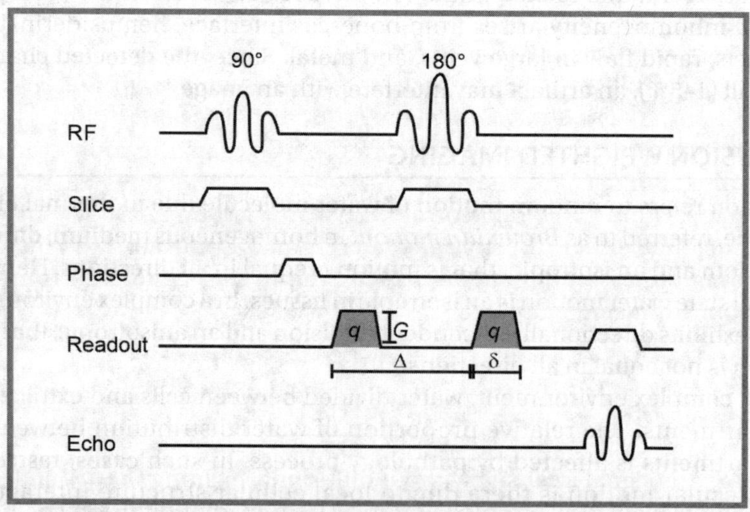

Fig. 14.19: Spin echo diffusion weighted image sequence. Though the both readout diffusion gradients are positive, the 180° RF pulse applied in between them reverses the gradient to negative.

relatively. First a T2* weighted image is obtained with no diffusion, it is known as, $b = 0$ image. The b value measures the degree of diffusion weighting applied, so that it indicates an amplitude (G), time of applied gradient (δ) and duration between the two paired gradients (Δ)t:

$$b = \gamma^2\, G^2\, \delta^2\left(\Delta - \frac{\delta}{3}\right)$$

where, γ is the gyromagnetic ratio. Next, the direction (X, Y and Z) in which water can diffuse easily is accessed. These diffusion gradients can be applied in any axis or in any combination. It is achieved by applying a strong gradient symmetrically on 180° pulse. The degree of diffusion weighting depends on an area under the diffusion gradients and on an interval between gradients. The combination of these factor generates b value. Higher the b value, more pronounced diffusion-related to signal attenuation.

Stationary water molecules (restricted diffusion) acquire phase information by the first gradient. After the 180° pulse, they are exposed to same gradient which nullify the effect of the first gradient. The spins are in phase and produce a strong echo signal.

Moving water molecule acquires phase information by first gradient but they are moving when they are exposed to second gradient. They are not in the same location hence not exposed to precisely the same gradient after 180° pulse. Hence, they are not rephased and they lose some of their signal. The further they move, lesser possibility of rephasing in turn lesser the signal. After the whole process four sets of images are generated:

❑ T2* b = 0
❑ T2* DWI, X-direction
❑ T2* DWI, Y-direction
❑ T2* DWI, Z-direction

These images are combined mathematically to generate maps, containing an isotropic-diffusion weighted images and an *apparent diffusion coefficient (ADC)* maps. ADC is a measure of magnitude of diffusion within tissue and its unit is mm²/s. To generate an isotropic DWI map, the geometric mean of the direction-specific images are calculated. ADC map is related to the natural logarithm (ln) of an isotropic DWI divided by T2* signal for which $b = 0$. It can be either directly calculated from an isotropic DWI images or by finding an arithmetic mean of ADC values (D_l) generated from each directional diffusion map:

$$D = \frac{1}{b}\ln\left(\frac{S_{DWI}}{S_{b=0}}\right)$$

$$D_l = \frac{D_x + D_y + D_z}{3}$$

where, $S_{b=o}$ is signal intensity without diffusion weighting ($b = 0$), and S_{DWI} is signal intensity of an isotropic DWI and D is apparent diffusion coefficient. The D_x, D_y, D_z are an isotropic ADC in X, Y and Z directions, respectively. The signal intensity decreases exponentially as b value increases. At least two DW images required to get a b value, usually first image with

$b = 0$ and another image with $b > 0$ is considered. The image with $b = 0$ provides same contrast as T2 weighted MR image:

DWI finds application in an ischemic stroke, differentiation of epidermoid cyst from an arachnoid cyst, differentiation of abscess from necrotic tumors, Creutzfeldt-Jakob disease (CJD), herpes encephalitis, gliomas, meningiomas, demyelination, grading prostate lesions and cholesteatoma and otitis media. ADC maps predicts pathophysiology in spine, early detection of an ischemic injury, and to measure multiple sclerosis, and structural integrity of certain tissues.

MRI IMAGE QUALITY AND ARTIFACTS

MRI image quality depends on many factors, namely magnetic field strength, pulse sequence, timing, number of excitations, slice thickness, slice separation, matrix size, FOV, presence of contrast and surface coils. MRI scan parameters have trade-off on contrast, noise, resolution, and an image acquisition time. Regular quality control is required to check the functional status of MRI and image quality. Image quality can be discussed under (1) spatial resolution, (2) signal-to-noise ratio, (3) contrast resolution, and (4) artifacts.

Spatial Resolution

Spatial resolution is an ability to differentiate two adjacent objects as an independent images, it is expressed in line pairs per mm (lp mm). It is controlled by matrix, field of view (FOV) and slice thickness. Pixel size depends on matrix size and FOV, e.g., a 25 cm FOV and 256×256 matrix, will have the pixel size of 1 mm for head and 1.4 mm for body images. MRI spatial resolution is about 1–2 lp mm which is 25–50 % of that of CT scan. Resolution is the size of the individual pixel in 2D and voxel in 3D.

$$\text{Pixel size} = \frac{\text{FOV}}{\text{Matrix size}}$$

$$\text{Voxel size} = \frac{\text{FOV}}{\text{Matrix size}} \times \text{Slice thickness}$$

Use of larger matrix size increases number of pixels, increases resolution for a fixed FOV. For example, increasing the matrix size from 4×4 to 8×8 will change the pixel size from 1 mm to 0.5 mm for a given FOV of 4 mm $\times$ 4 mm. Increasing the matrix size, increases spatial resolution due to smaller pixel, decreases signal due to few photons per voxel and increases scan time due to more voxels which requires more signals.

FOV refers to size of an area to be imaged, larger the FOV the larger the voxel size, for a fixed matrix size. For example, increasing the FOV from 4 mm $\times$ 4 mm to 6 mm $\times$ 6 mm will change the pixel size from 1 mm to 1.5 mm, for a given matrix size of 4×4. Increasing the FOV, increases the signal due to large voxel, decreases resolution due to large voxel and increases viewing area.

Increasing slice thickness, increases the signal, decreases resolution, increases partial volume effect, and covers larger imaging area. A slice gap is the amount of space between slices and it is expressed in percentage of slice thickness. Increased slice gap gives lesser crosstalk and increased coverage.

Signal-to-Noise Ratio

Higher signal-to-noise ratio (SNR) means lesser the noise and better the signal. Signal is increased by higher voxel size, decreasing TE, increasing TR, and using higher magnetic field. Noise is a random variation of the MR signal, and present in all frequencies in all time. Noise reduces contrast and it is worse with low proton density and low signal. Factors that influence noise are patient, scanner, and environment. Noise can be reduced by increasing an excitation, reducing bandwidth, reducing crosstalk, and reducing volume of tissue.

The higher the size of the pixel/voxel, more the signal per point and greater the SNR, but lower the resolution. SNR can be increased by scanning the area by number of times or number of acquisitions and taking an average signal to form an image. Increasing the number of acquisitions, increases signal, reduce noise, reduce artifacts, and increases scan time.

Contrast Resolution

Contrast resolution is an ability to distinguish the differences in an image intensity. Inherent contrast of a digital image is measured in pixel values and is defined as number of *bits per pixel value.* MRI has inherent contrast resolution that is an intrinsic which can be modified by scan parameters and use of contrast media. Fat suppression with STIR, will enhance contrast between lesions and an adjacent fatty tissue. T2 weighted image enhances contrast between normal and an abnormal tissue (brighter).

MRI contrast media is *Gadolinium-based contrast agents (GBCA)* which is used in contrast-enhanced MRI scans. Paramagnetic Gadolinium shortens T1, in adjacent tissues, increases an inherent contrast. Super paramagnetic, iron oxide (Fe_3O_4), and *dysprosium (Dy^{3+}) DTPA* produce large local magnetic field and shorten T2 and T2* and the area of uptake, and appear black. *Hyperpolarized (Xenon-129 exposed to laser)* gas as contrast dissolves in blood and shows large *chemical shift.* It can be used with low magnetic field, to give large SNR, e.g., lung, low field angiography and spectroscopy imaging.

MRI Artifacts

Image artifact is one that is visible on an image, but the structure is not actually present in the patient. It may be due to malfunction of software or hardware or patient body or an environment. They present as positive or negative intensities which can limit the diagnostic potential. Some artifacts affect the MRI image quality, and some do not, however may be confused with pathology. It should be compensated wherever possible to avoid pathology being misjudged. The physician and technologist must identify the artifacts and understand their causes to produce good quality images. Knowledge about impact of an acquisition protocols, an etiology of artifact production

Table 14.3: Various artifacts commonly occurring in MRI.

Source	Artifacts
Software	• Slice-overlap artifact (Crosstalk artifact) • Cross excitation
Hardware and room shielding	• Zipper artifact • Herringbone artifact • Zebra stripes • Moiré fringes • Central point artifact • RF overflow artifact • Inhomogeneity artifact • Shading artifact • Aliasing artifact (Wrap around artifact) • Starry sky artifact
Tissue inhomogeneity and foreign bodies	• Black boundary artifact • Magic angle effect • Magnetic susceptibility artifact ▪ Blooming artifact • Chemical shift artifact • Dielectric effect artifact
Patient and physiological motion	• Phase-encoded motion artifact ▪ Ventricular CSF pulsation artifact • Entry slice phenomenon
Fourier transform and Nyquist sampling theorem	• Gibbs artifact/Truncation artifact • Zero-fill artifact • Aliasing/Wrap around artifact

(*Courtesy:* Chikara Noda et al, 2022; Andrew Murphy 2023)

will enhance the goal of achieving good diagnostic images. Most artifacts can be eliminated or minimized by adjusting the imaging parameter.

MRI artifacts are caused by software, hardware and room shielding, pulse sequence, patient and physiological motion, tissue heterogeneity and foreign bodies, and Fourier transform and Nyquist sampling theorem **(Table 14.3)**. Some common artifacts are (1) aliasing artifacts, (2) motion artifacts, (3) susceptibility artifacts, (4) streak artifact, (5) zipper artifact, and (6) chemical shift artifact.

Aliasing Artifact

Aliasing or wraparound artifacts is quite common that occurs when FOV is smaller than the body part being imaged. The part of the body that lies outside the FOV is projected on the other side of an image, in the phase-encoding direction. The image appears fold-over or wrapround, hence the name wraparound artifact **(Fig. 14.20A)**. It can be corrected by oversampling the data twice as fast in the frequency direction. The number of phase-encoding steps can be increased but it increases scan time. If the FOV and matrix size is increased with reduction of an excitation to half, increase in an imaging time can be avoided.

Chemical Shift Artifact

Chemical shift artifact is due to difference in resonance frequency of fat and water. It occurs as displacement in the frequency encoding direction. It is due to the electron cloud which shields the nucleus from an external magnetic field. Precession frequency of Hydrogen differs in fat and water and different tissues will have slightly different Larmor frequency. Stronger the magnetic field the higher the chemical shift. Chemical shift may lead to spatial misregistration of the MR signal. It is common in MRI sequences used in magnetic resonance spectroscopy.

Chemical shift artifact can be controlled by reducing the magnetic field, increasing the gradient strength/receiver bandwidth, or decreasing the voxel size, fat suppression imaging and use of spin echo sequence instead of GE. This artifact more dominant in T2 weighted image than T1 weighted.

Gibbs Artifact

Gibbs or *Truncation artifact* refers to series of lines in MR image parallel to abrupt and intense changes in an object at this location. At high contrast boundaries the Fourier transform has an infinite number of frequencies whereas MR sampling is finite. This discrepancy manifests in the reconstructed image as series of lines. It appears in both phase and frequency directions.

Remedial measures are increasing the matrix size, use of smoothing filters and use of fat suppression if fat is at the boundary. Higher the encoding steps the less intense the artifacts.

Zipper Artifact

Zipper artifact is mainly due to RF interference signals contaminating received imaging data. It appears perpendicular to the frequency direction. It appears black and white signal band over an entire image **(Fig. 14.20B)**. Single frequency gives single band and multiple frequency gives multiple bands. Zipper is related to hardware or software problems in the scanner or in the shielding. It can be controlled by closing the room door during an acquisition so that RF from an electronic equipment cannot enter the scanning room.

Motion Artifact

Motion artifact is a patient related artifact that occurs due to voluntary and involuntary movement of tissue/fluid during an imaging. Motion artifacts cause blurring, reduce contrast, produce ghost images, and appear in the phase-encoding (slow event) direction. It is seen from an arterial pulsation, swallowing, breathing, peristalsis, and physical movement and can mimic pathology. Random motion like patient movement produces smear in the phase direction. Periodic motion like respiratory, or cardiac pulsation produce discreate, well defined ghosts. Motion artifacts can be differentiated from Gibbs or truncation since they extend over entire FOV.

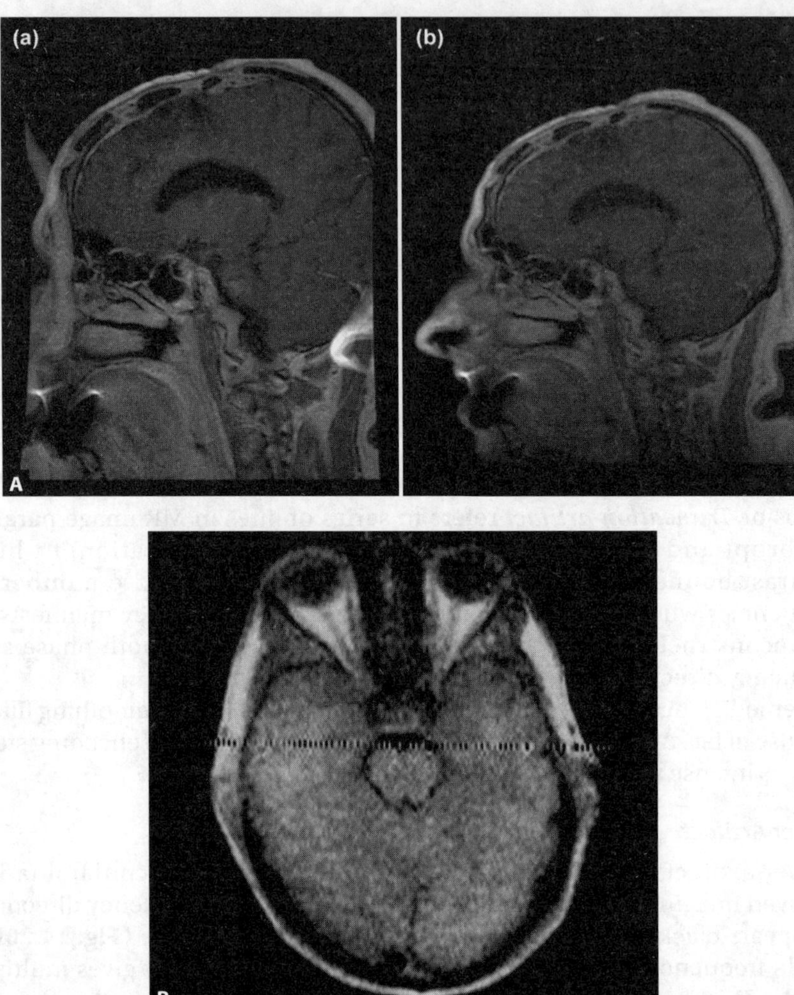

Figs. 14.20A and B: MRI artifacts: (A) Aliasing artifact (wraparound) in brain MRI: (a) FOV 24 cm × 18 cm, (b) FOV in increased to 24 cm × 24 cm to control artifact; (B) Zipper artifacts due to RF transmitter leakage.

Correction methods are cardiac/respiratory gating, spatial pre-saturation bands placed over moving tissues/outside the FOV, scanning prone to reduce an abdominal excursion, switching phase and frequency directions, increasing the number of signal averages and shorten the scan time.

Susceptibility Artifact

Susceptibility artifact arises while imaging near an orthopedic metallic hardware or dental work. It is displayed as localized signal loss, though high signal intensity is seen along the periphery of the signal void. It is due to local magnetic field inhomogeneity offered by the metallic objects. It depends on the property of the metal object being imaged. As a result, small lesion may appear more conspicuous, referred to as *blooming artifact*. Types of artifact include paramagnetic, diamagnetic and ferromagnetic.

Removal of metal can reduce such artifacts. However, cerebral artery clip, an embolic coil or pacemaker cannot be removed, and some degree of artifact remains in an image. Some time it is helpful in diagnosis, e.g., age of hemorrhage, since hemoglobin contains Iron, which is ferromagnetic. This artifact is more seen in GE than spin echo sequence.

QUALITY CONTROL

Quality assurance is a concept designed by the user to ensure that: given procedure is appropriate, information generated offer solution to the objective, correct interpretation of an image, and procedure is done with lower risk, low cost, and without much inconvenience to the patient. A quality assurance committee (QAC) is formed with radiologists, medical physicists, and senior technologists as members. They must realize their responsibilities and execute them properly.

Radiologists responsibilities include selecting a technologist, providing an orientation program for technologist, conduction quality control (QC) program, availability of test equipment and phantoms, selection of medical physicist, review of QC test results, oversee safety program and records and employing established protocols. Quality control is a part of quality assurance and consists of series of technical procedures that ensure the production of satisfactory high quality images:

- ❑ Acceptance testing during installation or after major repair
- ❑ Base line performance establishment
- ❑ Detection and diagnosis of changes in equipment performance before they become apparent in images
- ❑ Verification that causes of deterioration of equipment performance have been corrected.

Major repair includes replacement or repair of gradient amplifier, gradient coil, magnet, RF amplifier, digital boards, and signal processing boards.

Phantoms

Quality control test requires phantoms and test accessories. *American college of radiology (ACR)* MRI accreditation phantom is usually used which has two phantoms, large and small **(Fig. 14.21)**. Large phantom is used for whole body magnets and small phantom is used for an extremity magnet. A large phantom is a short, hollow cylinder of an *acrylic plastic* closed at both ends. Its inner dimensions are 148 mm length × 190 mm diameter. Phantom is filled with solution of *Nickal chloride and Sodium chloride (10mM NiCl$_2$ and 75 mM Nacl)*. In the outer, it is marked as NOSE and CHIN which is used for the orientation of the phantom. Small ACR phantom is same as that of large phantom except its dimension is 100 mm length × 100 mm diameter. Both

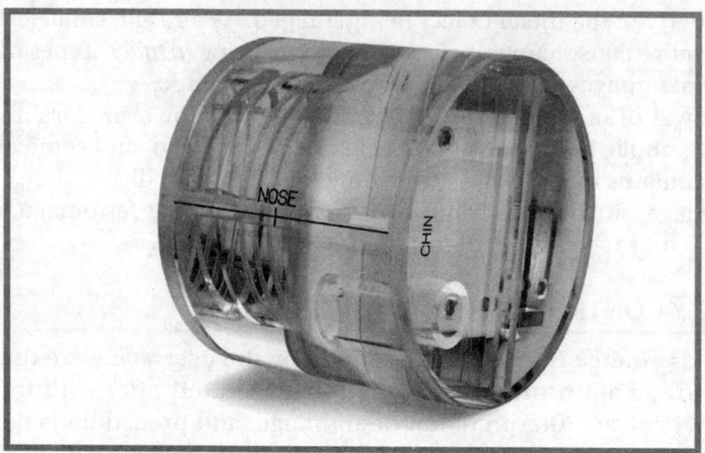

Fig. 14.21: ACR accredited MRI phantom.
(*Courtesy:* American College Radiology, 2015)

phantoms have a separate vial filled with 20 mM $NiCl_2$. Inside phantoms have structures that can perform the following tests:

☐ Geometric accuracy
☐ High-contrast spatial resolution
☐ Slice thickness accuracy
☐ Slice position accuracy
☐ Image intensity uniformity
☐ Percent signal ghosting
☐ Low-contrast detectability

ACR manual describes the various test parameters for performance evaluation, frequency of test and the procedure. Personnel should have enough training to use the QC gadgets. phantom QC test should be performed weekly and annually **(Table 14.4)**. Most of the test can be carried out by ACR

Table 14.4: Quality control test required for system performance evaluation with MRI test phantom.

S. No.	Test	Technologist/ Weekly	Medical physicist/ Annually
1.	Set-up and table position accuracy	Yes	Yes
2.	Center frequency	Yes	Yes
3.	Transmitter gain or attenuation	Yes	Yes
4.	Geometric accuracy measurements	Yes	Yes
5.	High-contrast spatial resolution	Yes	Yes
6.	Low-contrast detectability	Yes	Yes
7.	Artifact evaluation	Yes	Yes
8.	Fil printer quality control if any	Yes	Yes

Contd...

Contd...

9.	Visual check list	Yes	Yes
10.	Magnetic field homogeneity		Yes
11.	Slice position accuracy		Yes
12.	Slice thickness accuracy		Yes
13.	Radiofrequency coil checks • SNR • Percent image uniformity (PIU) • Percent signal ghosting (PSG)		Yes
14.	Soft-copy (monitor) quality control		Yes
15.	MR safety program assessment		Yes

(*Courtesy:* ACR, Quality Control, 2015)

test phantom. In addition, SMPTE phantoms is used and it is made by the *society of motion picture* and *television engineers*. It is used to evaluate display systems of medical diagnostic imaging. All measures data and test results are recorded in a log. The log should have the following:

❑ QC policy and procedures
❑ Data forms and results recorded
❑ Notes on QC problems and corrective measures

BIBLIOGRAPHY

1. Agazzi GM. MR Spectroscopy, Radiopaedia.org, 2023.
2. Allisy-Roberts PJ, Williams J. Farr's Physics for Medical Imaging, 2nd edn. Elsevier, 2008.
3. Bushong SC, Clarke G. Magnetic Resonance Imaging: Physical and Biological Principles, Elsevier, 2015.
4. Fussell D, Young RJ. Role of MRI in improving the treatment brain tumors: Imaging in Medicine, 2013; 5(5).
5. Graves MJ, Mitchell DG. Body MRI artifacts in clinical practice: A Physicist's and Radiologist's Perspective. J Magn Reson Imaging, 2013; 38:269-287.
6. https://www.scribd.com.
7. IMAIOS Inc. C/o Orbiss Inc, 1411 Broadway, Floor 16th, New York 10018, USA: Contact @imaios.com.
8. Joshua Yap Diffusion-weighted imaging. Radiopaedia, 2023.
9. Kozak BM, Jaimes C, Kirsch J, Gee MS. MRI techniques to decrease imaging times in children. RSNA RadioGraphics, 2020; 40(2).
10. Magnetic Resonance Imaging Quality Control Manual. American College of Radiology, 2015.
11. Murphy A. MRI Artifacts. Radiopaedia, Feb 6, 2023.
12. Navot B, Hecht EM, Lim RP, Edelman RR, Koktzoglou I. MR Angiography series: fundamentals of non-contrast-enhanced MR angiography. RadioGraphics 2021; 41:E157-E158.
13. Noda C, Venkatesh BA, Wagner JD, Kato Y, Ortman JM, Lima J AC. Primer on commonly occurring MRI artifacts and how to overcome them. RadioGraphics, 2022; Vol 42: E102-E103.
14. Wymer DT, Patel KP, Burke WF, Bhatia VK. Phase-contrast MRI: Physics, Techniques, and Clinical Applications. RadioGraphics, 2020;40(1).

Radiological Health and Safety

INTRODUCTION

Hazards of radiation were realized soon after the discovery of X-rays and gamma rays. *British X-ray* and *Radium protection committee* (1921) was renamed as *International Committee on X-ray and Radium Protection*, in turn the *International Commission on Radiological Protection (ICRP, 1928)*. ICRP reports form the basis for many National and International radiation protection programs. ICRP's latest report 103 (2007) provides recommendations for workers, patients and public. *International Commission on Radiological Units and Measurements* (ICRU) recommends units for radiation measurements.

In India, radiation protection was conceived by the formation of *Division radiological protection (DRP), Bhabha Atomic Research Center (BARC)*, Mumbai. *Atomic Energy Act, 1962* and *Radiation Protection Rules (RPR)-1977* formed the basis for radiation protection in India. Government of India established a competent authority, *Atomic Energy Regulatory Board (AERB, 1983)* to implement radiation safety both medicine and industry. *Atomic Energy (Radiation Protection) Rules, 2004*, provides necessary regulatory infrastructure for an effective implementation of radiation protection program in India.

DOSE PARAMETERS AND UNITS

Equivalent Dose

To account different biological effectiveness of different kinds of radiation, the *International Commission on Radiological Protection (ICRP)* have introduced the concept of an *equivalent dose* for radiation protection purposes. In this, an absorbed dose is weighed by a factor to account for its *relative biological*

Table 15.1: Radiation weighting factors (W_R), (ICRP-103, 2007).

Radiation type	W_R
Photons (X, γ)	1
Electrons and muons	1
Protons and charged pions	2
Alpha particles, fission fragments, heavy ions	20
Neutrons	Continuous curve as a function of neutron energy (2.5–20)

effectiveness (RBE). The above factor is known as *radiation weighting factor (W_R)*. The product of absorbed dose and radiation weighting factor is called an *equivalent dose (H)*:

$$H = D \times W_R$$

where, D is absorbed dose and W_R is weighting factor for a given radiation type. The weighting factor is 1 for X-rays, gamma rays and electron of all energies **(Table 15.1)**. High LET radiation may cause higher biological effect, hence, have higher radiation weighting factor.

SI unit of an equivalent dose is *sievert (Sv)* and 1 Sv = 1 J/kg, and its special unit is *rem*. Rem is a short form of *radiation equivalent men* and 100 rem is equal 1 Sv. In practice, milli sievert (mSv) and micro sievert (μSv) are used as units: 1 mSv = 100 mrem and 1 μSv = 0.1 mrem. For diagnostic radiology and radiation therapy, 1 roentgen (R) = 1 rad or 1 rem since the radiation weighting factor is unity.

Effective Dose

The relationship between probability of stochastic effect and an equivalent dose depends on an organ or tissue that is irradiated. ICRP defined a quantity which indicates relative sensitivity of different tissues correlated with total stochastic effects. This factor is known as *tissue weighting factor (W_T)*. It is used to weight equivalent dose in a tissue or an organ and represents its relative contribution to total detriment, resulting from an uniform irradiation of whole body. ICRP has established tissue weighting factors (W_T) for different tissues **(Table 15.2)**. *Bone marrow, colon, lung, stomach,* and *breast* the are most sensitive tissues towards radiation exposure. Organ of higher sensitivity carries a higher risk for a given radiation dose. Sum of all weighting factors is unity. Sum of the products of an equivalent dose to each tissue irradiated (H_T) and the corresponding weighting factor of tissue is called an *effective dose (E)*:

$$E = \sum W_T \times H_T$$

where, W_T is weighting factor of tissue T and H_T is mean equivalent dose received by the tissue T. Effective dose expresses an overall measure of health detriment associated with each irradiated tissue as a whole-body dose and considers radio sensitivity of each irradiated tissue. SI unit of an effective dose is Sv.

Table 15.2: Tissue weighting factors (W_T), (ICRP-103, 2007).

Tissue	W_T	Total contribution
Bone marrow, colon, lung, stomach (4 tissue)	0.12	0.48
Breast (1)	0.12	0.12
Gonads (1)	0.08	0.08
Bladder, esophagus, liver, thyroid (4)	0.04	0.16
Bone surface, skin (2)	0.01	0.02
Salivary gland, brain (2)	0.01	0.02
Remainder*	0.12	0.12
Total		1.0

*Remainder tissues: Adrenals, gallbladder, heart, kidneys, lymphatic nodes, muscle, oral mucosa, pancreas, prostate, small intestine, spleen, thymus, uterus, extrathoracic region.

SOURCES OF RADIATION

Every individual is exposed to radiation from sources such as (1) natural radiation sources or background, (2) artificial radiation sources (manmade), and (3) occupational exposures **(Fig. 15.1)**. Natural radiation sources include (1) cosmic rays, (2) terrestrial radionuclides and (3) internal radioisotopes. Annual average per capita total effective dose equivalent is 3.0 mSv **(Table 15.3)**. About 82% of the above exposure arises from naturally occurring sources, 18% arises from an artificial radiation sources, in which medical X-rays is a major contributor (58%). Background radiation involves both natural and manmade low level radiation exposure to all members of the public. This will vary with region, *Kerala* and *northern Iran* have high background levels of radiation of 12.5 and 260 mSv/year, respectively.

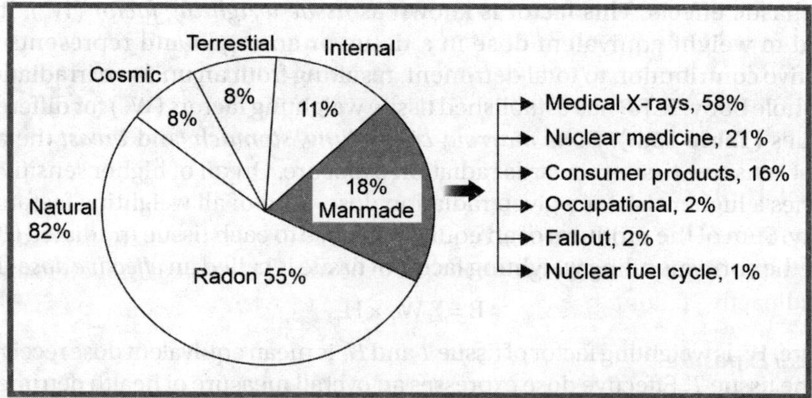

Fig. 15.1: Different sources of radiation (ICN) and their contribution in percentage (NCRP-93, US).

Table 15.3: Mean annual radiation exposure per person by ionizing radiation (IAEA, 2000).

Sources	Mean dose (range), mSv
Cosmic rays	0.4 (0.3–1.0)
Terrestrial	0.5 (0.3–0.6)
Inhalation (Radon)	1.2 (0.2–10)
Ingestion	0.3 (0.2–0.8)
Medical	0.4 (0.04–1.0)
Nuclear testing	0.15
Nuclear power production	0.0002
Total	2.95

Natural Radiation Sources

Cosmic Rays

Cosmic rays are energetic protons and alpha particles comes from the outer world, contributes about 0.4 mSv/year **(Table 15.3)**. Primary cosmic rays are protons (80%) that collide with an atmosphere, producing showers of secondary particles (electrons, muons) and electromagnetic radiations. Cosmic ray exposure increases with an altitude, it is doubling in every 1500 m, and it is greater at the earth poles than an equator. An air traveler of a transcontinental flight may be exposed to 5 mSv per year at a rate of about 10 μSv per hour. Cosmic ray's effective exposure is 20% lesser in an indoor than outdoor.

Terrestrial Radionuclides

Terrestrial radionuclides are present in the earth and contribute an external exposure *(K-40, U-238, and Th-232)*, inhalation, and ingestion. Biggest contributor of terrestrial radiation is *Radon gas (Rn-222)*, which is emitted from *U-238* in soil of the order of 2 mSv per year. Radon is an alpha emitter with half-life of 4 days, its daughters may attach to an aerosols and deposits in lungs. This may irradiate *bronchial mucosa* leading to an induction of *bronchogenic cancer*. Radon levels vary, it is high in low-raise and poorly ventilated buildings and its maximum limit is 160 Bq/m³. Internal radionuclide includes K-40 and C-14, present in human body from birth that contributes about 0.4 mSv/year.

Artificial Sources

Artificial or manmade sources of radiation include (1) medical exposure, (2) consumer products, (3) occupational exposure, (4) nuclear fuel cycle and (5) radioactive fallout.

Medical Exposure

Majority of medical exposure is from medical X-rays and Nuclear medicine. Both produce an annual average effective dose equivalent of 0.4 mSv/y, which is about 79% of an artificial radiation. Medical X-rays dose arises mainly from fluoroscopy and computed tomography. Effective dose in CT, interventional radiology and Nuclear medicine are 6.6 mSv, 8.6 mSv and 11.6 mSv per procedure, respectively. Effective doses from radiography, mammography and dental are 0.7 mSv, 0.1 mSv and <0.1 mSv per exposure, respectively which are much low. Population average dose increases mainly from CT scan use which increases at the rate 10% per year.

Consumer Products

Consumer products such as *tobacco, Radon gas dissolved in* domestic water supply, building materials such as *brick, concrete,* and *granite* which consists of Uranium, Thorium, and Potassium. To a lesser extent *smoke detector (Americium-241), gas lantern mantles (Thorium), dental prostheses, certain ceramics, optical lenses (Uranium),* televisions, and *computer screens.* Totally it accounts 0.1 mSv /y and accounts 16% of an artificial radiation.

Occupational Exposure

Occupational exposure of 2% arises from *Uranium mining, nuclear power operations, medical diagnosis* and *therapy, aviation and research, non-uranium mining, and agriculture.* Uranium miners, nuclear power operators, air crews, X-ray technologists and radiologists receive an annual effective dose equivalent of 12, 5, 1.7, 1.5 and 0.7 mSv/y respectively. Agricultural activity contributes to a lesser degree by fertilizers *(Uranium, Thorium decay products, and K-40).*

Nuclear fuel cycle and radioactive fallout contribute 0.004 mSv/y, and 0.01 mSv/y, respectively. Atmospheric testing of nuclear weapons gives out *Carbon-14* and radionuclides such as *H-3, Mn-54, Cs-136, 137, Ba-140, Ce-144, Plutonium* and *Transplutonium elements.*

BIOLOGICAL EFFECTS OF RADIATION

When radiation incident on human body, atoms and molecules absorbs energy and release electrons. Electrons transfer this energy to their surrounding by excitation, ionization, thermal heating, and production of δ rays, referred to as *physical stage* **(Fig. 15.2)**. Transfer of energy to molecules such as water gives free radicals which interact with *deoxyribonucleic acid (DNA),* resulting molecular alterations. Such structural changes include *Hydrogen bond leakage, molecular degradation,* and *inter-and intra-molecular cross-linking,* referred to as *chemical stage.*

Majority of lesions are repaired and lesions that are not repaired result in *cellular death or mutation in cells,* referred to as *biological stage.* Increased number of cell death may lead to an organ death and appear as clinical changes, e.g., *lethality, mitotic inhibition, division delay, chromosome aberration and induction of mutations.* Cells may take time to die and undergo *mitotic division* before death. This results two type of cell population, namely *dead cells and surviving cells.* A plot drawn with *dose vs survival fraction of cell* is known as *survival curve and it is an* exponential. Mutation can occur

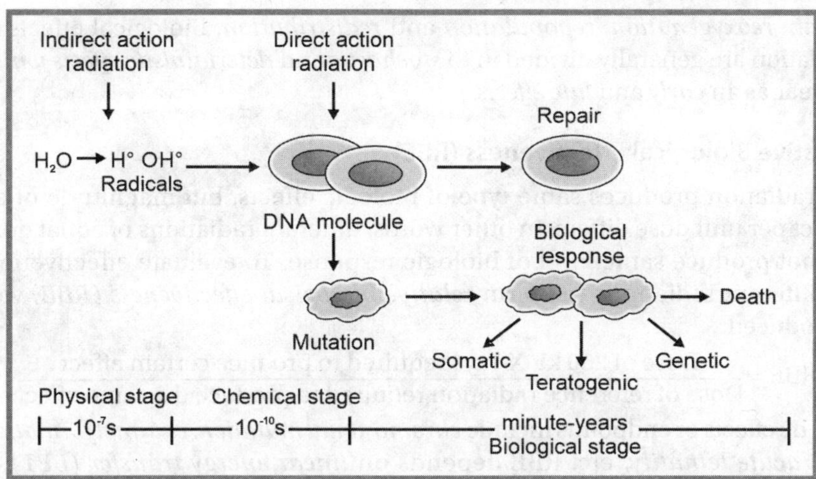

Fig. 15.2: Radiation interaction with cell: physical, chemical, and biological stages.

both in *germ cells* and *somatic cells.* Death of stem cell appear as *early effects*, mutation in germ cells leads to *hereditary effects* and mutation in somatic cells results *induction of cancer.*

Biological effects can be from direct and an indirect action of radiation. *In direction action*, radiation directly interacts DNA target and causes biological effects. It is common in high LET radiation which causes *rupture of cell membrane, breaking of chromosome structure resulting DNA strand breaks,* and *chromosome aberrations.* In an indirect action, radiation interacts with water molecule and forms *free radicals (H^*, OH^*, and HO_2^*)* which interacts with DNA and cause biological effects. Free radicals are an atom or molecule or an ion that has an unpaired electron in the outer shell. They are highly reactive and interacts strongly with biomolecules and is a major source of radiation damage. This is the most common and dominant in low LET radiation due to abundant of water in human body, e.g., X-and gamma rays.

Effects of radiation on cells depends on (1) radiation quality, (2) dose rate, (3) dose fractionation, (4) cell cycle stage, (5) Oxygen tension, (6) presence of chemical protectors and sensitizers, and (6) recovery and repair process. High LET radiations are much more effective in cell killing than low LET radiation. High dose rate or high dose per fraction are much effective in cell killing. Cells in the S-phase is more resistance than at G2 and M phase of the cell cycle. Oxygen is a best sensitizer which can increase cell killing by a factor of 3. Tumor with *hypoxic cells* tends to reduce radiation effects hence, radiation is fractionated.

Whole body radiation exposure is more critical than partial body irradiation. Radiation delivered in multiple fractions is less effective than that of single fraction (acute) radiation. Clinical radiotherapy treatments involving external beams follow multiple fractions as partial body irradiation. Justification of fractionation is well understood by 4Rs of radiobiology, namely *repair, reoxygenation, repopulation* and *redistribution*. Biological effects of radiation are generally divided in to *stochastic* and *deterministic effects which* appear as an *early* and *late effects.*

Relative Biological Effectiveness (RBE)

All radiation produces same type of biologic effects, but magnitude of an effect per unit dose differs. In other words, different radiations of equal dose do not produce same level of biologic response. To evaluate effectiveness of different radiations the term *relative biological effectiveness (RBE)* was introduced:

$$RBE = \frac{\text{Dose of 250 kV X-rays required to produce certain effect}}{\text{Dose of reference radiation required to produce the same effect}}$$

The effects or endpoints include *chromosomal mutation, cataract formation* and *acute lethality,* etc. RBE depends on *linear energy transfer (LET)* of radiation in a medium. LET is a parameter that describes an average energy deposition per unit path length of an incident radiation, and it is expressed in keV/μm. RBE also depends on total dose and dose rate of radiation. RBE values of X and gamma rays and electrons is 1, whereas it is 2, 2.5–20, and 20 for protons, neutrons, and heavy particles, respectively.

Stochastic Effect

A stochastic effect is one in which the probability of an occurrence increases with an increasing absorbed dose rather than its severity. It is due to changes in cell mutation after radiation exposure. It has no threshold dose and important at low doses, be seen only with *latent period* **(Fig. 15.3A)**, e.g., *carcinogenesis* and *hereditary effects.* Stochastic means random and severity of stochastic effect is an independent of radiation dose. For example, *leukemia, thyroid cancer, breast cancer, lung cancer, bone cancer* and *skin cancer* are radiation induced cancer in humans.

It is dependent of sex and age at the time of exposure. Even a smallest dose has probability to cause stochastic effect, which is significant in diagnostic energy X-ray range. Dose vs stochastic effect is a linear plot which is extrapolated from the response of higher doses from an atomic bomb survivors data. The plot reveals that stochastic effect starts from zero dose and confirm the statement that *no dose is a safe dose.* The dose-effect relationship <100 mSv is not verified hence, doses should be kept *as low as reasonably achievable (ALARA),* to minimize stochastic effects. Stochastic effects are also often classified into *somatic and genetic effects.*

Carcinogenesis

Radiation causes both benign and malignant tumor, carcinogenesis is a *stochastic effect.* It is a week carcinogen in medical exposures. *Bone marrow, colon, lung, female breast, stomach,* and *thyroid in children* are more radiosensitive for malignancy, whereas *bladder, liver* and *esophagus* are moderately sensitive. Time interval between time of an irradiation and an appearance of malignancy is referred as *latent field*. It indicates tissue sensitivity and inversely proportional to dose. Latent period varies with an age and gender of an exposed individual.

Latent period of leukemia is 2–3 years, whereas it is 5–40 years for solid tumors. Probability of an ovarian cancer is 3 times higher for 10 years old female than 50 years old. Probability of cancer induction increases with *dose, radiation quality, dose rate,* and *fractionation* without threshold. Low LET radiation causes less damage than high LET and it is easily repaired. High LET damages are irreparable and increases cancer incidence in *lung, thyroid,* and *bone.* Epidemiological and A-bomb survivor's studies have demonstrated an induction of *malignancy* in humans.

Hereditary Effects

Radiation effects due to irradiation of germ cells are referred to as *hereditary or genetic effects.* It is stochastic in nature without threshold dose, likely up to two generations of an exposed individual. It is from the result of radiation exposure to gonads, resulting in chromosome mutations. *There is no epidemiological evidence of genetic effect in humans* and *current estimates are based on animal experiments.* A-bomb survivors have not shown any increased hereditary effects.

Deterministic Effects

A deterministic effect is one in which severity of harm increases with an increasing absorbed dose due to degenerative changes in tissues in an individual. It has threshold dose (2 Gy) below which no radiation effect is seen, always appear at high doses. The dose vs deterministic effect is a *sigmoid plot* indicating a threshold and shoulder **(Fig. 15.3B)**. In this, radiation interacts with group of cells of tissue or an organ that end up with loss of tissue function, e.g., *skin erythema, cataract, epilation, organ atrophy, fibrosis, reduction of blood changes* and *sperm count, etc.*

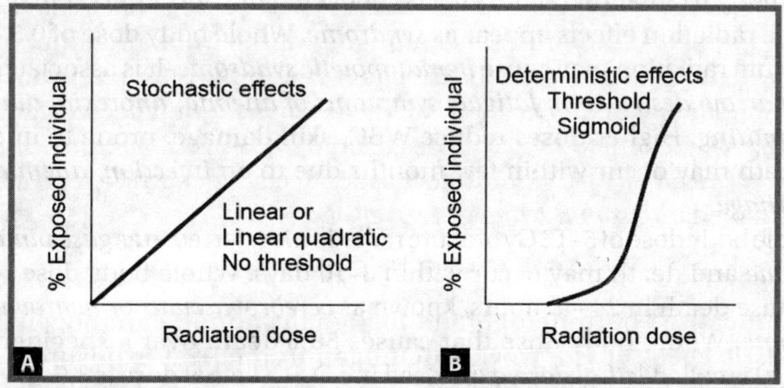

Figs. 15.3A and B: Dose response curves: (A) Stochastic effect; (B) Deterministic effect.

Early effects appear within a few weeks after radiation exposure as (1) injury of individual organ (local) due to partial body irradiation, (2) acute radiation syndrome (common) due to whole body exposure. *Late effects* appear within a few months-year after an irradiation, e.g., *radiation dermatitis, cataract, teratogenic effects on embryo* and *fetus.* Radiation protection aims to prevent all deterministic effects by keeping radiation exposure low.

Individual Organ Effects

Radiation effects on *skin* causes an *erythema, pigmentation, dermatitis, ulceration, necrosis* and *malignancy*, and deterministic threshold dose is 1 Gy. *Transient erythema* and *erythema* can occur at 2 Gy and 6 Gy, respectively. Doses for *dry desquamation* and *moist desquamation* are >10 Gy and 15 Gy, respectively. Threshold dose for an epilation is about 3 Gy. *Hematopoietic tissues (bone marrow, spleen liver)* and *stem cells* in circulating blood are sensitive to radiation. *Lymphocyte* is the most sensitive cell in the body and has threshold dose of 0.25 Gy as partial body radiation.

Cataract is opacification of an eye, appears at posterior pole of the lens. It depends on total dose and duration of time it is delivered. Threshold dose for an acute and fractionated radiation is about 0.5 Gy with latent period of 20 years. Gastrointestinal tract consists of *oral mucosa, esophagus, stomach, small* and *large intestine, small intestine* is most sensitive whereas an *esophagus* is radioresistant.

Exposure to *reproductive organs (testes, ovary) cause an impaired fertility,* tumor, and hereditary effects. Radiation exposure causes reduction in *fertility, temporary sterility,* and *permanent sterility.* An acute dose 0.5 Gy and 6 Gy can cause temporary and permanent sterility, respectively in *testes.* Fractionated radiation of about 2.5–3 Gy over 2–4 weeks may induce *permanent sterility.* In female, radiation can induce permanent an *ovarian failure* which is an age dependent. A dose of 12 Gy can cause *permanent sterility at prepuberty* whereas it is 2 Gy in *premenopausal women.*

Acute Radiation Syndrome

Whole body irradiation (acute effects) delivered in short interval may cause an acute radiation effects appear as *syndrome.* Whole body dose of 0.5–10 Gy of an acute radiation may cause *hematopoietic syndrome.* It is associated with *bone marrow destruction, fatigue, symptoms of anemia, anorexia, diarrhea,* and *vomiting.* Higher doses reduce WBC, skin damage, prone to infection and death may occur within few months due to an *infection, anemia, and hemorrhage.*

Whole body dose of 5–12 Gy of acute radiation is referred to as *gastrointestinal syndrome* and death may occur within 3–10 days. Whole body dose >30 Gy may cause death in 24–48 hours, known as *cerebrovascular or neurovascular syndrome.* Whole body dose that causes 50% death over a specified time (60 days) is called *lethal dose,* expressed in $LD_{50/60}$. Lethal dose is 3.5–4.5 Gy for young adults, and it is lower for children and aged.

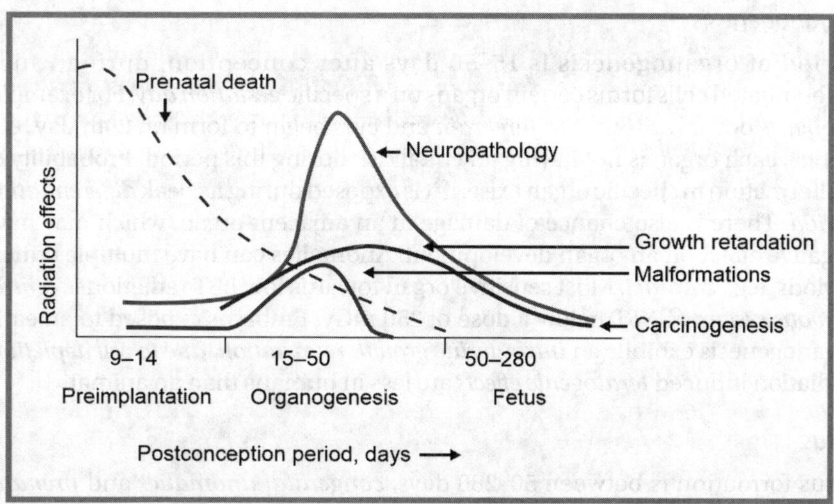

Fig. 15.4: Health effects of radiation exposure in utero at various stages of gestation.

Radiation Effects on Embryo and Fetus

Radiation exposure to pregnant women simulates the condition of in utero exposure that will affect an embryo and fetus. Human data is available from A-bomb survivors of *Hiroshima* and *Nagasaki* and mothers received pelvic radiotherapy before realizing that they were pregnant. Embryo has rapid cell proliferation and most sensitive to an ionizing radiation. Radiation response depends on *radiation quality, total dose, dose rate,* and *stage of development* at exposure. Radiation can produce *(1) lethal effects, (2) malformations,* and *(3) growth delay and retardation.*

Gestation period is divided into *(1) preimplantation, (2) organogenesis,* and *(3) fetal period* (**Fig. 15.4**). Preimplantation refers to time from fertilization to an attachment of *zygote* to an uterine wall, an organogenesis refers to period of an organ development, and fetus refers to growth of structures.

Preimplantation

Preimplantation stage is 9–14 days after conception, most sensitive, and cause lethal effects. However, for a radiation dose of <100 mGy, such lethal effects are low or negligible in humans (ICRP, 103). However, an irradiated embryo survives and grow normally, referred as an *all-or-nothing effect* of radiation. Embryo resistance to abnormalities is due to *repair capability, lack of cellular differentiation,* and *hypoxic state of embryo.* Most sensitive time in humans are (1) 12 hours after conception, during which the two pro-nuclei fuse to one cell stage, and (2) 30–60 hours when the first two cell division occur. Damage appears in the form of failure to implant or an undetected death in the conceptus. The women unable to realize that she is in preimplantation stage. Animal experiments have shown an increase of spontaneous abortion after a dose of 50–100 mGy, prenatal death after a dose of 250 mGy.

Organogenesis

Period of organogenesis is 15–50 days after conception, during which differentiated cells forms certain organs on a specific *gestation day*. For example, *neoblasts* occur on 18th day, *forebrain* and *eyes* begin to form on 20th day, etc. Hence, each organ is not having an equal risk during this period. Probability of malformation in specific organ exists if it is exposed during its peak *differentiation period*. There is also chance of damage in an adjacent organ, which may have negative effect on an organ development. Anomalies can have multiple critical periods, e.g., *cataract*. Most sensitive organ towards low LET radiation is *central nervous system (CNS)*, below a dose of 250 mGy. Embryos exposed to an early organogenesis exhibits an *intrauterine growth retardation, due to cell depletion*. Radiation induced *teratogenic effects* are less in humans than an animal.

Fetus

Fetus formation is between 50–280 days, *congenital anomalies* and *prenatal death* are unlikely during this period. Primary target for radiation is *nervous system* and *sense organs* relative to growth and development of organs. Damage of fetal growth may manifest as *behavioral alterations or reduced intelligence*. In the case of medical exposures, the radiation dose to fetus is about 25% of an entrance skin dose. Doses lower than 100 mGy generally carry negligible risk, comparable to normal risks of pregnancy.

Radiation Risk

Radiation risk is a probability that a given individual will incur a deleterious effect as result of a dose of radiation. Risk models such as an *absolute risk* and *relative risk* have been proposed to project risk for whole life span. Present risk estimate is based on *linear nonthreshold (LNT) model* suggested by *US National Academy of Sciences, Committee on the Biological Effects of Ionizing Radiation (BEIR repot VII)*. Age at the time of exposure is an important to estimate lifetime risk. Since A-bomb survivor study involves high doses, *Dose and Dose Rate Effectiveness Factor (DDREF)* is defined to convert the high-dose risk estimate into low-dose risk estimate, and it is 1.5 to 2. Radiation risk is quantified as *(1) somatic risk (cancer induction), (2) hereditary risk,* and *(3) fetal risk.*

However, it is worth to compare the radiation risks with risks in other industries. Safe industries are defined as "those having an associated annual fatality accident rate of 1 or less per 10,000 workers (average risk of 10^{-4}). The average fatal accident rate of radiation industry is less than 0.3×10^{-4}. Hence, the risk of radiation is comparable to safe industries such as trade, manufacturing, etc. However, the mining, agriculture and transport industries contribute higher risk than radiation industry.

Somatic Risk

Radiation effects, produced in an exposed individual during his lifetime is called *somatic effects*. Carcinogenesis is the main risk, which is a stochastic effect without threshold. It is likely below the threshold dose of deterministic effects, 2 Gy. Risk depends on sex and an age at the time of an exposure, and it is higher for children than an adult. Radiation induced thyroid cancer is more in children and women than men. Radiation induced cancer risk for public is 5.5% per Gy due to whole body, low dose, and dose rate irradiation (ICRP-103), whereas it is about 4.1% per Gy for radiation workers.

Genetic Risk

Hereditary risk depends on demographics (age, race, sex) of an exposed population. Older populations are having lower risks compared to younger population. ICRP-103 (2007) risk estimate is 0.2% per Gy up to two generations in general population. This means that an absorbed dose of 1 Gy to gonad may yield one genetic effect per 500 live births. For radiation workers, the risk is 0.1% per Gy of X-ray exposure. *Doubling dose* of gonad is 2 Gy, which likely to double the spontaneous mutation.

Fetal Risk

Fetal risk depends on stage of gestation period of pregnancy. Increased risk of malformation is seen during first 8 weeks. Mental retardation is a deterministic effect with threshold dose of 0.1 Sv and is about 40% per Sv for high dose rate exposures (ICRP). The embryo risk is about 10% per Sv from 16–25 weeks. In-utero exposure in third trimester will increase childhood cancer risk of the order of 0.1/Sv.

RADIATION HAZARDS, EVALUATION AND CONTROL

Radiation hazard arises from an external as well as internal. *External hazard* is caused when the source of radiation is outside the body. External hazard of beta rays is minimal and almost zero for alpha rays. X-rays and gamma rays are the major sources of an external hazards due to their penetrating power. In diagnostic radiology X-rays contribute an external hazards whereas gamma rays in nuclear medicine.

Internal hazard arises from an actual intake of radioactive material by a living organism. The possible routes of intake are *(1) inhalation of ontaminated air, (2) ingestion of contaminated food* and *water,* and *(3) entry of radionuclide directly into blood stream.* In case of fire, or an accident, there may be melting or an evaporation or dispersal of radionuclide, resulting in an internal hazard. Internal hazards to radiation workers are unlikely in diagnostic radiology since an unsealed source is used only in Nuclear medicine.

Hazard evaluation is necessary to take control measures in around radiation areas. It starts with design of radiation source or equipment. Manufacturer should ensure that an equipment meets the stipulated radiation safety standards. User of the radiation sources or equipment should also ensure the safety of patients, workers and public. It is essential to evaluate hazard likely to arise, under normal working conditions, as well as under potential accident conditions. It should be within the regulatory limits of national agency.

Principles of Radiological Protection

Aim of radiation protection is to prevent deterministic effects and minimize the probability of stochastic effects to levels deemed to be acceptable. This could be achieved, (1) by setting limits well below threshold dose to deterministic effects, and (2) the probability of stochastic effects could be reduced by limiting exposures *as low as reasonably achievable (ALARA)*. Radiation protection philosophy can be summarized as follows:

❑ **Justification of practice:** No practice involving radiation exposures shall be adopted unless it produces a net positive benefit.

❑ **Optimization:** Every effort shall be taken to reduce dose as low as reasonably achievable, considering the clinical, social, and economic factors.

❑ **Dose limits:** The effective doses to an individual shall not exceed limits recommended by the commission.

First principle emphasizes that all applications of radiation should be justified. Total detriment from a proposed practice involving exposure to radiation should be less than expected benefit. Since, deterministic effects exhibit threshold doses, they can be prevented by limiting exposures to levels lower than the threshold doses. However, stochastic effects do not have threshold dose hence, it is assumed that all radiation doses carry some risk.

Second principle aims at optimizing the risk level and cost of radiation protection. Thirdly, ICRP introduced the concept of permissible dose, defined as a dose of an ionizing radiation that, in the light of present knowledge, is not expected to cause an appreciable bodily injury to a person at any time during his lifetime **(Table 15.4)**.

Effective dose limit ensures an avoidance of deterministic effect in all body tissue and organ, except skin which may be subjected to localized exposures. Occupational dose limits exclude exposures from medical procedures and natural background.

Effective annual dose limit 20 mSv is because an aggregate *detriment* is 5% and it marginally exceeds the maximum mortality rate of 10^{-3} per year at an age of 65. Detriment is an overall harm due to stochastic effects arises from

Table 15.4: Recommended dose limits (ICRP-60, 1990).

Application	Occupational worker, mSv/year	Public, mSv/year
Effective dose (whole body)	20*	1*
Eye lens	20 (since 2011)	15
The skin	500	50
Hands and feet	500	50
Fetus, mean dose	2 after diagnosis**	—

* Averaged over a defined period of 5 consecutive years (1 mSv = 100 mrem). As per AERB, it should not exceed 30 mSv in a single year.

** After diagnosis, the limit to the surface of the women's abdomen is 1 mSv, for the remainder of the pregnancy.

radiation exposure. It assumes that the radiation exposure is low dose rate and the life expectancy is 75 years for the worker. The mean loss of life expectancy at 18 y is 0.5 y. Actual exposure to diagnostic radiology staff is relatively low, about 0.2 mSv/y for X-ray technologist. However, it is much lower for a radiation therapy technologist.

Dose limits for members of public are generally 10 times lower than those for an occupational exposure. Public includes children who get no direct benefit from an exposure. It is not the choice of public, they may be exposed to whole lifetime, in addition to their own occupational risk. Public is not a subject of selection, supervision, and monitoring.

A person may receive radiation dose from an external or internal sources. Radionuclides can enter the body through an *injection, inhalation, wounds, or absorption by skin*. The dose limit is same irrespective of an exposure route: internal or external or a combination of two. Accumulation of an internally deposited radionuclide will depend on their *concentration in air, water, rate of intake and metabolism*. Limits are, therefore, prescribed in terms an *annual limit of intake (ALI)* for different radionuclides.

Dose Limit to Pregnant Women

In the case of pregnant workers, the fetus is considered as a member of public. Once pregnancy is established, workers shall be monitored by an additional dosimeter worn on an abdomen under Lead apron. Conceptus shall be protected by applying a supplementary effective dose limit to her abdomen surface (lower trunk) of 2 mSv for the remainder of the pregnancy. A measured dose of 2 mSv to the surface of abdomen is normally considered equivalent to 1 mSv to the fetus.

Internal exposures shall be controlled by limiting an intake of radionuclides to about 1/20 of an *annual limit of intake (ALI)*. The employment shall be of such a type that it does not carry a probability of high accidental doses and an intake.

Dose Limit for Trainees

Trainee age limit should be above 16 years and an annual dose limit is 6 mSv. No person under an age of 18 years shall be allowed to work in controlled areas, unless supervised, and only for the purpose of training.

Personnel Monitoring

All personnel who are occupationally exposed to radiation should be monitored regularly. The monitoring frequency is three months, to ensure an uniform rate of personnel dose over the year. Hence, it is aimed to (1) monitor and control individual doses regularly, to ensure compliance with stipulated dose limits, (2) report and investigate over exposure and recommend necessary remedial measures urgently, and (3) maintain lifetime cumulative dose records of an user of the service.

Requirements of personnel monitoring system are: (1) appropriate range of dose measurement, accuracy, and reliability, (2) response independent of energy and type of radiation or ability to determine the same, (3) minimum fading of signal during the period of use, (4) environmental stability, (5) quick and simple readout system, and (6) rugged, light weight and economical.

Monitoring Dosimeters

Personnel monitoring dosimeters are classified into two types, namely *passive* and *active dosimeter*. Passive dosimeter stores radiation signal and later releases the same for dose analysis, e.g., film badge. Active dosimeter receives radiation and gives radiation induced signal as display of dose or dose rate directly, e.g., pocket dosimeter. Various personnel monitoring systems are *(1) thermoluminescen dosimeter (TLD), (2) film badge, (3) pocket dosimeter, (4) optically stimulated luminescence (OSL) dosimeter,* and *(5) radiophotoluminescent (RPL) dosimeter.*

The principle and function of thermoluminescent dosimeter, film dosimeter, pocket dosimeter and optically stimulated luminescence dosimeter have been explained in Chapter 5. RPL are glass dosimeters of accumulation type solid state dosimeters. They use *silver activated phosphate glass* and available in glass rods of small shape. It employs radiophotoluminescence phenomenon principle to measure radiation dose.

Personnel monitoring devices provide (1) occupational absorbed dose information, (2) assurance that dose limits are not exceeded and (3) trends in exposure to serve as check on working practice. In India, personnel monitoring program was started in 1959, currently more than 1,60,000 personnel are monitored, including medical, industry and nuclear facilities. The country wide personnel monitoring service is offered by private agencies, accredited by *Bhabha Atomic Research Center (BARC)* **(Table 15.5).**

Table 15.5: Accredited personnel monitoring agencies in India (AERB website).

S. No.	State/region	Name of the accredited agency
1.	Andhra Pradesh, Telangana, Tamil Nadu, Karnataka, Kerala, Puducherry, Andaman and Nicobar and Lakshadweep, (Southern Region)	Avanttec Laboratory Pvt Ltd, Plot No. 17, Arignar Anna Industrial Estate, Mettukuppam, Vanagaram, Chennai Pin-600095
2.	Maharashtra, Gujarat, Rajasthan, Goa, Dadra and Nagar Haveli and Diu (Western Region)	Renentech Laboratory Pvt Ltd, C-106, Synthofine Industrial Estate, Off Aarey Road, Goregaon (E), Mumbai, Maharashtra Pin-400063
3.	All other states in the central, Northern and Northeastern parts of the country	Ultra-Tech Laboratory Pvt Ltd, Cloth Market, G.E. Road, Kumhari, Bhilai, Durg, Chhattisgarh Pin-490042
4.	All Defense institutions of country	Defense Laboratory, Jodhpur

Thermoluminescent Dosimeter

Thermoluminescent dosimeter (TLD) is based on the phenomenon of *thermoluminescence*. When certain materials are heated after radiation exposure, emit light which is used to measure individual doses from X, beta, and gamma radiations. It gives much reliable results since no fading is observed under an extreme climatic conditions.

TLD Card

TLD card consists of 3 *CaSo$_4$: Dy-Teflon disc* of each 0.8 mm thick × 13.2 mm diameter, which are mechanically clipped over three symmetrical circular holes of diameter 12 mm, on a *Nickel-plated Aluminum plate* of dimension 52.5 mm × 29.9 mm × 1 mm **(Fig. 15.5)**. An asymmetric V cut provided at one end of the card ensures a fixed orientation of card in the TLD cassette. The card is enclosed by a *paper wrapper* in which user's personnel data and period of use is written. Thickness of wrapper is 12 mg/cm², makes measurements equivalent to 10 mm depth below skin surface in cassette. To protect TLD discs from mishandling, the card along with its wrapper is sealed in a thin *plastic (polythene) pouch*. The pouch also protects the card from radioactive contamination while working with open sources.

TLD Cassette

TLD cassette is made of high impact *plastic*. There are three filters in the cassette corresponding to each disc namely, *Cu + Al, Perspex and open*. When the TLD card is inserted properly in the cassette, the first disc (D1) is sandwiched between a pair of filter combination of *1 mm Al and 0.9 mm Cu (Thick:1000 mg/cm²)*, so that Al is facing the radiation. Second disc (D2) is sandwiched between a pair of 1.5 mm thick *plastic filters (180 mg/cm²)*. Third disc (D3) is positioned under a circular open window. A clip attachment affixes the badge to the users clothing or to the wrist.

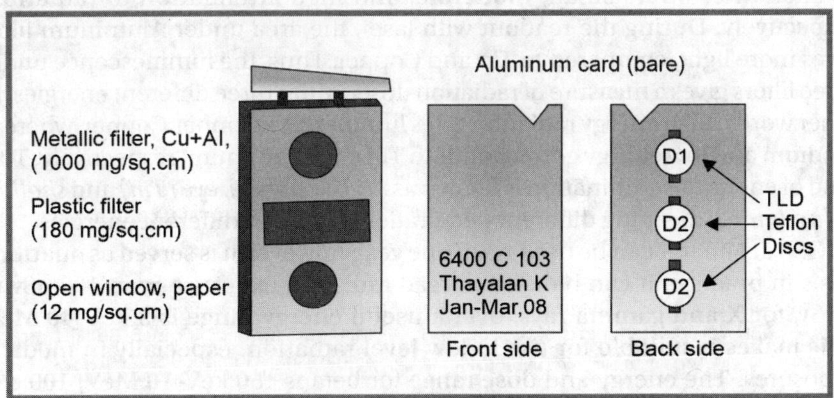

Fig. 15.5: TLD badge: Al cards with three filters in place.

Metallic filter is meant for X and gamma radiation, and *Perspex* is for beta radiation. The filters are mainly used to make the TLD discs energy independent. When the TLD disc is exposed to radiation, the electrons in the crystal lattice are excited and move from the *valence band to conduction band*. There, they form a trap just below the conduction band. The number of electrons in the trap is proportional to the radiation exposure and thus it stores an absorbed radiation energy in the crystal lattice.

Dose measurements are made by using a *TLD reader* (**Figs. 5.5 and 5.6**, Chapter 5) which has a heater, *photomultiplier tube (PMT)*, amplifier, and a recorder. The TLD disc is placed in the heater cup or *planchet* and heated. The electrons return to their ground state with emission of light which is measured by a PMT. The PMT converts light into an electrical current (signal) which is amplified and measured by a recorder. The reader is calibrated in terms of mR or mSv, so that one can get direct dose estimation. The disc is annealed and can be used again.

$CaSo_4$ TLD badge can cover a wide range of dose from 100 μSv to 100 Sv with an accuracy of ±10%. TLD badges are available as an extremity and finger dosimetry (ring) and do not provide permanent record. *Lithium fluoride (LiF)* can also be used as TLD phosphor, which has wide dose response range from 10 μSv to 1000 Sv. Its effective atomic number $(Z = 8.2)$ is close to that of tissue with an accuracy of ±2%

Optically Stimulated Luminescence Dosimeter

Optically stimulated luminescence (OSL) dosimeter is also used as personnel monitoring device which is replacing film badge and TLD. After radiation exposure the OSL is stimulated by a laser light during which light is emitted. Light emission is proportional to the given radiation exposure, is the principle of OSL. Emission of light can be plotted graphically, known as *glow curve*. OSL dosimeter consists of thin layer of *Aluminum oxide (Al_2O_3)* as detector (**Figs. 15.6A and B**). It has three filters, namely *(1) Aluminum, (2) Tin,* and *(3) Copper.*

Each filter offers small, moderate, and high attenuation to radiation, respectively. During the readout with laser, the area under Aluminum filter gives more light, compared to Tin and Copper. Thus, the luminescence under three filters gives a measure of radiation dose, under three different energies. In other words, high energy radiation gives luminescence under Copper, whereas medium and low energy corresponds to Tin and Aluminum, respectively. This kind of energy discrimination is known as *deep (Copper), eye (Tin)* and *shallow (Aluminum),* meaning different penetration depths or different energies.

OSL dosimeter can be used up to one year, however, it is served as quarterly basis in practice. It can be used to read radiation exposure from 100 μSv to 10 Sv, for X and gamma rays, over a useful energy range is 5 keV–40 MeV. This makes it suitable for use in low level radiation, especially in medical exposures. The energy and dose range for beta is 150 keV–10 MeV; 100 μSv –10Sv, and neutron is 40 keV–35 MeV; 200 μSv–250 Sv.

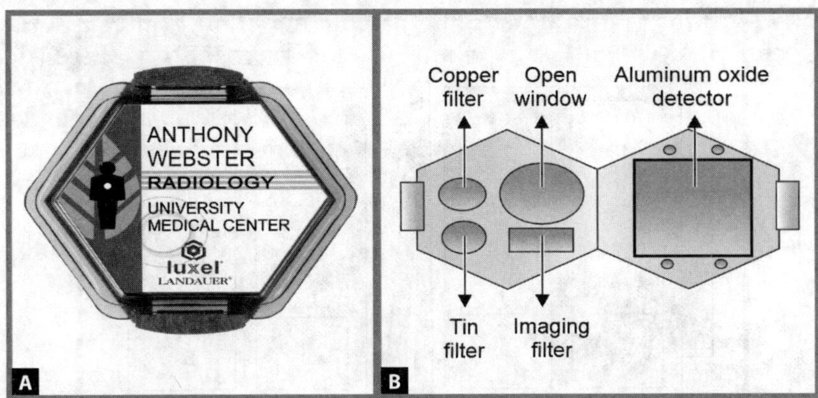

Fig. 15.6A and B: Optically stimulated luminescence dosimeter: (A) OSL Dosimeter; (B) OSL dosimeter composition.
(*Courtesy:* Luxel Landauer)

Advantages of OSL dosimeters are light weight, durable and simple. It is not affected by heat, moisture, and pressure since it is tamperproof. Reanalysis is possible if there is error in readout or any dispute. It can be worn for longer periods of time, compared to TLD and film dosimeter. OSL with in-house reader can be used for patient dose measurements. Nowadays, OSL comes with an open filter (bare) facility, to detect dynamic exposures.

Film Badge

Film badge is used to measure an external radiation dose of a person from *X*, *beta, gamma,* and *thermal neutron* radiations. It consists of a *film pack* loaded in a *film holder* which is made up of *plastic with stainless steel lining* (**Fig. 15.7**). It can hold one or more photographic films of size 4 × 3 cm, wrapped inside with a light tight *polythene* or paper cover. The film should be loaded in the film holder, so that the flap side of the film pack is always facing the body. Generally, the badge has two films, one is slow, and the other is fast and slow film is meant for recording high exposure.

The film holder has 6 filters namely *open, plastic, Cadmium, thin Copper, thick Copper,* and *Lead*. All the filters have 1 mm thick except thin Copper which is 0.15 mm thick. The filters are fixed on both sides of the holder, to identify type, energy, and penetrating power of an incident radiation. Thus, it will identify *alpha, beta, neutron, low energy X-rays, high energy X-rays* and *gamma rays*, over a range of energies from 10 keV to 2 MeV.

When the badge is exposed to radiation, it passes through filter and forms latent image in the film. After 4 weeks of use, it is returned for dose computation where the film is processed; optical densities under different filters are measured by a *densitometer*. Using standard calibration curves, the dose under each filter is evaluated. A control film is always needed to assess background level of radiation. Each institution should keep one film, loaded in a chest holder as control. This control badge should be kept in a cool,

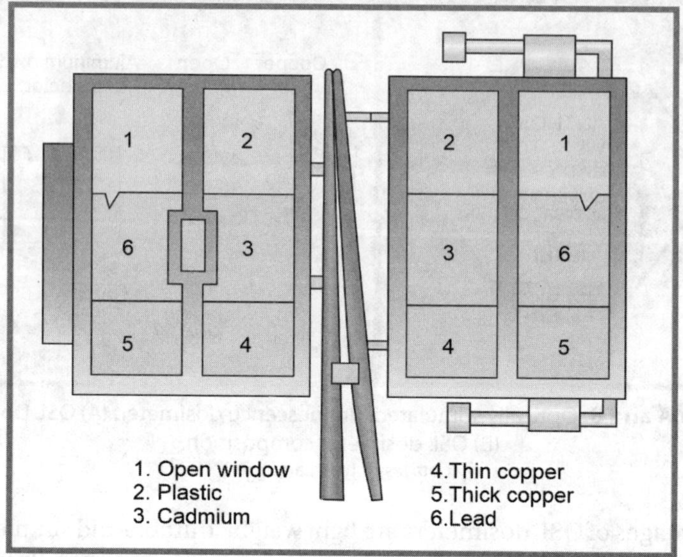

Fig. 15.7: Film badge personnel monitoring dosimeter.

dry, and radiation free area. Monthly dose reports are sent to an individual institutions after processing the film packs. These reports contain monthly doses and up-to-date cumulative doses of the current year. Film badge can be used to measure radiation from 10 μSv to 100 Sv with an accuracy of ± 10 percent.

Advantages of film badge are: (1) it is a permanent record, (2) nature of exposure, types of radiation and energy can be evaluated, and (3) is a least expensive device.

Guidelines for Using TLD Badge

TLD badges are used only by radiation workers. Every new radiation worker needs to fill up the *personnel data form (PDF)* and send to BARC accredited agency. TLD badge once issued to a person should not be used by any other person. A badge without filter or damaged filter should not be used and be replaced by a new holder. Every radiation worker must ensure that the badge is not left in radiation field or near hot plates, ovens, furnaces, burners, etc. All the used or unused TLD badges should be return, after every service period (quarterly) in one lot to reach 10th of next month. While leaving the hospital premises, workers should deposit their badges in storage area along with control TLD, which is kept in a radiation free zone. *TLD badge is used to measure radiation dose but does not protect the user from the radiation.*

Placement of TLD Badge

TLD badges are normally worn at chest level (torso) under Lead apron, so that it is expected to receive maximum and true whole body radiation exposure.

This ensures greater amount of radiation exposure received by most sensitive part of the body. However, Lead apron is not indicated for PET-CT work practice due to high energy photons. High energy photons interact through *Compton scattering* results in an increased scatter and an independent of Z. Additional wrist badge is advised for procedures involving nuclear medicine, and an interventional radiology.

During an interventional radiology or cardiology procedure, a collar level dosimeter is used to measure *thyroid and eye lens* dose. *Extremity dosimeter (ring)* under hand gloves is also used as an additional dosimeter. It enables the workers or physician to use their hands nearer to the primary radiation beam. A pregnant radiation worker can wear an additional dosimeter at *waist level* behind the Lead apron, to assess the fetal dose.

Methods of Radiation Control

Control of radiation hazard is an important step in radiation protection. Various methods of radiation control are (1) time, (2) distance, and (3) shielding. They are simply known as TDS, three pillars of radiological safety.

Time

Total dose received by a radiation worker is directly proportional to total time spent in handling the radiation source. *Lesser the time spent near the radiation source, lesser is the radiation dose.* As time spent in the radiation field increases, radiation dose received also increases. Hence, techniques or methods to minimize time in a radiation field should be recognized or practiced.

All radiation sources do not produce constant exposure rates. Diagnostic X-ray machines typically produce high exposure rates over brief time interval. Nuclear medicine procedure produces lower exposure rate for an extended periods of time. Hence, both knowledge of an exposure rate and how it changes with time are the important elements in reducing personnel exposures.

Time spent near a radiation source can be minimized by understanding the task to be performed and having suitable equipment to complete the task in short interval with safety. Hence, one must plan and practice radiation procedure, without much radiation. Essential duties are shared, to reduce radiation exposure.

Worked Example 15.1

A radiographer is performing Barium examination under fluoroscopy and the equipment is 'ON' for 5 minutes for each examination. Radiation level at the location of the radiographer is 30 mR/h. How many such procedures the radiographer can carry out per week?

Annual equivalent dose limit prescribed for
the radiographer is (occupational worker) 20 mSv = 2000 mrem = 2000 mR
Permitted weekly dose = 2000 mR/50 weeks   = 40 mR
(Assumed 1 year = 50 week for radiological occupancy)

Exposure rate at the location of radiographer = 30 mR/h

$$= (30/60)\, \text{mR/min} = 0.5\, \text{mR/min}$$

Exposure in each procedure

$$= (0.5\, \text{mR/min}) \times 5\, \text{min}$$

$$= 2.5\, \text{mR}$$

Hence, the number of procedures the
radiographer can associate within one week = 40 mR/2.5 mR = 16

The radiographer can perform 16 procedures without exceeding his dose
limit.

Worked Example 15.2

An operator is handling 5 mCi of I-131 source with 30 cm tongs. Within how
much time the technician will receive the weekly permissible equivalent
dose? (Assume 1R = 1 rad, $\Gamma_{20} = 2.18\, \dfrac{R.\,cm^2}{mCi.h}$ for I-131)

Exposure level at 30 cm from 5 mCi of I-131 source $= \dfrac{2.18 \times 5\, mCi}{30^2} = 0.012$ R/h

$$= 12\, \text{mR/h}$$

Permissible exposure is 2000 mR/50 weeks $= 40\, \text{mR,}$

Permissible time of work $= 40\, \text{mR}/12\, \text{mR/h}$

$$= 200\, \text{minutes or 3 h 20 min}$$

Distance

Radiation intensity (exposure rate) from a point source decreases with
distance, due to divergence of the beam. It is governed by an *inverse square
law*, which states that an exposure rate from a point source of radiation is
inversely proportional to the square of the distance (Chapter 1, **Fig. 1.4**). If an
exposure rate is X_1 at distance d_1, then an exposure rate X_2 at another distance
d_2 is given by:

$$X_2 = X_1 \left(\frac{d_1}{d_2}\right)^2$$

Larger the distance, lesser is the radiation dose. This is valid for point
sources only whose dimensions are much small compared to distance. This
relationship is not valid near a patient (<1 m), injected with radioisotopes
since an exposure rate decreases less rapidly than an inverse square law.

Hence, all personnel should stand as far away as possible from radiation
sources or X-ray procedures or behind a shielded barrier whenever possible.
Unshielded radiation sources never be manipulated by hand. Tongs or other
handling devices are used to increase the distance between source and hand.

Worked Example 15.3

Exposure rate from a fluoroscopic X-ray machine is 5 R/min at 50 cm. What
would be the exposure rates at (i) 40 cm, and (ii) 60 cm?

X_1 = 5 R/min, d_1 = 50 cm, d_2 = 40 cm, X_2 = ?

X_2 $= [X_1 \times (d_1)^2]/(d_2)^2$

$\qquad\ = [5\, \text{R/min} \times (50\, \text{cm})^2]/(40\, \text{cm})^2$

$$= 7.81 \text{ R/min}$$

$X_1 = 5 \text{ R/min}, d_1 = 50 \text{ cm}, d_2 = 60 \text{ cm}, X_2 = ?$

$X_2 = [5 \text{ R/min} \times (50 \text{ cm})^2]/(60 \text{ cm})^2$

$$= 3.47 \text{ R/min}$$

The exposure rate at 40 cm and 60 cm are 7.81 R/min and 3.47 R/min, respectively.

Shielding

When maximum distance and minimum time do not ensure an acceptably low radiation dose, an adequate shielding must be provided, so that radiation beam will be sufficiently attenuated. Material that attenuates radiation exponentially is called *shield* which reduce exposure to patients, workers, and the public. If I_o is the intensity of radiation at a point without shield and I is the intensity with a shield of thickness t, then:

$$I = I_o e^{-\mu t}$$

where, μ is the *linear attenuation coefficient* of the shielding material. The thickness of the shielding material that reduces an intensity to half is called *half value layer (HVL)* and it is related to μ :

$$\text{HVL} = \frac{0.693}{\mu}$$

Larger the shielding thickness, lesser is the radiation exposure.

X and gamma rays undergo an exponential attenuation in the shielding material. This means that even a large shielding material will not attenuate radiation to zero intensity. However, an optimal shielding thickness is required to bring down the radiation level below the permissible limit. *Brick, Concrete,* and *Steel* are used as shielding material to construct X-ray, and gamma rays shielding or barriers. *Lead* is used as protective material in Lead apron, thyroid shield, viewing window and gonad shield as well as in room door shielding.

Among time, distance, and shielding, distance is more effective in reducing radiation exposure.

REGULATORY REQUIREMENTS

Atomic Energy Regulatory Board

Atomic Energy Regulatory Board (AERB) constituted by the Government of India (November 1983), is entrusted with the responsibility of developing and implementing appropriate regulatory measures aimed at ensuring radiation safety in all applications involving ionizing radiations. Before the constitution of AERB, *division of radiological protection (DRP)* of BARC and *safety review committee of the department of atomic energy* were responsible for the implementation of radiation safety.

The mission of AERB is to ensure that the use of an ionizing radiation and nuclear energy does not cause undue risk to health and an environment. Its major objective is to develop and publicize specific codes and guides, which will deal the radiation safety aspects of various applications of ionizing

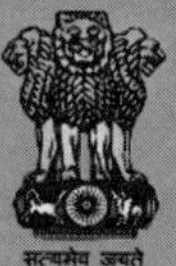

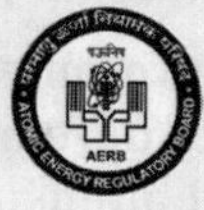

Fig. 15.8: AERB Safety code for diagnostic X-rays: CODE NO. AERB/RF-MED/SC-3 (Rev. 2), 2016.

radiations **(Fig. 15.8)**. AERB implements the safety provisions by the Atomic Energy (Radiation Protection) Rules, 2004, which provides necessary regulatory infrastructure for an effective implementation of radiation protection program in India.

Regulation for Diagnostic X-rays—For Users

General Requirements

Employer and licensee of an organization shall fulfill the responsibilities prescribed in the safety code.

Procurement of X-ray Equipment

Employer shall procure no objection certificate (NOC) validated/Type approved X-ray equipment from an authorized supplier and after obtaining procurement permission from the Competent Authority.

Operation of X-ray Equipment

No diagnostic X-ray equipment shall be operated for patient diagnosis unless license for operation is obtained from the Competent Authority.

Pre-requisites for Obtaining License for Operation of X-ray Equipment: X-ray Room Layout and Shielding Requirement

❑ X-ray room shall have an appropriate area for easy movement of staff and proper patient positioning. It should have an appropriate structural shielding for walls, doors, ceiling, and floor of the room **(Table 15.6)**. Radiation exposures received by workers and the members of the public are minimum and shall not exceed an annual dose limit.

❑ If mobile X-ray equipment is used as fixed X-ray, it should comply all the requirements of fixed X-ray installation. Movement of mobile X-ray equipment shall be restricted within the institution for which it is registered.

❑ **Vehicle mounted X-ray equipment:** X-ray equipment installed in a mobile van or vehicle, shall be provided with an appropriate shielding enclosure to ensure an adequate built-in protection for persons likely to be present in and around the vehicle. Shielding shall be provided around an equipment from all the sides up to a height of 2 m from an external ground surface. Radiation warning symbol shall be displayed on all sides of the vehicle.

Table 15.6: Reference shielding thickness required at 2 m for different X-ray rooms (AERB website).

Shielding material	Dental CBCT/OPG	Radiography & fluoroscopy*	Interventional radiology/ cardiac angiography*	Computed tomography*
Brick, cm	12	20	23	25
Concrete, cm	8	12	15	15
Steel, cm	—	2.0	2.0	2.5
Lead, cm	0.12	0.15	0.18	0.18
Any other material	1.4 TVT	1.8 TVT	2.0 TVT	2.8 TVT

*Ceiling thickness of concrete of 6–8 inch is adequate.

Staffing Requirements

X-ray installations shall have a radiologist/related medical practitioner/X-ray technologist with an adequate knowledge of radiation protection, to operate the X-ray equipment. They are considered as radiation workers, if qualified and shall comply with the duties and responsibilities as prescribed in the safety code.

Radiological Safety Officer (RSO)

X-ray department shall have RSO approved by the Competent Authority. The RSO may either be an employer himself/herself or an employee to whom the employer shall delegate the responsibility of ensuring compliance with an appropriate radiation safety/regulatory requirements applicable to his X-ray installation.

Radiation Protection Devices

Appropriate radiation protection devices such as *barriers, apron, goggles,* and *thyroid shields* shall be used during an operation of X-ray equipment. These devices shall be verified periodically for their shielding adequacy.

Personnel Monitoring Service

Personnel monitoring services shall be provided to all the radiation workers.

Quality Assurance (QA) Requirements

The end user shall ensure that periodic quality assurance (QA) of an equipment is carried out by an agencies authorized by the regulatory body.

Servicing

The end-user shall ensure that servicing of the X-ray equipment is carried out by an agencies authorized by the regulatory body.

Periodic Safety Reports

The user shall submit periodic safety reports in the format and frequency specified by the regulatory body.

Renewal of License

The license accorded by the Competent authority shall be renewed before its expiry.

Decommissioning of X-ray Equipment

Decommissioning of the X-ray equipment shall be carried out by authorized agencies with prior intimation to the Competent Authority.

Responsibilities of the Employer

❑ The ultimate responsibility of ensuring radiation safety in handling the X-ray equipment shall rest with an employer and is the custodian of X-ray equipment in his possession.

- ❑ No person under the age of 18 years shall be employed as a worker. No worker under the age of 16 years shall be taken as trainee or employed as an apprentice for radiation work.
- ❑ Prior to employment of a worker, obtain the dose records from his former employer, where applicable.
- ❑ Every employer shall designate, with the written approval of the Competent Authority, a person having an appropriate qualifications as a Radiological Safety Officer (RSO).
- ❑ Employer shall designate those of his employees as classified workers, who are likely to receive an effective dose more than three-tenths of an average annual dose limits notified by the Competent Authority and shall forthwith inform those employees that they have been so designated.
- ❑ Employer shall provide facilities and equipment to the licensee, RSO, and other worker(s) to carry out their functions effectively in conformity with the provisions of the safety code, directives and guidelines issued by the Competent Authority from time-to-time.
- ❑ Ensure that provisions of the Atomic Energy (Radiation Protection) Rules 2004 are implemented by the licensee, RSO and radiation workers.
- ❑ Health surveillance of classified workers and radiation surveillance of all radiation workers shall be carried out as specified in Atomic Energy (Radiation Protection) Rules, 2004.
- ❑ Upon termination of service of worker, provide to his new employer on request his dose records.
- ❑ Inform the Competent Authority if the licensee and/or the RSO leaves the employment.
- ❑ Comply with the terms and conditions of license.

Responsibilities of the Licensee

- ❑ Establish written procedures and plans for controlling, monitoring and assessment of exposure for ensuring adequate protection of workers, members of the public, environment, and patients, wherever applicable.
- ❑ Ensure periodic training in radiation safety for radiation workers towards performing their intended task.
- ❑ Subject the radiation workers to personnel monitoring and maintain dose record.
- ❑ In consultation with the RSO, investigate any case of exposure more than prescribed regulatory limits received by individual workers, implement the follow-up actions, take steps to prevent recurrence of such incidents and promptly inform the Competent Authority of the same. The licensee shall also maintain records of such investigations.
- ❑ Arrange for or conduct quality assurance tests of an equipment and arrange for preventive maintenance of radiation protection equipment, and monitoring instruments.
- ❑ Advise the employer about the modifications in working condition of a pregnant radiation worker.

- ❑ Ensure that the workers are familiar with the contents of the relevant safety documents issued by the Competent Authority.
- ❑ Inform the Competent Authority when he/she leaves the employment.
- ❑ Comply with the terms and conditions of license.

Responsibilities of Radiological Safety Officer

- ❑ Carry out routine measurements and analysis on radiation safety of the radiation installation and maintain records of the results thereof.
- ❑ Investigate any situation that could lead to potential exposures.
- ❑ Prepare and make available periodic reports on safety status of the radiation installation to an employer and the licensee for reporting to the Competent Authority.
- ❑ Prepare and make available the reports on all hazardous situations along with details of any immediate remedial actions taken to an employer and the licensee for reporting to the Competent Authority.
- ❑ Verify the performance of radiation monitoring systems, safety interlocks, protective devices such as Lead (equivalent) aprons, and other safety systems such as structural shielding in the radiation installation if any.
- ❑ Advise the employer and the licensee regarding:
  - ❑ Necessary steps to ensure the dose of radiation workers are well within the dose limits prescribed by the Competent Authority.
  - ❑ The good work practices that ensure radiation doses are maintained as low as reasonably achievable (ALARA).
  - ❑ Initiation of suitable remedial measures in respect of any situation that could lead to potential exposures.
  - ❑ Carrying out periodic QA tests as prescribed by the regulatory body.
  - ❑ Promptly carrying out servicing and maintenance of an equipment, which can impact radiation safety.
  - ❑ Ensuring periodic calibration of monitoring instruments.
  - ❑ Modifications in working conditions of a pregnant worker.
- ❑ Assist the employer and licensee in instructing the workers on hazards of radiation, suitable safety measures and work practices aimed at optimizing exposures.
- ❑ Inform the Competent Authority when he leaves the employment.

Responsibilities of Operators and Other Radiation Workers

- ❑ Provide the employer information about his previous occupations including radiation work, if any.
- ❑ Undergo training provided by the supplier, towards appropriate exposure parameters and dose reduction protocols.
- ❑ Use an appropriate exposure parameters for adults and children X-ray examinations.
- ❑ Use protective devices during an operation of X-ray equipment.
- ❑ Use personnel monitoring devices appropriately within the facility and monitor dose received.

❑ Inform the RSO and the licensee of any accident or potentially hazardous situation that may come to his notice.
❑ Female workers shall, on becoming aware of her pregnancy, notify the employer, licensee, and RSO in order that her working conditions may be modified if necessary.

Responsibilities of Students/Trainees

❑ Medical students/trainees shall not operate X-ray equipment except under direct supervision of an authorized operating personnel.
❑ They shall not receive an effective dose more than as stipulated by regulatory body.

Responsibilities of Medical Practitioner

The medical practitioner shall undertake an X-ray examination based on medical requirement. The medical practitioner shall:

❑ Be satisfied that the necessary clinical information is not available from radiological examinations already done or from any other medical tests or investigations.
❑ Be conscious of the patient dose and for any given examination shall attempt to be in line with an international reference levels or those recommended by the regulatory body.
❑ Evaluate medical procedures continuously for possible reduction of doses, especially for pediatric procedures.
❑ Customize an exposure protocol as per his expectation for an optimum image quality for new installations.

Health Surveillance of Workers (Rule 25)

❑ Every employer shall provide the services of a physician with an appropriate qualifications to undertake an occupational health surveillance of classified workers.
❑ Every worker, initially on employment, and classified worker, thereafter at least once in *three years* until an individual is employed, shall be subjected to the following: (a) general medical examination, and (b) health surveillance to decide on the fitness of each worker for an intended task.
❑ The health surveillance shall include (a) special tests or medical examinations as specified by order by the competent authority, for workers who have received dose more than regulatory constraints; and (b) counseling of pregnant workers.

Overexposure

Radiation worker is said to be over exposure, if he receives a whole-body effective dose of >10 mSv, in quarterly period. All over exposure cases will be examined by an overexposure committee, AERB. The AERB will investigate the reported overexposure and the same will be reported promptly to the institution and the individual. The RSO of the institution must investigate the causes of overexposure and submit an elaborate investigation report in the prescribed format within the stipulated period as per the directive of AERB. The individual also should make a statement regarding the causes of the overexposure to AERB. This is to take preventive steps to avoid such exposure in future.

The RSO should re-construct the incident which might have resulted an overexposure and initiate measures to prevent such an occurrences in future. A detailed report of an incident shall be submitted to the competent authority by the RSO. If it is not genuine, it may be due to misplacement of badge or wrong storage of badge, etc. If the overexposure is genuine, an individual will be subjected *chromosome aberration assay (CAA)*, by recognized laboratory to confirm the overexposure, if the exposure >100 mSv.

PLANNING A DIAGNOSTIC X-RAY INSTALLATION

General Requirements

Location

Rooms housing the diagnostic X-ray units and related equipment should be located as far away as feasible from areas of high occupancy and general traffic, such as maternity and pediatric wards and other departments of the hospital that are not directly related to radiation and its use.

Layout

Layout of rooms in an X-ray department should aim at providing integrated facilities so that handling of X-ray equipment and related operations can be conveniently performed with an adequate protection. The doors and passages leading to the X-ray installation should permit safe and easy transport of an equipment and nonambulatory patients. The number of doors for entry and windows should be kept minimum. Normally, X-ray room should be provided with only one door.

Unnecessary doors and windows present in an existing room, where X-ray machine is installed should be bricked off and if not possible should be provided with an adequate Lead lining of 2 mm and kept permanently closed. Whenever Lead lining is provided, care should be taken to provide an adequate overlapping in the shielding. The darkroom should be so located that the primary X-ray beam cannot be directed on it.

Room Size

Room housing the X-ray equipment must be spacious enough to permit installation and servicing and operation of equipment with safety and convenience for patients, servicing personnel and operators. It should facilitate the wheeling in of patients in and around the couch of the X-ray unit. Proper grouping of the rooms comprising the installation should be done bearing in mind their dependence on each other.

Shielding

Appropriate structural shielding shall be provided for the walls, ceilings, and floors, so that the doses received by an occupational workers and members of public are kept to a minimum and shall not exceed an annual effective dose limit. The current limits are 20 mSv and 1 mSv for an occupational workers and members of public, respectively. The doors of the X-ray room shall provide the same shielding as that of adjacent walls in case persons are likely to be present in front of them when the X-ray unit is energized.

Appropriate shielding must be provided for dark room to ensure that an undeveloped X-ray films stored in it will not be exposed to more than an air kerma rate of 10 µGy per week (about 1.13 mR per week). Thickness equivalent to 2.0 mm Lead (15 cm/6-inch concrete or 23 cm/9-inch brick walls) with plaster will provide an adequate protection outside the X-ray room against both primary and secondary radiation in most of the diagnostic X-ray installation.

Opening and Ventilation

Un-shielded openings, if provided in the X-ray room for ventilation/exhaust or natural light, must be located above a height of 2.1 m from the finished floor level/ground outside the X-ray room.

Equipment Layout

X-ray equipment must be installed in such a way that in normal use, the useful beam is not directed towards control panel, doors, windows, dark room, and areas of high occupancy. The useful beam should preferably be directed towards an unoccupied areas and away from the dark room. For example, chest stand shall be installed in the X-ray room such that dose limits to radiation worker and members of public are not exceeded. Sufficient area should be left all around the X-ray table for safe and free movements of equipment/trolley, staff, and service personnel. More than one examination should not be conducted simultaneously in the same room hence, the installation of more than one X-ray equipment in the same room is discouraged.

Control Panel

Diagnostic X-ray units operating below 125 kV, control panel should be located away from the primary beam inside a stationery/mobile protective barrier. The protective barrier should have sufficient Lead equivalence (1.5 mm). Both control console and machine can be housed in the same room.

For equipment operating at 125 kV or above, the control panel must be installed in a separate control room, located outside but contiguous to the machine room and provided with appropriate shielding. Computed tomography and an interventional radiology equipment shall be installed with a separate control console with an appropriate shielding. The operator can view of the patient through viewing window (1.5 mm Lead equivalence) along with an oral communication.

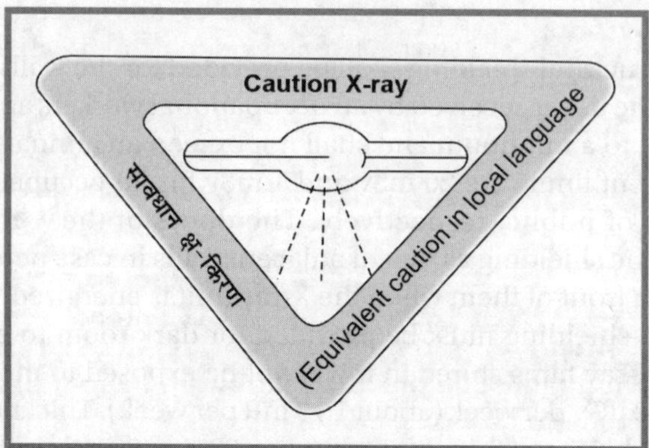

Fig. 15.9: X-radiation warning inverted triangle placard.

Waiting Area

To avoid crowding of patients and relatives near the entrance door, a waiting area must be provided outside and an adjacent to the X-ray room. It should have sufficient area to match the patient workload with toilet facility.

Warning Light and Placard

A suitable warning signal such as the *red light* must be provided at a conspicuous place outside the X-ray room and kept ON when the X-ray equipment is energized to prevent an inadvertent entry of persons not connected with an examination into the diagnostic room. An appropriate warning *placard* should be posted outside the diagnostic room **(Fig. 15.9)**. A permanent radiation warning symbol and instructions for pregnant/likely to be pregnant women shall be pasted on the entrance door of the X-ray installation, illustrating that an equipment emits X-radiation.

Other Specifications

X-ray room may be an air-conditioned to control temperature, pressure, and humidity. Suitable monitors should be provided to indicate the above parameters. It will ensure long-term, trouble free, safe operation of an equipment. Spilt AC with sufficient capacity to suit the room size is preferable than window AC's. Suitable electrical interlocks between door, equipment and control panel must be provided, wherever it is necessary. There should be an exclusive room for preparing patients for special procedures, post scan recovery and handling an emergency. In addition, space must be provided to accommodate trolly and wheelchairs, etc.

Approval of Diagnostic X-ray Facility

The site and layout plan of diagnostic radiology facility is prepared in 1:200 scale and submitted through *e-LORA* by the user and get approved from AERB. Plan should indicate various rooms along with their dimensions, positions of doors, windows, type of occupancy around, etc. Cross-sectional views may be required for CT scan. To start a radiology department, an institution get registered with AERB and obtain USERNAME and PASSWORD. Further details can be obtained from AERB website: www.aerb.gov.in.

MODEL LAYOUT FOR DIAGNOSTIC X-RAY INSTALLATIONS

Radiography X-ray Installation

Radiography X-ray units are operated in the range of 50–125 kV applied voltage. Objects that are irradiated are considered as primary barriers. Additional shielding must be provided for a wall behind the chest stand. Provisions are made to observe and communicate with the patient on the table. The operator should be in the control area. The shield at the control (protective barrier) must be a permanent/mobile one with 2.1 m height. It should not be used as primary barrier. The viewing window (VW) of suitable size must be there at the control barrier which is centrally placed. Chest stand is positioned away from the control panel or door, preferably on the opposite direction. If dark room is adjacent, Lead lined *pass-box* is provided for easy movement of cassette **(Fig. 15.10)**.

Walls of the X-ray room on which scattered X-ray fall is (are) not less than 23 cm or 9-inch thickness brick or equivalent, and primary X-ray beam falls is (are) not less than 35 cm or 14-inch thickness brick or equivalent. The ceiling must have a thickness of concrete (density 2.35 g/cc), not less than 6 inches or 15 cm. There is a shielding equivalent to at least 23 cm or 9-inches

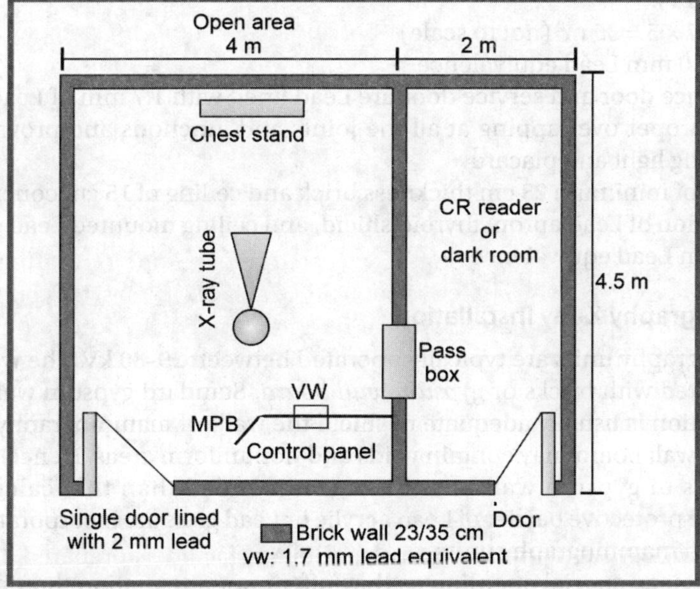

Fig. 15.10: Model layout of a general radiography X-ray installation.

thickness brick or 1.7 mm Lead in front of the door (s) and windows of the X-ray room to protect the adjacent areas, either by public or not under possession of the owner of the X-ray room. The density of the normal masonry brick is considered as 1.6 g/cc:

❑ Area: 18 m² (Not to scale)
❑ Mobile protective barrier (MPB) of 1.7 mm Lead equivalence
❑ VW of 45 × 45 cm size and 1.7 mm Lead equivalence
❑ Window or ventilator (W) at a height of 2.1 m from the finished floor level outside the X-ray room
❑ Entrance door Lead lined with 1.7 mm of Lead sheet with proper overlapping at all the joints, and provision of warning light and placard
❑ Provision of Lead apron of 0.25 mm and gonad shield of 0.5 mm Lead equivalence

Fluoroscopy X-ray Installation

Fluoroscopic imaging or an interventional radiology/cardiac angiography systems are usually operated at potentials ranging from 60–120 kV. A primary barrier is incorporated into the fluoroscopic image receptor. Therefore, a protective design for a room containing only a fluoroscopic unit, consider only secondary protective barriers against leakage and scattered radiations. However, provisions are made with primary barriers so that the function of the room can be changed later date without the need to add an additional shielding. Most modern fluoroscopic X-ray imaging systems also include a radiographic X-ray tube. The shielding requirements for such a room are based on the combined workload of both units **(Fig. 15.11)**:

❑ Area: 7 × 5 = 35 m² (not to scale)
❑ VW: 2.0 mm Lead equivalence
❑ Entrance door and service door are Lead lined with 1.7 mm of Lead sheet with proper overlapping at all the joints and junctions and provision of warning light and placard
❑ Walls of minimum 23 cm thickness brick and ceiling of 15 cm concrete
❑ Provision of Lead apron, thyroid shield, and ceiling mounted Lead glass of 0.5 mm Lead equivalence

Mammography X-ray Installation

Mammography units are typically operated between 25–30 kV. The walls are constructed with bricks or *gypsum wall board.* Standard gypsum wallboard construction is usually adequate to shield the walls of mammography room. Gypsum wall board may contain voids and nonuniform areas. Hence, higher thickness of gypsum wall board is recommended than that calculated. Adequate protective barrier of Lead acrylic or Lead glass are incorporated into dedicated mammography units.

Doors need special attention as they offer poor attenuation than brick or gypsum wall board. Solid core wooden door (5 cm thick) leading to corridors

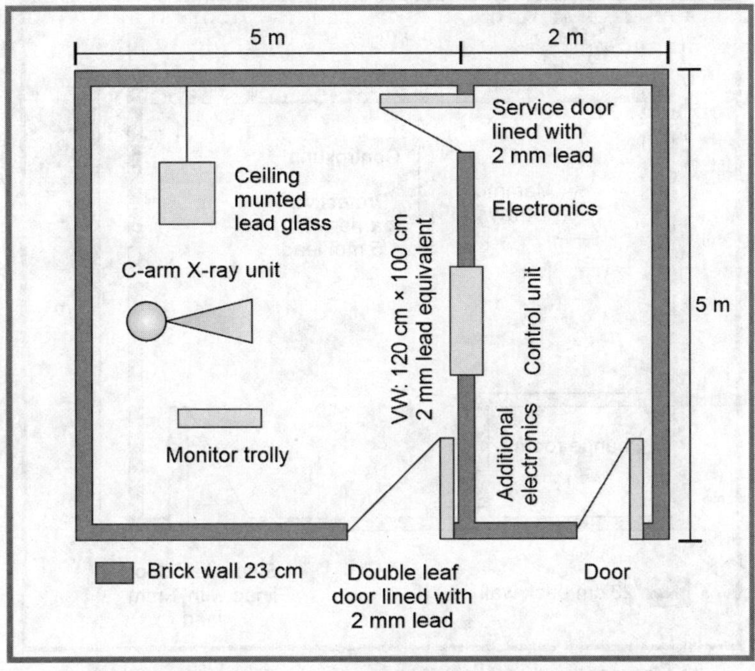

Fig. 15.11: Model layout of a fluoroscopy X-ray installation.

outside a mammography room provide an adequate shielding. Standard wooden doors may not be sufficient if the shielded area has significant occupancy. Standard concrete construction provides an adequate barriers above and below mammographic facilities. *Lead lined walls* and *doors* are usually not required **(Fig. 15.12)**:

❑ Area: $3 \times 3.5 = 10.5$ m² (Not to scale)
❑ Window or ventilator (W) at a height of 2.1 m from the finished floor level outside the X-ray room
❑ Entrance door Lead lined with 1.0 mm of Lead sheet with proper overlapping at all the joints, and provision of warning light and placard.
❑ Walls of minimum 23 cm thickness brick and ceiling of 15 cm concrete
❑ Provision of Lead glass shield of 1.5 mm Lead equivalent

Computed Tomography Installation

Computed tomography (CT) employs a collimated X-ray fan-beam that is intercepted by the patient and by the detector array. Consequently, only secondary radiation is incident on protective barriers. The operating potential, typically in the range of 80 to 140 kV, as well as the workload are much higher than for general radiography or fluoroscopy. Due to the potential for a large amount of secondary radiation, floors, walls, and ceilings need special consideration. Additionally, scattered and leakage radiations from

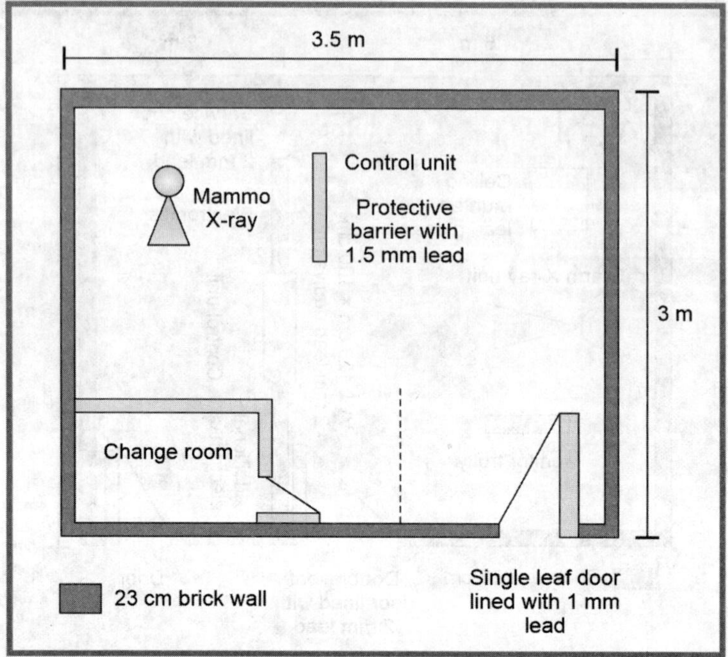

Fig. 15.12: Model layout of a mammography X-ray installation.

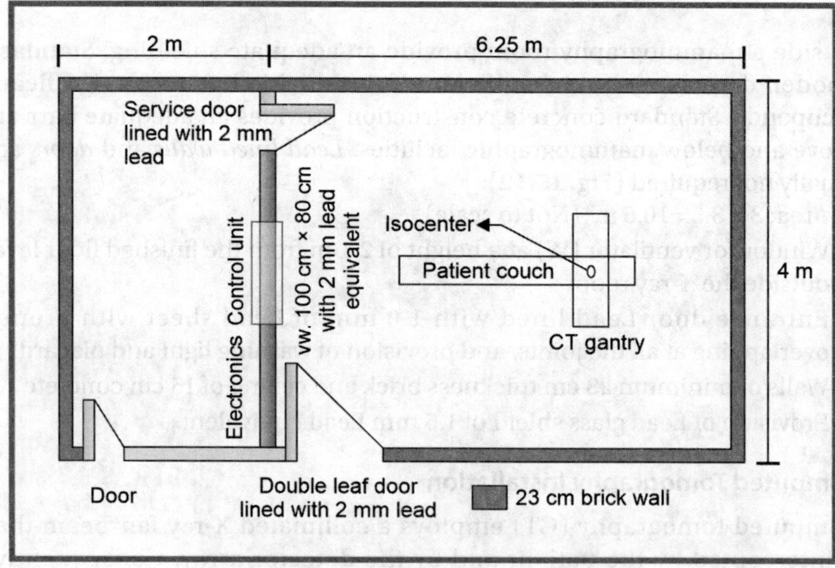

Fig. 15.13: Model layout of a computed tomography installation.

CT systems are not an isotropic. The radiation levels in the direction of the gantry are much less than the radiation levels along an axis of the patient table **(Fig. 15.13):**

- Area: $4 \times 8.25 = 33$ m² (not to scale)
- VW of 2 mm Lead equivalent
- Entrance door and service doors are Lead lined with 1.7 mm Lead sheet with proper overlapping at all the joints and junctions, and provision of warning light and placard
- Walls of minimum 23 cm thick brick and ceiling 15 cm concrete

Other X-ray Installations

Bone mineral densitometer (BMD) dose rate at 1 m is less than allowable dose limit for public hence, no structural shielding is needed even with the smallest room **(Fig. 15.14)**. Dental X-rays uses cone beam CT (CBCT), an orthopantomogram (OPG), and an intraoral radiography. Normal wall thickness is sufficient to offer protection to such units and the suggested shielding are recommendary in nature. However, if the installation is not on the ground floor, a 6–8 inches thickness of concrete is required for the ceiling. Mobile C-arm and lithotripsy equipment can be used in an operation theater (OT) with normal wall thickness of 9" brick/6" concrete and should have 1.0 mm Lead lined doors/windows.

SHIELDING CONCEPTS FOR DIAGNOSTIC X-RAY FACILITY

Workload

Workload (W) is a measure of X-ray tube's use, and it is the time integral of tube current, over certain period, expressed in mA.min/week **(Table 15.7)**. In diagnostic X-ray unit, it is obtained by multiplying the maximum mAs/

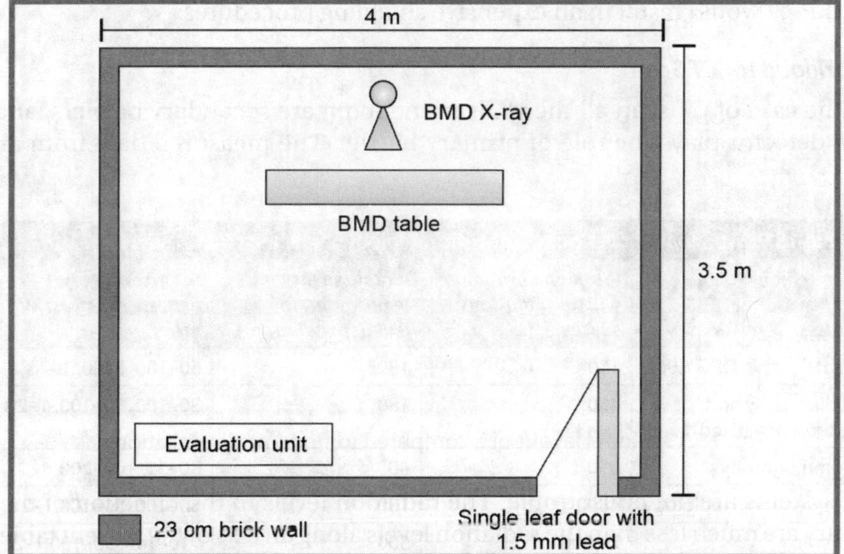

Fig. 15.14: Model layout of a bone mineral densitometer (BMD) installation.

exposure with beam ON time in minutes/week (mAs/60). For example, the workload of a hospital with 20 patients per day, 3 films per patient, and 60 mAs per film is calculated as follows:

$$W = (20 \text{ patients/day}) \times (5 \text{ days/week}) \times (3 \text{ films/patient}) \times (10 \text{ mAs/film}) \times (1 \text{ min/60s})$$

$$= 50 \text{ mA-min/week}$$

Higher kV settings always go with decreased workload due to an increase of output (mR/mAs). It also has reduced mA, that increases beam penetration and reduces X-ray attenuation in the patient.

Workload Per Patient

NCRP-147 suggested normalized workload per patient (W_{norm}). It conveys the average workload per patient, including various procedures of the patient. The total workload (W_{tot}) is the product of normalized workload, and an average number of patients per week (N):

$$W_{tot} = N \times W_{norm}$$

This makes the workload as a function of kV rather than magnitude of workload. This is much useful to design shielding thickness since attenuation of radiation by primary barrier depends on kV. Workload distribution varies widely, and it is specific to radiography, fluoroscopy, and CT scans.

The NCRP-49 (1976) describes the structural shielding design and an evaluation for medical use of X-rays and gamma rays of energies up to 10 MeV. When the report was made single phase generator was in use, an annual dose limit is 100 mrem per year, report neglected an image receptor attenuation, and considered low speed film-combination. Hence, strict adherence of NCRP-49 would result in an expensive shielding procedures.

Workload for CT Scan

In the case of CT scan all the walls in the room are secondary barriers, and the detector plays the role of primary barrier. The measured data from an

Table 15.7: Workload for various diagnostic radiology X-ray units (AERB website).

Types of X-ray units	Workload (mA.min/wk) for radiation survey	Workload (mA.min in one hour) for leakage radiation	Approximate exposure factors: kV, mA, s
Dental X-rays, OPG/CBCT	150	180*	60–100, 8–20, 1–2 s
Radiography and fluoroscopy (fixed)	400	180	80–100, 50–100, 1–2 s
Mammography	650	40	30–35, 100–200, 1–2 s
Interventional radiology	4800	180	80–100, 50–100,1–2 s
CT scan	20,000	500	110–140, 50–100,1–2s

*Workload for intraoral X-rays is 20 mA.min/wk

individual CT scan is required to determine an amount of scattered radiation, arising from the gantry. Normally, these measured data are provided as exposure lines from an isocenter of the gantry on a per slice basis for a given mAs **(Fig. 15.15)**. Workload of a CT scan is calculated from an average number of patients per week, fraction of head verses body scans, and an average mAs per patient.

The workload of a head CT scan having 20 abdominal scan per day, 40 slices per scan with 200 mAs per slice can be calculated as follows (Assume 50% of the scans are with contrast, and 50% are without any contrast = 1.5 studies/patient).

Total number of slices

= (20 patients/day) × (5 day/wk) × (40 slices/study) × (1.5 studies/patient)

= 6000 slices/wk

$$W = 6000 \frac{\text{slices}}{\text{week}} \times \frac{200 \text{ mAs}}{\text{slice}} \times \frac{1}{60 \text{ min}} = 20,000 \text{ mAmin/week}$$

Nowadays helical CT is more common it is difficult to estimate number of slices exactly, hence a workload of 20,000 mA.min per week is used for barrier calculations and radiation survey (AERB). In the case of leakage radiation calculation, it is about 500 mA.min in one hour.

Occupancy Factor

Occupancy factor (T) of an area is an average fraction of time (8 hours/day) that an individual stays at that area while the X-ray machine is ON. It can be full, partial, and an occasional occupancy **(Table 15.8)**. Radiation workers who spent an entire time in controlled areas will have occupancy factor of 1.

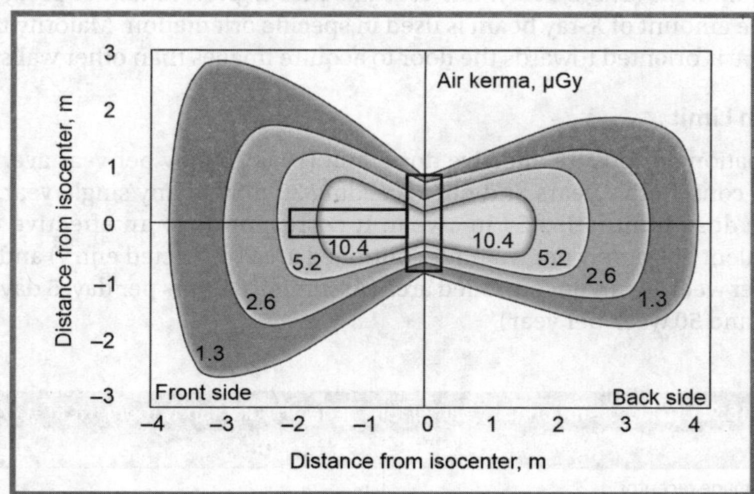

Fig. 15.15: CT scan layout: Secondary radiation distribution from an isocenter in a 32 cm PMMA phantom, measured in air kerma, μGy (140 kV, 100 mA, 1s). Horizontal dose distribution includes both scatter and leakage. Front side radiation levels are higher than that of back side levels and minimum near the gantry.

Table 15.8: Occupancy factors for diagnostic X-rays (NCRP-147).

Location	Occupancy level	Occupancy factor
Administrative or clerical offices; laboratories, pharmacies and other work areas fully occupied by an individual; receptionist areas, attended waiting rooms, children's indoor play areas, adjacent X-ray rooms, film reading areas, nurse's stations, X-ray control rooms	Full	1
Rooms used for patient examinations and treatments	Partial	½
Corridors, patient rooms, employee lounges, staff rest	Partial	1/5
Corridor doors	Partial	1/8
Public toilets, unattended vending areas, storage rooms, outdoor areas with seating, unattended waiting rooms, patient holding areas	Occasional	1/20
Outdoor areas with only transient pedestrian or vehicular traffic, unattended parking lots, vehicular drop off areas (unattended), attics, stairways, unattended elevators, janitor's closets		1/40

Occupancy factor modifies shielding design objective at a point by 1/T or barrier attenuation lower the radiation level by P/T ratio, where P is an effective dose limit.

Use Factor

Use factor (U) is a fraction of primary beam workload that is directed towards a primary barrier. It depends on the type of X-ray room and an orientation of the equipment **(Table 15.9)**. It is estimated for a given nature of procedure and the amount of X-ray beam is used in specific orientation. Majority times the tube is oriented towards the floor to acquire images than other walls.

Design Limit

Occupational exposure effective dose limit (P) is 20 mSv per year averaged over 5 consecutive years and not exceeding 30 mSv in any single year. The public dose limit is 1 mSv in a year. It corresponds to an effective dose equivalent of 0.4 mSv per week for controlled area (restricted entry) and 0.02 mSv per week for an uncontrolled area (Assuming 8 hours per day, 5 days per week, and 50 week per year).

Table 15.9: Use factors for primary barrier for a general radiography room (NCRP-147).

Barrier	Use factor (U)
Chest image receptor	1
Floor	0.89
Cross-table lateral walls	0.09
Unspecified wall	0.02

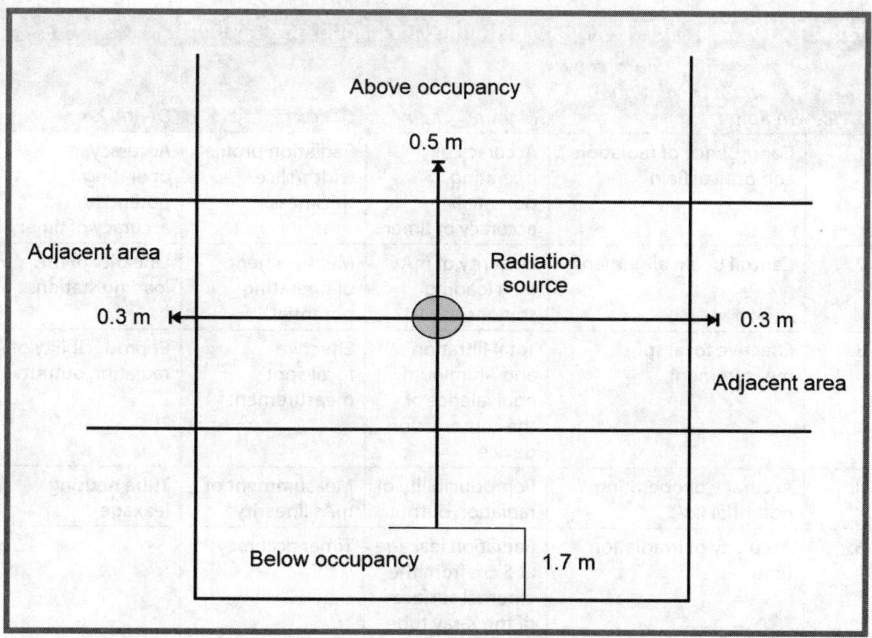

Fig. 15.16: Point of dose measurements for barrier calculation showing below the radiation source, above the ceiling and lateral occupancies.

NCRP 147, recommends a weekly shielding design limit of 0.1 mGy air kerma for controlled areas (10 times lesser than NCRP 49). In case of an uncontrolled area, weekly shielding design limit of 0.02 mGy air kerma (5 times lesser than NCRP 49).

Distance

NCRP recommends distances (d) to the points of measurement. If an occupancy is below the X-ray/radiation source, sensitive organs of the person below can be assumed not more than 1.7 m above the floor. If an occupancy is above the X-ray/radiation source, the distance can be measured to a point 0.5 m above the floor. Lateral distances to be measured at a point not less than 0.3 m from the far side of a barrier (**Fig. 15.16**).

SAFETY IN DIAGNOSTIC RADIOLOGY

Quality Assurance

Quality assurance (QA) describes a set of policy that is designed to control and maintain the standard of quality of patient care. It ensures that the X-ray machine is up to the specification of the vendor. The goal of QA in diagnostic radiology is to obtain an optimal image with minimum radiation dose with minimum cost. In general, the mechanical characteristics, the control panel display/indicators and the tube housing details are checked initially, and

Table 15.10: Various QA tests to be performed for diagnostic X-ray units.

S. No.	Radiography/fluoroscopy (C-arm/interventional radiology)	Mammography	CT scan	Dental X-ray
1.	Congruence of radiation and optical field	Accuracy of operating potential/ accuracy of timer	Radiation profile width/slice thickness	Accuracy of operating potential/ accuracy of timer
2.	Central beam alignment	Linearity of mA/ mAs loading stations	Measurement of operating potential	Linearity of mA loading stations
3.	Effective focal spot measurement	Total filtration and Aluminum equivalence of the compression device	Effective focal spot measurement	Reproducibility of radiation output
4.	Accuracy of operating potential (kV)	Reproducibility of radiation output	Measurement of mAs linearity	Tube housing leakage
5.	Accuracy of irradiation time	Radiation leakage at 5 cm from the external surface of the X-ray tube housing	Timer accuracy	—
6.	Total filtration/HVL	Imaging performance evaluation	Measurement of computed tomography dose index (CTDI)	—
7.	Linearity of mA/mAs loading stations	Effective focal spot measurement	Low contrast resolution	—
8.	Output consistency	—	High contrast resolution	—
9.	Low contrast sensitivity (Only for Fluoro/C-arm)	—	Radiation leakage levels from X-ray tube housing at 1 M from the focus	—
10.	High contrast sensitivity (Only for Fluoro/C-arm)	—	Output consistancy	—
11.	Exposure rate at tabletop (Only for Fluoro/C-arm)	—	Total filtration	—
12.	Tube housing leakage	—	—	—

it is followed by set of tests. The test varies with type of X-ray machine, and it should be carried out during commissioning/installation, and later once in two years. Radiography, mammography, fluoroscopy/radiography, and computed tomography require separate QA tests **(Table 15.10)**.

Test gadgets with suitable phantoms and *ion chamber, pocket dosimeter* and *all in one meter* are required to perform the QA. QA test providers, accredited by AERB should be only employed to perform QA tests. Each test has its own tolerance value which is available at the AERB website. QA test of a X-ray machine is completed before registering or renewing an X-ray machine with AERB.

Radiation Survey

Radiation survey of the installation is performed after completing QA test. The radiation levels in and around the X-ray machine is measured (radiation survey) with suitable phantom and it should be within permissible limits.

The assessment of radiation levels at different locations in the vicinity of radiation installation is known as *area monitoring or radiation survey*. These measurements will give an idea about the radiation status of an installation. Based on measurements taken, one could confirm an adequacy or inadequacy of an existing radiation protection status. If the radiation levels are found to be higher than the permissible levels, suitable remedial measures can be taken. Hence, an objective of the above measurement is to ensure radiation safety and minimize personnel exposure. Devices used for the above purpose is referred to as *radiation survey meter*. Survey meter and *zone monitors* have been discussed in Chapter 5. All QA test details, including radiation survey is recorded and a register is maintained.

Testing Protective Shields

Lead apron, gonad shield, thyroid shield are used as protective shields in diagnostic radiology. They should be stored properly with serial numbers so that no damage happens while folding. They should be kept in wall mounted hangers at each workplace. However, Lead apron weight concentrates at the bottom due to gravity in such hangers. They can be placed horizontally one over the other on a table, if available. Even than there may be cracks and damage in the Lead apron over age. It should not be used by the worker and needs testing since not providing full protection.

Lead apron can be tested either in a C-arm or CT scan. Superior part of Lead apron is placed under a C-arm and pulled slowly while the beam is ON. Cracks if any may appear as white lines in an image. In the same way, upper surface of the Lead apron is kept at an isocenter of the CT scan on the table and couch is moved like one does for a scout image. The defective apron appears with white lines or spots **(Fig. 15.17)**. The damaged aprons are isolated and should not be kept in use. The digital image of the damaged apron is stored for NABH inspection as document. Relevant records of Lead apron and test with dates needs to be maintained. The damaged Lead aprons are handed over to biomedical department towards disposal. It should be disposed to a licensed hospital waste disposal company or firm. Receipt of the same kept for future records. Since, Lead is toxic it should be disposed to an ordinary vendor.

Radiation and Pregnancy

Pregnant women should not be given an unnecessary radiation exposures. If exposed, fetal and embryo dose must be evaluated to estimate risk. If the

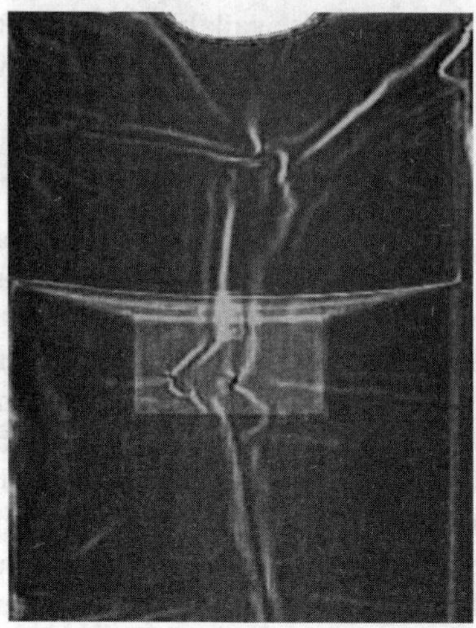

Fig. 15.17: Testing the Lead apron in a CT scan. Image shows cracks in the apron as white lines.

embryo is not directly irradiated the dose will be low, except from scatter radiation. Generally, it is implemented on risk vs benefit, where benefit always outweighs the risk.

Ten-day and 28-day Rule

Earlier 10-day rule is recommended by the WHO for women of reproductive age. It states that "whenever possible, one should confine the radiological examination of the lower abdomen and pelvis to the 10-day interval following the onset of menstruation." Later evidence suggests that the 10-day rule puts too much restriction on radiological examination of patients. This is because that the number of cells in the conceptus is small and their nature is not yet specialized. The effect of damage to these cells is most likely to take the form of failure to implant, or of an undetectable death of the conceptus; malformations are unlikely or much rare. Since an organogenesis starts 3 to 5 weeks postconception, it was felt that radiation exposure in early pregnancy could not result in malformation. Based on this, it was suggested to do away with the 10-day rule and replace it with a 28-day rule.

As per 28-day rule, if the *last menstrual period (LMP)* is within 28-day, all radiological examinations can be carried out, if justified. If the LMP is >28 days, no examination should be carried out and needs further discussion, including the pregnancy test, consulting the patient, and the referring physician. This means that examinations can be carried out throughout the cycle, except the missing period. Thus, now the focus is more on the missed period and the possibility of pregnancy.

Pregnant Radiation Worker

In general, all radiation workers including pregnant employee should wear Lead aprons during their occupational work. Pregnant employee should wear an additional TLD badge at an *umbilical level,* to assess the fetal dose. The fetus dose is about 50% of the TLD reading at 1 cm. Those who are working in fluoroscopy guided interventional work should wear wraparound Lead apron and thyroid shields. This will provide an adequate shielding to the breast tissue, thyroid, and the conceptus, during pregnancy. Such aprons should have a thickness of 0.25–0.5 mm Lead equivalent.

In the case of pregnant staff working in Nuclear medicine, there is no need to take any additional precautions, other than limiting their direct contact of patients. Exposure from patients, who have been administrated radiopharmaceuticals, is quite low and hence the pregnant staff can continue imaging procedures. Pregnancy shall not be considered a reason to exclude a female worker from work, as per an international basic safety standards. The use of Lead apron is preferred while imaging with Gamma camera using Tc-99m (140 keV) and not indicated for PET-CT, since it uses F-18, which has higher energy of 0.55 MeV.

Termination of Pregnancy

Thousands of pregnant women are undertaking diagnostic X-ray procedures daily in the world. Lack of knowledge is responsible for great anxiety and an unnecessary termination of pregnancy. Studies on hospital patients has stated that the conceptus dose from radiographic, fluoroscopic, CT examinations of an abdomen and pelvis and from nuclear medicine procedures rarely exceed 25 mGy. They also suggested that risk of fetal effects, including childhood cancer induction are small at conceptus doses of 100 mGy and negligible at doses of <50 mGy.

American College of Obstetricians and Gynecologists (ACOG) recommend that "women should be counseled that X-ray exposure from a single diagnostic procedure does not result in harmful fetal effects. Specifically, exposure to <50 mGy has not been associated with an increase in fetal anomalies or pregnancy loss. *National Council on Radiation Protection and Measurements (NCRP)* has stated that the risk is considered to be negligible at 50 mGy or less when compared to other risks of pregnancy, and risk of malformation is significantly increased above control levels only at doses above 150 mGy.

According to *ICRP (Repot-84), termination of pregnancy at fetal doses of less than 100 mGy is not justified based upon radiation risk.* The reason for the above is that induction of childhood malignancy or leukemia at 100 mGy is 1 in 170, whereas the natural frequency is much lower. However, fetal doses between 100 and 500 mGy, at 7–13 weeks, the decision of termination of pregnancy is based on an individual circumstance that should be considered in consultation with the referring physician. At fetal doses between 100 and 500 mGy, at 7–13 weeks, the decision should be based upon an individual circumstance. Of course, this is a guideline value and other parameters must be accounted with parental decision in consultation with referring physician. This includes pregnancy hazard to mother, an expectancy of parents, their mental outlook, and an ethnic and religious family background. It also requires the provision of counseling for the patient and her partner.

Operational Safety in Radiography

Equipment Operation

Personnel monitoring devices shall be used by all radiation workers, while on duty. Before making an exposure, the doors of the X-ray room must be closed. The X-ray beam should not be directed towards windows, control panel or dark room wall. Medical students/trainees must not be allowed to operate a X-ray unit. When performing portable examinations, an operator should stand at least 2 m away from the patient.

Protective Shield

All radiation workers must wear Lead apron of 0.5 mm thickness, which reduces radiation exposure by a factor of 10. Use of Leaded glass and Lead gloves must be encouraged in fluoroscopy type of work. Repeat X-rays must be avoided to reduce patient dose. *Gonad shield, eye shield* and *thyroid shields* should be used, to protect the patient organ, during radiography.

Field Area

Minimum field size to cover the patient's volume should be used. Field size reduction reduces the scatter thereby reducing the dose to an adjacent organ. The scatter incident on the detector also decreases, resulting in an improved image contrast. Hence, the rule of thumb is *always use smallest, possible field size* and *good collimation*.

Source to Object Distance

Higher the source to object distance (SOD) and source to image distance (SID) the lesser the patient dose. Increase of SOD/SID ratio, reduces beam divergence, in turn reduces volume of patient irradiation. This will enable us to decrease an integral dose. Increased SOD also facilitates reduction of patient exposure due to tube leakage since the tube is away from the patient.

In radiography with stationary X-ray equipment, the SOD should be not less than 45 cm. When the SID is less than 100 cm, the quality of the diagnostic information becomes poorer hence, longer SID has clinical advantages. Chest radiography should be performed with a SID of at least 180 cm. In the case of C-arm units, fixed SID is used, therefore increase of SOD is the only way of reducing patient dose. In fluoroscopy, the minimum distance between source and the patient must be not less than 30 cm.

Occupancy in the Room

Only person whose presence is necessary should be in an imaging room during exposure and overcrowding should be avoided. All such persons in the room must be protected with Lead aprons/shields. The X-ray room shall be kept closed during radiation exposure.

Assistance to Patients

Holding of children or infirm patients for X-ray examination shall be done only by an adult relative or escort of the patient. Hospital personnel should not hold the patients during an imaging procedure. No person should routinely hold patients during diagnostic examinations, certainly not those who are pregnant or under the age of 18 years. Such person shall be provided with *protective aprons* and *gloves.* In no instance shall the holder's body be in the useful beam and should be as far away from the primary beam as possible. In no case should the film or X-ray tube be held by hand.

Patient Motion

Patient motion may cause *motion artifacts,* which may increase repeat X-rays and patient dose. To reduce patient motion (1) short exposure times, (2) use of immobilization or sedation, and (3) entertainment, or distracting devices should be applied and adopted. Immobilization devices prevent movement of children during an exposure.

Pregnant Women

Radiological examination of the lower abdomen and pelvis of a pregnant woman must be conducted only when considered essential. One or two X-rays may be performed if the last mensural period (LMP) is within 28 days. For other X-ray examinations away from pelvis, an abdomen and the pelvis must be covered with a protective Lead shield.

Log Book and Records

Each X-ray equipment must have a separate logbook, which provides an information about an equipment manufacturer, model, serial number, date of purchase, cost, repair, down time, etc.

Records of all radiological examinations should be maintained. Reports and radiographs should be given to the patient for future reference.

Patient Safety and Dose Reduction in Radiography

Diagnostic X-ray contributes the highest radiation dose to the patients. The radiation dose received by a patient is specified in terms of an *entrance skin dose (ESD).* Effective dose in general radiography ranges from 0.1–1 mSv. ESD for chest radiograph is 0.1 to 0.2 mGy and for an abdominal radiograph is 0.7 mGy. ESD increases with short focus to skin distance. The patient exposure is proportional to mAs and kV_p squared, and inversely related to the square of the distance from the focal spot. *A rule of thumb is that a technique of 100 kV and 100 mAs produces an exposure of about 1R at a distance 1m.* Hence, an optimal technique must be used to reduce patient dose. The following are the important steps which will protect the patient from radiation dose:

❑ New diagnostic X-ray equipment must not be used unless quality assurance tests have been performed satisfactorily.

- Any X-ray examination should be prescribed only after a critical evaluation of the patient's condition, to avoid an unnecessary exposure.
- No fluoroscopic or CT examination should be conducted if the required information can be obtained from radiography.
- Transfer of radiographs from one institution to another should be encouraged to avoid repeat examination.
- All efforts shall be made to keep the patient dose as low as technically achievable.
- Use of rare earth intensifying screens will reduce the patient dose significantly.
- Repeat X-rays must be avoided to reduce patient dose.
- Use of high kV reduce radiation due to increased penetration of X-rays.

Operational Safety in Fluoroscopy

Since, an interventional procedure involve an angiography and angioplasty procedures. It causes higher radiation exposures of 1–100 mSv to the patients, all the personnel involved in the procedure should address the following for operational safety:

- Use of *Lead apron, couch flaps, Lead gloves,* and *ceiling suspended Lead screen* must be encouraged during fluoroscopy. *Wraparound Lead apron* is beneficial, however *skirt type Lead apron* is preferrable to distribute weight.
- Along with TLD chest badge additional *wrist badge* for procedures involving hands closer to the primary beam is advisable.
- X-ray tube should be positioned as close to the patient as possible.
- Personnel should be in an opposite direction to the X-ray tube during an oblique orientation.
- During C-arm procedures standing on the side of an image intensifier is safest because there is more scatter produced at an entrance skin side of the patient.
- Table height is positioned as high as possible so that it is comfortable for an operator.
- Over workers should not be there in the fluoroscopy room if not necessary.
- Restriction of X-ray beam size (collimation) to being as small as necessary for the clinical purpose.
- Preventive maintenance and QA of the equipment are performed periodically.
- Update with current regulatory requirements.

Patient Safety and Dose Reduction in Fluoroscopy

- Select suitable exposure factors (kV, mA), e.g., higher kV (> 60) is much effective in dose reduction.
- Anti-scatter grid should be removed when imaging small patients of thin body parts.

- ❑ Use heavy X-ray beam filtration.
- ❑ Time of exposure must be shorter.
- ❑ Use largest FOV suitable for the given clinical study.
- ❑ Utilize radiation only when imaging is necessary to support clinical care.
- ❑ Vary the imaging beam angle to minimize an exposure to any one skin area of interest.
- ❑ Monitor radiation dose in real time to assess patient risk/benefit during procedure.
- ❑ Direction of X-ray beam should be far away from the fetus, if pregnant women is examined.
- ❑ Keep patient's extremities out of the beam.
- ❑ Minimize use of steep angles of X-ray beam
- ❑ Minimize the use of cine mode.
- ❑ Magnification technique should be avoided or kept lower.
- ❑ Use of low frame rate, especially in digital subtraction angiography (DSA).
- ❑ Use of low dose rate pulsed fluoroscopy.
- ❑ Use of lower-dose automatic brightness control (ABC) options.
- ❑ Use of last frame hold features.
- ❑ Patient dose, dose length product (DLP) is recorded in the case sheet.

Patient Safety and Dose Reduction in Computed Tomography (CT)

- ❑ Employ well collimated X-ray beam.
- ❑ Set minimum field of view (FOV) and an optimal slice thickness.
- ❑ Use heavily filtered X-ray beam.
- ❑ Employ X-ray tube current modulation and adoption for patient body habitus.
- ❑ Ensure body imaging protocols, do not use an automatic mA modulation techniques.
- ❑ Employ peak voltage optimization.
- ❑ Verify last mensural period (LMP) for pregnant or likely to be pregnant patients.
- ❑ Scan only the Z-axis for the required length
- ❑ Use higher pitch in helical scanning.
- ❑ Avoid radiation directly to the eyes.
- ❑ Use iterative reconstruction, if possible.
- ❑ Use of noise reduction algorithms.
- ❑ Create low dose protocols (chest, kidney stone)
- ❑ Use of pediatric protocols.
- ❑ Number of multiple scans with contrast material is reduced.
- ❑ Only scan the contrast phases necessary for diagnosis and vary mA according to contrast phase.
- ❑ Use CT fluoroscopy shall be used very rarely.
- ❑ Ensure $CTDI_{vol}$ does not exceeds 0.5 Gy in brain perfusion study.
- ❑ Record the patient radiation dose.

BIBLIOGRAPHY

1. ACOG Committee on Obstetric Practice. Guidelines, for diagnostic imaging during pregnancy. ACOG Committee opinion no. 299, September 2004. Obstet Gynecol 2004;104:647-651.
2. Dauer LT et al. Occupational Radiation Protection of Pregnant or Potentially Pregnant Workers in IR: A Joint Guidelines of the Society of Interventional Radiology and the Cardiovascular and Interventional Radiological Society of Europe. J Vasc Interv Radiol 2015; 26:171-181.
3. htttps://www.aerb.gov.in
4. International Commission of Radiological Protection. Pregnancy and Medical radiation, ICRP publication 84, Elsevier, New York; Ann. ICRP, 2000; (30)1.
5. Kelsey CA et al. Radiation biology of medical imaging; Wiley Blackwell, New Jersey, 2014.
6. McCollough CH et al. Radiation exposure and pregnancy: When should we be concerned? Radiographics 2007; 27:909-918.
7. National Council on Radiation Protection and Measurements. Medical radiation exposure of pregnant and potentially pregnant women, NCRP report no. 54, Bethesda, Md: National Council on Radiation Protection and Measurements,1977.
8. Structural shielding design for medical X-ray imaging facilities. National council on radiation protection and measurements (NCRP), report No.147, Bethesda, 2015.
9. Thayalan K. Basic radiological physics, 2nd ed Jaypee Brothers Medical Publishers (P) Ltd, New Delhi, 2017.

APPENDIX

REVIEW OF MATHEMATICS

Numbers and Fractions

Numbers we use are decimal system **(Hindus, 600–900 AD)** and have 10 digits, namely 0, 1, 2, 3, 4, 5, 6, 7, 8, 9. It can be written in single or multiple numbers. A real number is divided into rational number and irrational number. An *irrational number* is a nonterminating type, e.g., value of $\pi = 3.14159265$. A *rational number* is a terminating or repeating decimal type, and it is divided into integers (–2, –1, 0, 1, 2), whole numbers (0, 1, 2), natural numbers (1, 2), and prime numbers. The *prime numbers* are divisible only by 1 and themselves, e.g., 2, 3, 5, and 7. A positive or negative number is called *signed number* and the sign is either + or –, e.g., +2, and –2. An *absolute number* is a measure of deviation from 0, irrespective of sign, e.g., $|2| = -2$ to +2. An *imaginary number* is denoted by i and its square is equal to –1. A *complex number* consists of real and imaginary number.

Fraction is a quotient of two numerical values, e.g., 1/2, number 1 is called *numerator* and 2 is called *denominator*. If the numerator is small compared to denominator it is called *proper fraction*. If the numerator is larger than the denominator it is called *improper fraction*. A common fraction is one which has whole number and proper fraction.

Base and Exponent

A physical quantity (a) is often written as either a^1, or a^2 or in general a^n. Here, a is the base and n is the exponent or power. It refers to repeated multiplication provided the exponent is positive integer as follows:

$$a^2 = a \times a, \quad a^3 = a \times a \times a,$$
$$a^n = a \times a \times a \dots a \,(n\ times).$$

If $n = 1/2$, it is not a positive integer then, $a^{1/2} = \sqrt[2]{a}$ or simply $\sqrt{a}$. If $n = 0$, then $a^0 = 1$, provided, $a \neq 0$.

An exponent can have minus sign, e.g., $a^{-n} = \dfrac{1}{a^n}$. Two exponential can be multiplied or divided or raised to a power as follows:

$$a^m \times a^n = a^{m+n}$$
$$(a^m)^n = a^{mn}$$
$$(ab)^n = a^n b^n.$$

The term a^n is often called an exponential term and if the exponent is 1, it is simply written as a, since it has no repeated multiplication. If the exponent is *0*, the value is *1*, provided the base number is not 0 or infinity.

Base e

Number e is often used in radioactive decay, radiation attenuation and cell survival curve, etc. It is an irrational number having a constant value

Table A.1: Binary and equivalent decimal numbers.

Binary number	0	1	10	11	100	101	110	111	1000	1001	1010
Decimal number	0	1	2	3	4	5	6	7	8	9	10

of 2.71828. It is like number π, which was discovered by **Leonhard Euler**, Swiss mathematician, referred as *Euler's number* (1736). Base e is often used with exponent like +x and –x, and e^{+x} refers to rapid growth of the value. Alternatively, e^{-x} refers to rapid decline of the value towards zero. Logarithms to base e is called *natural logarithm* and the value of $e^0 = 1$.

Decimal and Binary Numbers

We generally use decimal numbers which has a base of 10 and involves digits 0 to 9. In a binary number, the value of a digit in a position is 2 times than it is in right. In a decimal number, it is 10 times than it is in right. Decimal point is allowed in decimal system, whereas it is not allowed in binary. For example, the value of a binary number 10 is written as below: $(1 \times 2) + (0 \times 2) = 2$.

Similarly, one can convert any binary number into a decimal number by raising powers of 2 in a series and then adding them. **Table A.1** gives the equivalence of binary and decimal numbers. Digital memory and storage use the terms like *bit, byte,* and *word* etc. A bit is a small portion of a disk or tap that can be magnetized for data storage. Bits are grouped into bytes and words and 1 byte (B) is equal to 8 bits. Number of bits in a word may be 16 or 32 or 64, depending on the computer system. Normally, kilobytes ($2^{10}=1024$ bytes), megabytes ($2^{20} = 1048$ kB), and gigabytes ($2^{30} = 1073$ MB) are commonly used.

Logarithms

Logarithm of a decimal number is the exponent to which the base must be raised to produce the number. For example, the logarithm of 1000 to base 10 is 3, because 1000 is 10 to the power of 3: $1000 = 10^3 = 10 \times 10 \times 10$. More generally, if $x = b^y$, then y is the logarithm of x to base b, and is written as $log_b(x)$, so $log_{10}(1000) = 3$. Logarithm is denoted by the notation log:

$$log(ab) = log(a) + log(b)$$
$$log(a/b) = log(a) - log(b)$$
$$and \qquad log(an) = n\, log(a).$$

Reversal of logarithm is called *antilogarithm*, denoted by antilog and logarithm of a negative number is zero. There are three types of logarithms, namely *common logarithm* (log_{10}), *natural logarithm* (ln_e), and *binary logarithms* (log_2). In common logarithm, $log_{10}2 = 0.30$, the base must raise to power of 0.30; $10^{0.301} = 2$. In natural logarithm, $log_e2 = 0.693$, the base e must be raised to power of 0.693, $e^{0.693} = 2$, and the value of $e = 2.71828$.

Logarithm is used to simply calculations and solving equations. Nowadays computer and calculators are used for the above task. Measurements of optical density and sound intensity are expressed in logarithm to base 10. Radioactive decay, and X-ray attenuation uses logarithm to base *e*, which is denoted by natural logarithm ($\ln_e$). Logarithmic scales reduce wide-ranging quantities to smaller scales. The survival curve in radio biology and characteristics curve of X-ray film are plotted in logarithmic scales. It is useful to describe many radiation events such as X-ray absorption, radioactive decay etc.

Trigonometry

Trigonometry is a mathematics which deals with triangles and relation between angle and sides **(Fig. A.1A)**. A triangle is made by the intersection of three nonparallel lines. Shape of a triangle is determined by its angles and sum of the angles is 180°. If one of its angles is 90°, it is called *right triangle,* the remaining two acute angles are referred as *complementary angles.* Sides of a right triangle are *adjacent side (base), opposite side (perpendicular), and hypotenuse.* Hypotenuse is the side opposite to 90° angle and it is the longest side of a triangle. If the length of one side is known, the other two sides can be determined. Side ratio is determined by angle of the triangle regardless of its overall size and expressed in terms of trigonometric functions of known angle θ, where *a*, *b* and *c* refer to lengths of the sides in a triangle. The sine function (sin) is the ratio of opposite side to hypotenuse, Cosine function (cos) is ratio of adjacent side to hypotenuse, and Tangent function (tan) is the ratio of opposite side to adjacent leg:

$$Sin\,\theta = \frac{Opposite\ side}{Hypotenuse} = \frac{a}{c},\ Cos\,\theta = \frac{Adjacent\ side}{Hypotenuse} = \frac{b}{c},\ \text{and}\ Tan\,\theta = \frac{Opposite\ side}{Adjacent\ side} = \frac{a}{b}$$

Few more useful relations are, *sin* 0° = 0, *cos* 0° = 1, and *tan* 0° = 0, *sin* 90° = 1, *cos* 90° = 0, and *tan* 90° = ∝. *Pythagorean theorem* states that the square of the length of hypotenuse of a right triangle is equal to sum of the squares of adjacent and opposite sides: $c^2 = a^2 + b^2$.

Similar Triangle

Similar triangles have same corresponding angles and shape but different size. Two triangles in **Figure A.1B** are called similar triangles since one is

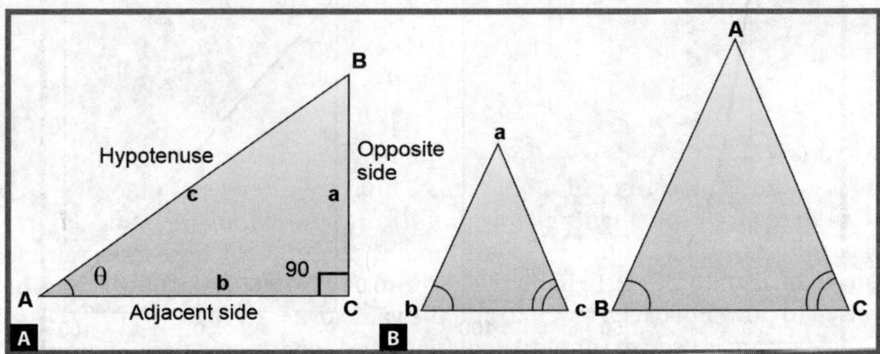

Figs. A.1A and B: (A) Relation between angles and sides in a triangle; (B) Similar triangles.

just bigger version of the other, while retaining the shape. The corresponding angles of the two triangles are equal, but lengths of the corresponding sides are not equal. In a similar triangle, the lengths of the sides are in proportion to one another, or the side ratios are equal as given below:

$$\frac{BC}{bc} = \frac{AB}{ab} = \frac{AC}{ac}.$$

This means that, if one side has a length which is double that of the corresponding side of the other triangle, then all the sides will be doubled, compared to the other triangle. Similar triangle concept is used to follow a divergent radiation beam and to calculate field size at a given distance. It has role in inverse square law too.

Semilog Graph

Graph gives the relationship between physical quantities, plotted as series of points or lines with reference to set of axes. A Cartesian graph has two axes, namely x-axis called *abscissa* and y-axis called *ordinate*. x-axis contains independent variable (e.g., time, distance), and y-axis contains dependent variable (e.g., velocity, exposure). If a physical quantity y varies with x in a proportional way, then it is a straight-line graph or linear plot that obeys the relation: $y = mx + c$ where, m is the slope of the line, and c is the intersection with the y axis. The logarithmic functions such as e^{+x}, and e^{-x} can also be plotted as curve, where a rapid increase or rapid decrease exists. A *semilog* graph is used to visualize such data in which one axis is plotted in logarithmic scale and the other is in linear scale (log-lin). Spacing of scale on the y-axis is proportional to logarithm of number, not number itself **(Figs. A.2A and B)**.

This kind of plot is useful when one of the variables being plotted covers a large range of values and the other has only a restricted range. Advantage being that it can bring out features in the data that would not easily be seen if both variables had been plotted linearly. Semilog plot requires only few measurements of the exponential function.

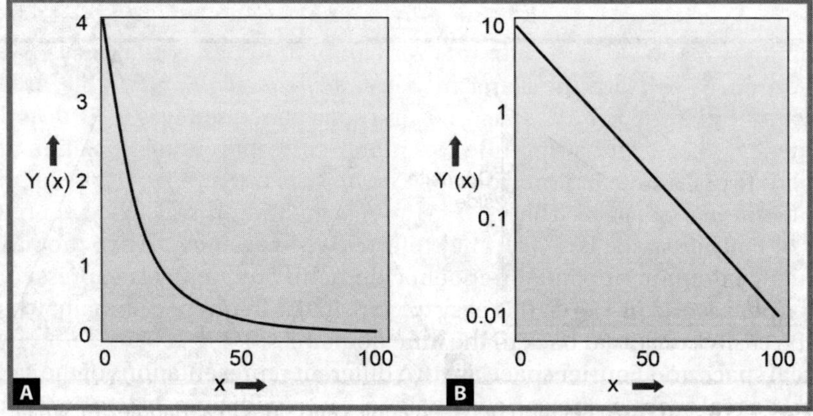

Figs. A.2A and B: (A) Linear graph (lin-lin); (B) Semilog graph (log-lin).

Fourier Transform

Fourier transform (FT) is one of many transforms in mathematics (**Jean Baptiste Joseph Fourier,** France). It is basically a mechanism, which converts a mathematical function from one domain into another domain. For example, mathematical data from a *spatial domain* can be converted into *frequency domain* with the help of *Fourier transform*. The frequency can be angular or linear. Let f(x) is an image intensity profile in object space or distance space. The profile can be represented as a sum of sine and cosine functions of different frequencies (k). Fourier transform, f(x) can be written as:

$$F(k) = FT\,[f(x)]$$

where, FT denotes Fourier transform operation, F(k) refers to image intensity profile in k space or spatial frequency space, while f(x) is in object space. F(k) represents the amplitudes for different spatial frequencies. Fourier is also applicable for two dimensional functions such as f (x, y) and the corresponding FT is also a 2-D function:

$$F\,(k_x, k_y) = FT\,[f\,(x, y)]$$

where, k_x and k_y refers to x, and y orthogonal axis in *k* space. The function and its FT are equal and either one can be derived from each other. Conversion of FT of a function back into the original function are called *inverse FT*:

$$FT^{-1}F\,(k_x, k_y) = f\,(x, y)$$

where FT^{-1} denotes the inverse of FT operation. It plays an important role in tomographic reconstruction and convolutions in computer. Computer consists of image and signal processing software, which can perform FT quickly. It is also used for image analysis and image processing, e.g., modulation transfer function. It is useful to converts a signal from an imaging device into a diagnostic image, e.g., MRI. FT can be presented in terms of graphs of functions, so that one can see how FT changes the shape of these graphs. For example, FT can change a square wave into a sine function and 1/FT (inverse) of sine function can yield a square wave.

Let us consider a sin wave signal whose intensity is varying with time (**Fig. A.3A**). The signal is basically a time domain in *real space*. Wave form's amplitude and phase vary with time with amplitude 1 and frequency 1 cycle per second. FT converts the signal intensity into *frequency domain* (**Fig. A.3B**). Now the amplitude is 1 at k space = 0, and special frequency is 1. FT decodes frequency, phase, and amplitude variations, corresponding to position and amplitude of the data in time domain. The unit of Fourier space is the inverse of the unit in real space. That is, if *s* (time) is the unit in real space, then the unit of Fourier space is s^{-1} (1/time) referred as frequency, hence the name frequency domain or spatial frequency domain. Frequency is expressed in cycles per second or Hertz. It is easy to work in the frequency domain, which can be easily converted back to the time domain.

Real space and Fourier space are two different representations of the same data. In a real space, it shows how the signal varies with time. In Fourier space, one can see how the signal varies with frequency or how many frequencies are

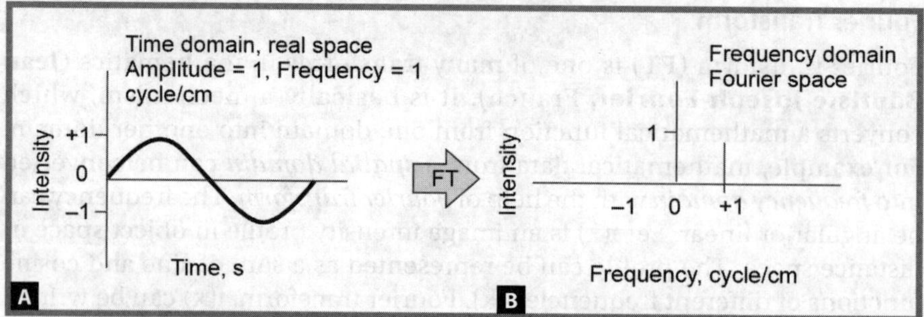

Figs. A.3A and B: Fourier transform application: (A) Signal is in time domain; (B) Signal is in frequency domain, after Fourier transform.

there in the signal. FT does not change the information present in a function but offers newer viewpoints on the data.

Fourier transform can be performed either two dimensional (2D) or three dimensional (3D), which finds application in *Magnetic resonance imaging* and *nuclear medicine.* 2D Fourier transform is applied in length and width of an image matrix. 3D Fourier transform is applied for each column, row, and depth axis in the image matrix cube which is used in 3D image acquisition of MRI.

STATISTICS

Statistics is a mathematical manipulation of numerical data. It is used to analyze and formulate population characteristics by way of sampling, which saves time and money. The types of sampling are: (1) *random sampling,* and (2) *stratified sampling.* Random sampling is one in which sample is obtained independently from each other and each sample has the same probability of being selected. If heterogeneity is present in the data and it influences the study, the data set is said to be *strata.* Random sample selected from such strata data set is called *stratified ample.*

Source of Errors

There are three types of errors in measurements, namely *systemic error, random error,* and *blunder.* Systemic error occurs when measurements differ from the correct values in a systemic fashion. Random error is caused by random fluctuations in the measurement process itself. The processes by which radiation is emitted and by which radiation interacts with matter are random in nature. Hence, all radiation measurements are subject to random error. Counting statistics helps us to judge the validity of measurements.

Accuracy and Precision

If a measurement is close to the correct value, it is said to be *accurate.* If measurements are reproducible, they are said to be *precise,* and precision does not imply accuracy. If a set of measurements differ from the correct value in a systematic fashion, the data are said to be *biased*.

Mean, Median, and Standard Deviation

Mean ($\bar{x}$) is an arithmetic average of a set of measurements as defined:

$$\bar{x} = \frac{x_1 + x_2 + x_3 + \cdots x_N}{N} = \frac{\sum x_i}{N}$$

where, N is the number of measurements. *Median* is measure of central tendency and is the value that separates the data in half and defines 50%. It is the middle most measurement if the number of measurements is odd. It is the average of the two middle most measurements, if the number measurements are even. For example, the median of the five measurements 5, 8, 9, 12 and 14 is 9. *Mode* of a sample is the value that often appears in the sample. *Range* refers to maximum variation of the values in the sample. *Standard deviation* (σ) of a sample describes precision or reproducibility of measurements. It is used to describe the spread of a data set:

$$\sigma_x = \sqrt{\frac{\sum_{i=1}^{N} (x_i - \bar{x})^2}{N-1}}$$

Standard deviation of mean value of the sample is called *standard uncertainty*.

The term *percentile (P)* is used to understand test scores and biometric measurements. It is calculated from the relation:

$$n = (p/100) \times N$$

where, N = number of values in a data set and n is the ordinal rank of a given value. In diagnostic radiology, 75th percentile is used to set reference doses. 75% percentile is the value at which 25% of the answers lie above that value and 75% of the answers lie below that values.

Variance (σ^2_x) is a measure of variability of a set of measurements and obtained from the relation:

$$\sigma^2_x = \frac{(x_1 - \bar{x})^2 + (x_2 - \bar{x})^2 + \ldots \ldots (x_N - \bar{x})^2}{N-1} = \frac{\sum_{i=1}^{N} (x_i - \bar{x})^2}{N-1}$$

where, N is the total number of measurements and $\bar{x}$ is the sample mean. The *standard deviation* is the square-root of the variance, $\sigma_x = \sqrt{\sigma_x^2}$. When samples are taken from a large population, there is uncertainty between the sample mean and the actual population mean. It is measured by *fractional standard deviation or fractional error* = $\frac{\sigma_x}{\bar{x}}$. Coefficient of variation (COV) is a measure of spread within the samples, given in percentage:

$$COV = \left(\frac{\sigma_x}{\bar{x}}\right) \times 100$$

where, $\sigma_x/\bar{x}$ is the *fractional error* in the measurements. If the sample size is large, then probability distribution function is used to describe the outcome.

The various probability distribution functions are *binomial distribution, Poisson distribution* and *normal distribution.*

Probability Distribution Functions

A trail is an event, which may have more than one outcome. One outcome is called a success. A binary process is a process in which a trail can only have two outcomes. A toss of a coin is a binary process. Whether a particular nucleus decays during a specified time interval is a binary process. Whether a particular gamma ray is detected by a radiation detector is a binary process.

The probability of obtaining each outcome from a measurement is described by the probability function. There are three probability functions: *binomial, Gaussian,* and *Poisson.* The binomial distribution describes exactly the probability of each outcome from a measurement of a binary process:

$$P(X) = \frac{N!}{X!(N-X)!} P^X (1-P)^{N-X}$$

where, N is the total number of trials in a measurement, P is the probability of success in a single trial and X is the number of success. For example, the probability of obtaining 2 heads in a toss of four coins, X = 2, N = 4, and P = 0.5:

$$P(2\,\text{heads}) = \frac{4!}{2!(4-2)!}\, 0.5^2 (1-0.5)^{4-2} = 0.375$$

The mean and standard deviation of the binomial are $X = PN$ and $\sigma = PN\sqrt{(1-P)}$. In radiation measurements the probability of a success in a trial is <1 (P << 1), $\sigma \approx \sqrt{PN} = \sqrt{X}$. In a single measurement, the value is close to the mean and hence, $\sigma = \sqrt{X}$ for example, a single measurement of a radioactive source gives 1256 counts. The standard deviation is given by: $\sigma = \sqrt{1256} = 35.4$ counts, and fractional error is $\sigma/X = 35.4/1256 = 0.028 = 2.8\%$.

The Gaussian (normal) distribution curves are bell shaped and represent a normal probability distribution. They are symmetrical around a central mean value (m) with a standard deviation (σ). All Gaussian curves have the same mean, median and mode value **(Fig. A.4)**. By the definition, 68% of the data fall within 1σ of the mean ($m \pm \sigma$), 95% of the data fall within 2σ of the mean ($m \pm 2\sigma$), and 99% of the data fall within 3σ of the mean ($m \pm 3\sigma$).

The Poisson distribution is used to model the probability distribution of uncommon events such as radiation decay. Poisson distribution is not symmetrical for low average values (m) of counts. It approaches a Gaussian distribution for values of m >10.

Statistical Tests

Data collected in the field of medicine is either quantitative or qualitative. For example, in quantitative data, height, weight, serum cholesterols are measurement data which are continuously variable. To analyzes these data, *Student's t-test* and *Analysis of Variance* is employed. Example for qualitative

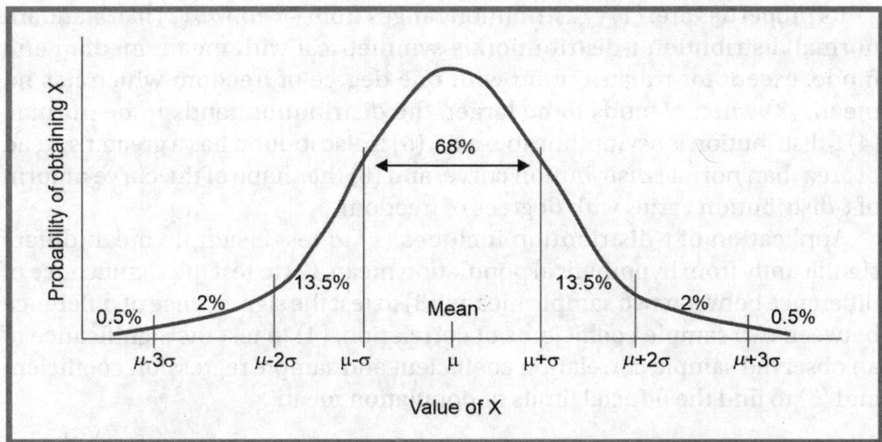

Fig. A.4: Gaussian probability distribution (normal curve).

data is, disease symptom (presence/absence), degree of severity of a disease (mild, moderate, severe), pregnancy risk (high risk, low risk). These counts or proportion or enumeration data are discontinuous or random in nature. To analyze these data, the appropriate test is *chi-squared* (χ^2) *test*. Hence, the χ^2 test meant for testing whether random variables in a set of measurements are consistent with what is expected for a *Poisson distribution*. Readers are advised to refer relevant textbooks for detailed information on the above subject.

Student t-test

It was introduced by **WS Gosset** (1905) under the pen name *student* and it is popularly known as *t-test or t-distribution or student's distribution*. It is used when sample size is small, and the population standard deviation is unknown. It is a symmetrical distribution similar in shape to the normal distribution and in fact it approaches the normal distribution as N, the sample size, increases. It can be used to test the statistical significance difference between the means of two different groups. In t test, the logic examined as:

$$t = \frac{\text{difference in sample means}}{\text{standard error of difference of sample means}}$$

When this ratio is small, it concludes that the data are compatible with the hypothesis that both samples were drawn from a single population. When the ratio is large, it concludes that it is unlikely that the samples were drawn from a single population and ensure that the treatment has produced an effect. Types of t-tests are *independent t-test/unpaired t-test and dependent/matched/paired t-test*. Condition for application of t-test is, small sample test (Sample size is <30), samples are drawn from normally distributed population, population standard deviation is not known, and it should be quantitative data.

Its properties are: (1) t-distribution ranges from $-\infty$ to $+\infty$, (2) like standard normal distribution t-distribution is symmetrical with mean, median and mode, except for t-distribution with one degree of freedom which has no mean, (3) when N tends to be larger, the distribution tends to be normal, (4) t-distribution is asymptotic to x-axis, (5) t-distribution has a greater spread of area than normal distribution curve, and (6) the shape of the curve or form of t-distribution varies with degrees of freedom.

Application of t-distribution includes (1) to test a sample mean differs significantly from hypothetical population mean, (2) to test the significance of difference between two sample means, (3) to test the significance of difference between two sample coefficients of correlation, (4) to test the significance of an observed sample correlation coefficient and sample regression coefficient and (5) to find the fiducial limits of population mean.

The Chi-Square Test

The Chi-square test (**Karl Pearson**) is a nonparametric test of proportions. It is used to test a hypothesis. If the *association* between two variables is to be tested, this test is commonly used. The quantity of χ^2 is defined as:

$$\chi^2 = \frac{\Sigma(O-E)^2}{E}$$

where O is observed frequencies, and E is expected frequencies. If the calculated value of χ^2 is greater than the value at certain level of significance, usually 5%, the difference between theory and observation is significance i.e., the hypothesis is rejected. If the computed value of χ^2 is less than the table value at a certain degree of level of significance, it is said to be nonsignificant. This implies the discrepancy between the observed and expected frequencies may be due to fluctuations in simple sampling method. Characteristics of χ^2 test are: (1) test is based on events or frequencies or counts, (2) to draw inferences, the test is applied specially testing the hypothesis, but not useful for estimation and (3) the test can be used between the entire set of observed and expected frequencies.

Conditions for Chi-square test are: (1) there must be large number of observations (say >50), (2) all the observations must be independent, (3) values/categories on independent and dependent variables must be mutually exclusive and exhaustive, (4) the sample must be randomly drawn from the population, (5) calculations must be based on actual numbers of observations and not on percentages, ratios, observed values etc.), and (6) when overall total is between 20 and 40, all expected values are at least 5.

Uses of Chi-square test is (1) to test the goodness of fit, (2) to test the independence of attributes, (3) to test the homogeneity of independent estimates of the population variance, and (4) to test the homogeneity of independent estimates of the population correlation coefficient.

Linear Regression

Linear regression is an analysis of relationship between one variable to another along with prediction of future events. Usually, the data is available as paired variables (x, y) which are plotted on a graph to get *best straight line*. A method referred as *least squares linear regression* is used to determine the best straight line. It minimizes the sum of the squares of the data points deviation from the straight line and is described by the relation y = mx + c. The slope m and y intercept can be evaluated. *Correlation coefficient (R)* is used to measure how best straight line is fitted to the data:

$$R = \frac{m\sigma_x}{\sigma_y},$$

where σ_x, and σ_y are the standard deviation of x and y respectively.

INDEX

Page numbers followed by *f* refer to figure and *t* refer to table.

A

Abdomen 326
   imaging 439
   lower 535
Abdominal excursion 486
Abscess, differentiation of 482
Absorption
   differential 85, 100
   edge 84
   rate, specific 445
   unsharpness 166
Absorptive collimation 331
Accelerating voltage 60
Accredited agency 504
Acetic acid 127, 161
Acoustic
   absorber 377
   energy 375
   enhancement 406*f*
   impedance 371
   lens 390
   matching 372
   noise 444, 445
   power 409
   properties 371*t*
   radiation force impulse 414
   shadowing 405, 406*f*
Acoustic-optical modulator 155
Actinium series 30
Activated target nucleus 43
Active matrix liquid crystal display 205
Active shield 432
   magnet 434
Acute radiation
   exposure 128
   syndrome 498
Adaptive array detector 314
Additives 124
Adenosine triphosphate 52
Adhesive layer 115, 116, 151, 152
Adipose tissue 219
Adrenal gland, right 344*f*
Afterglow 121
Air 101, 106, 141, 289, 371, 455
   calibration scans 292
   filled microspheres 413
   gap technique 146
   instead of 112
   physical characteristics of 140*t*
Al window 251
Albumin 53
Alcohol 163

Algebraic reconstruction technique 293, 338
Aliasing 400
Alignment coils 257
Alkali 163
   hydroxide 380
Allyl sucrose 380
Alpha particle 39, 43, 45, 491
Alpha-bombardment 39
Alumina resin 48
Aluminum 24, 42, 76, 144, 147, 228, 300, 431,
     506
   alloy of 18
   box 211
   chloride 162
   oxide 119, 506
   wall cylindrical ion chamber 132
Alzheimer's disease 354
Americium-241 494
Ammonium
   molybdenite 48
   thiosulfate salts 161
Amniotic fluid 425, 427
A-mode display 392*f*
Amorphous microcalcifications 238
Amorphous selenium 126, 191*f*, 194, 235
Amorphous silicon 188, 191*f*, 234, 266
   photodiode 191, 268
Amplifier 118, 383
Amplitude 370, 387
   mode 392
Analog-to-digital converter 315, 333
Anaphylactoid reactions 447
Anemia 498
   symptoms of 498
Aneurysm clips 443, 447
Angiography 157, 315
   phase contrast 476
Angular frequency 419
Angular momentum 417
Annealing 119
   oven 119
Annihilation coincidence detection 346, 346*f*,
     349, 356
Annotation 208
Annular transducer 391
Anode 64, 70, 74, 76, 220, 253
   angle 65, 66
      effective 220
      large 66
   electrode 64
   stem 65, 74
   tubes, rotating 72